Reverse Shoulder Arthroplasty

Stefano Gumina
Federico Alberto Grassi • Paolo Paladini
Editors

Reverse Shoulder Arthroplasty

Current Techniques and Complications

Springer

Editors
Stefano Gumina
Department of Orthopaedics and Traumatology
Sapienza University of Rome
Rome
Italy

Paolo Paladini
Department of Shoulder and Elbow Surgery
Ospedale Cervesi di Cattolica
Cattolica
Italy

Federico Alberto Grassi
Department of Orthopaedics and Traumatology
University of East Piedmont,
Hospital "Maggiore della Carità"
Novara
Italy

ISBN 978-3-319-97742-3 ISBN 978-3-319-97743-0 (eBook)
https://doi.org/10.1007/978-3-319-97743-0

Library of Congress Control Number: 2018961568

This Springer imprint is published by the registered company Springer Nature Switzerland AG
The registered company address is: Gewerbestrasse 11, 6330 Cham, Switzerland

To Prof. Randelli and Prof. Perugia, founding fathers of the Italian Society for the Shoulder and Elbow Surgery.

To Paul Grammont, inventor of the modern reverse shoulder prosthesis.

Foreword

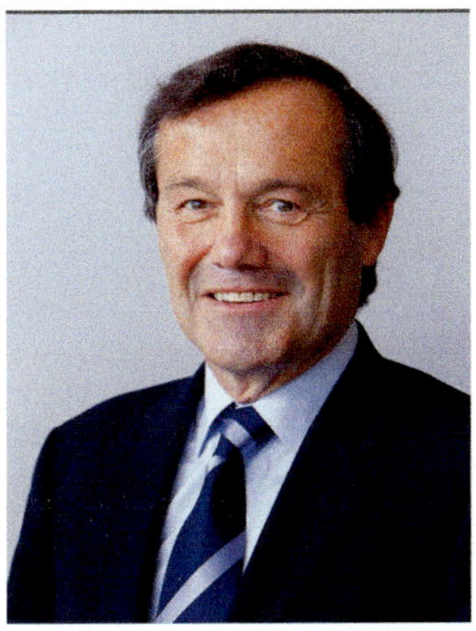

The Italian Society of Shoulder and Elbow Surgery is to be congratulated for this excellent work on the reverse shoulder replacement. Professors Mario Randelli and Lamberto Perugia were able, by creating this society, to inspire Italian surgeons to dedicate themselves to subspecialization in shoulder surgery, thereby promoting Italy as a flagship nation in Europe and throughout the world.

Paolo Paladini, Stefano Gumina, and Federico Grassi are the three engines that drive this new Italian generation. They have gathered around them the most active members of their society to create a body of work that will permit all surgeons–new and veteran alike–to learn more about the reverse shoulder prosthesis. This prosthesis was invented by Paul Grammont, the Lyonnaise surgeon from the school of Professor Trillat, who spent his career as professor at the University of Dijon. In 1985, Paul Grammont designed his first prototype of the reverse prosthesis, which incorporated the critical idea of transferring the center of rotation of the glenohumeral joint to the glenoid surface in order to avoid component loosening. The second prototype in 1987 and then the definitive Delta prosthesis in 1991 were not immediately recognized as the greatest advances in shoulder surgery of the twentieth century.

The lack of clinical evaluation and rigorous follow-up of patients operated on by Dr. Grammont and his team had long delayed the success of this prosthesis. Widely used in France and then in Italy after 1995, it would take nearly 10 years for this prosthesis to gain its current recognition when it was finally authorized for use in the United States by the FDA (2004). For 15 years now, the reverse shoulder prosthesis has achieved the same level of success and acceptance in the world as has the anatomic prosthesis designed by C.S. Neer.

Neer and Grammont are and will remain two giants in the field of Shoulder and Elbow surgery, the fathers of the prosthetic surgery that has allowed thousands of injured or debilitated patients to rediscover their shoulder function.

This truly excellent book perfectly analyzes the biomechanics of the reverse prosthesis and the etiologies that lead to its implantation. Initially proposed for the treatment of arthritis in the setting of massive rotator cuff tears, the excellent results obtained have led to the gradual expansion of indications to include massive rotator cuff tears without concomitant arthritis, fractures of the proximal humerus in the elderly, fracture sequelae, treatment of rheumatoid arthritis, tumors, and to numerous other circumstances in which other satisfactory options are not available to relieve patients.

Preoperative planning, surgical technique, complications, and postoperative rehabilitation are perfectly detailed and constitute a veritable bible for shoulder surgeons.

I encourage all shoulder surgeons to read this wonderful book and I congratulate once more Paolo Paladini, Stefano Gumina, and Federico Grassi for this success.

Lyon, France Gilles Walch

Preface

In 1985, Paul Grammont proposed adapting the principle of medialization to the reverse design previously implanted a new prosthesis, during the 1970s. He called his prototype the "Trompette." It was composed of a glenoid component, consisting of 2/3 of a 44-mm-diameter sphere, with its COR set in a specific, medialized location facing the glenoid. This ceramic glenoid component was cemented onto the glenoid. On the humeral side, a concave, monoblock polyethylene cone was also cemented. Deries tested this prototype; results were described in his graduate thesis in 1986.

Initially, reverse prosthesis was indicated for low demanding elderly patients with cuff tear arthropathy; nowadays it is commonly implanted in patients with irreparable cuff tear, glenohumeral arthropathy with healthy cuff, complex fractures of the humeral head, inflammatory arthropathies, failures of anatomical prosthesis and hemiarthroplasty, proximal humerus fracture sequelae, humeral head neoplasm, and avascular necrosis of the proximal humerus. This expansion of the surgical indication, associated with good functional results, led the reverse to exceed 75% of all types of shoulder prostheses in many specialized centers.

In the last decade, the reverse prosthesis has passionate hundreds of shoulder surgeons who, with their studies, have tried to reduce possible complications, such as scapular notching and mobilization of the components, and to increase function and stability.

This book was written by experts and affirmed Italian shoulder surgeons; all members of the prestigious Italian Society for the Shoulder and Elbow Surgery, founded in 1992. The monograph is aimed at all the lovers of this subject, residents and young specialists who are passionate about this sector of surgery, and physiotherapists who will find useful indications to set up a proper rehabilitation program.

We are proud to see the realization of this monograph; it represents the result of passion, seriousness, and scientific rigor of our countrymen.

Rome, Italy — Stefano Gumina
Novara, Italy — Federico Alberto Grassi
Cattolica, Italy — Paolo Paladini

About the Editors

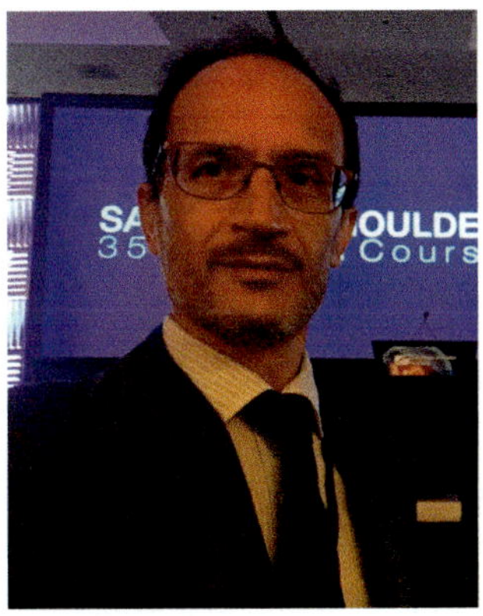

Stefano Gumina, MD, PhD is Professor of Orthopedics and Traumatology in the Department of Anatomy, Histology, Legal Medicine and Orthopedics and Traumatology at the Sapienza University of Rome, Italy. Since 2008 he has worked as an orthopedic surgeon, specializing in shoulder surgery, at the same university. In 2000 and 2001 he spent periods as a fellow at the University of Texas Health Science Center at San Antonio, the Cleveland Clinic Foundation, and the Rush-Presbyterian-St Luke's Hospital at Chicago. In 2003 he obtained his doctorate in Physiopathology of the Skeletal Apparatus, focusing his attention on shoulder disorders. Associate member of the European Society for the Surgery of the Shoulder and Elbow (ESSSE/SECEC) since 1997, he was nominated as an ordinary member in 2001. In 2006 he was nominated as a corresponding member of the American Shoulder and Elbow Surgeons. His interest in shoulder disorders and surgery dates back to 1990 and is reflected by the publication of numerous papers in Italian and international journals. He is President of the Italian Society of Shoulder and Elbow Surgery (SICSeG).

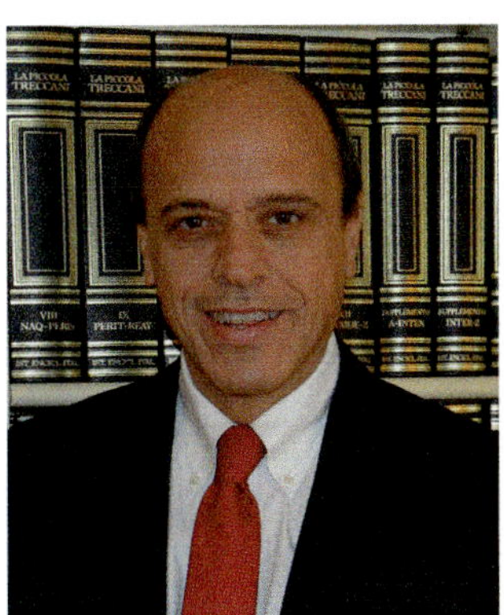

Federico Alberto Grassi is Professor and Chairman of the Department of Orthopedics and Traumatology at the University of East Piedmont, Hospital "Maggiore della Carità" (Novara, Italy). He was educated at the University of Pavia (Italy), qualifying as a doctor in 1986 and specialist in orthopedics in 1991. He then completed a Shoulder Fellowship at the University of Texas in San Antonio with Charles A. Rockwood (1991–1992). Between 1992 and 2000 he served as Assistant Professor of Orthopedics and Traumatology at the University of Insubria (Varese, Italy), where he progressed to the position of Associate Professor (2001–2005) and Full Professor (2006–2008) under the direction of Paolo

Cherubino. Prof. Grassi's clinical and surgical practice has always been dedicated to shoulder problems, with a special interest in arthroplasty and trauma. He is the author of several publications on different topics concerning the shoulder and editor of an Italian textbook of Orthopedics and Traumatology for medical students and junior residents. He served as President of the Italian Society of Shoulder and Elbow Surgery (SICSeG) during the 2015–2016 biennium.

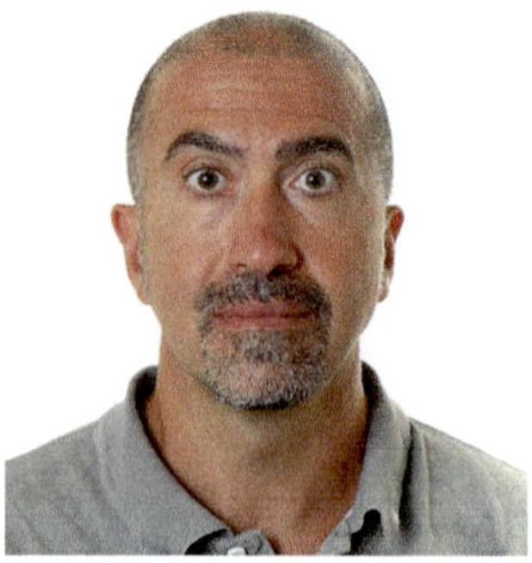

Paolo Paladini is chief of the Unit of Shoulder and Elbow Surgery of Cervesi Hospital in Cattolica (RN, Italy). He was educated at the Catholic University of Rome (Italy), qualifying as a doctor in 1993 and specialist in orthopedics in 1999 at Ancona University. During his residency he completed a Shoulder Fellowship at the Epsom General Hospital under Dr. D.H. Mok. (1995). In 2000 he founded, with Dr. Giuseppe Porcellini, a Unit of Shoulder and Elbow Surgery at Villa Serena Private Clinic in Forlì (Italy). His clinical and surgical practice has always been dedicated to shoulder and elbow problems. Author of several international publications on different topics concerning the shoulder and elbow, Dr. Paladini is involved with important international societies in the field: member of Italian Society of Orthopedics (SIOT), board member of Italian Society for Shoulder and Elbow Surgery (SICSeG), corresponding member of the American Shoulder and Elbow Society (ASES), ordinary member of European Society for Shoulder and Elbow Surgery (SECEC-ESSSE), and former member of its East European Support Committee and actual member of Educational Committee.

Contents

Part I

Basic Science

1 History of Reverse Shoulder Arthroplasty

Giuseppe Fama and Assunta Pozzuoli

1.1 Introduction

Degenerative and traumatic shoulder arthroplasty, with combined massive and irreparable rotator cuff tear, may lead to a painful and pseudo-paralyzed shoulder. The management of these conditions has long been challenging. It has been well addressed with the use of an anatomical, non-constrained total shoulder arthroplasty but with limited functional results or even contraindications.

The first introduction of such implants was by Charles Neer [1]. However, the problem of damaged or absent periarticular structures remained unsolved. Then, semi-constrained or constrained prostheses were tested in both anatomical and reverse types, but all these implants failed due to loosening of the glenoid component and poor functional outcomes [2, 3].

In 1985, Paul Grammont introduced a revolutionary design of reverse prosthesis that replaced the traditional glenoid socket with a "glenosphere" component fixed to the scapular neck and a small cup in the humeral component [4]. Grammont defined new biomechanical principles of medialization and lowering of the center of rotation. This medialization of the center of rotation in reverse shoulder prosthesis was crucial in successfully overcoming implant failures of previous designs mainly due to loosening.

The new ingenious idea of Paul Grammont has been decisive for all the next reverse shoulder arthroplasties in the treatment of degenerative arthropathies of the shoulder associated with an irreparable tear of the rotator cuff.

Since 1985, many new models, designed on the basis of Grammont reverse shoulder prosthesis, are now available with good clinical outcomes.

In this chapter, we present a historical review of the evolution of reverse shoulder arthroplasty, the biomechanical variations and the complications from the early models, through the development of Grammont's prosthesis, to the more recent ideas and designs to face the controversies and challenges that still remain.

1.2 Historical Review

The first shoulder arthroplasty was performed in 1893 by a French surgeon Jules Emile Péan to treat the tuberculous arthritis shoulder of a 37-year-old baker. Jean Porter Michaels, a Parisian dentist, designed for him a prosthesis

G. Fama (✉)
Orthopaedic Clinic, Azienda Ospedaliera-University of Padova, Padova, Italy
e-mail: giuseppe.fama@aopd.veneto.it

A. Pozzuoli
Department of Orthopaedics and Orthopaedic Oncology, University of Padova,
Padova, Italy

S. Gumina et al. (eds.), *Reverse Shoulder Arthroplasty*,
https://doi.org/10.1007/978-3-319-97743-0_1

with the humeral stem made of platinum and leather and a head made of rubber coated with paraffin [3, 5, 6]. It had moderate and short-lived functional results because the prosthesis was removed 2 years later for a recurrence of the infection.

Then, no references to the shoulder prostheses were done until 1955 when Neer [7] performed the first non-constrained humeral prosthesis which was a one block implant made of Vitallium which reproduced the anatomy of the superior part of the humerus (Neer I). He treated seven patients with fracture-dislocations of the shoulder by replacement of the humeral head and repair of the avulsed tuberosities and five patients with old fractures of the humeral neck complicated by avascular necrosis. He reported pain relief in 11 of 12 patients. In 1974, Neer [8] subsequently extended the use of his proximal humeral arthroplasty for the treatment of glenohumeral osteoarthritis. He reported excellent and satisfactory clinician results in 40 of 44 patients. Although pain relief was reliably obtained with hemiarthroplasty, Neer [8] reported variable strength and function in patients with irreparable rotator cuff tears. Superior humeral head migration was often seen postoperatively in patients who had lost the stabilizing function of the rotator cuff.

In fact, between 1950 and 1970, together with the widening of the indications for shoulder arthroplasty, many surgeons noticed poorer function in patients with a deficient rotator cuff. They recognized the stabilizing role of the rotator cuff and increased awareness that the development of glenohumeral prosthesis had to solve the challenges of balancing joint stability with the range of motion (ROM) impaired by tear and deficiency of the cuff [8–11].

Nevertheless, over the next years, a number of other studies followed reporting the use of hemiarthroplasty for traumatic and degenerative changes in the glenohumeral joint [8, 12–14].

However, the early attempts were unable to consistently alleviate pain and restore function in cases of rotator cuff tear arthropathy. Such unsatisfactory outcomes led surgeons to use designs that compensated for severe rotator cuff deficiency with a convex glenoid and a concave humerus, replicating the biomechanical design of other weight-bearing joints [10, 15–18]. Inspired by the success of total hip arthroplasty, several subsequent shoulder implant designs attempted to increase the conformity and constraint of the prosthesis [19].

In 1972, Neer and Averill, RG [1] designed three different types of fixed-fulcrum arthroplasty. The first of these reversed shoulder prostheses, Mark I (Fig. 1.1), included a large anatomical glenoid used to stabilize the prosthesis and prevent proximal humeral migration.

The second version, the Mark II, was modified to a smaller ball to allow rotator cuff repair but, unfortunately, with a decreased excursion and motion [20]. The Mark II and similar implants, including the English-MacNab prosthesis and

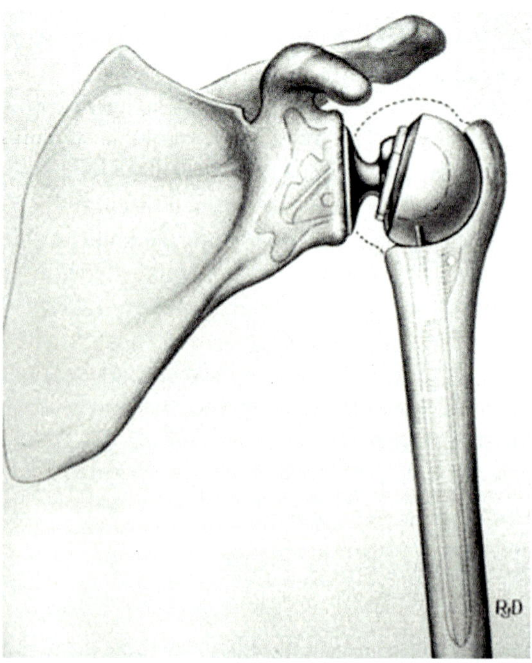

Fig. 1.1 The Mark I system. A large glenoid implant to allow more motion and a large head (Reprinted with permission from Flatow EL, Harrison AK. A history of reverse total shoulder arthroplasty. Clin Orthop Relat Res. 2011;469:2432–2439)

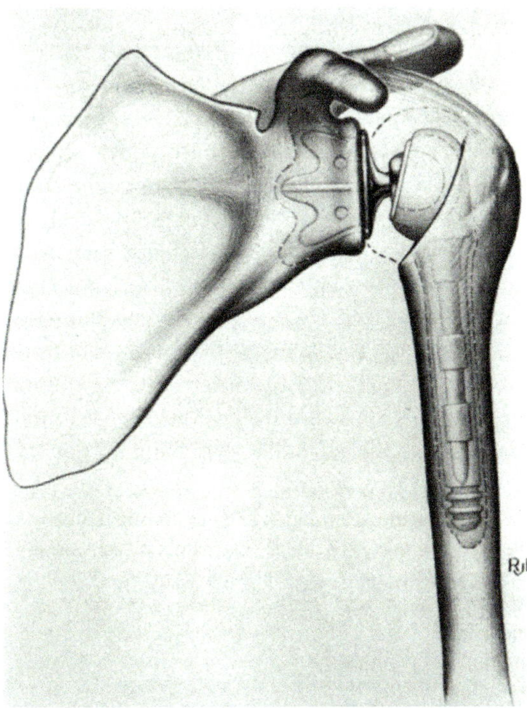

Fig. 1.2 The Mark III reverse prosthesis. Smaller ball and rotating metallic stem within a polyethylene sleeve (Reprinted with permission from Flatow EL, Harrison AK. A history of reverse total shoulder arthroplasty. Clin Orthop Relat Res. 2011;469:2432–2439)

the DANA shoulder prosthesis, were quickly abandoned, secondary to high rates of loosening of the glenoid component [18, 21].

The third version, the Mark III, was subsequently developed with a new design that allowed axial rotation between the humeral stem and the diaphysis to limit constraint and to improve ROM (Fig. 1.2) [22]. Dislocation, loosening, and scapular fixation were still major concerns with this implant [23]. Therefore, Neer abandoned his constrained prosthesis designs, concluding that constraint alone cannot adequately compensate for a nonfunctional rotator cuff [22]. However, other surgeons continued to explore the reverse shoulder concepts.

In fact, new total shoulder arthroplasty designs in the 1970s reversed the normal anatomy by placing the socket in the proximal humerus and the prosthetic ball on the glenoid with different scapular fixations in order to improve motion and strength without increasing the risk of dislocation and loosening (Table 1.1) [4, 10, 18, 24–29].

Table 1.1 Reverse shoulder arthroplasty models pre-Grammont

Prosthesis name/author	Year of introduction	Main characteristics
Mark I, Mark II, Mark III/Neer and Averill	1972	Reverse ball-and-socket joint with a fixed-fulcrum. Mark I with a oversized ball to allow increased motion. Mark II modified to a smaller ball to permit rotator cuff reconstruction. Mark III with a small ball and an axial rotation in the humeral stem to regain motion
Leeds/Reeves	1972	Glenoid component with a divergent threaded peg; center of rotation coinciding with the anatomic center
Gerard and Lannelongue	1972	A central screw with an articulating sphere was placed through a base plate along with two more screws
Kölbel and Friedebold	1973	The glenoid fixation was secured with a central screw and two plates with the screws directed to the base of the scapular spine
Kessel	1973	Fixation of the scapula with a single large central glenoid screw; center of rotation placed laterally; cemented humeral stem
Bayley-Walker	1973	Implant similar to Kessel design with a large hydroxyapatite-coated glenoid screw; the center of rotation placed medially and distally. "Snap-fit" components to enhance stability
Jefferson/Fenlin	1975	Large polyethylene glenosphere to improve deltoid function. The glenosphere articulated with a large cup on a metallic humeral stem
Liverpool/Beddow	1975	Similar to hip prosthesis. The glenoid component has a stem fixed into the scapular pillar to achieve a secure fixation. This model mimics the anatomic center of rotation outside the scapula
Buechel-Pappas-DePalma	1978	Double glenosphere decreased in size realizing a "floating fulcrum" that increases shoulder motion over the anatomic limits
Trispherical/Gristina	1978	Two small ball joints on both humeral and scapular sides articulating with a third larger central polyethylene sphere

1.2.1 1972: The Leeds/Reeves Prosthesis

This shoulder arthroplasty had the normal anatomic center of rotation. The glenoid component was fixed with a divergent threaded peg. It demonstrated higher pullout strength than other designs in *in vitro* testing. This implant was only experimental (Fig. 1.3) [10, 29].

1.2.2 1972: The Gerard and Lannelongue Prosthesis

Gerard and Lannelongue reported in 2 papers the results of 22 cases, in which this model was used. This system showed many complications (four implant breakages, three dislocations, and two infections) not only related to the prosthesis design. In fact, the cases were particularly complicated and challenging because they included reconstruction following tumor resection or post-traumatic and revision surgery [17, 30].

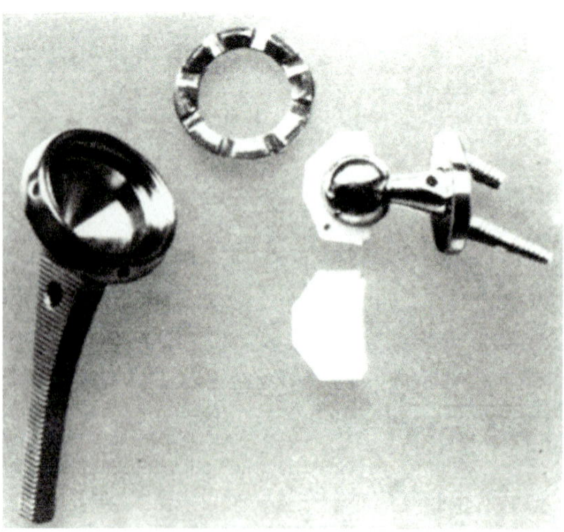

Fig. 1.3 The Leeds/Reeves reverse shoulder system. It included a divergent threaded peg glenoid component. It had an instant center of rotation that recreated the normal anatomic center (Reprinted with permission from Flatow EL, Harrison AK. A history of reverse total shoulder arthroplasty. Clin Orthop Relat Res 469:2432–2439, 2011)

1.2.3 1973: The Kölbel and Friedebold Prosthesis

This constrained implant was designed to reduce the marked bone removal from the glenoid vault for implantation of the glenoid component, characteristic of the earlier constrained designs. Kölbel and Friedebold [18] introduced a new system to improve scapular fixation with a flange bolted to the base of the scapular spine and functioned in stress transfer. The glenoid implant was fixed with a central screw and two plates with the screws directed toward the coracoid process and/or the base of the scapular spine (Fig. 1.4). It was especially used for the reconstruction of bone loss after tumor resection [18, 21, 31]. Its use was reported in six cases, for resection of malignancy from the humerus, the glenoid, or both.

1.2.4 1973: The Kessel Prosthesis

In this model the glenoid component was fixed to the glenoid by a large and single central screw which was placed laterally, while the humeral stem was cemented. Both components were snap-fit coupled (Fig. 1.5).

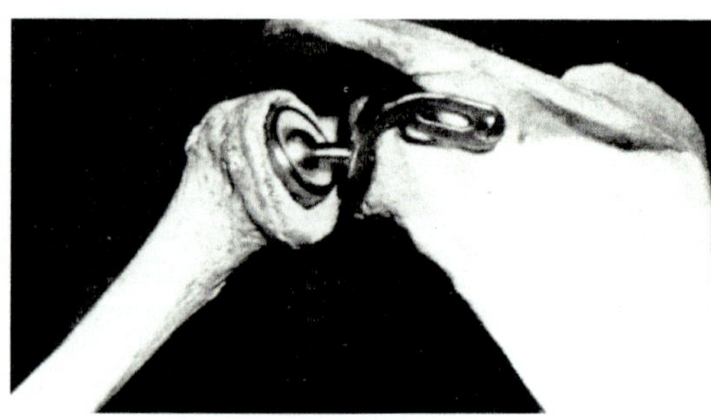

Fig. 1.4 The Kölbel reverse shoulder prosthesis. The glenoid component is fixed with a flange bolted to the base of the scapular spine (Reprinted with permission from Matsen FA, Rockwood CA, Wirth MA, Lippitt SB: Artropatia gleno-omerale e suo trattamento. In: Rockwood CA, Matsen FA. La Spalla. eds. Roma: Verduci; 2000:823–944)

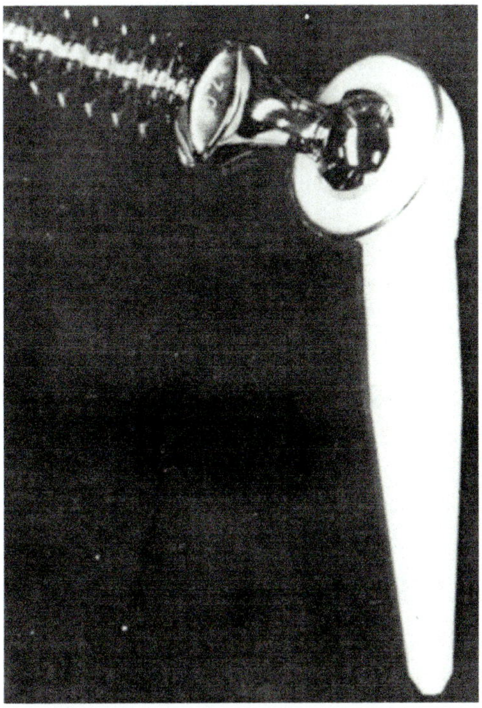

Fig. 1.5 The Kessel reverse shoulder prosthesis. The glenoid component is screwed to the glenoid, while the humeral stem is cemented (Reprinted with permission from Matsen FA, Rockwood CA, Wirth MA, Lippitt SB: Artropatia gleno-omerale e suo trattamento. In: Rockwood CA, Matsen FA. La Spalla. eds. Roma: Verduci; 2000:823–944)

Bodey described decreased pain and some improvement in function [32].

Also, Broström et al. reported a series of 23 shoulders (all with rheumatoid arthritis), with a follow-up of 87 months, in which pain relief was good in over 90%, but average gain in active elevation was poor (35%) and the reoperation rate was high (26%). Moreover, all shoulders had radiolucent lines around the glenoid screw within a year [33]. Seven years later, Wretenberg confirmed this finding on the same series of patients [34]. Of the 22 patients, 13 were not available for the study (11 died and 2 had serious illness), and 1 had revision surgery after 2 years. The remaining 8 patients had a low functional level but were able to manage daily hygiene. Five patients were pain-free. The radiographs showed no radiolucent zones around scapular components in two of eight patients. No radiolucent zones were detected around the humeral components [34].

1.2.5 1973: The Bayley-Walker Prosthesis

In 1973, the Bayley-Walker system was developed on Kessel's model improving both design and fixation. A central glenoid screw coated with hydroxyapatite was introduced to achieve a secure glenoid fixation without a concomitant increase in loosening. In this prosthesis the center of rotation was moved medially and distally to increase the abductor muscle lever arm. Ahir reported no loosening and radiolucencies after 5 years of follow-up in 81 non-tumor cases and 43 cases of malignancy [24].

1.2.6 1975: The Jefferson Prosthesis of Fenlin

Fenlin developed a new model of reverse shoulder arthroplasty to increase the deltoid function. He introduced a large glenosphere with an enlarged ball-and-socket construct to compensate the absent rotator cuff [27]. The glenosphere was made of polyethylene to lighten the implant weight, while the humeral cup was metallic (Fig. 1.6).

In 1975, Fenlin described the early satisfactory results, and concluded that the right indication of this prosthesis was rotator cuff arthropathy [27]. However, in 1985 he reported implant mechanical breakage, prosthesis loosening, and anterior instability in a long-term follow-up [35].

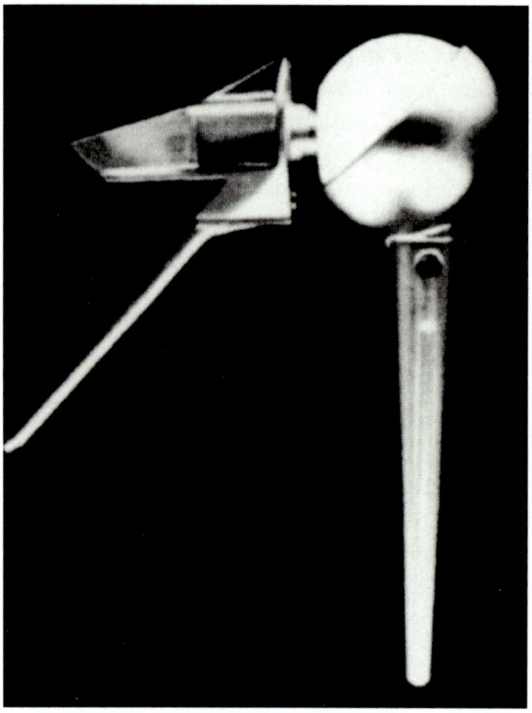

Fig. 1.6 The Fenlin JM Jr. reverse shoulder prosthesis. It is characterized by a large polyethylene glenosphere to increase deltoid lever arm. A wedge is inserted to fix the scapula, and a column is placed along the axillary border of the scapula (Reprinted with permission from Matsen FA, Rockwood CA, Wirth MA, Lippitt SB: Artropatia gleno-omerale e suo trattamento. In: Rockwood CA, Matsen FA. La Spalla. eds. Roma: Verduci; 2000:823–944)

1.2.7 1975: The Liverpool Prosthesis of Beddow

This prosthesis was initially designed in 1969 by Beddow and Elloy and was similar to a Charnley hip prosthesis (Fig. 1.7) [25]. The glenoid component (ball diameter 20 mm) and the stem were fixed into the scapular pillar with the polyethylene socket cemented into the proximal humerus. This design mimicked the anatomic center of rotation outside the scapula. Nineteen prostheses were implanted, and 16 had a 5-year follow-up; 11 patients experienced almost pain-free, and 4 patients showed loosening of the scapular component [36].

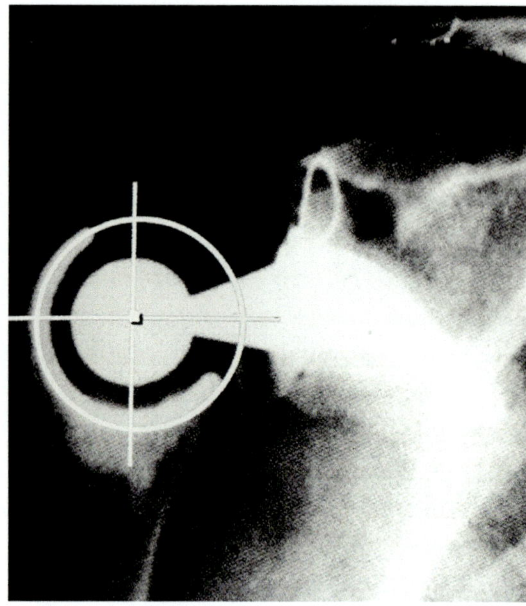

Fig. 1.7 The Liverpool reverse shoulder prosthesis. The glenoid component has a stem fixed in the scapular pillar to a depth of about 50 mm and with the polyethylene socket cemented into the proximal humerus (Reprinted with permission from Boileau P, Walch G, et al. Shoulder Concepts. Reverse Shoulder Arthroplasty. eds. Montpellier: Sauramps Medical; 2016)

1.2.8 1978: The Buechel-Pappas-DePalma Prosthesis

In 1978, Buechel et al. [26] designed a prosthesis similar to the Neer Mark III (Fig. 1.8). This model was based on a supporting system with two spheres to realize a "floating fulcrum." It was characterized by a small glenosphere articulated with a larger and mobile intermediate polyethylene cup and with the humeral head to allow supraphysiologic motion [26, 37]. The early results in few patients were promising. They reveal superior fixation strength of both glenoid and humeral components and functional adaptation of the prosthesis without fracture of fixturing bone or prosthetic dislocation [26]. However, Buechel et al. [26] hypothesized that, at a longer follow-up, the muscle forces across the glenohumeral joint would lead to loosening at the bone-cement or humerus-glenoid interfaces of the prosthesis.

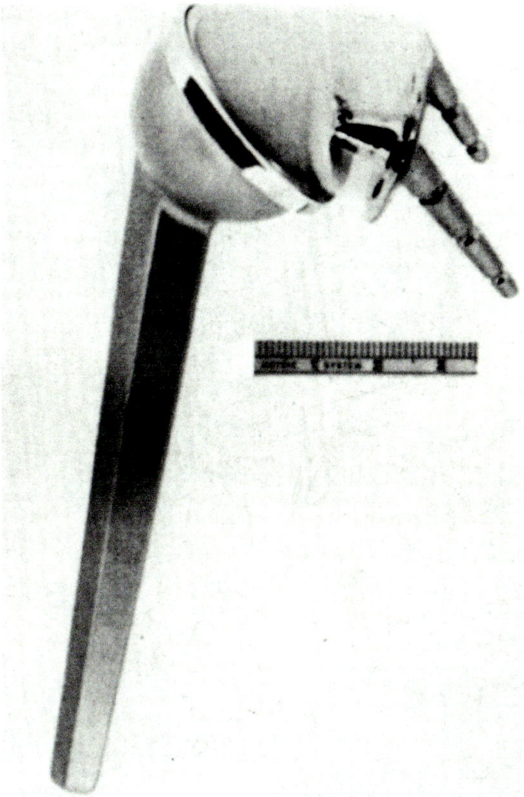

Fig. 1.8 The Buechel reverse shoulder arthroplasty. This implant includes a supporting device with double spheres that functions as a "floating fulcrum." This system allows shoulder motion over the anatomic limits (Reprinted with permission from Matsen FA, Rockwood CA, Wirth MA, Lippitt SB: Artropatia gleno-omerale e suo trattamento. In: Rockwood CA, Matsen FA. La Spalla. eds. Roma: Verduci; 2000:823–944)

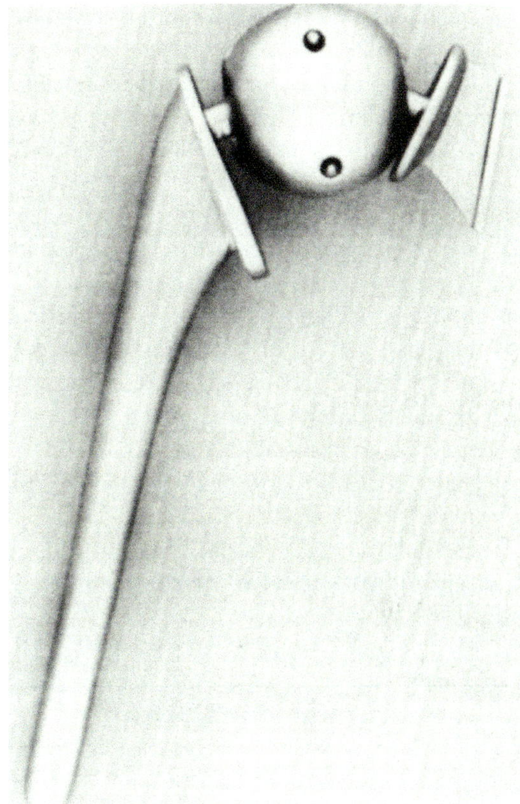

Fig. 1.9 The trispherical total shoulder of Gristina and Webb. It consisted of Vitallium humeral and glenoid small balls, both incorporated in a larger polyethylene sphere (Reprinted with permission from Matsen FA, Rockwood CA, Wirth MA, Lippitt SB: Artropatia gleno-omerale e suo trattamento. In: Rockwood CA, Matsen FA. La Spalla. eds. Roma: Verduci; 2000:823–944)

1.2.9 1978: The Gristina Trispherical Prosthesis

In 1978, Gristina and Webb designed a system similar to Buechel's prosthesis [28] (Fig. 1.9). The name "trispherical" was related to the presence of a unique double ball-and-socket configuration. These two small ball joints, on both humeral and scapular sides, are articulated with a central polyethylene sphere inserted in a separate metallic socket [37]. This system was successful in improving pain and ROM but experienced several dislocations of the humeral sphere and glenoid component fracture.

These previous constrained reverse shoulder prostheses (reverse ball-and-socket designs) tended to fail because their center of rotation was lateral to the scapula with limited motion and, thus, they produced excessive torque and shear forces at the glenoid component-bone interface leading to early loosening (Fig.1.7). In most cases, the functional active elevation was limited, less than 90 degrees, and especially related to scapulothoracic motion. Many models remained experimental and were abandoned because of the failures, particularly for the prosthetic instability and loosening [27, 33, 38–41].

The challenge of finding a compromise among mobility, stability, mechanical efficiency, and resistance to loosening in the prosthesis design was considered impossible.

In 1985, Paul Grammont, unlike the previous reverse models, first introduced a new reverse shoulder prosthesis characterized by two major and revolutionary innovations: a large glenoid hemisphere without the neck and a small humeral cup almost horizontally inclined and covering less than half the hemisphere. In Grammont reverse prosthesis, the center of rotation was medialized and stabilized, minimizing torque on the glenoid component and recruiting more fibers of the anterior and posterior deltoid which led to an increase of the abduction force [39].

These innovations represent the main causes of the worldwide success of this prosthesis design.

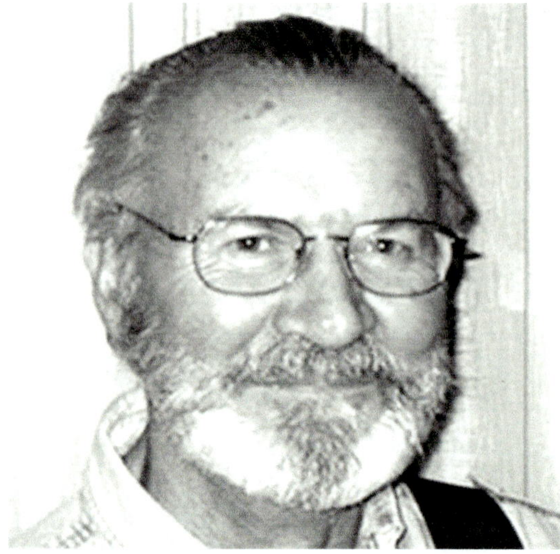

Fig. 1.10 Dr. Paul-Marie Grammont is shown in 2011 (Reprinted with permission from Boileau P. Biographical Sketch. Clin Orthop Relat Res. 2011;469:2422–2423)

1.3 Paul Grammont Biography

Paul Grammont was born on April 12, 1940 in Salins-les-Bains (Fig. 1.10). His father was a teacher and his mother was trained as a physicist. His father taught in different schools in Besançon, Alès, Quimper, Lons-le-Saunier, Troyes, and finally in Lyon, where Grammont took the baccalaureate in "Elementary Math," in 1957. After graduating from secondary school, he began his medical studies in Lyon as a resident in general and osteoarticular surgery. In Lyon, he worked as a university assistant in Michel Latarjet's anatomy laboratory from 1968 to 1971. From March 1972 to April 1974, he was a fellow and then a senior registrar in Professor Albert Trillat's orthopedic department in Lyon specializing in knee and shoulder surgery. He did his military service in French Guiana where he treated many difficult cases. In 1974, when he was 34, he became an Associate Professor of Orthopedic Surgery and Traumatology (Fig. 1.11). Then, he became the Chairman of the Orthopedic Department of the University Hospital in Dijon, in September 1974. It was in Dijon that he began his biomechanical experiments on the knee and the shoulder in his own garage before having the opportunity to work in the anatomical and biomechanical labs in the Medical University of Dijon. Innovation was Paul-Marie Grammont's keyword and he was really creative; besides developing the reverse shoulder prosthesis [4, 42], he also developed an early patellofemoral prosthesis [43] and one of the first nails with a self-advancing mechanism designed to lengthen long bones like the tibia and

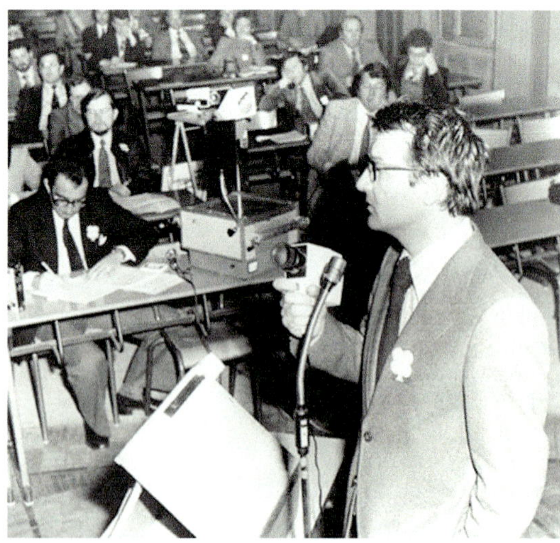

Fig. 1.11 Dr. Paul-Marie Grammont is shown about in 1970 (Reprinted with permission from Boileau P. Biographical Sketch. Clin Orthop Relat Res. 2011;469:2422–2423)

the femur (Albizia nail) [44]. The shoulder was the joint that he mostly studied. He firstly proposed a procedure named "Bristow-Trillat" for the anterior instability explaining its biomechanical rationale. But, his ingenious mind was developed in the degenerative pathology and prosthetic surgery of the shoulder. In 1985, Grammont designed a reverse prosthesis for arthritic shoulders with insufficient rotator cuff. In 1987, he published his first paper on the reverse prosthesis in the French literature [4, 45]. Six years later, in 1993, he summarized the results of his biomechanical studies in the English language [42].

In 1997, at 57 years old, he had a stroke with right hemiplegia and aphasia. Despite functional deficits, he continued his carpentry and plumbing activities in his home and became a painter using his left hand. Paul-Marie Grammont died on March 30, 2013 [45, 46].

1.4 The Principles of Grammont's Reverse Prosthesis

In 1981, Professor Paul-Marie Grammont directed two engineers in a study with a theoretical and mathematical approach entitled *Study of a Mechanical Model for a Shoulder Total Prosthesis: Realization of a Prototype* [47]. Grammont observed that, when the cuff is absent, the solution is to intrinsically balance the middle deltoid to strengthen its abduction component and lessen the elevation component responsible for loosening stress on the glenoid. Moreover, regarding the center of rotation, he said: "medializing the center of rotation of the scapulohumeral joint, and so increasing the deltoid lever arm, will compensate for the lack of activity of the supraspinatus muscle. In this way, we would move the mobile joint against the scapula without allowing a change in the position of the humerus in reference to the scapula. Indeed, if at the same time, we medialized the humerus itself, the deltoid lever arm would remain unchanged instead of being increased… In a first step, we'll have to lower the center of rotation" [47]. This is the concept of medializing the center of rotation.

The above method of strengthening the deltoid abduction component was consistent with, and validated by, the experience of the translation-rotation-elevation osteotomy of the scapular spine, described in 1975 [48–51]. After all, the increase of the middle deltoid lever arm induced by the acromial lateralization through this osteotomy was measurable [50]. Therefore, the deltoid can be affected in the same way by two different means: lateralizing the acromion without moving the center of rotation or medializing the center of rotation without moving the acromion [52].

1.4.1 1985. The First Version of Grammont's Arthroplasty, the Delta™ Reverse Prosthesis

This *first model* of Grammont's prosthesis was the *Delta™ reverse prosthesis* (Delta for deltoid, the only motor of this design) as it relied solely on the strength of the deltoid muscle for both movement and stability [42, 53] (Table 1.2). It was designed by Grammont in 1985.

This prosthesis, also named "Trompette," had only two components (Fig. 1.12). The glenoid component was a metallic or ceramic ball without a neck, initially two-thirds of a sphere, and 42 mm in diameter. It was designed to fit over the glenoid like a glove and fixed with cement. The humeral component was a polyethylene socket. Its concave surface was a third of a sphere, and its stem was trumpet-shaped for cementing into the humeral medullary canal. A "bell saw" was used to prepare the glenoid, and two broaches were used to prepare the different parts of the humerus, one for the epiphysis and one for the diaphysis. The initial Grammont reverse prosthesis was cemented on both humeral and glenoid sides.

The underlying principles which differentiate this prosthesis from the failed reverse semi-constrained designs of the past include (Fig. 1.5):

1. A fixed center of rotation with congruent large joint surfaces (cup on sphere instead of sphere on a "flat" surface) to compensate for the deficient rotator cuff muscles and increase stability

2. A medialized center of rotation (so that it actually lies at the glenoid bone-prosthesis interface) in order to:
   (a) Increase the deltoid lever arm.
   (b) Reduce the torque at the point of fixation of the glenoid component.
3. Lowering of the humerus relative to the glenoid to increase deltoid tension to overcome the weak/absent rotator cuff muscles

To achieve this, Grammont used a reverse ball-and-socket prosthesis, but he introduced two majors design innovations: (1) a large ball and no neck on the glenoid side and (2) a small cup, oriented with a nonanatomical inclination of 155°, and that covers less than half of the hemisphere on the humeral side. Almost all reversed prostheses designed before the Delta had a small prosthetic head and a neck and/or a more vertically oriented and covering cup, which created a very different biomechanical environment [3, 8, 18, 28, 34].

In 1987, Grammont et al. [54] reported a study on eight patients with his first design: three cases of post-radiotherapy necrosis, one case of inflammatory osteoarthritis, and four revisions of failed prostheses. The mean age was 70 years, and cuff was absent or destroyed in all cases. The mean follow-up was only 6 months. A transacromial approach (with osteotomy of the lateral acromion) was used in all but one case. Revision osteosynthesis of acromial nonunion was required in three of these cases. All shoulders were pain-free, but mobility was variable. In three cases, active anterior elevation was 100–130°, but in the three other cases, it was less than 60°. Unsatisfied with these results, Grammont made further modifications to progress to the current design. Since he experienced several

Table 1.2 Reverse shoulder prosthesis of Grammont and post-Grammont

Prosthesis name/author	Year of introduction	Main characteristics
Grammont prostheses		
First prototype	1985	The humeral component was a polyethylene socket with a trumpet shape; the glenoid component was metallic or ceramic ball with a press-fit central peg; center of rotation medialized but lateral to native glenoid surface
Delta III—first generation	1991	The glenoid components included a circular glenoid baseplate with a central peg for press-fit impaction, reinforced with two divergent screws to resist initial shear forces. The glenosphere was directly screwed onto the peripheral edge of the plate
Delta III—second generation	1991	Morse taper with a central countersunk screw
Delta III—third generation	1994	A diaphyseal stem screwed onto a modular metaphyseo-epiphyseal block; the polyethylene cup fitted over the epiphyseal end
Post-Grammont prostheses		
Aequalis® reversed	1998	The metaglenoid is fixed with divergent locking screws and implanted lower on the glenoid with a small amount of inferior tilt
Encore Reverse®/ Frankle	1998	Placed less medially than the Delta prosthesis; the center of rotation was closer to its usual anatomic location
Duocentric® reverse prosthesis	2001	Inferior extension of the glenosphere to avoid scapular notching and fixation peg to preserve the glenoid bone stock
Universal Arrow System	2002	Placed less medially than the Delta prosthesis; the COR is in the glenoid; the humeral cup has an inbuilt medial notch to avoid friction against the pillar of the scapula
Lima Corporate SMR™	2003	The central peg is made of a Trabecular Titanium™ technology
TESS (Total Evolutive Shoulder System)—Biomet	2006	Uncemented glenoid baseplate secured by a full hydroxyapatite central peg with titanium plasma spray; the humeral implant is based on the short reverse corolla
Aequalis Ascend™ Flex	2012	Short, uncemented, and convertible humeral stem to preserve bone stock; 145° angle to avoid scapular notching. Onlay design

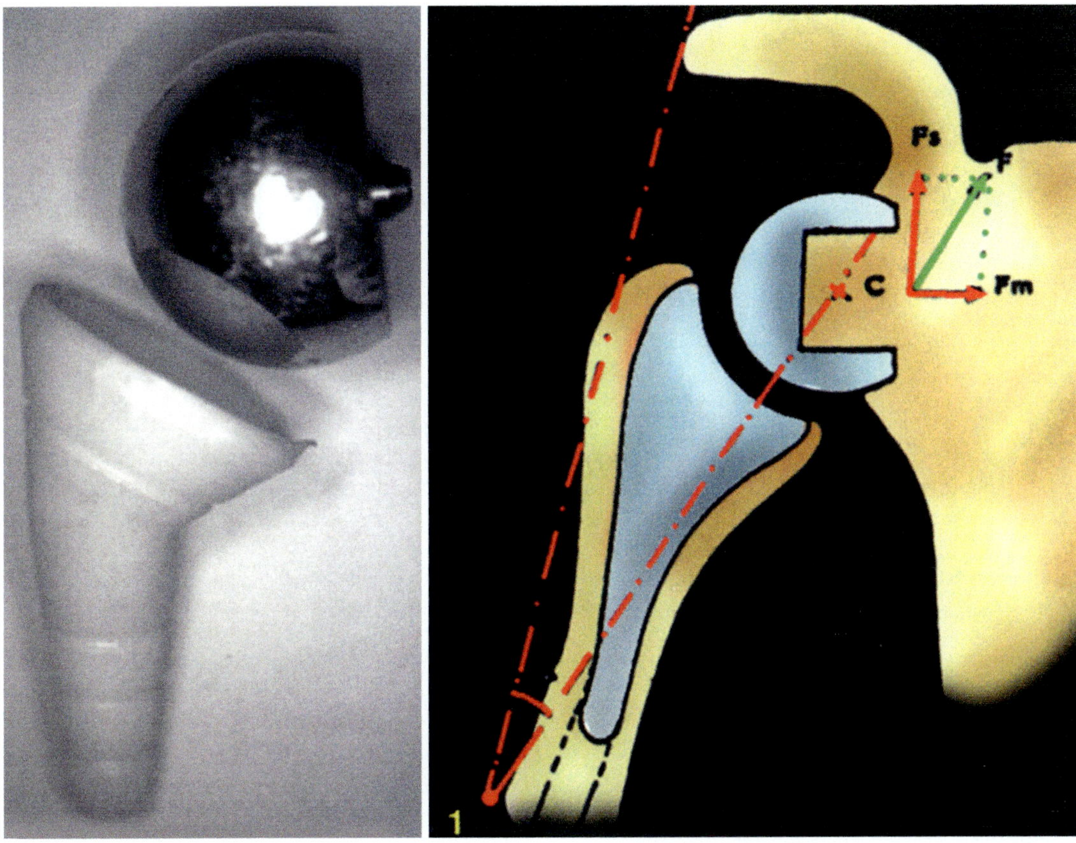

Fig. 1.12 The first model of Grammont reverse prosthesis named "Trompette," designed by Grammont in 1985 and first implanted in 1986. This prosthesis included a polyethylene humeral component and an alumina ceramic glenoid component with a volume equivalent to 2/3 of a sphere of 44 mm (Reprinted with permission from Boileau P, Walch G, et al. Shoulder Concepts. Reverse Shoulder Arthroplasty. eds. Montpellier: Sauramps Medical; 2016)

failures with the cemented glenoid component, he decided to change the glenoid to an uncemented system fixing the glenoid component with a central peg and some screws of divergent direction to counteract the initial shearing forces [53]. He also abandoned the idea of having two-thirds of a sphere and opted for a design based on half of a sphere in order to place the center of rotation directly in contact with the glenoid surface, decreasing lateral offset at the glenohumeral articulation and thus decreasing shearing forces.

Later, Grammont and his collaborators observed loosening of the cemented large sphere (2/3 of sphere), and they moved to a press-fit glenoid baseplate with a smaller hemisphere [52]. However, some of these early Grammont reverse prostheses are still surviving at more than 15 years of follow-up. Notably, this Trompette prosthesis has been associated only with small and nonprogressive notches on the scapular pillar [52].

1.4.2 1991: The Second Model of Grammont's Prosthesis: The Delta III

The Delta III prosthesis came on the market in 1991 and is still available.

The Delta III has five parts: the glenoid baseplate (metaglenoid), the glenosphere, the polyethylene humeral cup, the humeral neck, and the humeral stem (Fig. 1.13a, b).

In the first generation, the metaglenoid was a circular plate with a long and uncemented central

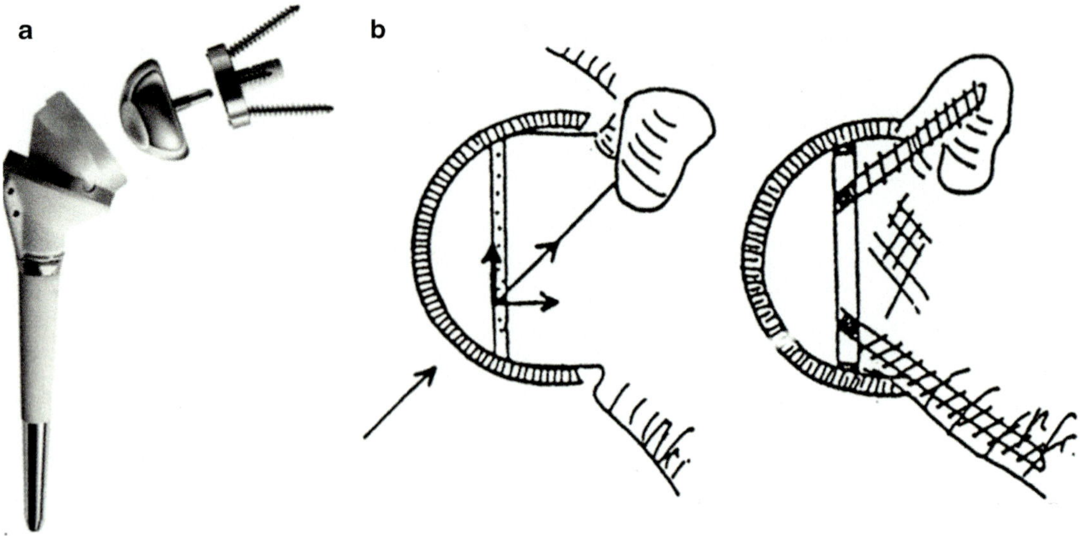

Fig. 1.13 (**a**) The Delta ™ reverse prosthesis has five components: the glenoid baseplate (metaglenoid), the glenosphere, the polyethylene cup, the humeral neck, and the humeral stem. (**b**) The change from a cemented to an uncemented glenoid with divergent screws to resist initial shear forces (Reprinted with permission from Boileau P, Walch G, et al. Shoulder Concepts. Reverse Shoulder Arthroplasty. eds. Montpellier: Sauramps Medical; 2016)

peg. It was fixed with two divergent 3.5 mm screws superiorly and inferiorly in order to resist to the shearing forces at the bone-implant interface. The glenosphere was screwed directly onto the peripheral edge of the plate, but this peripheral screwing was abandoned due to secondary loosening of the screws [20].

In the second generation, the metaglenoid was conical and smooth in the periphery with a Morse taper effect. The metaglenoid was coated with hydroxyapatite on its deep surface to improve bony fixation. The center of the metaglenoid was hollow to securely fix the glenosphere with a central screw. The humeral component was a monobloc with a cup of standard thickness [20].

The third generation became available in 1994 with a new humeral component. A diaphyseal stem was screwed on to a metaphyseo-epiphyseal block of one of three available sizes in order to obtain a better fit. The polyethylene cup (a third of a sphere) was fitted over the epiphyseal end, but it was too small and rapidly deteriorated due to medial impingement. The cup was, therefore, replaced by a lateralized cup of two diameters of 36 mm and 42 mm. A metallic wedge is available to allow correction of length problems in the cases with loss of metaphyseal bone. A retentive cup can be used in cases of major instability [20].

The choice of a large humeral stem came from the idea developed in hip arthroplasty of maximizing the contact area between the stem and the host bone [20].

The Delta III prosthesis (DePuy International Limited, Leeds, England) has been used for the last 20 years worldwide, and its results have been extensively reported [55–60]. In cases of pseudoparalytic shoulders with massive irreparable cuff tears and glenohumeral arthritis, all series have shown a recovery of active abduction of between 120 and 130 degrees.

1.4.3 Complications of Grammont Reverse TSA

The persistent problems and high complication rate with this procedure have been described extensively in the current literature with complications including [55, 59–62] hematoma formation [63], infection [55, 59, 63–66], scapular notching [59, 66–68], instability [63, 65, 66], acromial complications [63, 64], glenoid component failures (loosening, disassembly) [10, 28, 35, 59], intraoperative fractures, and neurological complications.

Deep infection has been reported in up to 5.1% of primary reverse TSA. This is likely related to the large subacromial "dead space" that allows the formation of a hematoma [69].

Scapular notching is a direct consequence of both the absence of a prosthetic neck of the glenosphere and the horizontal orientation of the humeral cup. It is caused by the impingement of the medial aspect of the polyethylene humeral cup on the scapular neck inferiorly but also posteriorly. This repetitive contact can lead to bone loss under the inferior aspect of the glenoid with incidence of up to 50–96% [58, 63, 67, 68] (Fig. 1.14a) and in polyethylene wear (Fig. 1.14b). Moreover, the polyethylene particle disease may cause local osteolysis with progression of the notch [60, 62, 70]. This is supported by the finding of polyethylene particles in the pseudomembrane in the osteolytic area [71].

A series from Nice reported this complication in 74% of cases (45 cases) [55] and another from Sirveaux in 65% (77 cases) [59]. Gerber et al. [72] studied the passive range of motion in prosthesis with superior fixation of the glenosphere. This confirmed previous reports [61, 62] that contact between the humeral cup and the pillar of the scapula is much more significant when the metaglenoid is fixed high on the glenoid.

Instability. Proper deltoid tensioning can be another source of complications with inadequate tension leading to instability [69].

Acromial complications like fracture are due to the high tensioning of the deltoid [69].

Glenoid loosening. Although intraoperative glenoid complications are uncommon, *glenoid loosening* has been observed in up to 4.1% of Grammont reverse prostheses [69].

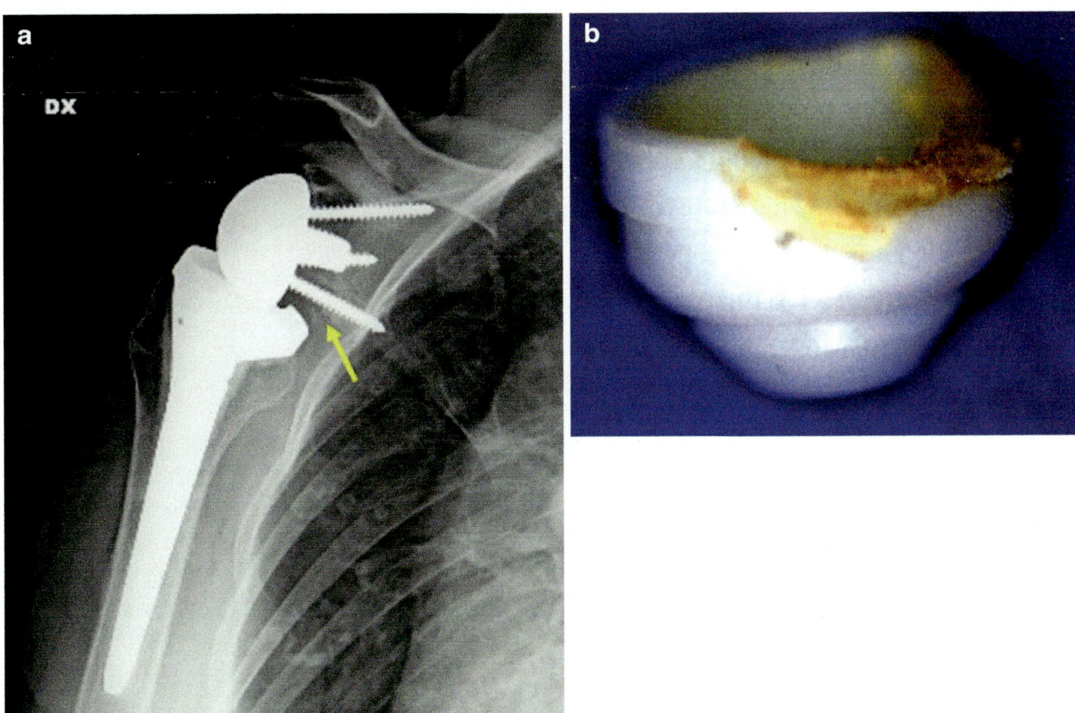

Fig. 1.14 The scapular notching. (**a**) The yellow arrow shows the scapular notching that results from a mechanical conflict between the medial border of the humeral implant and the inferior rim of the glenoid. This conflict leads to a polyethylene wear of the glenoid component. (**b**) Retrieved glenoid component with polyethylene wear (Reprinted with permission from Boileau P, Walch G, et al. Shoulder Concepts. Reverse Shoulder Arthroplasty. eds. Montpellier: Sauramps Medical; 2016)

A *limited external rotation,* despite the good elevation, achieved by the reverse shoulder prosthesis was reported due to the medialization of the humeral component that increases the medial impingement against the scapula. It also accounts for the medial notch [55, 61, 62].

Moreover, the medialization of the center of rotation reduces the strength of the posterior deltoid fibers. Injury to the suprascapular nerve while fixing the metaglenoid may also be a cause of lack of external rotation [62].

Limitation of internal rotation was also noticed. It is caused by the prosthesis design, the medialization that reduces the strenght of the anterior fibers [30], and the state of the subscapularis. Active medial rotation will be improved if part of subscapularis remains intact.

1.5 Post-Grammont Reverse Shoulder Arthroplasty

Several new models were developed based on Grammont's principles [64, 73, 74] to overcome all the complications of the previous reverse shoulder prostheses (Table 1.2).

The Tornier Company (Montbonnot-Saint-Martin, France) has developed the Aequalis® reversed prosthesis, based on the biomechanical principles described by Grammont, but with some innovations. The metaglenoid is fixed with divergent locking screws. Wedges and polyethylene cups of varying thickness are used to correct the tension of the deltoid and metaphyseal bone loss. Users of the Delta and Tornier prostheses, following the work of Gerber [72], have recommended that the metaglenoid be implanted lower on the glenoid with a small amount of inferior tilt (Fig. 1.15).

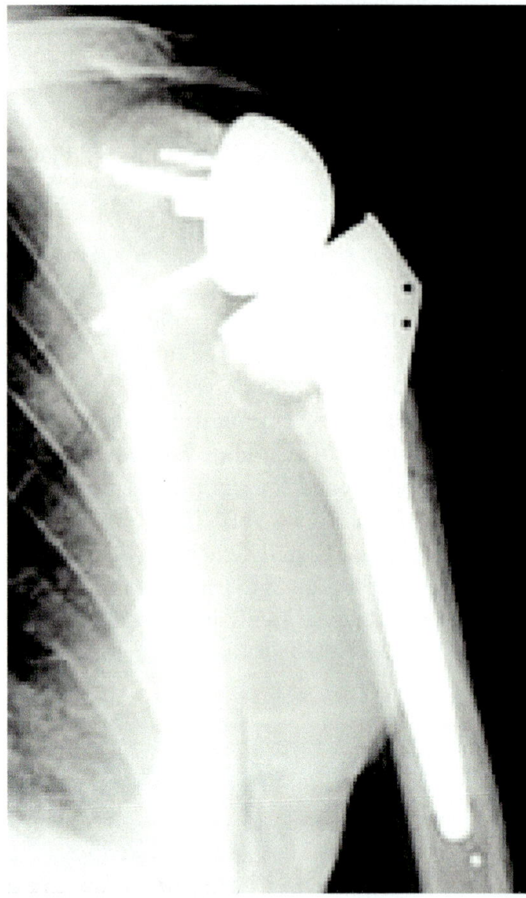

Fig. 1.15 The Aequalis reversed shoulder prosthesis ™ (Tornier Company, Montbonnot Saint Martin, France). The metaglenoid is fixed with divergent locking screws with inferior tilt (Reprinted with permission from Boileau P, Walch G, et al. Shoulder Concepts. Reverse Shoulder Arthroplasty. eds. Montpellier: Sauramps Medical; 2016)

In *1998*, Frankle designed the reverse prosthesis (ENCORE Medical, Austin, Texas, USA) (Fig. 1.16). It was placed less medially than the Delta, and the center of rotation was closer to its usual anatomical location [64]. In his series of 60 patients with more than 2 years follow-up, less abduction than in the Delta series was observed but with a better range of rotation. However, the design of the glenosphere, which was two-thirds of a sphere, increased shearing of the screwed metaglenoid. Several complications of the glenoid component were noted, including loosening (seven cases) and breakage of the platinum and screws. Frankle's biomechanical studies concluded that a concave metaglenoid was better than a flat one [74].

In *2001*, the Duocentric® reverse prosthesis (Aston Medical) was designed and developed until a third generation based on the "Trompette" and Delta® (DePuy). It was first implanted in 2003. This system was characterized by three main features: spherical inferior overhang to avoid scapular notching, fixation peg of various

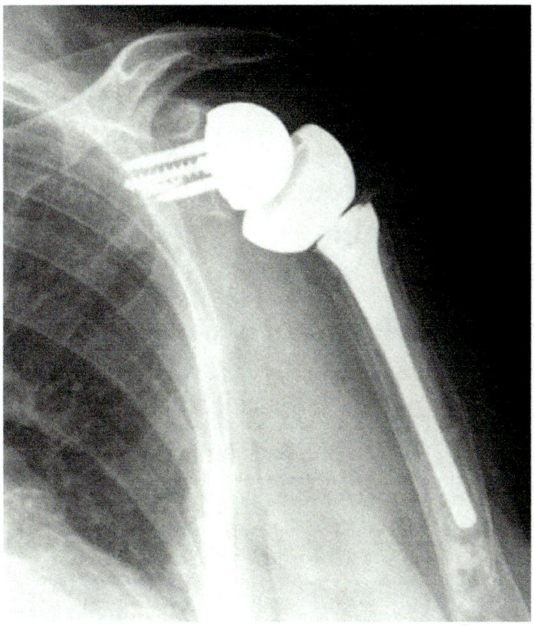

Fig. 1.16 The Encore reverse prosthesis (Encore Medical, Austin, Texas, USA). The glenosphere is placed less medially than the Delta and the center of rotation is similar to the anatomical position (Reprinted with permission from Boileau P, Walch G, et al. Shoulder Concepts. Reverse Shoulder Arthroplasty. eds. Montpellier: Sauramps Medical; 2016)

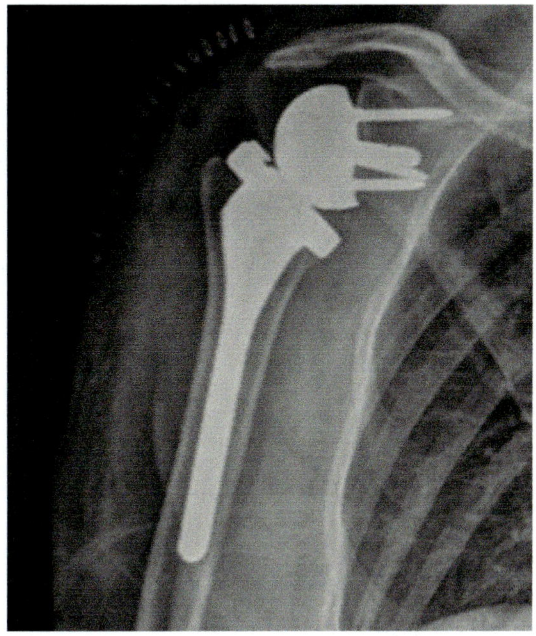

Fig. 1.17 The Duocentric® reversed shoulder prosthesis with uncemented stem

sizes to preserve the glenoid bone stock, and adjustable length to reinforce the fixation if needed (Fig. 1.17). After more improvements, the Duocentric® Expert reversed prosthesis became available in 2007 [75].

In *2002*, the Universal Arrow System (FH orthopedics, Heimsbrunn, France) was developed in France and became available commercially in Europe. This model was based on Grammont's principles with the center of rotation lying at the level of the glenoid unlike Encore reverse prosthesis. The center of rotation was in the glenoid, and the prosthesis was placed less medially than the Delta prosthesis (Fig. 1.18). Thus, the range of rotation (poor in Grammont's design) was improved, and the risk of medial impingement was eliminated. In addition, the humeral cup had an inbuilt medial notch to avoid friction against the pillar of the scapula. The metaglenoid was concave, adapting to the normal curvature of the glenoid fossa.

De Wilde [73] confirmed that medialization and lowering the implant affect the moment arm of the deltoid and improve the arc of rotation, which is essential in daily activities.

A retrospective study was presented at the French Congress of Orthopedic Surgery in Paris in November 2006 which compared the results of 40 Delta and 40 Arrow prostheses. Radiologically, it was shown that Arrow System allowed for less medialization, but that the extent of humeral lowering was the same with both systems.

In *2003*, Lima Corporate introduced a reverse shoulder prosthesis with a modular shoulder replacement system (SMR™) [76]. This system also allows the conversion to a reverse shoulder arthroplasty without changing the humeral stem, and the glenoid metal back avoids the risk of sacrificing the bone [77]. At a mean follow-up of 32.3 months, all patients improved in terms of range of motion, and no signs of loosening of the implant were reported.

In the SMR Axioma TT Metal Back implant (Lima Corporate SMR™), a wide range of modular pegs are provided to manage bone deficiency. This system is made of a Trabecular Titanium™

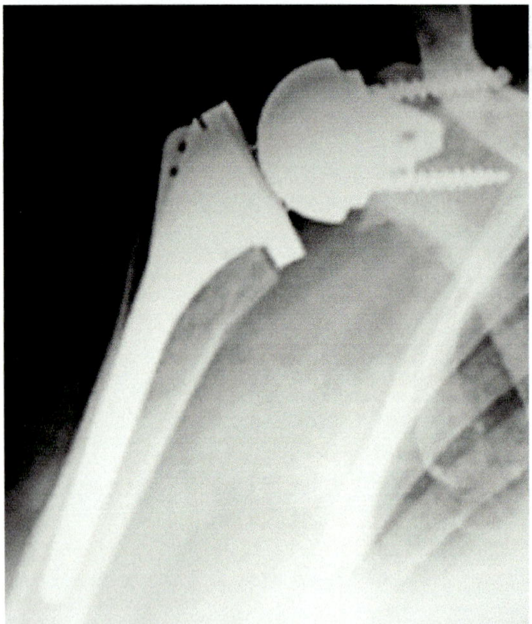

Fig. 1.18 The Universal Arrow System (FH Orthopedics, Heimsbrunn, France). This prosthesis is placed less medially than the Delta; the center of rotation is in the glenoid unlike Encore reverse prosthesis; the humeral cup has an inbuilt medial notch to avoid friction against the pillar of the scapula

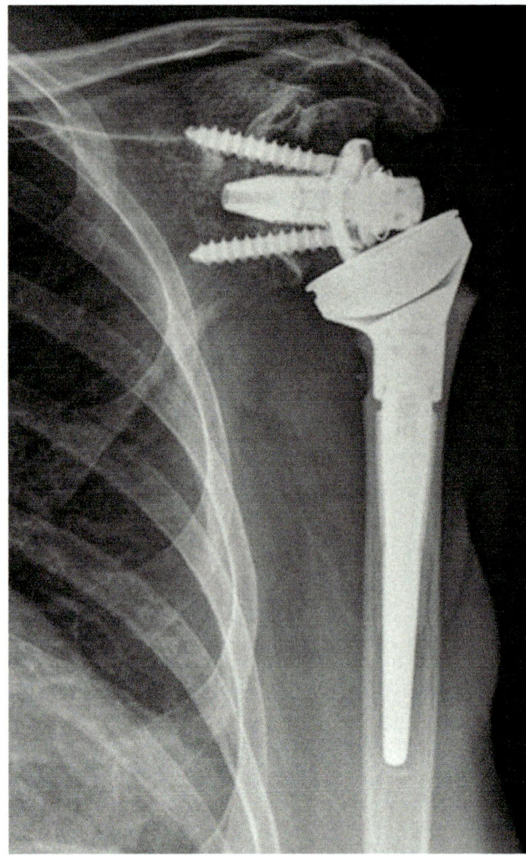

Fig. 1.19 SMR Axioma TT Metal Back implant (Lima Corporate SMR™). The central peg is made of a Trabecular Titanium™ technology

technology that provides significant osseointegration with high bone ingrowth percentage both in cancellous and cortical bone in sheep model [78] (Fig. 1.19).

In *2012*, Tornier Company designed a new reverse shoulder prosthesis with an onlay design, the Aequalis Ascend™ Flex (Tornier SAS-Wright Medical Inc., Bloomington, MN, USA). It is characterized by a new short, uncemented, and convertible humeral stem to comply with these specifications: bone stock preservation with a short stem, avoiding scapular notching utilizing a 145° angle through a summation of the stem and polyethylene liner angles and making the humeral revision easier. This angle has been shown to minimize scapular impingement while optimizing elevation, internal, and external rotation through virtual implantation studies completed by Tornier, Inc. [79, 80] (Fig. 1.20). Goetzmann et al. presented the preliminary results of 24 reversed shoulder arthroplasty at 2 years of follow-up. The average CS improved from 21 preoperatively to 63 postoperatively ($P < 0.0001$). Anterior active elevation and active external rotation improved from 79° and 10° preoperatively to 139° and 28° postoperatively. The mean active internal rotation improved significantly from the sacrum to L3 ($P < 0.0001$). SSV improved from 34 to 73%. No mechanical complication (migration, fracture, instability, or loosening), loosening, and radiolucent lines around the stem were reported [80].

Recently, new models of reverse shoulder prostheses without stem were proposed.

The TESS (Total Evolutive Shoulder System) (Biomet, Warsaw, IN, USA) has an uncemented glenoid baseplate secured by a full

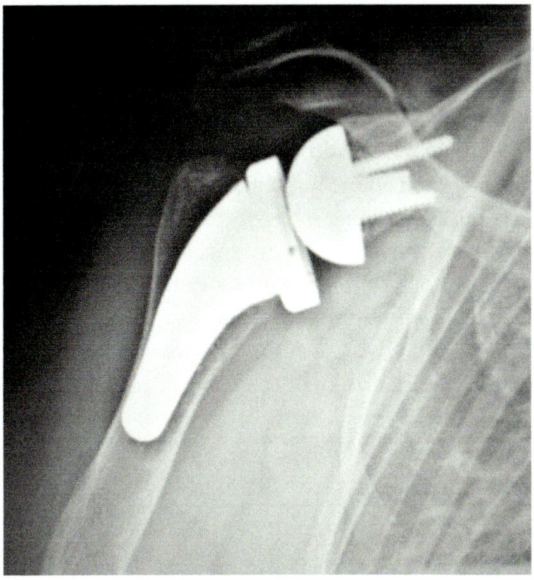

Fig. 1.20 The Aequalis Ascend™ Flex (Tornier SAS-Wright Medical Inc., Bloomington, MN, USA). This prosthesis has an onlay design and a short, uncemented, and convertible humeral stem to preserve bone stock; 145° angle to avoid scapular notching

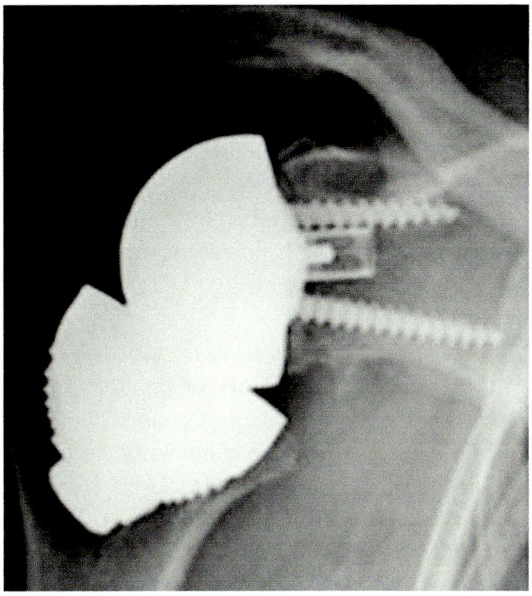

Fig. 1.21 TESS stemless reverse shoulder arthroplasty. Glenoid baseplate is uncemented and secured by a hydroxyapatite central peg with titanium plasma spray. The humeral implant is based on the anatomic RCo (Reprinted with permission from Boileau P, Walch G, et al. Shoulder Concepts. Reverse Shoulder Arthroplasty. eds. Montpellier: Sauramps Medical; 2016)

hydroxyapatite central peg with titanium plasma spray, as well as two superior and inferior locked screws. The glenosphere is eccentric, with a 3 mm lateralization, and is placed inferiorly. The humeral implant based on the short reverse corolla is an uncemented metaphyseal-epiphyseal implant, made of chrome cobalt, with a titanium plasma spray, and full hydroxyapatite coating. Six wings on the surface of the reverse corolla optimize the rotational stability. Teissier et al. found a significant improvement in pain relief, flexion, abduction, and external rotation, no infections or neurologic lesions, no humeral loosening of the corolla despite the lack of a stem, as well as no component dissociation; scapular notching in medium-term follow-up study was about 19% [81] (Fig. 1.21).

In *2015*, also Lima LTD produces a stemless reverse shoulder prosthesis, the Lima shoulder modular replacement (SMR) stemless shoulder system. This is a convertible system with four parts for anatomic configuration (humeral core component, double male Morse taper, locking screw, and humeral head) and two parts for reverse configuration (humeral core component and reverse liner). The humeral core component is composed of Trabecular Titanium designed for bone ingrowth and is seated by impaction. When utilized in reverse configuration, a metallic reverse liner is impacted into the humeral core component. This metallic liner, manufactured out of CoCrMo, then articulates with an all-polyethylene glenosphere [82].

1.6 Indications and Contraindications

Reverse shoulder arthroplasty represents primary indication for elderly patients with cuff tear arthropathy and a cuff-deficient shoulder demonstrating predictable outcomes [58, 83].

As surgeons have acquired more experience, indications have been extended to include revision arthroplasty, proximal humeral nonunion [84], acute fractures [84, 85], pseudo-paralysis due to massive and irreparable cuff tear without arthritis [27, 53, 60], severe fracture sequelae (type 3 or type 4) with tuberosity migration and osteolysis [39, 56, 86], prosthetic revision in a cuff-deficient shoulder [39, 61, 87], and tumor surgery [88, 89].

There are two major contraindications for a reversed prosthesis: a history of previous infection and a nonfunctional deltoid muscle.

As the study of reverse shoulder arthroplasty has advanced and varying systems have developed, vibrant controversies have arisen. Debate exists over the medialization of the center of rotation, with some proposing a more lateral offset pointing to a lower rate of scapular notching and an increase in impingment-free motion [89, 90]. Others suggest notching may also be minimized with appropriate positioning of the more medial glenoid component [68]. These issues require additional high-quality studies and must continue to be explored and debated [91].

1.7 Conclusion

The design of the reverse shoulder prosthesis was introduced about 50 years ago, but the initial models, introduced in the early 1970s, failed due to many complications, particularly instability and loosening of the glenoid component. To overcome these concerns, Paul Grammont first introduced two major revolutionary innovations in reverse shoulder prosthesis: a fixed and medialized center of rotation minimizing torque on the glenoid component and a lowered humerus improving the power of the deltoid for elevation/abduction. The pioneering concepts of Grammont and the development of the Delta III prosthesis have been fundamental to all subsequent shoulder arthroplasty systems. After more than 20 years of follow-up of these reverse prostheses, glenoid loosening and impingement of the humeral cup on the scapular neck are still present.

Despite these problems, the Grammont reverse prosthesis is, today, the main available surgical option in severe shoulder pathologies where the rotator cuff and proximal humerus are destroyed or absent and have become an essential part of shoulder prosthetic surgery.

Actually, many designs of reverse shoulder prosthesis have been introduced on the market, all based on the innovative Grammont concepts.

Other studies will be necessary to improve and develop new designs of reverse shoulder prosthesis to minimize the complications associated to these prostheses.

References

1. Neer CS 2nd, Watson KC, Stanton FJ. Recent experience in total shoulder replacement. J Bone Joint Surg Am. 1982;64(3):319–37.
2. Sanchez-Sotelo J, Cofield RH, Rowland CM. Shoulder hemiarthroplasty for glenohumeral arthritis associated with severe rotator cuff deficiency. J Bone Joint Surg Am. 2001;83-a(12):1814–22.
3. Wirth MA, Rockwood CA Jr. Complications of total shoulder-replacement arthroplasty. J Bone Joint Surg Am. 1996;78(4):603–16.
4. Grammont PM, Trouilloud P, Laffay JP, Deries X. Etude et réalisation d'une nouvelle prothèse d'épaule. Rhumatologie. 1987;39:407–18.
5. Bankes MJ, Emery RJ. Pioneers of shoulder replacement: Themistocles Gluck and Jules Emile Pean. J Shoulder Elb Surg. 1995;4(4):259–62.
6. Lugli T. Artificial shoulder joint by Pean (1893): the facts of an exceptional intervention and the prosthetic method. Clin Orthop Relat Res. 1978;133:215–8.
7. Neer CS 2nd. Articular replacement for the humeral head. J Bone Joint Surg Am. 1955;37-a(2):215–28.
8. Neer CS 2nd. Replacement arthroplasty for glenohumeral osteoarthritis. J Bone Joint Surg Am. 1974;56(1):1–13.
9. Cofield RH. Status of total shoulder arthroplasty. Arch Surg. 1977;112(9):1088–91.
10. Reeves B, Jobbins B, Flowers F, Dowson D, Wright V. Some problems in the development of a total shoulder endo-prosthesis. Ann Rheum Dis. 1972;31(5):425–6.
11. Severt R, Thomas BJ, Tsenter MJ, Amstutz HC, Kabo JM. The influence of conformity and constraint on translational forces and frictional torque in total shoulder arthroplasty. Clin Orthop Relat Res. 1993;292:151–8.
12. Kenmore PI, MacCartee C, Vitek B. A simple shoulder replacement. J Biomed Mater Res. 1974;8(4 Pt 2):329–30. https://doi.org/10.1002/jbm.820080412.

13. Marmor L. Hemiarthroplasty for the rheumatoid shoulder joint. Clin Orthop Relat Res. 1977;122:201–3.
14. Tanner MW, Cofield RH. Prosthetic arthroplasty for fractures and fracture-dislocations of the proximal humerus. Clin Orthop Relat Res. 1983;179:116–28.
15. Coughlin MJ, Morris JM, West WF. The semiconstrained total shoulder arthroplasty. J Bone Joint Surg Am. 1979;61(4):574–81.
16. Franklin JL, Barrett WP, Jackins SE, Matsen FA 3rd. Glenoid loosening in total shoulder arthroplasty. Association with rotator cuff deficiency. J Arthroplasty. 1988;3(1):39–46.
17. Gerard Y, Leblanc JP, Rousseau B. A complete shoulder prosthesis. Chirurgie; memoires de l'Academie de chirurgie. 1973;99(9):655–63.
18. Kölbel R, Friedebold G. Shoulder joint replacement. Archiv fur orthopadische und Unfall-Chirurgie. 1973;76(1):31–9.
19. Jazayeri R, Kwon YW. Evolution of the reverse total shoulder prosthesis. Bull NYU Hosp Jt Dis. 2011;69(1):50–5.
20. Katz D, O'Toole G, Cogswell L, Sauzieres P, Valenti P. A history of the reverse shoulder prosthesis. Int J Shoulder Surg. 2007;1:108–13.
21. Burkhead W. History and development of shoulder arthro-plasty. In: Arthroplasty of the shoulder. New York: Thieme; 1994. p. 838–53.
22. Neer CS. Shoulder reconstruction. Philadelphia: WB Saunders Co; 1990.
23. Khazzam MF. History and development of shoulder arthroplasty. Shoulder arthroplasty. New York, NY: Thieme Medical Publishers, Inc.; 2008. p. 1–9.
24. Ahir SP, Walker PS, Squire-Taylor CJ, Blunn GW, Bayley JI. Analysis of glenoid fixation for a reversed anatomy fixed-fulcrum shoulder replacement. J Biomech. 2004;37(11):1699–708. https://doi.org/10.1016/j.jbiomech.2004.01.031.
25. Blauth W, Donner K. Notes on the history of arthroplasty (author's transl)Zeitschrift fur Orthopadie und ihre Grenzgebiete. 1979;117(6):997–1006.
26. Buechel FF, Pappas MJ, DePalma AF. "Floating-socket" total shoulder replacement: anatomical, biomechanical, and surgical rationale. J Biomed Mater Res. 1978;12(1):89–114. https://doi.org/10.1002/jbm.820120109.
27. Fenlin JM Jr. Total glenohumeral joint replacement. Orthop Clin North Am. 1975;6(2):565–83.
28. Gristina AG, Webb LX. The Trispherical total shoulder replacement. In: Bayley IKL, editor. Shoulder surgery. New York: Springer-Verlag; 1982. p. 153–7.
29. Reeves B, Jobbins B, Dowson D, Wright V. A total shoulder endo-prosthesis. Eng Med. 1972;1(3):64–7. https://doi.org/10.1243/EMED_JOUR_1971_001_028_02.
30. Gerard Y. Is a retentive total shoulder prosthesis possible? Acta Orthop Belg. 1985;51(4):616–24.
31. Kölbel R. Stabilization of shoulders with bone and muscle defects. In: Kölbel R, Helbig B, Blauth W, editors. Shoulder replacement. Berlin, Heidelberg: Springer Berlin Heidelberg; 1987. p. 189–95.
32. Bodey WN, Yeoman PM. Prosthetic arthroplasty of the shoulder. Acta Orthop Scand. 1983;54(6):900–3.
33. Broström L-Å, Wallensten R, Olsson E, Anderson D. The Kessel prosthesis in total shoulder arthroplasty: a five-year experience. Clin Orthop Relat Res. 1992;277:155–60.
34. Wretenberg PF, Wallensten R. The Kessel total shoulder arthroplasty. A 13- to 16-year retrospective follow-up. Clin Orthop Relat Res. 1999;365:100–3.
35. Fenlin JM Jr. Semi-constrained prosthesis for the rotator cuff deficient patient. Orthop Trans. 1985;9:55.
36. Wolff R, Kölbel R. The history of shoulder joint replacement. In: Kölbel R, Helbig B, Blauth W, editors. Shoulder replacement. Berlin, Heidelberg: Springer Berlin Heidelberg; 1987. p. 3–13.
37. Ungethum M, Blomer W. Endoprosthetic replacement of the shoulder joint. Possibilities and their analysis. Zeitschrift fur Orthopadie und ihre Grenzgebiete. 1986;124(1):50–6. https://doi.org/10.1055/s-2008-1044523.
38. Bayley J, Kessel L. The Kessel total shoulder replacement. In: Springer, editor. Shoulder surgery. Berlin Heidelberg New York: Springer; 1982.
39. Boileau P, Walch G, Molè D, Favard L, Levigne C, Sirveaux F, Kempf JF, Clavert P, Collin P. Shoulder concepts 2016. In: Reverse shoulder arthroplasty 20-year anniversary. Montpellier: Sauramps Medical; 2016.
40. Lee DH, Niemann KM. Bipolar shoulder arthroplasty. Clin Orthop Relat Res. 1994;304:97–107.
41. Perry J. Biomechanics of the shoulder. In: Roockwood CA, Martsen FA, editors. The shoulder. Philadelphia: Saunders; 1990.
42. Grammont PM, Baulot E. Delta shoulder prosthesis for rotator cuff rupture. Orthopedics. 1993;16(1):65–8.
43. Renard JF, Grammont P. La prothèse autocentrique de rotule. Technique et résultat après 7 ans de recul. Rhumatologie. 1989;41:241–5.
44. Guichet JM, Grammont PM, Trouilloud P. A nail for progressive lengthening. An animal experiment with a 2-year follow-up. Chirurgie; memoires de l'Academie de chirurgie. 1992;118(6–7):405–10.
45. Boileau P. Biographical sketch: Paul M. Grammont, MD (1940). Clin Orthop Relat Res. 2011;469(9):2422–3. https://doi.org/10.1007/s11999-011-1959-y.
46. Baulot E. Paul-Marie Grammont. Orthop Traumatol Surg Res. 2013;759–60.
47. Grammont PM, Bourgon J, Pelzer P. Study of a mechanical model for a shoulder total prosthesis: realization of a prototype [in French]. Dijon: Université Dijon; 1981.
48. Baulot E, Cavaille A, Grammont P. Ostéotomie de translation rotation élévation de l'épine de l'omoplate dans les conflits antérieurs et les lésions fonctionnellement incomplètes de la coiffe des rotateurs. Orthopédie Traumatologie. 1993;3(3):221–6. https://doi.org/10.1007/BF01796521.
49. Grammont PM, Lelaurin G. Osteotomy of the scapula and the acropole prosthesis (author's transl)Der Orthopade. 1981;10(3):219–29.

50. Grammont PM, Trouilloud P, Sakka M. Translation-rotation osteotomy. 1975–1985 experiences with anterior impingement and incomplete lesions of the rotary cuff. Revue de chirurgie orthopedique et reparatrice de l'appareil moteur. 1988;74(4):337–40.
51. Grammont PM. Place de l'ostéotomie de l'épine de l'omoplate avec translation, rotation, élévation de l'acromion dans les ruptures chroniques de la coiffe des rotateurs. Lyon Chir. 1979;55:327–9.
52. Baulot E, Sirveaux F, Boileau P. Grammont's idea: the story of Paul Grammont's functional surgery concept and the development of the reverse principle. Clin Orthop Relat Res. 2011;469(9):2425–31. https://doi.org/10.1007/s11999-010-1757-y.
53. Grammont PM, Baulot E, Chabernaud D. Résultats des 16 premiers cas d'arthroplastie totale d'épaule inversée sans ciment pour des omarthroses avec grande rupture de coiffe. Rev Chir Orthop Reparatrice App Mot. 1996;82(Suppl. 1):169.
54. Grammont PM, Trouilloud P, Laffay JP, Deries X. Concept study and realization of a new total shoulder prosthesis [French]. Rhumatologie. 1987;39:407–18.
55. Boileau P, Watkinson DJ, Hatzidakis AM, Balg F. Grammont reverse prosthesis: design, rationale, and biomechanics. J Shoulder Elb Surg. 2005;14(1 Suppl S):147s–61s. https://doi.org/10.1016/j.jse.2004.10.006.
56. Boulahia A, Edwards TB, Walch G, Baratta RV. Early results of a reverse design prosthesis in the treatment of arthritis of the shoulder in elderly patients with a large rotator cuff tear. Orthopedics. 2002;25(2):129–33.
57. Renaud P, Wahab H, Bontoux L, Dauty M, Richard I, Brégeon C. Prothèse totale inversée de l'épaule et insuffisance de la coiffe des rotateurs : évaluation et approche de paramètres anatomiques prédictifs d'une bonne fonctionnalité à propos de 21 cas. Ann Readapt Med Phys. 2001;44(5):273–80.
58. Rittmeister M, Kerschbaumer F. Grammont reverse total shoulder arthroplasty in patients with rheumatoid arthritis and nonreconstructible rotator cuff lesions. J Shoulder Elb Surg. 2001;10(1):17–22. https://doi.org/10.1067/mse.2001.110515.
59. Sirveaux F, Favard L, Oudet D, Huquet D, Walch G, Mole D. Grammont inverted total shoulder arthroplasty in the treatment of glenohumeral osteoarthritis with massive rupture of the cuff. Results of a multicentre study of 80 shoulders. J Bone Joint Surg. 2004;86(3):388–95.
60. Valenti PH, Boutens D, Nerot C. Delta 3 reversed prosthesis for osteoarthritis with massive rotator cuff tear: long-term results (>5 years). In: Walch GBP, Mole D, editors. 2000 shoulder prostheses: two to ten year follow-up. Montpellier: Sauramps Medical; 2001. p. 253–9.
61. Delloye C, Joris D, Colette A, Eudier A, Dubuc JE. Complications mechanical prosthesis reversed the shoulder. Revue de chirurgie orthopedique et reparatrice de l'appareil moteur. 2002;88:410–4.
62. Nyffeler RW, Werner CM, Simmen BR, Gerber C. Analysis of a retrieved delta III total shoulder prosthesis. J Bone Joint Surg. 2004;86(8):1187–91.
63. Werner CM, Steinmann PA, Gilbart M, Gerber C. Treatment of painful pseudoparesis due to irreparable rotator cuff dysfunction with the Delta III reverse-ball-and-socket total shoulder prosthesis. J Bone Joint Surg Am. 2005;87(7):1476–86. https://doi.org/10.2106/jbjs.d.02342.
64. Frankle M, Siegal S, Pupello D, Saleem A, Mighell M, Vasey M. The reverse shoulder prosthesis for glenohumeral arthritis associated with severe rotator cuff deficiency. A minimum two-year follow-up study of sixty patients. J Bone Joint Surg Am. 2005;87(8):1697–705. https://doi.org/10.2106/jbjs.d.02813.
65. Guery J, Favard L, Sirveaux F, Oudet D, Mole D, Walch G. Reverse total shoulder arthroplasty. Survivorship analysis of eighty replacements followed for five to ten years. J Bone Joint Surg Am. 2006;88(8):1742–7. https://doi.org/10.2106/jbjs.e.00851.
66. Wierks C, Skolasky RL, Ji JH, McFarland EG. Reverse total shoulder replacement: intraoperative and early postoperative complications. Clin Orthop Relat Res. 2009;467(1):225–34. https://doi.org/10.1007/s11999-008-0406-1.
67. Levigne C, Boileau P, Favard L, Garaud P, Mole D, Sirveaux F, et al. Scapular notching in reverse shoulder arthroplasty. J Shoulder Elb Surg. 2008;17(6):925–35. https://doi.org/10.1016/j.jse.2008.02.010.
68. Simovitch RW, Zumstein MA, Lohri E, Helmy N, Gerber C. Predictors of scapular notching in patients managed with the Delta III reverse total shoulder replacement. J Bone Joint Surg Am. 2007;89(3):588–600. https://doi.org/10.2106/jbjs.f.00226.
69. Mole D, Favard L. Excentered scapulohumeral osteoarthritis. Revue de chirurgie orthopedique et reparatrice de l'appareil moteur. 2007;93(6 Suppl):37–94.
70. Vanhove B, Beugnies A. Grammont's reverse shoulder prosthesis for rotator cuff arthropathy. A retrospective study of 32 cases. Acta Orthop Belg. 2004;70(3):219–25.
71. Roberts CC, Ekelund AL, Renfree KJ, Liu PT, Chew FS. Radiologic assessment of reverse shoulder arthroplasty. Radiographics. 2007;27(1):223–35. https://doi.org/10.1148/rg.271065076.
72. Nyffeler RW, Werner CM, Gerber C. Biomechanical relevance of glenoid component positioning in the reverse Delta III total shoulder prosthesis. J Shoulder Elb Surg. 2005;14(5):524–8. https://doi.org/10.1016/j.jse.2004.09.010.
73. De Wilde LF, Audenaert EA, Berghs BM. Shoulder prostheses treating cuff tear arthropathy: a comparative biomechanical study. J Orthop Res. 2004;22(6):1222–30. https://doi.org/10.1016/j.orthres.2004.03.010.
74. Harman M, Frankle M, Vasey M, Banks S. Initial glenoid component fixation in "reverse" total shoulder arthroplasty: a biomechanical evaluation. J Shoulder Elb Surg. 2005;14(1 Suppl S):162s–7s. https://doi.org/10.1016/j.jse.2004.09.030.

75. Trouilloud P, Gonzalvez M, Martz P, Charles H, Handelberg F, Nyffeler RW, et al. Duocentric® reversed shoulder prosthesis and personal fit(R) templates: innovative strategies to optimize prosthesis positioning and prevent scapular notching. Eur J Orthop Surg Traumatol. 2014;24(4):483–95. https://doi.org/10.1007/s00590-013-1213-2.
76. Young SW, Everts NM, Ball CM, Astley TM, Poon PC. The SMR reverse shoulder prosthesis in the treatment of cuff-deficient shoulder conditions. J Shoulder Elb Surg. 2009;18(4):622–6. https://doi.org/10.1016/j.jse.2009.01.017.
77. Castagna A, Delcogliano M, de Caro F, Ziveri G, Borroni M, Gumina S, et al. Conversion of shoulder arthroplasty to reverse implants: clinical and radiological results using a modular system. Int Orthop. 2013;37(7):1297–305. https://doi.org/10.1007/s00264-013-1907-4.
78. Devine D, Arens D, Burelli S, Bloch HR, Boure L. In vivo evaluation of the osteointegration of new highly porous trabecular Titanium™. J Bone Joint Surg Br. 2012;94-B(Suppl XXXVII):201.
79. Bradley Edwards T, Morris BJ, Hodorek B. Tornier Aequalis ascend™ flex convertible shoulder system. Reverse shoulder arthroplasty. Cham: Springer; 2016.
80. Goetzmann T, Molé D, Aisene B, Neyton L, Godeneche A, Walch G, et al. A short and convertible humeral stem for shoulder arthroplasty: preliminary results. J Shoulder Elbow Arthroplasty. 2017;1:1–9. https://doi.org/10.1177/2471549217722723.
81. Teissier P, Teissier J, Kouyoumdjian P, Asencio G. The TESS reverse shoulder arthroplasty without a stem in the treatment of cuff-deficient shoulder conditions: clinical and radiographic results. J Shoulder Elb Surg. 2015;24(1):45–51. https://doi.org/10.1016/j.jse.2014.04.005.
82. Churchill RS, Athwal GS. Stemless shoulder arthroplasty-current results and designs. Curr Rev Muscoskelet Med. 2016;9(1):10–6. https://doi.org/10.1007/s12178-016-9320-4.
83. Drake GN, O'Connor DP, Edwards TB. Indications for reverse total shoulder arthroplasty in rotator cuff disease. Clin Orthop Relat Res. 2010;468(6):1526–33. https://doi.org/10.1007/s11999-009-1188-9.
84. Martin TG, Iannotti JP. Reverse total shoulder arthroplasty for acute fractures and failed management after proximal humeral fractures. Orthop Clin North Am. 2008;39(4):451–7., vi. https://doi.org/10.1016/j.ocl.2008.06.006.
85. Wall B, Walch G. Reverse shoulder arthroplasty for the treatment of proximal humeral fractures. Hand Clin. 2007;23(4):425–30., v–vi. https://doi.org/10.1016/j.hcl.2007.08.002.
86. Boileau P, Trojani C, Walch G, Krishnan SG, Romeo A, Sinnerton R. Shoulder arthroplasty for the treatment of the sequelae of fractures of the proximal humerus. J Shoulder Elb Surg. 2001;10(4):299–308. https://doi.org/10.1067/mse.2001.115985.
87. De Wilde L, Mombert M, Van Petegem P, Verdonk R. Revision of shoulder replacement with a reversed shoulder prosthesis (Delta III): report of five cases. Acta Orthop Belg. 2001;67(4):348–53.
88. De Wilde LF, Plasschaert FS, Audenaert EA, Verdonk RC. Functional recovery after a reverse prosthesis for reconstruction of the proximal humerus in tumor surgery. Clin Orthop Relat Res. 2005;430:156–62.
89. De Wilde LF, Van Ovost E, Uyttendaele D, Verdonk R. Results of an inverted shoulder prosthesis after resection for tumor of the proximal humerus. Revue de chirurgie orthopedique et reparatrice de l'appareil moteur. 2002;88(4):373–8.
90. Gutierrez S, Comiskey CA, Luo ZP, Pupello DR, Frankle MA. Range of impingement-free abduction and adduction deficit after reverse shoulder arthroplasty. Hierarchy of surgical and implant-design-related factors. J Bone Joint Surg Am. 2008;90(12):2606–15. https://doi.org/10.2106/jbjs.h.00012.
91. Flatow EL, Harrison AK. A history of reverse total shoulder arthroplasty. Clin Orthop Relat Res. 2011;469(9):2432–9. https://doi.org/10.1007/s11999-010-1733-6.

Shoulder Anatomy

2

Stefano Gumina, Vittorio Candela, Giovanni Ziveri, and Carlo Felice De Biase

2.1 Subacromial Space

This is the space delimited above by the coracoacromial arc (anterior-inferior margin of the acromion, coracoacromial ligament, apex, and distal third of the posterior surface of the coracoid) and below by the humeral head, by the tendons of the rotator cuff, and of the long head of the biceps (Fig. 2.1a, b). The area between the tendons of the supraspinatus and the subscapularis is called the rotator interval.

2.2 Coracoacromial Arc

2.2.1 Acromion

The acromion is flat in shape and extends laterally, then anterolaterally. We distinguish an upper surface, in close contact with the skin, bearing rough scores and vascular orifices; an inferior concavity, which forms the tip of the glenohumeral joint; a lateral margin, the bundles from which the deltoid muscle originates; and a medial margin where the surface of the acromioclavicular joint is.

In the last 30 years, the shape of the acromion has been the object/topic of several studies because it was considered the cause of predisposing aliments such as subacromial impingement and rotator cuff tendon tears [1]. In an anatomical study, Bigliani et al. [2] have classified the acromion as types I, II, and III based on the orientation and shape of their lower surface and identified the type likely to cause a reduction in the anatomical space between the acromion and the humeral head. According to this classification, the lower surface of the type I acromion is flat (flat acromion), while in the II and III acromion type, it is curvilinear (curved acromion) and hooked (hooked acromion), respectively (Fig. 2.2a–c). Shoulders with a type III acromion are more prone to have a narrow subacromial space. Other studies have confirmed the correlation between subacromial impingement and rotator cuff tear [3–5].

In a study of ours, during which we examined 500 dry scapulae belonging to Caucasians, we evaluated the shape (on the basis of the Bigliani's classification) [2] and some morphometric features of the acromion. The shape of the acromia was flat in 38.9%, curvilineous in 39.4%, and hooked in 21.7% of the scapulae examined. The percentage of hooked acromia was higher in the

S. Gumina
Department of Orthopaedics and Traumatology, Sapienza University of Rome, Rome, Italy

V. Candela (✉)
Department of Anatomy, Histology, Legal Medicine and Orthopedics, Sapienza, University of Rome—Istituto Chirurgico Ortopedico Traumatologico (ICOT), Latina, Italy

G. Ziveri · C. F. De Biase
Shoulder and Elbow Surgery Unit, Humanitas Clinic, Rozzano, Milan, Italy

S. Gumina et al. (eds.), *Reverse Shoulder Arthroplasty*, https://doi.org/10.1007/978-3-319-97743-0_2

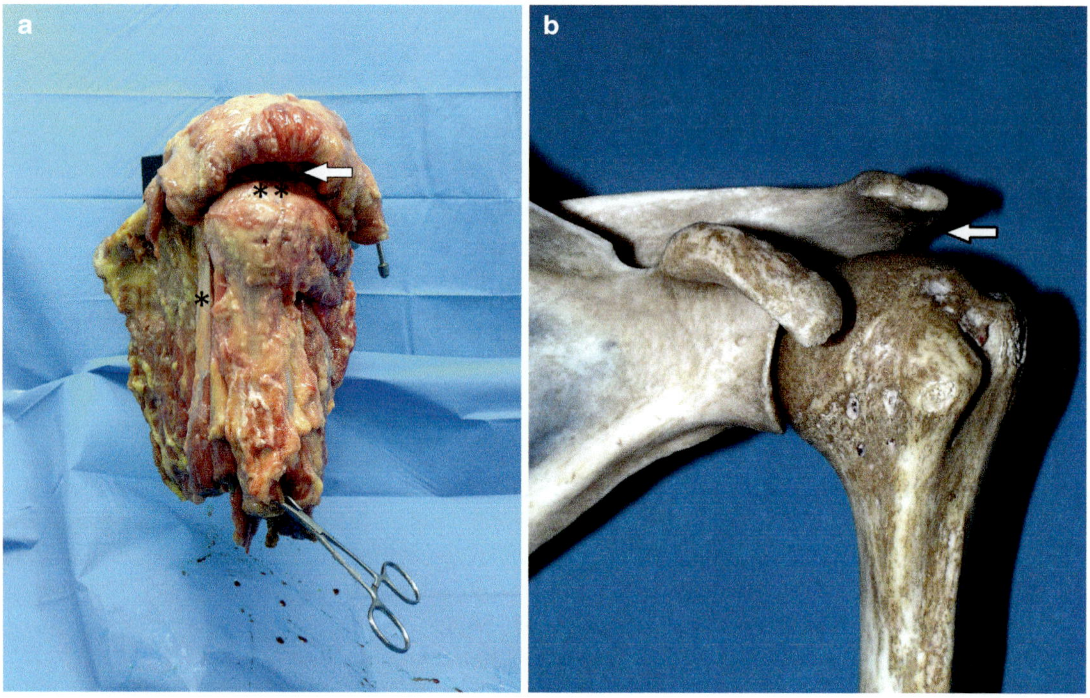

Fig. 2.1 (**a**–**b**) Lateral (**a**) and anterior (**b**) view of a left shoulder. The arrows indicate the subacromial space. *The long head biceps tendon. **Rotator cuff

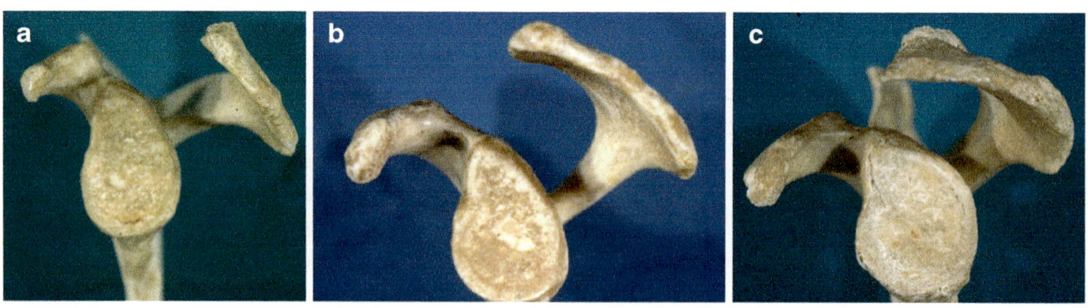

Fig. 2.2 (**a**–**c**) (**a**) Type I (flat) acromion; (**b**) type II (curved) acromion; (**c**) type III (hooked) acromion

scapulae of those aged over 60 (26%); thus, the hook-shaped acromion is currently considered as being acquired (ossification of the coracoacromial ligament) and not as something that is genetically determined. This observation seems to be confirmed by the studies of Natsis et al. [6] and Schippinger et al. [7] Other kinds of acromion recently described are the type IV (convex) [8] and the chiglia-like [9]. In an anatomical study, Zuckerman et al. [10] have not been able to identify the three types of acromia described by Bigliani. The authors concluded that the correlation between type of acromion and cuff tear is not clear and further studies are needed to support the role of extrinsic factors in the genesis of cuff tear [10]. Chang et al. [11], after having performed a three-dimensional analysis of the acromion with MRI, came to the conclusion that impingements of any kind caused by the acromion are not the primary cause of cuff tendon rupture.

In our study [12], the average thickness of the acromion was 8.5 mm; in addition, there was a direct linear correlation with the size of the scapula [12]. The acromia of the scapulae as well as the type III acromion belonging to male subjects were significantly thicker than those of females. The torsion

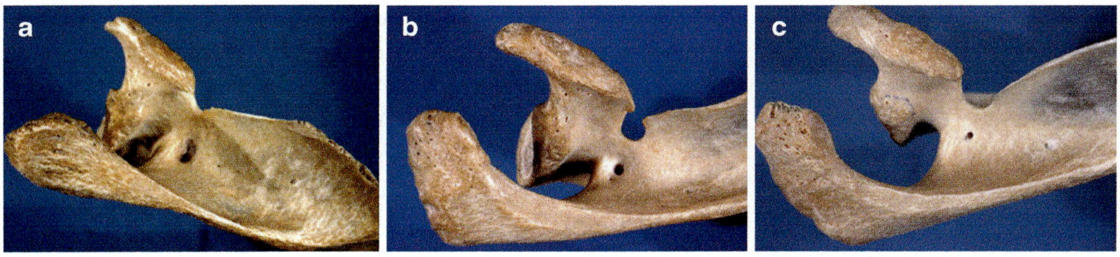

Fig. 2.3 (**a–c**) (**a**) Cobra head acromion; (**b**) squared acromion; (**c**) intermediate acromion

angle of the acromion is between 0° and 40° that of inclination between 20° and 70° [13].

In another study we conducted on 200 dry scapulae [13], the acromia were distinguished on the basis of Edelson's classification [14] that differentiates them according to the position of the articular facet with respect to the acromioclavicular joint tip. In 33% of the acromia, the facet of the acromioclavicular joint was at a distance from the apex of the acromion (type "cobra head"), 22% were on the apex (type "squared"), and 45% in an intermediate position (such as "intermediate") (Fig. 2.3a–c). The average length of the scapular facet of the acromioclavicular joint was 12.7 mm (range, 8–22 mm). Two forms of facet were identified: one to "drop" (31%) and "elliptical" (69%). The "drop" type belonged to elderly subjects; the edge of the veneer often presented degenerative changes. No dependency between the form and the spatial arrangement of the facet was discovered/found.

The lack of fusion of one or more growth centers located in the apex of the acromion (os acromialis) occurs in about 8% of scapulae (Fig. 2.4) [15]. When the unfused core is found at the apex of the acromion, it is defined as preacromion; instead, when it is found more distally, it is named, respectively, mesacromion, metacromion, and basiacromion [16]. The correlation between os acromialis and subacromial impingement is still a matter of discussion [17–19]. A study of ours has shown that the longer the distance between the acromioclavicular joint and the apex of the acromion, the higher the possibility that fusion of the growth nuclei will not occur [20].

Baechler and Kim [21] have observed that there is a relationship between the degree of humeral coverage by the lateral margin of the acromion and rupture of the rotator cuff. This association is thought to be due to the friction that is likely to occur during abduction. Nyffeler et al. [22] consider that the sum of the forces brought to bear in flexion/abduction favors humeral proximal migration in cases of greater degrees of acromial coverage. Torrens et al. [23] observed that the prevalence of acromia with higher degrees of humeral coverage was greater in patients with cuff tears than in those belonging to the control group.

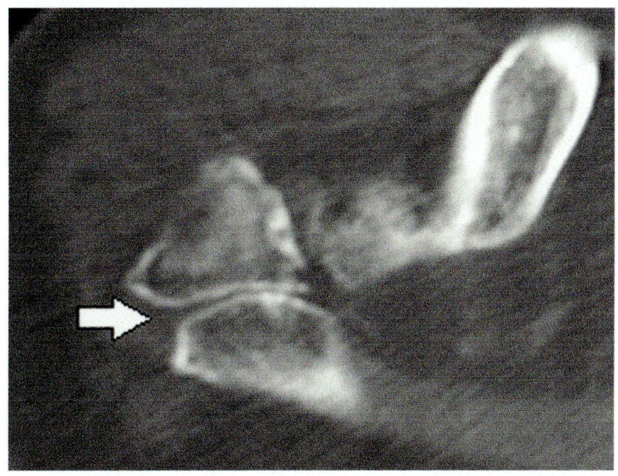

Fig. 2.4 MR scan of a left shoulder. Axial view. The arrow indicates the os acromialis

2.2.2 Coracoacromial Ligament (CAL)

It is located between the base of the coracoid and the inferomedial surface of the acromion (Fig. 2.5). It fits on top of the acromion, right in front of the acromioclavicular joint's surface and along the entire lateral section of the coracoid. An artery (a branch of the suprascapular) is

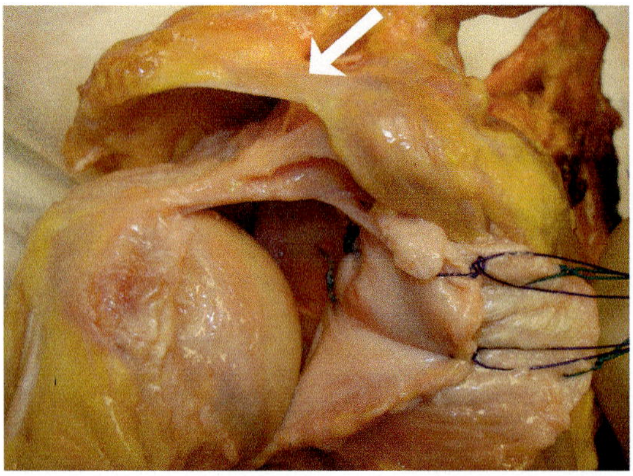

Fig. 2.5 Cadaveric right shoulder. The arrow indicates the coracoacromial ligament

constantly present on the posterior surface of the ligament. Macroscopically, it presents no homogeneous morphological characteristics.

An anatomic study revealed that 60% of the shoulders had a bipartite coracoacromial ligament, a single ligament in 25%, and tripartite in 15% of the cases [24]. In the latter case, the coracoid insertion of the third band was more medial and may not be visible until a resection of the lateral third of the clavicle is performed. Kesmezacar et al. [25] argued that there are five possible anatomical variants of the CAL (type I, Y-shape; type II, single broadband; type III, quadrangular; type IV, V-shape; and type V, multiband). The Y-shape inserts itself in a unique manner into the acromion. The two bands of the "Y", which are inserted on the coracoid, are separated by a thin membrane. Of the two bands, one side is thicker and wider. The width of the two insertions of the single broadband variation (type II) is similar [26]. The ligament maintains its width along its entire extension. In type III, the width of the insertion on the coracoid is wider than that of type II. Type IV differs from type I because of the two arms that appear to be separate after the acromial insertion. Even in this case, the side of the higher band is thicker and wider. Type V does not present homogeneous morphological features. Of all the variants, the most common type is the "Y" (41%); the rarest are types IV and V (both 11%). For the authors, none of the variants predisposes rupture of the cuff more than the others. However, CALs with the greatest number of bands seem to have a significant association with the degeneration of the cuff. Kopuz et al. [27] conducted an anatomical study on neonatal CALs and observed that the variants at birth are simply three: square, single broadband, and "U." This observation suggests that the final shape of the ligament is acquired over time. In rare cases, where the pectoralis minor muscle inserts on the capsule of the glenohumeral joint rather than on the coracoid, the tendon passes through the bands of the CAL [28].

In an anatomical study, Fremery et al. [29] observed that shoulders with cuff tears have CAL bands shorter compared to those without tendon rupture and that the CAL changes its morphological and biomechanical features over time. The insertional areas are constituted by fibrocartilage [30]. With aging, the fibrocartilage is also present in the middle portion of the ligament [30].

It was observed [31] that the CAL contains four types of nerve endings: free, Pacinian corpuscles, and Ruffini and Golgi receptors. In addition to these typical endings, other "atypical" ones were observed. All these endings are equally distributed on the surface of the subacromial side of the ligament and in correspondence with the acromial and coracoid insertion [30, 31]. The number of nerve endings decreases in older subjects and in those with subacromial impingement. This observation suggests that in these two categories of persons, the proprioceptive activity of the shoulder is reduced.

With aging, the portion of the ligament that fits onto the acromion may experience ossification (enthesopathy) [30]. The new bone can modify the profile of the anteroinferior acromion, increasing the downward curvature. This explains why the percentage of the hooked acromion increases with aging. In the case of two-part ligament (anterolateral and posteromedial band), spur formations occur predominantly on the anterolateral band [32]. This has led to the hypothesis that of the two bands, the anterolateral is that subjected to greater functional stresses [32]. Ogata and Uhthoff [33] argued that the development of enthesopathy is the result of the transmission of tensile forces within the ligament and that the formation of this spur determines transition from a dysfunctional syndrome to an organic stenosis. Kijima et al. [34] observed that the modulus of elasticity of the CAL of patients with cuff tear is higher than that recorded in the ligaments of subjects without tendon rupture. This shows that physiological tissue degeneration causes progressive rigidity of the ligament. Even Sarkar [35] and Schiavone-Panni [36] observed that tissue disorganization and loss of normal orientation of the collagen fibers are more common in the CAL of patients with subacromial impingement, especially in the deep layer of the ligament.

The CAL is perhaps the only ligament subtended between two transverse processes belonging to the same bone. It has been speculated that this reduces the movement which both the acromion and the coracoid face during the action, respectively, of the deltoid and the conjoint tendons/pectoralis minor [37]. The CAL opposes the upward migration of the humeral head in the case of massive cuff tears [38, 39]. In a study of cadavers, Fagelman et al. [40] have shown that reinsertion of the CAL prevents upper static instability and contributes to refocusing the humeral head inside the coracoacromial arch.

2.2.3 Coracoid

Anterior to the glenoid and lateral to the scapular notch, there is an apophysis that due to its shape, like a crow's beak, was formerly called coracoid (χ ο ρ α ξ = *chorax* = crow).

The coracoid apophysis originates from the anterior-upper extremity of the neck of the scapula and protrudes at first upward and forward from the side and subsequently arranges itself almost horizontally. The conjoint tendons (short head of the biceps and coracobrachialis) fit onto the anterior apex of the coracoid, further back and laterally onto the coracohumeral and the coracoacromial ligament; medially, onto the tendon of the pectoralis minor muscle (Fig. 2.6a); and superiorly, onto a rough surface of the coracoclavicular ligaments (conoid and trapezoid) (Fig. 2.6b).

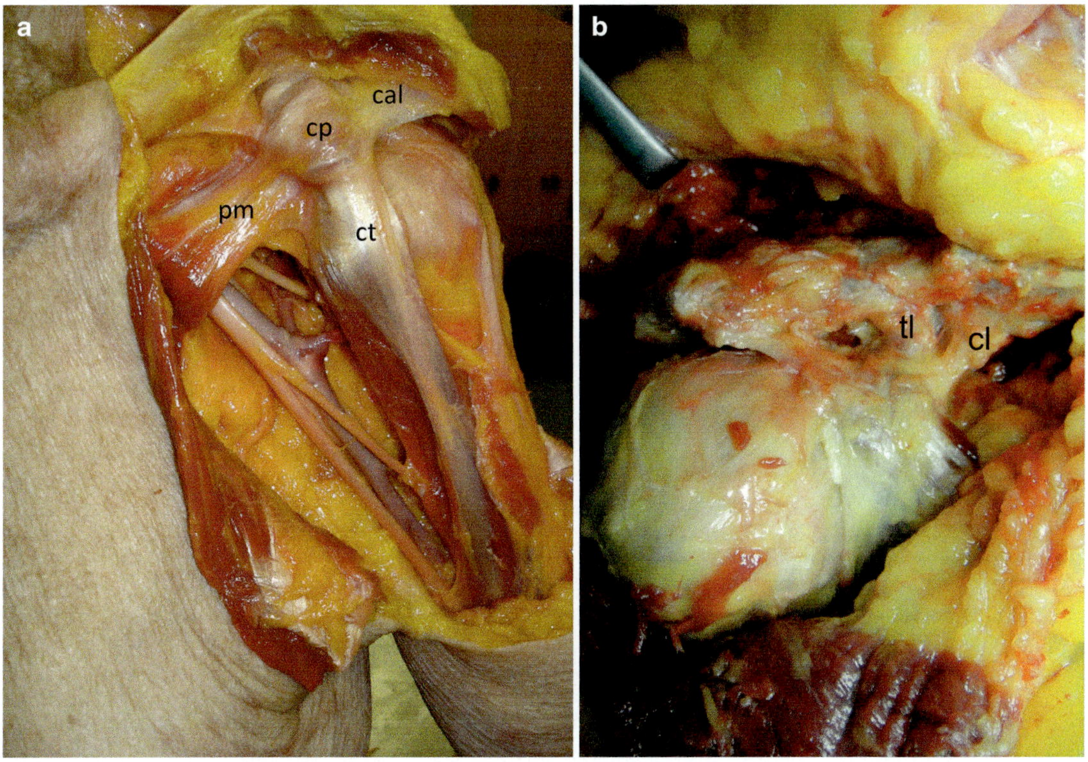

Fig. 2.6 (**a–b**) (**a**) Left shoulder of a cadaver. *cs* coracoid process, *pm* pectoralis minor, *ct* conjoint tendons, *cal* coracoacromial ligament. (**b**) Right shoulder. *cl* conoid ligament, *tl* trapezoid ligament

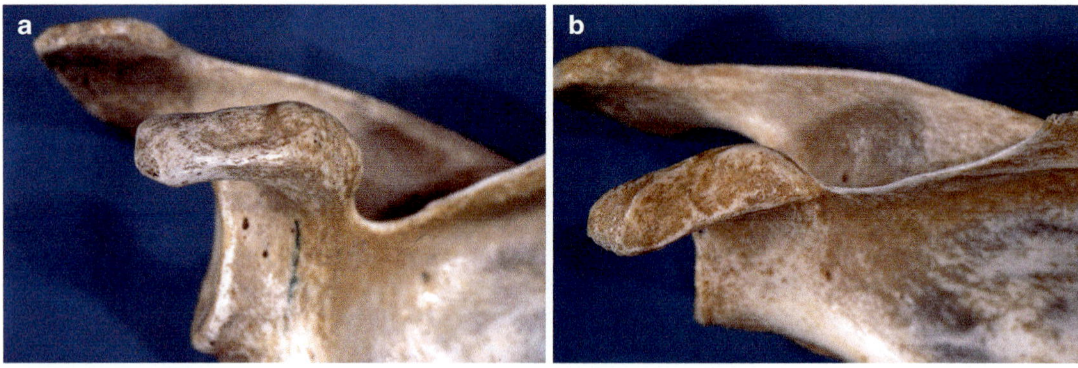

Fig. 2.7 (**a**–**b**) Coracoid processes (right samples) with different inclination

In a study conducted on 204 dry blades [41], we carried out measurements of the length of the coracoid (L) and the thickness of the coracoid tip (T), the apex of the coracoid prominence over the glenoid plane (cp), the minimum distance between the coracoid tip and the anterior-superior margin of the glenoid (cgd), the distance between the horizontal plane, tangential to the lower edge of the coracoid tip, and the horizontal plane tangential to the cranial glenoid (d). The inclination of the coracoid (cs) (Fig. 2.7a, b), in the cranial-caudal direction, was measured using Edelson and Taitz's method [14]. Then, we analyzed the shape of the space delimited by the posterolateral margin of the coracoid and the anterior-superior edge of the glenoid.

The range, the mean, and the standard deviation of L, T, cp, cs, cgd, and d were:

	L (mm)	T (mm)	cp (mm)	cgd (mm)	cs (°)	d (mm)
Max	50	10.2	22	22.1	42	12
Min	31	5	11	11.8	19	0.5
Mean	38.15	7.19	14.62	16.23	25.57	7.11
SD	3.97	1.04	1.96	1.7	4.71	1.23

Three types of configuration of the coraco-glenoid space were identified (Fig.2.8a–c). In the type I configuration, this space had a "round parenthesis" shape, while in types II and III, respectively, the shape was that of a "bracket" and a "hook." The configuration of type I was observed in 45% of the shoulder blades and types II and III in 34% and 21%, respectively. The minimum coraco-glenoid distance was found in the shoulder blades with a type I configuration. In a study of cadavers, Ferreira Neto et al. [42] observed that in females the distance between the apex of the coracoid and lesser tuberosity is lower than that measured in males. Therefore, women appear to be more likely to develop a syndrome of subcoracoid impingement. Richards et al. [43] availing of MRI scans measured the coracohumeral distance and observed that patients with a lesion of the subscapularis present a significantly smaller distance than the people in the control group. The possible morphological and morphometric correlation between the coracoid and the subcoracoid impingement was challenged instead by Radas and Pieper [44] who correlate the development of this syndrome to anterior glenohumeral joint instability.

Schulz et al. [45] correlated the position of the apex coracoid to rupture of the rotator cuff. Employing true anteroposterior radiographs, the authors divided coracoids into two classes: those whose apex is projected into the lower half of the glenoid (type I) and those which project their peak into the mid-upper glenoid (type II). The study found that type I coracoids are more frequently found in patients with rupture of the supraspinatus, while those of type II are more frequently observed in patients with injury to the subscapularis tendon.

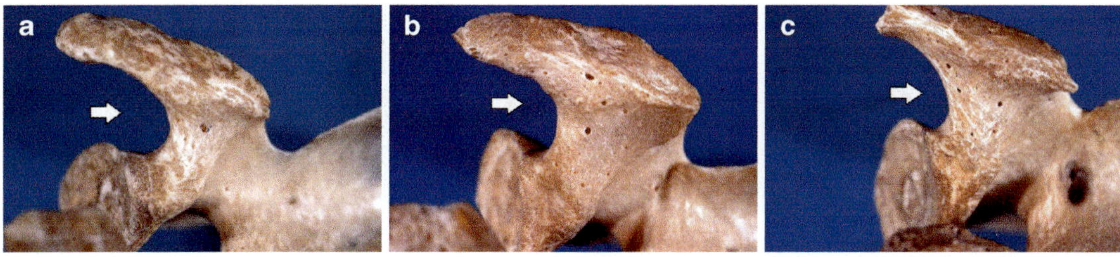

Fig. 2.8 (**a–c**) Three types of configuration of the coraco-glenoid space (arrows)

2.3 Humeral Tuberosities and Bicipital Groove

The greater tuberosity represents the posterolateral region of the humeral head (Fig. 2.9). On it, there are three areas onto which the tendon of the supraspinatus, the infraspinatus, and the teres minor (see rotator cuff) may be fixed. The bone mineral density of the two tuberosities is an important factor in the surgical treatment of cuff lesions. Osteopenia of the greater tuberosity may, in fact, complicate surgical repair of the supra- and infraspinatus and hinder the healing of the two tendons. The tendon of the subscapularis muscle is inserted instead onto the lesser tuberosity that is placed anteromedially. Along with the greater tuberosity, the lesser tuberosity helps to delimit the bicipital groove within which the tendon of the long head of the biceps brachii and the arcuate artery, a branch of the anterior humeral circumflex, slide (Fig. 2.9). Proximally, it is wide and deep and is lost, gradually, on the front face of the shaft, mingling with the roughness of the bone corresponding to the insertional area of the teres major. Data regarding the morphological and morphometric features of the groove emerging from studies of dry shoulders are mixed. This has been attributed to the extreme variability of the ethnogeographical origin and age of the samples examined (Fig. 2.10a–c). A radiographic study performed on 200 humeri [46], of which the sex and approximate age were known, showed that the average value of the opening angle (Fig. 2.11a) of the groove is 102° (extreme 28°–160°), while the medial angle (Fig. 2.11b) is 46° (range 16°–78°). The depth and the average width of the groove are, respectively, 4.3 and 12.2 mm. Statistically significant differences between the sexes were found only for values regarding the average width (M,13.1–F,10.2).

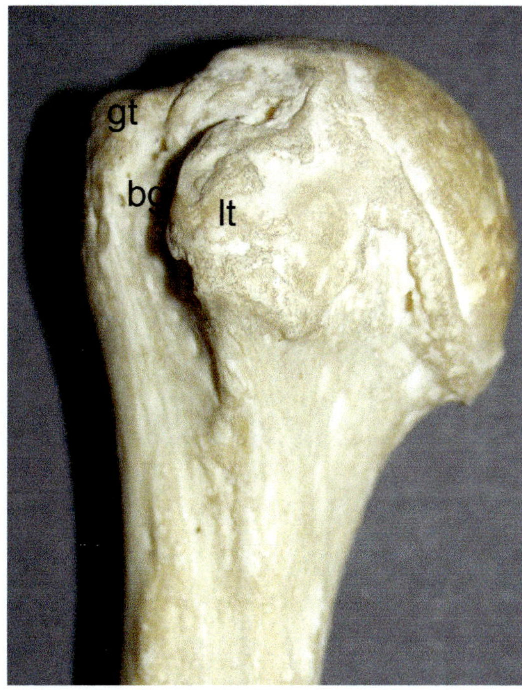

Fig. 2.9 Dry (right) humeral head. *gt* greater tuberosity, *lt* lesser tuberosity, *bg* bicipital groove

2.4 Rotator Cuff

This consists of the supraspinatus, infraspinatus, teres minor, and subscapularis tendons (Fig. 2.12). The first three (external rotators) are fixed onto the greater tuberosity, the other (internal rotator)

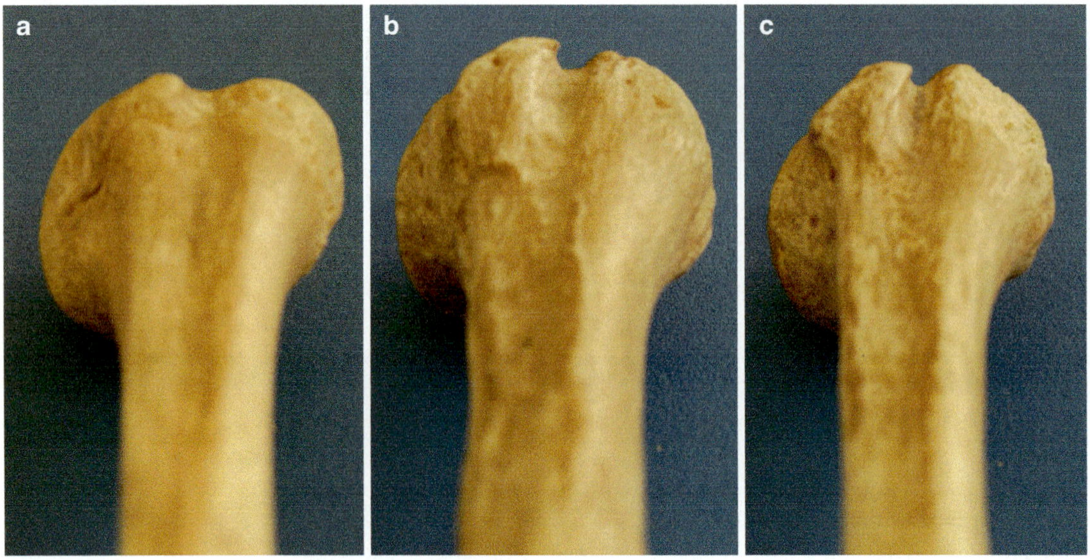

Fig. 2.10 (**a**–**c**) Dry humeri. Bicipital grooves with different depth and width

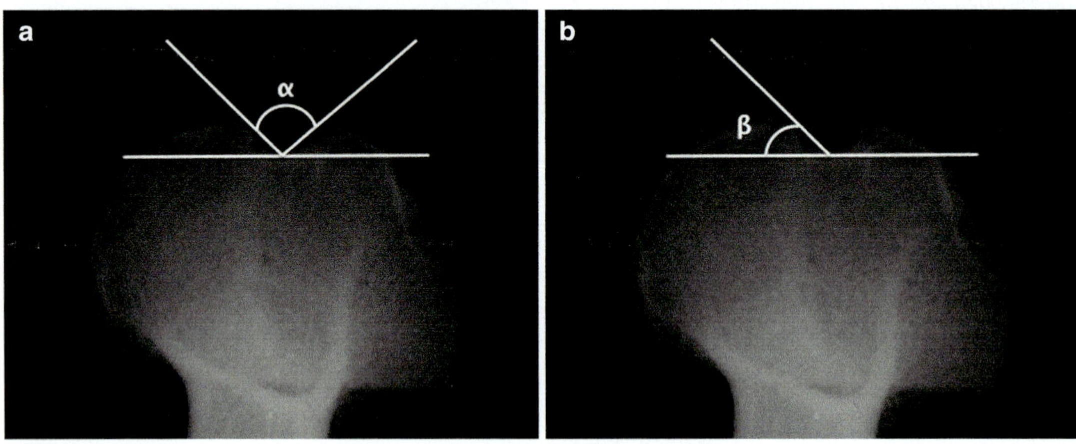

Fig. 2.11 (**a**–**b**) Radiograms of dry humeri. Opening (**a**) and medial (**b**) angle of the bicipital groove

on the lesser tuberosity. At about 15 mm from the insertion on the humerus, the external rotator tendons are seemingly fused together, in particular those of the supra- and infraspinatus. However, if the coracohumeral ligament and connective tissue that overhang the two tendons near their insertion are removed, the front edge of the infraspinatus is more easily highlighted, and the boundary between the two muscles becomes more apparent. The front edge of the infraspinatus is slightly more prominent than that of the adjacent rear supraspinatus. This is because the front of the infraspinatus partially covers the portion of the posterolateral supraspinatus.

If the infraspinatus is removed, leaving the capsule below intact, we note that the greater tuberosity is constituted by three distinct areas (the higher, middle, and lower) [47]. Mochizuki et al. [48] observed that the insertion of the infraspinatus occupies about half of the higher and the whole of the middle area. The anteriormost region of the humeral insertion of the infraspinatus almost reaches the anterior margin of the highest part of the greater tuberosity. Because the infraspinatus

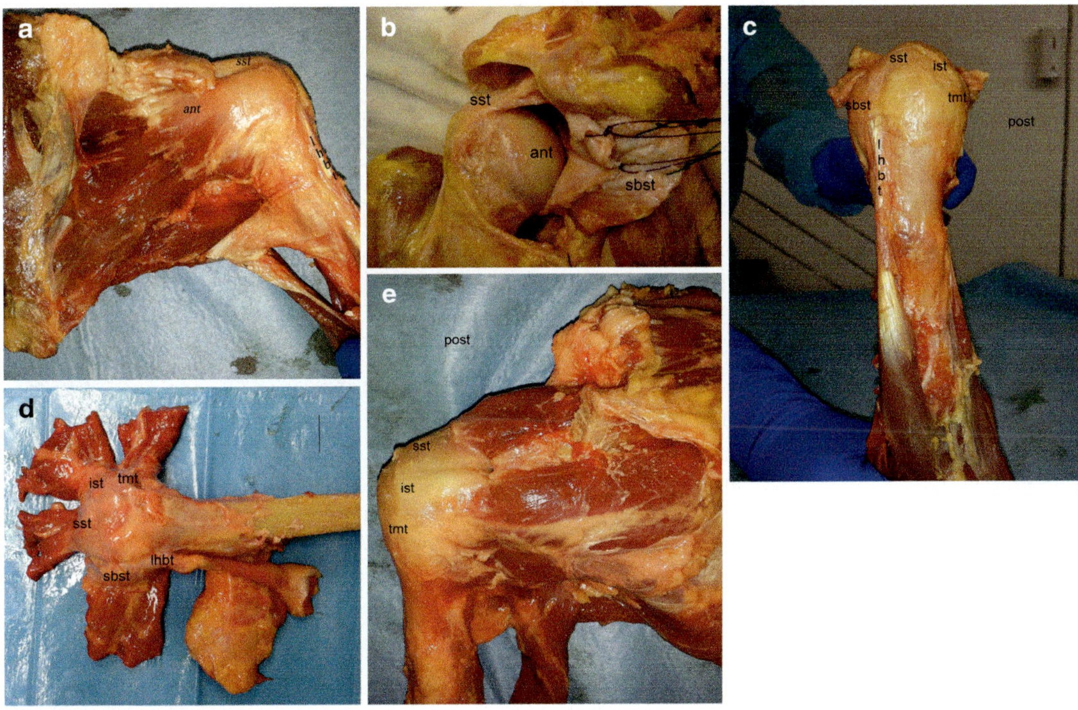

Fig. 2.12 (**a**–**e**) Rotator cuff tendons. (**a**–**b**) Anterior views. (**c**–**d**) Lateral views; (**e**) posterior view; the scapular spine was removed. *sbst*, subscapularis tendon, *sst* supraspinatus tendon, *ist* infraspinatus tendon, *tmt* teres minor tendon, *lhbt* long head biceps tendon, *ant* anterior, *post* posterior

fits laterally, it can be argued that it can also play an important role in abduction. These new acquisitions concerning insertion of the infraspinatus suggest that the frequent atrophy of the infraspinatus muscle, visible in MRI scans on the occasion of apparent isolated lesions of the supraspinatus, are not attributable to lesions of the suprascapular nerve (due to traction caused by supraspinatus retraction) [49] but to a direct involvement of the infraspinatus itself in the lesion.

Upon removing the supraspinatus, it can be noted that it fits onto the highest anteromedial part of the greater tuberosity.

The footprint of the supraspinatus is triangular in shape, with the longer side toward the articular surface; it is wider at the front and narrower at the back. The supraspinatus also fits onto the lesser tuberosity in 21% of cases. In these cases, the anteriormost part of the tendon covers the top of the bicipital groove.

Mochizuki et al. [48] measured the maximum length (from medial to lateral) and width (front to rear) of the footprints of the supra- and infraspinatus. That of the supraspinatus is triangular in shape. The maximum length was 6.9 ± 1.4 mm. Instead, the maximum width of the medial margin was 12.6 ± 2.0 mm, while the lateral measured 1.3 ± 1.4 mm. The footprint of the infraspinatus is trapezoidal, wider laterally and medially. Its maximum length was 10.2 ± 1.6 mm. The maximum medial width was 20 ± 6.2 mm; the lateral was 32.7 ± 3.4 mm.

Previous studies assumed that the footprint of the supra- and infraspinatus was longer [50–52] probably because the joint capsule was included in the measurements.

The tendon of the supraspinatus is composed of two portions: the anterior half is long and thick and the posterior short and thin. Itoi et al. [53, 54] arbitrarily divided the tendon into three portions (anterior, middle, and posterior) and observed that the anterior third is significantly stronger and tougher than the other two portions. However, the anterior portion, which fits onto the greater tuberosity for an extension corresponding to only 40% of the tendon insertion, bears proportionately higher mechanical stress, which makes it more vulnerable and predisposed to rupture [55, 56]. In view of these findings, during the repair of the supraspinatus tendon, considerable attention should be paid to reinsertion of the anterior portion.

The so-called critical zone of the supraspinatus tendon is that at about an inch from the insertion of the middle third of the tendon [57]. Nakajima et al. [58] performed a histological and biomechanical study of tendons of the supraspinatus and identified four independent structural subunits. The "real tendon" extends from the myo-tendinous junction to about 2 in. from the insertion on the greater tuberosity. It consists of parallel collagen dossiers oriented along the stress axis. The "fibrocartilage" extends from the tendon to the greater tuberosity and is mainly composed of intertwined collagen fibers. The "rotator cable" extends from the coracohumeral ligament to the infraspinatus, lying between the surface layer and the depth of the true tendon. The "capsule" is composed of thin collagenous sheets, each consisting of fibers with the same orientation. The combination of these subunits provides the supraspinatus with dispersive load and compression stress resistance properties [59].

The term "cable" (Fig. 2.13) is commonly used to indicate the ropelike thickening consisting of fibers oriented perpendicularly to the axis of the tendon of the supraspinatus; arthroscopically it becomes visible by pointing the camera lens at the intra-articular tendon insertion. Clark and Harryman [60] assumed the cable to be a deep extension of the coracohumeral ligament. It is believed that the task of this structure is to bypass the mechanical stresses to which the supraspinatus tendon insertion (crescent) would be subjected. This explains why, arthroscopically, it is possible to observe a kneeling of the cuff next to the insertional area in the presence of a well-represented cable. It has been suggested that some shoulders may be defined as "cable dominant," others as "crescent dominant." The former seems to preserve the tendon insertion from excessive mechanical stress; the others seem more prone, therefore, to tendon injuries. Burkhart [61] suggested that lesions of the crescent, in the presence of an intact and well-represented cable, might even be considered functional and therefore manageable by availing of conservative treatment.

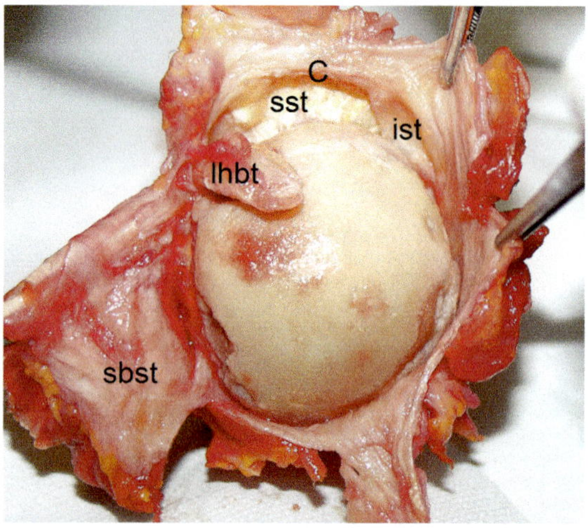

Fig. 2.13 Right shoulder of a cadaver. *C* cable, *sbst* subscapularis tendon, *sst* supraspinatus tendon, *ist* infraspinatus tendon, *lhbt* long head biceps tendon

Clark and Harryman [60] observed that the supra- and infraspinatus tendons are composed of five layers. The first (1 mm) is represented by fibrous expansions of the coracohumeral ligament; the second (3–5 mm), by bands of tendon fibers crossed by fine arterioles; and the third (3 mm) by bands formed by smaller tendon bundles arranged in a disorderly manner. The arterioles present in this layer have an even smaller diameter than those closer to the surface. The underlying layer (the fourth) is formed by connective tissue with thick collagen fibers lying on the surface layer of the articular capsule (therefore, they are extra-articular). Finally, the last layer (2 mm) is formed by the joint capsule.

The tendon of the teres minor runs obliquely, from the bottom upward, and is particularly adherent to the articular capsule of the glenohumeral joint. Much of the tendon is inserted into the so-called low area of the greater tuberosity; a small portion, instead, is inserted directly below this area.

The tendon of the subscapularis is made up of tendon and collagenic bands arranged in a parallel fashion. Only close to the insertion on the lesser tuberosity, the bands differ in range. On the surface, they are close to one another; deeper down (near the joint capsule), they are separated by abundant connective tissue. Expansions of the subscapularis rise to cover the greater tuberosity, between the first and third layer of the "fibrous plate" of the rotator interval, on the floor of the bicipital groove.

Cooper et al. [62] observed that the upper portion of the subscapularis is intra-articular (IASS = intra-articular subscapularis). The IASS is only 86% of the sagittal diameter of the entire subscapularis and 25% of the upper part of the tendon [28–63]. The tendon inserts onto the lesser tuberosity forming a "comma." The footprint has an average length of 40 mm (range 35–55 mm) and an average width of 20 mm (range, 15–25) [50]. Like other tendons, with aging, the rotator cuff grows progressively thinner, with degeneration and reduction of its tensile properties. This predisposes to stress failure and progressively lower loads.

2.5 Rotator Cuff Muscles

The muscles of the rotator cuff of the shoulder are the supraspinatus, infraspinatus, teres minor, and subscapularis. The first three act predominantly as external rotators of the shoulder, while the subscapularis is an internal rotator. They are also dynamic stabilizers of the glenohumeral joint with other muscles of the shoulder [64]. In fact, the shoulder muscles because of their extensive mutual connection and insertion generate rotational movements. If you wish to perform a movement without rotation, this requires a partial neutralization by other muscles. For example, to perform an internal rotation, the latissimus dorsi needs to be neutralized by the headset and the deltoid; otherwise this too would generate adduction.

Supraspinatus. It originates from the supraspinatus fossa of the scapula and extends anteriorly and laterally toward the greater tuberosity into which it fits with a tendon located between that of the infraspinatus (posterolateral) and the coracohumeral ligament (front) (Fig. 2.14). There are two muscular corpora: the first and forwardmost (anterior muscle belly) is essentially fusiform and originates entirely from the supraspinatus fossa. Along its front runs an intramuscular tendon (intramuscular core), the thickness of which increases progressively close to its insertion. The second muscle corpus (posterior muscle belly) is smaller, a single band devoid of intramuscular tendon cores. It originates mainly from the spine of the scapula and the neck of the glenoid.

The supraspinatus is innervated by the suprascapular nerve (C5–C6) which enters the muscle

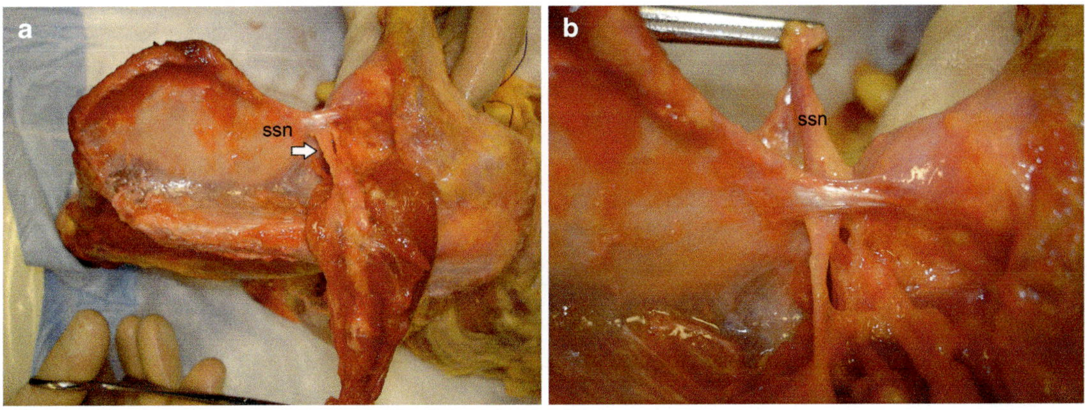

Fig. 2.14 (**a–b**) (**a**) View from above of the right shoulder of a cadaver. The supraspinatus muscle was detached from the scapular supraspinatus fossa and overturned laterally. Suprascapular nerve (ssn) as it passes through the scapular notch. (**b**) Particular of the nerve

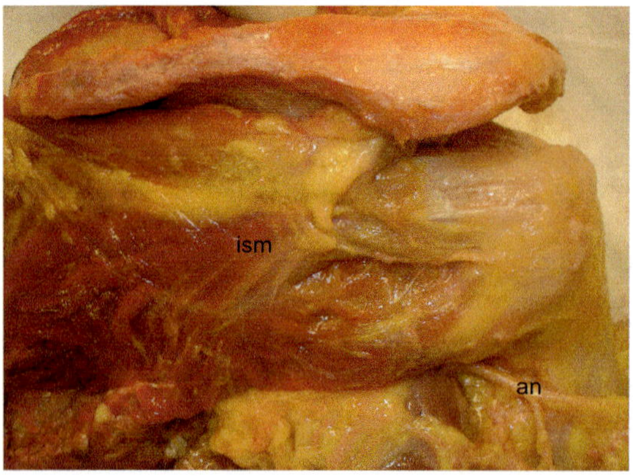

Fig. 2.15 Rear view of the right shoulder of a cadaver. Double band infraspinatus muscle (ism). *an* axillary nerve

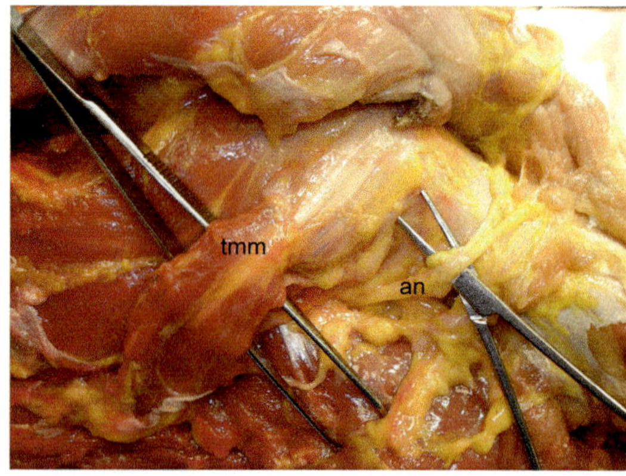

Fig. 2.16 Rear view of the right shoulder of a cadaver. Teres minor muscle (tmm). *an* axillary nerve

near the coracoid base, after passing through the scapular notch. The vascular supply is mainly ensured by the suprascapular artery, which passes over the notch and penetrates into the muscle in proximity to the homonymous nerve and, to a lesser extent, the scapular dorsal artery. The muscle is involved in elevation movements of the shoulder [65, 66].

Infraspinatus. It originates from the infraspinatus fossa of the scapula (Fig. 2.15). It is a tri-band muscle in 80% of cases and a double-single band one in the remaining 20%. The median raphe can easily be confused with a cleavage plane between the infraspinatus and the teres minor. It inserts onto the greater tuberosity, posteriorly and laterally to the tendon of the supraspinatus. Like the supraspinatus, it is innervated and vascularized, respectively, by the suprascapular nerve and artery. An anatomical study, however, has also revealed a vascular supply from the dorsal artery and subscapular circumflex branch [67]. The nerve penetrates the muscle after passing the spino-glenoid notch of the scapula. Here, it can be pulled during movements of abduction and external rotation and injured if this action is repeated sharply for professional reasons or sport. The muscle is predominantly an external rotator. It has been calculated that it produces 60% of the strength in cases of external rotation [65]. During internal rotation, it opposes posterior dislocation, while during abduction and external rotation, it opposes the anterior subluxation [68].

Teres minor. This muscle originates from the middle portion of the lateral margin of the scapula and from the thick end of the infraspinatus (Fig. 2.16). It passes anterolaterally and inserts itself onto the lower part of the greater tuberosity. With its lower margin, the muscle belly delimitates the quadrilateral space laterally and the triangular one medially. It is innervated by the posterior branch of the axillary nerve (C5); the vascular supply is provided by several vessels, but the main contribution is provided by the posterior humeral circumflex artery [67]. The teres minor is predominantly an external rotator (45% of the entire strength), and it opposes, along with the infraspinatus, anterior dislocation [65].

Subscapularis. The subscapularis constitutes the anterior portion of the rotator cuff and originates from the subscapularis fossa covering a large area (Fig. 2.17). It fits predominantly onto the lesser tuberosity and, with a small contingent of musculotendinous fibers, to the bottom of the lesser tuberosity. The subscapularis muscle is multi-branched and rich in collagen fibers arranged in parallel formation on the surface layer and in a disorderly manner in the deep one. The upper portion of the fibers of this layer is inserted along the groove of the biceps.

Anteriorly, the subscapularis is bounded by the axillary space and by the coracobrachialis pouch, above the coracoid. In depth with respect to the muscle, in the quadrilateral space, the axillary nerve and the posterior humeral circumflex

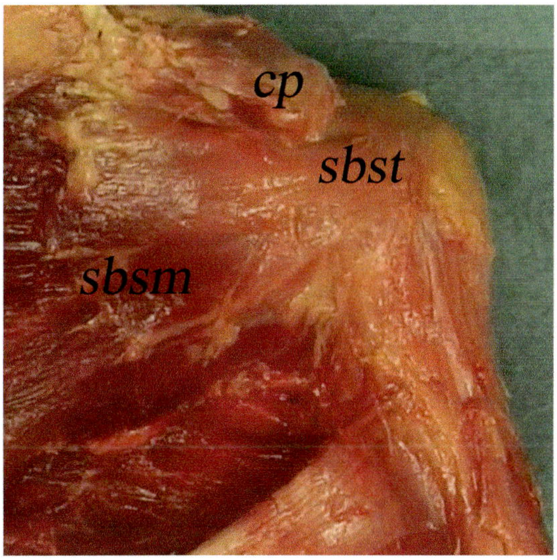

Fig. 2.17 Front view of the left shoulder of a cadaver. Subscapularis muscle (sbsm). *sbst* subscapularis tendon, *cp* coracoid process

artery pass. In a more medial position within the triangular space, the circumflex artery of scapula starts. The subscapularis' deeper surface covers the glenohumeral articulation joint. The relationship with the capsule is such as to make it difficult to find a cleavage plane. The middle glenohumeral ligament begins near the upper end of the subscapularis; the anterior band of the inferior glenohumeral ligament is placed lower down.

The upper (C5) and lower (C5–C6) subscapular nerves innervate the upper and lower portion of the muscle, respectively. The vascular supply comes from the axillary artery and from the circumflex (subscapular artery branches) and dorsal scapula artery [67, 69, 70].

Due to its close relationships with the glenohumeral joint, the subscapularis is considered one of the passive stabilizers in cases of sub-dislocating stresses of the humeral head [71, 72]. It is predominantly an internal rotator, but it contributes, along with the deltoid, to the elevation of the shoulder. The upper musculotendinous portion withstands greater mechanical stresses than those recorded for the lower portion. This explains why lesions of the subscapularis most frequently involve the upper third of the tendon [73].

2.6 Deltoid

This muscle has a conical shape and is the widest of the scapulohumeral muscles (Fig. 2.18). The deltoid consists of three parts: the front, midway, and back. The first (mono-branched) originates from the lateral third of the clavicle, the middle part (multi-branched) and posterior (mono-branched), respectively, from the acromion and the spine of the scapula. The insertion of the three parts is located on the deltoid tuberosity of the humerus.

The three parts of the deltoid differ in their internal structure. The anterior and posterior have parallel fibers and a longer excursion; the middle section is multi-branched and stronger. Of the three portions, the medial has the highest collagenic content [28].

Medially, it is in contact with the edge of the pectoralis major muscle. The triangular space between the two muscles constitutes the deltopectoral interval through which the surgeon reaches the subscapularis tendon and the front face of the glenohumeral joint. The muscular interval contains the cephalic vein and smaller vessels from the thoracoacromial artery (Fig. 2.19).

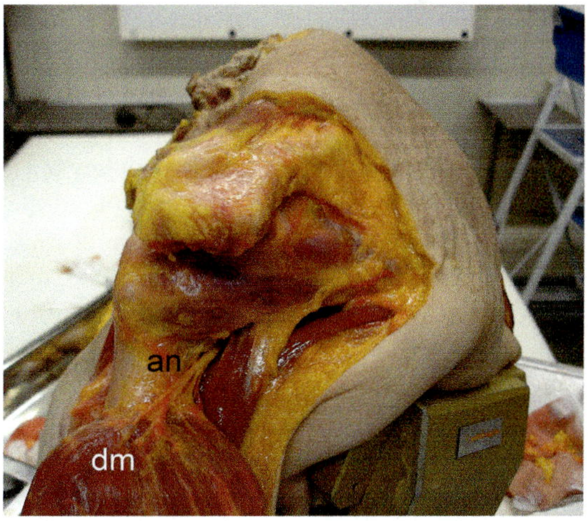

Fig. 2.18 Lateral view of the left shoulder of a cadaver. The deltoid muscle (dm) has been detached from the clavicle and scapula and lower overturned. *an* axillary nerve

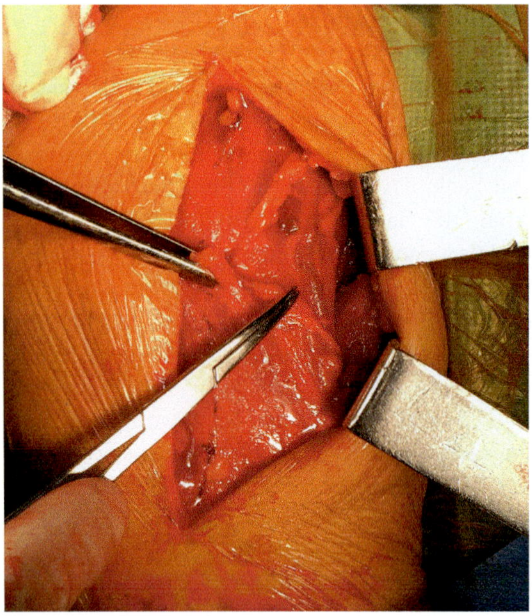

Fig. 2.19 The cephalic vein

Deep down, a very thick band covers the muscle belly; this structure must be reinserted necessarily with the deltoid when detached from the acromion; otherwise, a subcutaneous depression which is accentuated and painful during abduction against resistance will appear.

The front and midway fibers ensure elevation movement on the scapular plane [74]. During abduction, the contribution of the anterior fibers decreases while that of the posterior fibers increases. The decrease implies the triple action of the front and midway fibers and combined fibers of the pectoralis major and the biceps. It has been calculated that the deltoid supplies 60% of all abduction force [65] and that the role of the deltoid in the stability of the glenohumeral joint is still a matter of debate. Motzkin et al. [75], in a study of cadavers, showed that the contribution made to lower stability of the shoulder by the deltoid is irrelevant. The same conclusion was reached by Markhede et al. [76] who observed that patients devoid of the deltoid due to deltoid cancer do not suffer from a severe impairment of the stability of the glenohumeral joint. A study by Kido et al. [77] has demonstrated, instead, how this muscle contributes toward the anterior stability of the shoulder. It has been hypothesized that contributions toward stability happen thanks to four mechanisms: tension produced by the muscle mass itself, compression due to the contraction of the muscle, ligament tension secondary to the movement, and a barrier effect caused by muscle contraction [78].

The deltoid is innervated by the axillary nerve (circumflex) (C5–C6) and vascularized by the posterior circumflex artery [79].

2.7 Long Head of the Biceps Tendon (LHBT)

The long head of the biceps tendon (LHBT) originates with different individual characteristics from the labrum (45%) and glenoid tuberculum (30%) (Fig. 2.20). In the remaining cases (25%), the tendon originates from both the labrum and

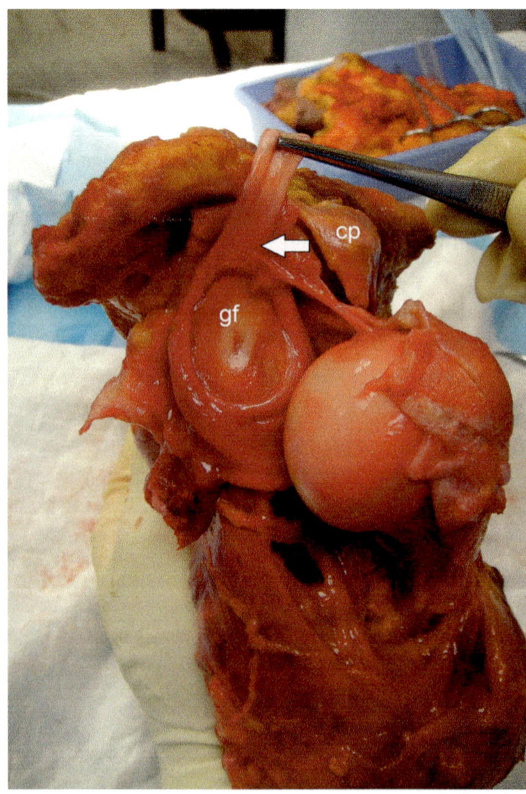

Fig. 2.20 Lateral view of the right shoulder of a cadaver. The arrow shows the long head of the biceps tendon insertion and its continuity with the labrum. *cp* coracoid process, *gf* glenoid fossa

tuberculum [28, 80]. In a study of 100 shoulders, Vangsness et al. [81] divided insertion of the tendon into four types: posterior (22%), predominantly posterior (33%), central (37%), and anterior (8%). The thickness of the tendon is greatest close to the glenoid insertion. In an ecographic study [82], it was observed that thickness depends on gender and on sporting activities. Near to the insertion, the average diameter is 8.4 mm × 3.4 [83].

The intermediate section is the area with the lowest resistance to mechanical stresses. It runs obliquely downward and laterally as far as the entrance of the bicipital groove (Fig. 2.21), and thereafter, it passes in a straight line along the volar facet of the humerus. Its average length is 10 cm (range, 9.0–14.5 cm, depending on the sex), with no major differences between the two limbs. It seems to be true that the taller the subject, the longer the tendons.

The CLB is intra-articular but extrasynovial; in fact, the synovial sheath is folded back on itself and covers the tendon. Classically, the CLB was divided into two parts: the intra-articular and that within the bicipital groove (Fig. 2.22). However, this classification is incorrect. It is known that the fibrocartilaginous shower slips onto the tendon and not vice versa; therefore, the extension of the intra-articular portion of the tendon varies depending on the position of the arm.

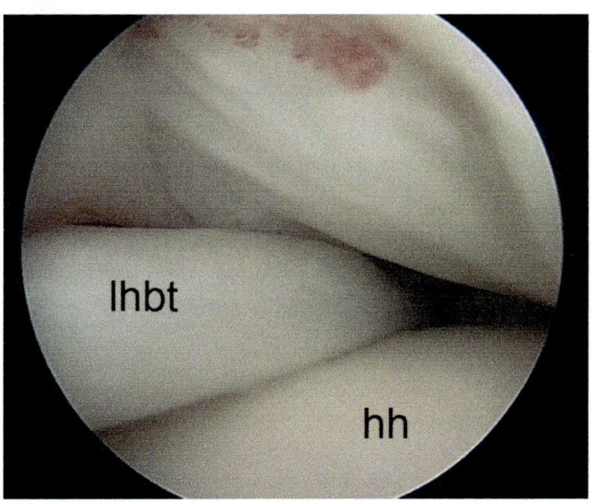

Fig. 2.21 Right shoulder. Arthroscopic view of the long head of the biceps tendon (lhbt). *hh* humeral head

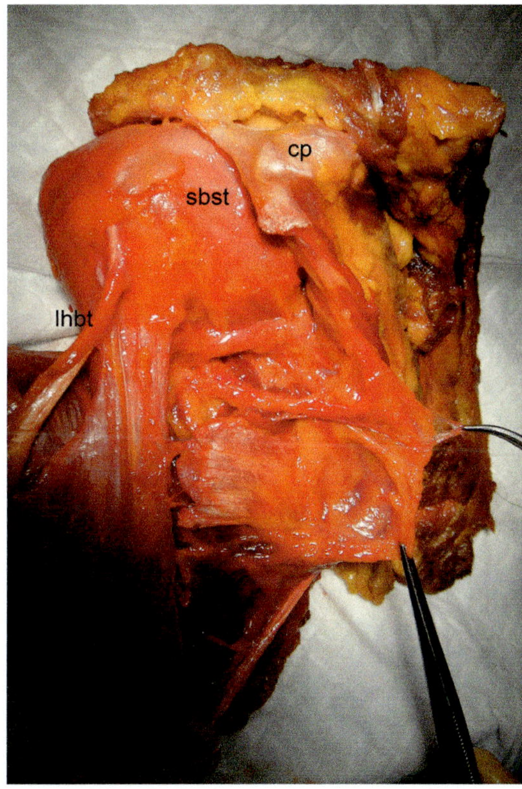

Fig. 2.22 Front view of the right shoulder of a cadaver. The long head of the biceps tendon (lhbt). *cp* coracoid process, *sbst* subscapularis tendon

The intra-articular portion of the tendon is highest when the arm adducts.

The CLB is maintained inside the groove thanks to the coracohumeral ligament, the superior glenohumeral ligament, and expansions of the supraspinatus and subscapularis tendon (Fig. 2.23). A mesotendon containing ascending branches of the anterior humeral circumflex artery constrains the CLB to shower in the proximal segment. Little is known, however, of the stabilizing function of the transverse ligament. A histological study [46] of ours showed that the surface layer of the transverse ligament is in contact with the expansions of the subscapularis tendon and of the coracohumeral ligament that constitute the second layer of the lateral portion of the rotator interval (Fig. 2.24). For this reason, we believe that the transverse ligament is part of the ligament-tendinous complex of the rotator interval. After resection of the other stabilizers,

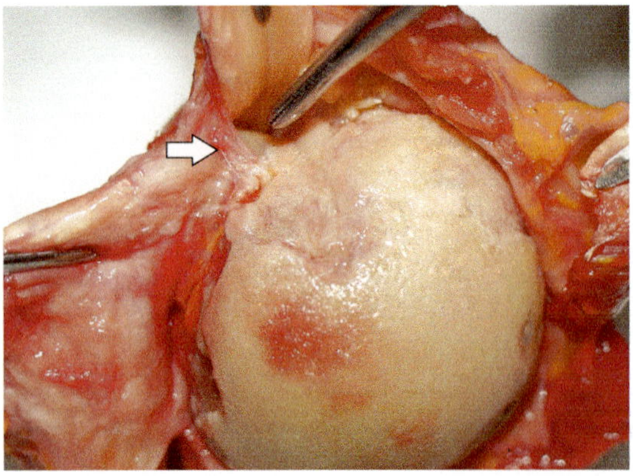

Fig. 2.23 Front view of the right shoulder of a cadaver. The arrow shows the medial vincula of the long head of the biceps tendon. They are mainly represented by the superior glenohumeral ligament and coracohumeral ligament. Supraspinatus and subscapularis tendon expansions contribute to stabilize the tendon

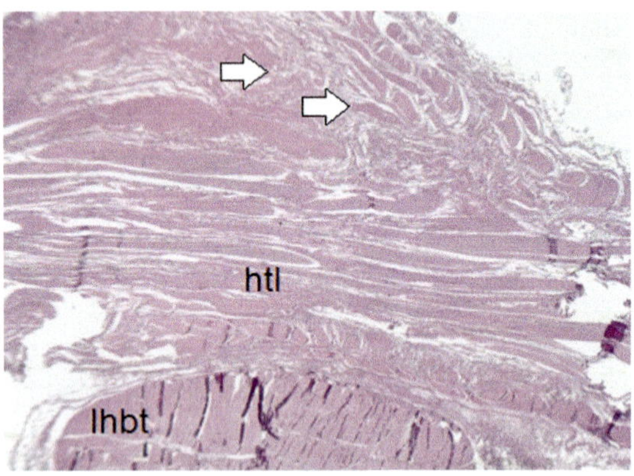

Fig. 2.24 Histological study. Humeral transverse ligament (htl) is in contact with the expansion of the subscapularis tendon and of coracohumeral ligament (arrows). *lhbt* long head of the biceps tendon

the transverse ligament is able to oppose the medial displacement of the CLB (Fig. 2.25a, b). Recently, MacDonald et al. [84] have suggested that the transverse ligament is not a distinct structure, but formed, rather, by the union of the fibers of the tendon of the subscapularis, supraspinatus, and pectoralis major. In an anatomical study of 20 shoulders, Arai et al. [85] argued that to maintain a stable biceps tendon in its groove, the integrity of the superior glenohumeral ligament and of the upper portion of the subscapularis tendon is essential.

The function of the biceps is that of flexing and supinating the forearm. Recently, its role as depressor of the humeral head, through the long head, has been revised. Our studies of patients with inveterate rupture of the long head of the biceps have shown that the absence of the tendon does not prepare systematically for a rupture of the cuff due to secondary subacromial impingement [86]. The rupture of the long head results in a reduction of strength during supination, but this reduction is not felt by the patient.

The muscle is innervated by the musculocutaneous nerve (C5–C6) and vascularized mainly by the biceps branch of the brachial artery [47].

In case of rotator cuff tear, subacromial biceps stability is strongly compromised (Fig. 2.25c–e).

2.8 Interval Rotator

The interval rotator is the space between the front edge of the supraspinatus tendon and the upper end of the subscapularis. Fealy et al. [87] stated that this space is already observable in a 14-week-old fetus. The interval is triangular in shape (Fig. 2.26). The base of the triangle is formed by the coracoid and by the coraco-glenoid ligament; laterally, it is bounded by the bicipital groove, the transverse humeral ligament (assuming this ligament as a structure distinct from the coracohumeral ligament), and the oblique fascicle. It is delimited above by the coracohumeral ligament and superior glenohumeral ligament and below by the middle glenohumeral ligament. Gohlke et al. [88] have pointed out that the capsular floor of the interval is composed of the coracohumeral and superior glenohumeral ligaments. Abe et al. [89] have suggested that the shape of the interval changes over time depending on the mechanical stresses it undergoes; thus, anatomical reconstructions after lesions of the anterior-superior cuff should take the specific individual requirements into due account.

Arthroscopically, this space is formed by the superior and the middle glenohumeral ligament and corresponds to that formerly known as Weitbrecht's foramen. Therefore, in common practice, the term "rotator interval" may refer

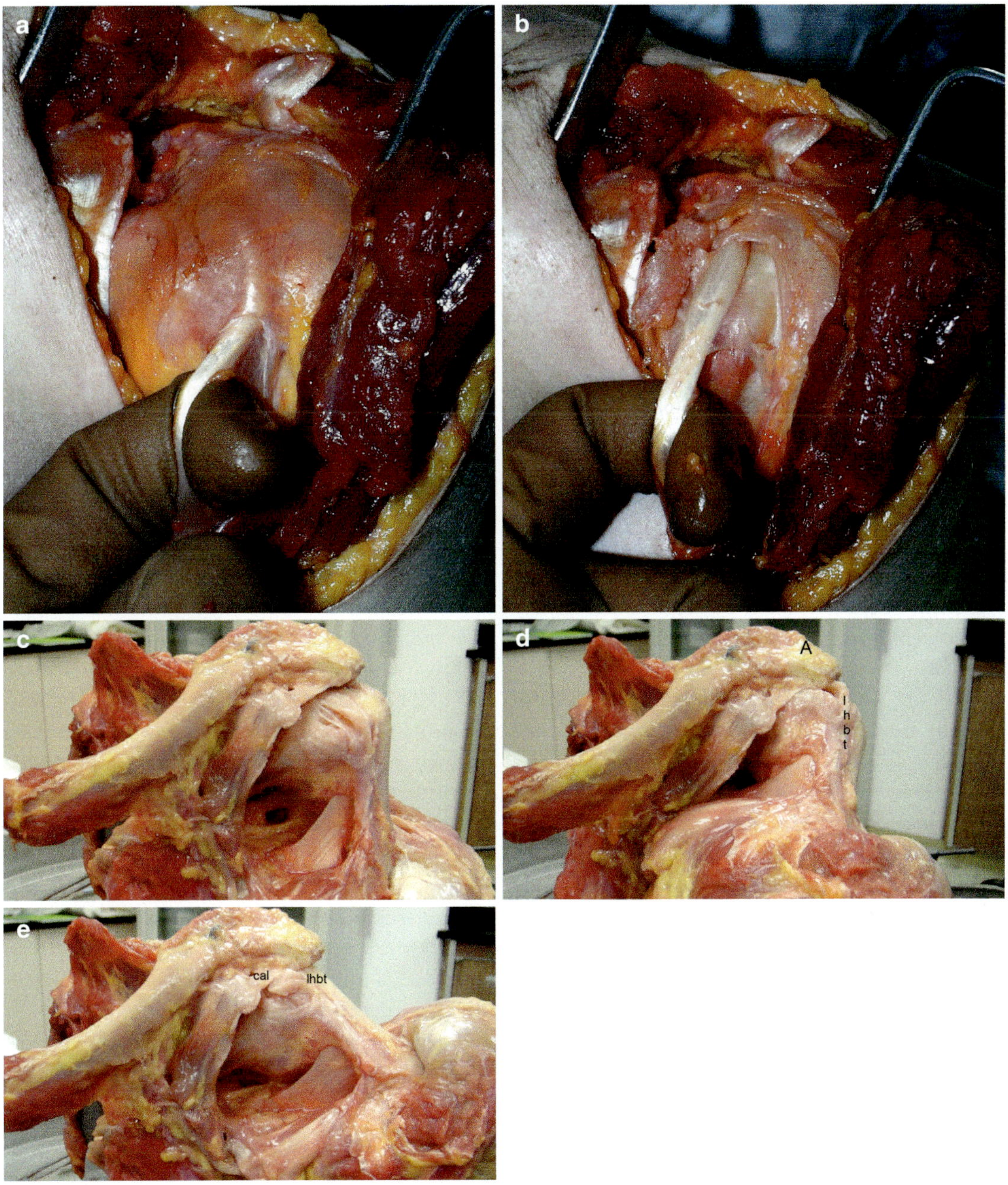

Fig. 2.25 (**a**–**e**) (**a**) The humeral transverse ligament is still able to maintain the stability of the biceps tendon alone even when coracohumeral ligament is detached. (**b**) In the absence of the transverse ligament, the medial traction of the tendon causes its dislocation. When the anterior-superior cuff is torn (**c**) and the shoulder is flexed (**d**) or abducted (**e**), the unstable biceps tendon (lhbt) comes in contact with the lateral margin of the acromion (**a**) and with the coracoacromial ligament (cal), respectively

either to the tissue anatomically connecting the supraspinatus and the subscapularis (if we are treating an anterior-superior cuff tear) or the triangular capsular space between the superior and middle glenohumeral ligaments (if we are dealing with unstable glenohumeral joint).

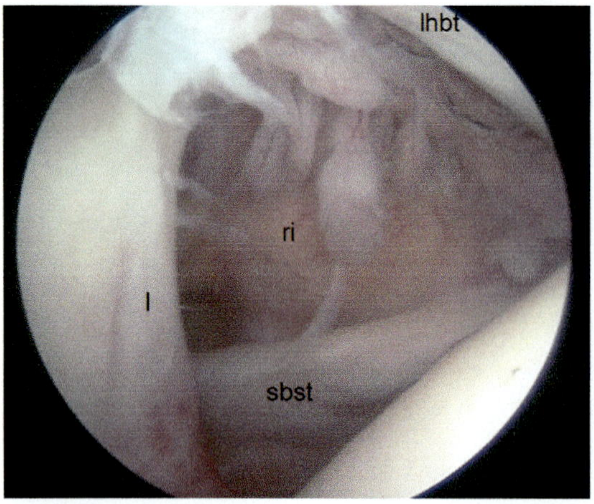

Fig. 2.26 Arthroscopic view from the posterior portal of a right shoulder. The rotator interval (ri) is defined by the labrum (l); long head of the biceps tendon (lhbt); and upper portion of the subscapularis tendon (sbst)

During internal rotation of the arm, the interval is the almost obliterated, while it is large during external rotation.

Jost et al. [90] divided the rotator interval into two ends, lateral and medial, formed, respectively, by two to four layers. The surface layer of the lateral end is formed by fibers of the coracohumeral ligament that intersect with those of the supraspinatus and subscapularis tendons. Cross fibers of these tendons form the second layer. Through the bicipital groove, some fibers of the supraspinatus reach the lesser tuberosity insertion of the subscapularis, while others from the subscapularis arrive at the greater tuberosity. The third layer is formed by fibers of the coracohumeral ligament fitted predominantly onto the greater tuberosity and to a lesser extent onto the lesser tuberosity. The fourth layer consists of the glenohumeral ligament and the superior articular capsule. The two layers of the medial end are represented, respectively, by the coracohumeral ligament, closer to the surface, and by a combination of superior glenohumeral ligament and joint capsule, more in depth. The first three layers of the lateral end form the so-called fibrous plate which limits the external rotation when the arm is adducted. Instead, the medial end limits lower translation and external rotation. Neer et al. [91] observed that the resection (in cadavers) of the coracohumeral ligament results in an average increase of 32° in external rotation.

Kolts et al. [92] conducted a study of cadavers and found that the range of the cuff is composed of three parts, each of which is represented by macroscopic anatomical structures. The lateral portion is reinforced by the presence of the semicircular humeral ligament (cable) and the anterior fibers of the supraspinatus. The mid-upper part is composed of the coracohumeral and coraco-glenoid ligaments. The middle-lower portion is reinforced by the superior and middle glenohumeral ligament.

2.9 Bone Anatomy

2.9.1 Proximal Humerus

The proximal epiphysis of the humerus has a roundish shape and consists of a medial joint portion and two tuberosities separated by an intertuberosity groove. The boundary between the articular surface and the tuberosities is delimited by the anatomical neck, which appears distinct in the upper anterior region (Figs. 2.9 and 2.12a).

Distal to the tuberosities, the surgical neck separates the head from the humeral diaphysis.

The articular portion represents about a third of a sphere; it appears flattened on the frontal plane and is covered by articular cartilage whose thickness decreases with age and is close to the tuberosities. With respect to the diaphyseal axis, it is inclined approximately 130°–150° (Fig. 2.9) [93], while the center of the sphere is located medially 6 and 3 mm posteriorly [93].

With the arm in anatomic position, the humeral head is 25°–30° retroverted with respect to the interepicondyloid axis. However, extremes of 18° and 40° of retroversion were found in anatomical studies [93, 94].

The greater tuberosity is placed posterolaterally. On it, three facets are recognized on which, from top to bottom, the tendons of the supraspinatus, infraspinatus, and teres minor are inserted. The tendon of the subscapularis muscle is inserted, instead, on the lesser tuberosity which is placed anteromedially. Together with the greater tuberosity, the lesser tuberosity delimits the bicipital groove, inside which the long head biceps tendon and the arched artery, branch of the anterior humeral circumflex artery, are present. It is broad and deep in the proximal part of the groove and is progressively lost on the anterior face of the diaphysis, confusing itself with the bone roughness corresponding to the insertion area of the teres major. The data concerning morphological and morphometric characteristics of the groove, obtained from studies on dry humerus, are contrasting. It was due to the extreme racial variability and age of the samples examined. A radiographic study [46] performed on 200 dry humeri, of which gender was known and, roughly, the age, showed that the mean value of the total opening angle of the groove is 102° (extremes 28° -160°) while that of the medial angle is 46° (extremes 16°–78°). The depth and average width of the groove are 4.3 and 12.2 mm, respectively. Statistically significant differences between the gender were detected according to the average width (13.1 M–10.2F) (see Figs. 2.10a–c and 2.11a, b).

2.9.2 Scapula

The scapula is a flat bone, placed against the posterior and upper thorax; inappropriately this relationship is identified with the term "scapulothoracic joint." Grossly, it has a triangular shape; therefore there are three margins, two faces, and three corners. Proximally, the scapula rises up until the first intercostal space; the lower angle corresponds to the seventh or eighth space.

The medial margin is on average 7 cm from the dorsal spine apophysis. It has a straight course in the tract corresponding to the three distal quarters and deviates laterally in the proximal quarter, near the spine of the scapula. The margin is bordered by a front and a back lip. On the first one, the serratus, the levator scapulae, and the rhomboid muscles insert and on the second, the supraspinatus and infraspinatus muscles.

The upper margin is delimited medially from the upper corner and laterally from the suprascapular notch. The latter is transformed into a hole by the suprascapular ligament, whose width is proportional to the size of the incision. Within the hole the suprascapular nerve and the transverse vein of the scapula run. The corresponding artery (transverse artery of the scapula) runs above the ligament; however, in rare cases, it can start with the vein and the nerve. An anatomical study [95–97] highlighted six possible configurations of the notch: in the first type the incision is wide and deep, and in the sixth the transverse ligament is ossified; therefore, the notch is transformed into a foramen. Together, types III and IV are found in over half of the population. The omohyoid muscle is inserted posteromedially to the notch.

The lateral margin is thin and has a vertical course in the upper half; in the lower one, however, it is medially oblique. It ends proximally with a triangular and wrinkled face on which the long portion of the triceps tendon is inserted.

The anterior face is concave, furrowed by two or three ridges with an oblique and ascending direction on which the subscapularis muscle is inserted, hence the name of "subscapular fossa." This face is very thin and sometimes, in the center of the face, an irregularly shaped hole connects the infraspinous and subscapular fossae. Near the medial margin, two small triangular surfaces are designed for the insertion of some bundles of serratus muscle.

The back face is convex. In correspondence with its upper quarter, the spine of the scapula emerges which divides the posterior face into two fossae: superior (supraspinous) and inferior (infraspinous). The spine of the scapula has a triangular shape. Therefore, two faces (upper and lower) and a rear edge are distinguished. The latter, broad and rough, consists of two lips: the upper one is the insertion of the trapezius muscle and the lower one of the posterior deltoid. Medially the spine assumes a triangular shape; its surface is smooth and gradually merges with the medial margin of the scapula. The infraspinous and supraspinous fossae are the insertion of the homonymous muscles. The lower one is further divided by a wrinkled crest, on which the teres minor and teres major are inserted. Laterally, the two fossae communicate widely through an incised digging between the lateral edge of the spine and the posterior margin of the neck of the scapula. Through this spino-glenoid notch, the suprascapular nerve runs; due to the close proximity to the bone and to the particular course imposed by the shape of the notch, it can be crushed during the repeated movement of abduction and external rotation. From the lateral end of the spine of the scapula, the large acromial apophysis originates.

2.9.3 Glenoid Fossa

The glenoid cavity is connected to the scapular body by the neck. It has an oval or pear shape (inverted comma) and is slightly concave, due to the presence of two rough surfaces (supra-glenoid and infra-glenoid tubercles). The glenoid labrum, which is inserted for a large part of the entire glenoid circumference, contributes to increase the concavity (see Fig. 2.20). The glenoid surface is coated with articular cartilage whose thickness is very small in its center; its dimensions are lower than those of the humeral head; in fact the glenoid receives only a third or a quarter of the opposing articular surface. Anatomical and radiographic studies showed that the glenoid retroversion is about 4°–12° [98, 99].

Anterior to the glenoid cavity, an apophysis, which, due to its shape, similar to a crow's beak, was formerly called coracoid, detaches.

References

1. Neer CS II. Anterior acromioplasty for the chronic impingement syndrome in the shoulder. J Bone Joint Surg Am. 1972;54:41–50.
2. Bigliani LU, Morrison DS, April EW. The morphology of the acromion and its relationship to the rotator cuff tears. Orthop Trans. 1986;10:228.
3. Flatow E, Coleman W, Kelkar R. The effect of anterior acromioplasty on rotator cuff contact: an experimental computer simulation. J Shoulder Elb Surg. 1995;4:S53–4.
4. Wang J, Horner G, Brown E, Shapiro M. The relationship between acromial morphology and conservative treatment of patients with impingement syndrome. Orthopedics. 2000;23:257–559.
5. Gill T, McIrvin E, Kocher M, Homa K, Mair S, Hawkins R. The relative importance of acromial morphology and age with respect to rotator cuff pathology. J Shoulder Elb Surg. 2002;11:327–30.
6. Natsis K, Tsikaras P, Totlis T. Correlation between the four types of acromion and the existence of enthesophytes: a study on 423 dried scapulas and review of the literature. Clin Anat. 2007;20:267–72.
7. Schippinger G, Bailey D, McNally E, Kiss J, Carr A. Anatomy of the normal acromion investigated using MRI. Langenbecks Arch Chir. 1997;382:141–4.
8. Vanarthos W, Monu J. Type 4 acromion: a new classification. Contemp Orthop. 1995;30:227–9.
9. Tucker T, Snyder S. The keeled acromion: an aggressive acromial variant- a series of 20 patients with associated rotator cuff tears. Arthroscopy. 2004;20:744–53.
10. Zuckerman J, Kummer F, Panos S. Characterization of acromial concavity: an in vitro computer analysis. Bull Hosp J Dis. 2000;59:69–72.
11. Chang E, Moses D, Babb J, Schweitzer M. Shoulder impingement: objective 3D shape analysis of acromion morphologic features. Radiology. 2006;239:497–505.
12. Gumina S, Albino P, Carbone S, Arceri V, Passaretti D, Candela V, Vestri A, Postacchini F. The relationship between acromion thickness and body habitus: practical implications in subacromial decompression procedures. Musculoskeletal Surg. 2012;96:41.
13. Gumina S. Morfometria ossea della spalla. Atti del Congresso sulle: Fratture e fratture-lussazioni della spalla. Roma 25–27 Marzo, 1999. pp. 9–12.
14. Edelson JG, Taitz C. Anatomy of the coraco-acromial arch. J Bone J Surg. 1992;74-B:589–94.
15. Sammarco VJ. Os acromiale: frequency, anatomy and clinical implication. J Bone Joint Surg. 2000;82-A:394–400.
16. Liberson F. Os acromiale – a contested anomaly. J Bone Joint Surg. 1937;19:683–9.
17. Boehm T, Rolf O, Martetschlaeger F, Kenn W, Gohlke F. Rotator cuff tears associated with os acromiale. Acta Orthop. 2005;76:241–4.
18. Mudge M, Wood V, Frykman G. Rotator cuff tears associated with os acromiale. J Bone Joint Surg Am. 1984;66:427–9.
19. Park J, Phelps C. Os acromiale associated with rotator cuff impingement: MR imaging of the shoulder. Radiology. 1994;193:255–7.
20. Gumina S, De Santis P, Salvatore M, Postacchini F. Relationship between os acromilale and AC joint anatomical position. J Shoulder Elb Surg. 2003;12:6–8.
21. Baechler M, Kim D. Uncoverage of the humeral head by anterolateral acromion and its relationship to full-thickness rotator cuff tears. Mil Med. 2006;171:1035–8.
22. Nyffeler R, Werner C, Sukthankar A, Schmid M, Gerber C. Association of large lateral extension of

the acromion with rotator cuff tears. J Bone Joint Surg Am. 2006;88:800–5.
23. Torrens C, Lopez J, Puente I, Caceres E. The influence of the acromial coverage index in rotator cuff tears. J Shoulder Elb Surg. 2007;16:347–51.
24. Pieper HG, Radas CB, Krahl H, Blank M. Anatomic variation of the coracoacromial ligament: a macroscopic and microscopic study of cadavers. J Shoulder Elb Surg. 1997;6:291–6.
25. Kesmezacar H, Akgun I, Ogut T, Gokay S, Uzun I. The coracoacromial ligament: the morphology and relation to rotator cuff pathology. J Shoulder Elb Surg. 2008;17:182–8.
26. Holt EM, Alibone RO. Anatomic variants of the coracoacromial ligament. J Shoulder Elb Surg. 1995;4:370–5.
27. Kopuz C, Baris S, Yildirim M, Gülman B. Anatomic variations of the coracoacromial ligament in neonatal cadavers: a neonatal cadaver study. J Pediatr Orthop Part B. 2002;11:350–4.
28. Di Giacomo G, Pouliart N, Costantini A, De Vita A. Atlas of functional shoulder anatomy. Milan: Springer-Verlaged; 2008. p. 50.
29. Fremery R, Bastian L, Siebert W. The coracoacromial ligament: anatomical and biomechanical properties with respect to age and rotator cuff disease. Knee Surg Sports Traumatol Arthrosc. 2000;8:309–13.
30. Milz S, Jaob J, Büttner A, Tischer T, Putz R, Benjamin M. The structure of the coracoacromial ligament: fibrocartilage differentiation does not necessarily mean pathology. Scand J Med Sci Sports. 2008;18:16–22.
31. Morisawa Y. Morphological study of mechanoreceptors on the coracoacromial ligament. J Orthop Sci. 1998;3:102–10.
32. Fealy S, April E, Khazzam M, Armengol-Barallat J, Bigliani L. The coracoacromial ligament: morphology and study of acromial enthesopathy. J Shoulder Elb Surg. 2005;14:542–8.
33. Ogata S, Uhthoff HK. Acromial enthesopathy and rotator cuff tear: a radiologic and histologic postmortem investigation of the coracoacromial arch. Clin Orthop. 1990;254:39–48.
34. Kijima H, Minagawa H, Saijo Y, Sano H, Tomioka T, Yamamoto N, Shimada Y, Okada K, Itoi E. Degenerated coracoacromial ligament in shoulders with rotator cuff tears shows higher elastic modulus: measurement with scanning acoustic microscopy. J Orthop Sci. 2009;14:62–7.
35. Sarkar K, Taine W, Uhthoff HK. The ultrastructure of the coracoacromial ligament in patients with chronic impingement syndrome. Clin Orthop. 1990;254:49–54.
36. Schiavone-Panni A, Milano G, Lucania L, Fabbriciani C, Logroscino CA. Histological analysis of the coracoacromial arch: correlation between age-related changes and rotator cuff tears. Arthroscopy. 1996;12:531–40.
37. Tillmann B. Functional anatomy of the shoulder. Presented at the Fourth Congress of the European Society of Knee Surgery and Arthroscopy Stockholm 25–30 June, 1990.
38. Moorman CT, Deng XH, Warren RF. Role of the coracoacromial ligament in normal shoulder function. Presented at the American Academy of Orthopaedic Surgeons, 62nd Annual Meeting, 16–21 February 1995, Orlando, FL.
39. Lazarus MD, Ynung SW, Sidles JA. Anterosuperior humeral displacement: limitation by coracoacromial arch. Presented at the American Academy of Orthopaedic Surgeons, 62nd Annual Meeting, 16–21 February 1995, Orlando, FL
40. Fagelman M, Sartori M, Freedman KB, Patwardhan AG, Corandang G, Marra G. Biomechanics of coracoacromial arch modification. J Shoulder Elb Surg. 2007;16:101–6.
41. Gumina S, Postacchini F, Orsina L, Cinotti G. The morphometry of the coracoid process – its aetiologic role in subcoracoid impingement syndrome. Int Orthop. 1999;23:198–201.
42. Ferreira Neto A, Almeida A, Maiorino R, Zoppi Filho A, Benegas E. An anatomical study of the subcoracoid space. Clinics. 2006;61:467–72.
43. Richards D, Burckhart S, Campbell S. Relation between narrowed coracohumeral distance and subscapularis tears. Arthroscopy. 2005;21:1223–8.
44. Radas C, Pieper H. The coracoid impingement of the subscapularis tendon. A study of cadavers. J Shoulder Elbow Surg. 2004;13:154–9.
45. Schulz C, Anetzberger H, Glaser C. Coracoid tip position on frontal radiographs of the shoulder: a predictor of common shoulder pathologies. Br J Radiol. 2005;78:1005–8.
46. Gumina S. Il capo lungo del bicipite: anatomia ossea e del legamento trasverso. Atti del Congresso: Il capo lungo del bicipite. 2002, Abano Terme (PD). p. 36.
47. Clemente CD. Gray's anatomy. 30th ed. Philadelphia: Lea & Febiger, 1984; 233–235., 370, 375, 512–528.
48. Mochizuki T, Sugaya H, Uomizu M, Maeda K, Matsuki K, Sekiya I, Muneta T, Akita K. Humeral insertion of supraspinatus and infraspinatus. New anatomical findings regarding the footprint of the rotator cuff. J Bone Joint Surg. 2008;90:962–9.
49. Albritton MJ, Graham RD, Richards RS 2nd, Basamania CJ. An anatomic study of the effects on the suprascapular nerve due to retraction of the supraspinatus muscle after a rotator cuff tears. J Shoulder Elb Surg. 2003;12:497–500.
50. Minagawa H, Itoi E, Konno N, Kido T, Sano A, Urayama M, Sato K. Humeral attachment of the supraspinatus and infraspinatus tendons: an anatomic study. Arthroscopy. 1998;14:302–6.
51. Dugas JR, Campbell DA, Warren RF, Robie BH, Millet PJ. Anatomy and dimensions of rotator cuff insertions. J Shoulder Elb Surg. 2002;11:498–503.
52. Curtis AS, Burbank KM, Tierney JJ, Scheller AD, Curran AR. The insertional footprint of the rotator cuff: an anatomic study. Arthroscopy. 2006;22:603–9.

53. Itoi E, Berglund LJ, Grabowski JJ, Schultz FM, Growney ES, Morrey BF, An KN. Tensile properties of the supraspinatus tendon. J Orthop Res. 1995;13:578–84.
54. Itoi E, Berglund LJ, Grabowski JJ. Tensile properties of the supraspinatus tendon. J Musculoskelet Res. 2004;8:29–34.
55. Sano H, Ishii H, Yeadon A, Backman DS, Brunet JA, Uhthoff HK. Degeneration at the insertion weakens the tensile strength of the supraspinatus tendon: a comparative mechanical and histologic study of the bone-tendon complex. J Orthop Res. 1997;15:719–26.
56. Uhthoff HK, Sano H. Pathology of failure of the rotator cuff tendon. Orthop Clin North Am. 1997;28:31–41.
57. Cooper DE, O'Brien S, Warren R. Supporting layers of the Gleno-humeral joint: an anatomic study. Clin Orthop. 1993;289:144–59.
58. Nakajima T, Rokuuma N, Hamada K. Histologic and biomechanical characteristics of the supraspinatus tendon: reference to rotator cuff tearing. J Shoulder Elb Surg. 1994;3:79–87.
59. Fallon J, Blevins FT, Vogel K, Trotter J. Functional morphology of the supraspinatus tendon. J Orthop Res. 2002;20:920–6.
60. Clark JM, Harryman DT. Tendons, ligament and capsule of the rotator cuff. Gross and microscopic anatomy. J Bone Joint Surg. 1992;74-A:713–25.
61. Burkhart SS. Arthroscopic treatment of massive rotator cuff tears: clinical results and biomechanical rationale. Clin Orthop. 1991;267:45–56.
62. Cooper DE, Arnoczky SP, O'Brien SJ. Histology and vascularity of the glenoid-labrum- an anatomic study. J Bone Joint Surg. 1992;74-A:46–52.
63. Pearsall AW, Holovacs TF, Speer KP. The intra-articular component of the subscapularis tendon: an anatomic and histological correlation in reference to surgical release in patients with frozen shoulder syndrome. Arthroscopy. 2000;16:236–42.
64. Matsen FA, Arntz CT, Lippitt SB. La cuffia dei rotatori. In: Rockwood CA, Matsen FA, editors. La spalla. Roma: Verduci; 2000. p. 733–821.
65. Colachis SC Jr, Strohm BR, Brecher VL. Effects of axillary nerve block on muscle force in the upper extremity. Arch Phys Med Rehabil. 1969;50:645–7.
66. Howell SM, Imobersteg AM, Seger DH, Marone PJ. Clarification of the role of the supraspinatus muscle in the shoulder function. J Bone Joint Surg. 1986;68-A:398–404.
67. Salmon M. Anatomic studies: arteries of the muscles of the extremities and the trunk and arterial anastomotic pathways of the extremities. St Louis: Quality Medical Publishing Inc.; 1994. p. 11–7.
68. Cain PR, Mutschler TA, Fu FH, Lee SK. Anterior stability of the glenohumeral joint. A dynamic model. Am J Sports Med. 1987;15:144–8.
69. Bartlett SP, May JW, Yaremchuk MJ. The latissimus dorsi muscle: a fresh cadaver study of the primary neurovascular pedicle. Plast Reconstr Surg. 1981;65:631–6.
70. Huelke DF. Variation in the origins of the branches of the axillary artery. Anat Rec. 1959;132:233.
71. Oversen JO, Nielsen S. Stability of the shoulder joint. Cadaver study of stabilizing structure. Acta Orthop Scand. 1985;56:149–51.
72. Symeonides PP. The significance of the subscapularis muscle in the pathogenesis of recurrent anterior dislocation of the shoulder. J Bone Joint Surg. 1972;54-B:476–83.
73. Halder A, Zobitz ME, Schultz E, An KN. Structural properties of the subscapolaris tendon. J Orthop Res. 2000;18:829–34.
74. Alpert SW, Pink MM, Jobe FW, McMahon PJ, Mathiyakom W. Electromyographic analysis of deltoid and rotator cuff function under varying loads and speeds. J Shoulder Elb Surg. 2000;9:47–58.
75. Motzkin NE, Itoi E, Morrey BF. Contribution of passive bulk tissues and deltoid to static inferior glenohumeral stability. J Shoulder Elb Surg. 1994;3:313–9.
76. Markhede G, Monastyrski J, Stener B. Shoulder function after deltoid muscle removal. Acta Orthop Scand. 1985;56:242–4.
77. Kido T, Itoi E, Lee SB, Neale PG, An KN. Dynamic stabilizing function of the deltoid muscle in shoulders with anterior instability. Am J Sports Med. 2003;31:399–403.
78. Morrey B, Itoi E, An K. Biomechanics of the shoulder. In: Rockwood Jr C, Matsen III FA, editors. The shoulder. 2nd ed. Philadelphia: Saunders; 1998. p. 890–6.
79. Jobe CM. Gross anatomy of the shoulder. In: Rockwood CA, Matsen FA, editors. The shoulder. Philadelphia: WB Saunders; 1990. p. 34–97.
80. Habermeyer P, Kaiser E, Knappe M, Kreusser T, Wiedemann E. Functional anatomy and biomechanics of the long biceps tendon. Unfallchirurg. 1987;90:319–29.
81. Vangsness CT, Jorgenson SS, Watson T, Johnson DL. The origin of the long head of the biceps from the scapula and glenoid labrum. J Bone Joint Surg Br. 1994;76:951–3.
82. Van Holsbeek M, Introcaso JH. Musculoskeletal ultrasound. 1st ed. St. Louis: Mosby-Year Book; 1991. p. 265–84. 316
83. Refior HJ, Sowa D. Long tendon of the biceps brachii: sites of predilection for degenerative lesions. J Shoulder Elb Surg. 1995;4:436–40.
84. MacDonald K, Bridger J, Cash C, Parkin L. Transverse humeral ligament: does it exist? Clin Anat. 2007;20:663–7.
85. Arai R, Mochiziki T, Yamaguchi K, Sugaya H, Kobayashi M, Nakamura T, Akita K. Functional anatomy of the superior glenohumeral and coracohumeral ligaments and the subscapularis tendon in view of stabilization of the long head of the biceps tendon. J Shoulder Elb Surg. 2010;19:58–64.

86. Gumina S, Carbone S, Perugia D, Perugia L, Postacchini F. Rupture of the long head biceps tendon treated with tenodesis to the coracoid process. Results at more than 30 years. Int Orthop. 2011;35:713–6.
87. Fealy S, Rodeo SA, DiCarlo EF, O'Brien SJ. The developmental anatomy of the neonatal glenohumeral joint. J Shoulder Elb Surg. 2000;9:217–22.
88. Gohlke F, Essigkurg B, Schmitz F. The pattern of collagen fiber bundles of the capsule of the glenohumeral joint. J Shoulder Elb Surg. 1994;3:111–27.
89. Abe S, Nakamura T, Rodriguez-Vazquez JF, Murakami G, Ide Y. Early fetal development of the rotator interval region of the shoulder with special reference to topographical relationships among related tendons and ligaments. Surg Radiol Anat. 2011;33:609–15.
90. Jost B, Koch PP, Gerber C. Anatomy and functional aspects of the rotator interval. J Shoulder Elb Surg. 2000;9:336–41.
91. Neer CS 2nd, Satterlee CC, Dalsey RM, Flatow EL. The anatomy and potential effects of contracture of the coracohumeral ligament. Clin Orthop. 1992;280:182–5.
92. Kolts I, Busch LC, Tomusk H, Raudheiding A, Eller A, Merila M, Russlies M, Pääsuke M, Leibecke T, Kühnel W. Macroscopical anatomy of the so called "rotator interval". A cadaver study on 19 shoulder joints. Ann Anat. 2002;184:9–14.
93. Testut L. In: Anatomia Umana, vol I. Torinese; 1942. p. 301.
94. Pearl ML, Volk AG. Retroversion of the proximal humerus in relationship to prosthetic replacement arthroplasty. J Shoulder Elb Surg. 1995;4:286–9.
95. Rengachary SS, Burr D, Lucas S. Soprascapular entrapment neuropathy: a clinical, anatomical and comparative study. Part. 2: anatomical study. Neurosurgery. 1979;5:446–51.
96. Rengachary SS, Burr D, Lucas S, Brackett CE. Soprascapular entrapment neuropathy: a clinical, anatomical and comparative study. Part. 3: comparative study. Neurosurgery. 1979;5:452–5.
97. Rengachary SS, Neff JP, Singer PA, Brackett CE. Soprascapular entrapment neuropathy: a clinical, anatomical and comparative study. Part. 1: Clinical study. Neurosurgery. 1979;5:441–5.
98. Rothman RH, Marvel JP, Heppenstal RB. Anatomic considerations in the glenohumeral joint. Orthop Clin North Am. 1975;6:341–52.
99. Das SP, Ray GS, Saha AK. Observations on the tilt of the glenoid cavity of the scapula. J Anat Soc India. 1966;15:114–8.

3 Biomechanic Principles of Reverse Shoulder Prosthesis

Raffaele Russo, Michele Ciccarelli, and Giuseppe Della Rotonda

Reverse total shoulder arthroplasty (RTSA) is used to reduce pain and to improve function in cases of rotator cuff arthropathy, four-part proximal humeral fractures, inflammatory arthritis, and revision shoulder arthroplasty [1–4]. This new design of total shoulder arthroplasty was introduced in the 1970s with a reversion of the normal anatomy by placing the socket in the proximal humerus and the prosthetic ball on the glenoid. Proponents for this design argued this change would allow improved motion and strength without the increased risk of dislocation and loosening. A number of reverse implant systems were designed beginning in the 1970s with variable designs for scapular fixation [5–7] (Table 3.1). These prostheses created a foundation for reverse shoulder arthroplasty and made important contributions to our understanding of the reverse concept.

Initial devices were constrained and had high rates of clinical failure, mostly from component loosening [8, 9]. These early failures led to the development of a semiconstrained prosthesis by Grammont and Baulot in 1985 [10] evolved in 1991 to the Delta III prosthesis (DePuy International Ltd., Warsaw, IN) (Fig. 3.4) with a pain decrease and improvement in function [11].

R. Russo (✉) · M. Ciccarelli · G. Della Rotonda
Department Orthopedics and Traumatology, Institution Pineta Grande Hospital, Castelvolturno, Italy

Table 3.1 Reverse shoulder arthroplasty designs

Prosthesis name	Year	Prosthesis features
Leeds shoulder/ Reeves et al. Fig. 3.1	1972	Glenoid component with divergent threaded peg; anatomic center of rotation recreated
Kessel	1973	Single central glenoid screw; center of rotation placed laterally
Kolbel and Friedebold Fig. 3.2	1973	Flange bolted glenoid component to scapular spine; designed to allow dislocation at lower forces
Bayley-Walker	1973	Large hydroxyapatite-coated screw; center of rotation moved medially and distally
Fenlin Fig. 3.3	1975	Glenosphere enlarged to increase deltoid lever arm
Liverpool/ Beddow and Elloy	1975	Glenoid component included a stem fixed into the scapular pillar to improve glenoid fixation
Buechel et al.	1978	A "floating fulcrum"; glenosphere decreased in size to increase shoulder motion
Trispherical/ Gristina and Webb	1978	A glenosphere and a small sphere on the humerus, both articulating in a larger polyethylene cup
Grammont Version 1	1985	Center of rotation medialized but remained lateral to native glenoid surface; glenoid baseplate had a press-fit central peg
Delta III/ Grammont Fig. 3.4	1991	Center of rotation further medialized to the native glenoid face; glenoid baseplate coated with hydroxyapatite to improve fixation

S. Gumina et al. (eds.), *Reverse Shoulder Arthroplasty*,
https://doi.org/10.1007/978-3-319-97743-0_3

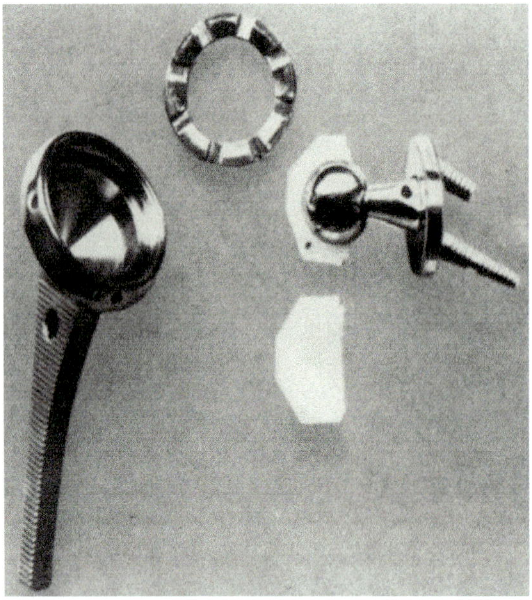

Fig. 3.1 Reverse total shoulder system designed by Reeves

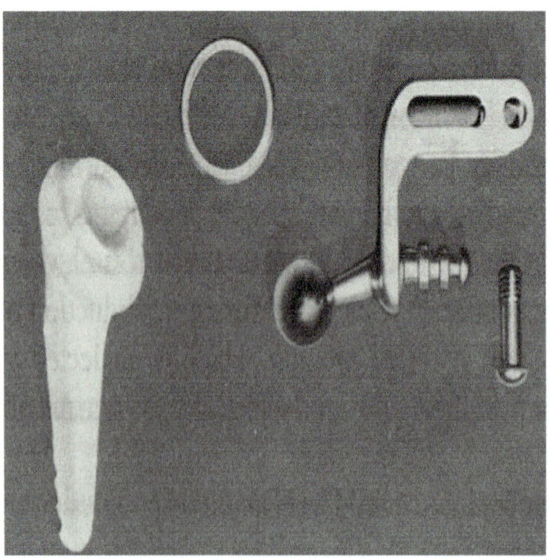

Fig. 3.2 Shoulder prosthesis designed by Kolbel

The Grammont's prosthesis was based on four principles necessary to give stability and allow the deltoid to compensate an absent rotator cuff:

- The center of rotation must be fixed, distalized, and medialized to the level of the glenoid surface.
- The prosthesis must be inherently stable.

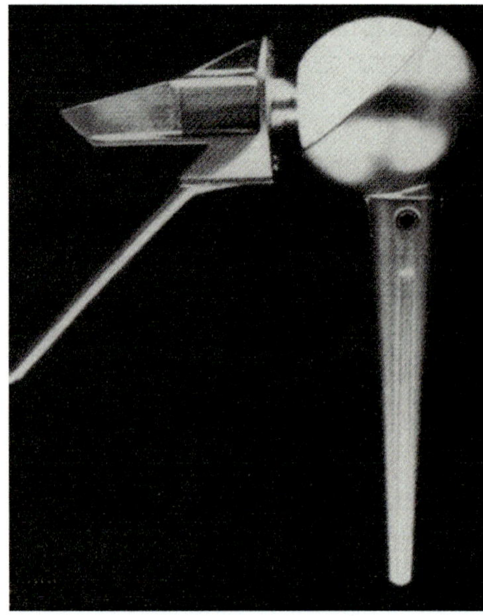

Fig. 3.3 The prosthesis designed by John M. Fenlin

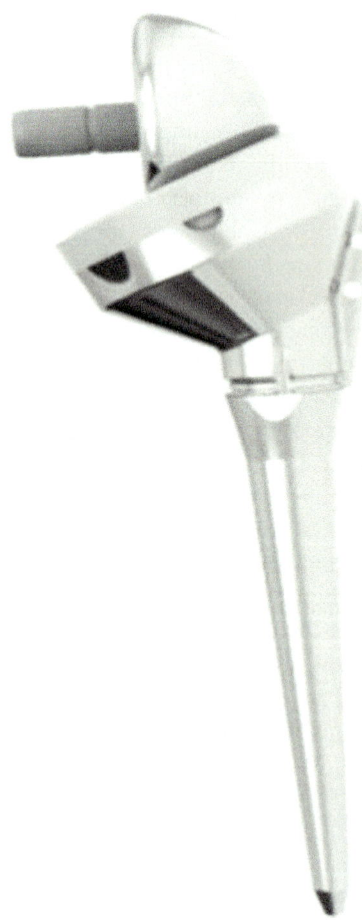

Fig. 3.4 Delta III prosthesis

- The lever arm of the deltoid must be effective from the start of movement.
- The glenosphere must be large and the humeral cup small to create a semiconstrained articulation.

In the initial Grammont's design, the center of rotation was medialized but remained lateral to the native glenoid surface, and in order to solve this problem in the Grammont's second-generation prosthesis, the Delta III, the glenosphere was changed from two thirds of a sphere to a hemisphere, the baseplate had a central press-fit peg and two divergent 3.5 mm screws specifically angled to resist the shear forces at the bone-implant interface, and the humeral component featured a small cup, covering less than half of the glenosphere, oriented almost horizontally with a nonanatomic neck-shaft angle of 155° [10].

Following the four basic principles introduced by Grammont, there are eight important points to analyze in order to understand the biomechanics of this complex system:

- Glenosphere position
- Inclination
- Lateral offset
- Neck-shaft angle and humeral component version
- Stability
- Deltoid and teres minor function
- Prosthesis design

The function of a native shoulder is characterized in a variable center of rotation throughout the arc of motion, and the movement of the humeral head on the glenoid is around two main centers of rotation [12] with a resultant force vector, composed of both compressive and shear forces, that varies throughout the range of motion but that consistently passes through the joint's fixed center of rotation. Reverse total shoulder arthroplasty (RTSA) components create a new fixed center of rotation secondary to increased constraint and matched radii of curvature with a maximization of compressive forces and reduction of shear ones at the bone-implant interface. By creating a glenoid component shaped as a hemisphere, Grammont reduced the system's center of rotation directly to the bone-implant interface, and the medialization of the joint's center of rotation stabilized the bone-implant interface by converting the shear forces into compressive [13]. However, medialization of the shoulder's center of rotation has been associated with scapular notching [14], the most common RTSA complication, caused by the mechanical impingement of the superomedial humeral prosthesis against the inferior scapular neck during adduction. More recently, notching has been recognized as a three-dimensional phenomenon, with acknowledgment of the possible rotational impingement that occurs between the liner and the scapular neck [15]. In order to reduce and avoid the incidence of scapular notching, there are some technical and biomechanical notes to follow during a glenosphere implant:

(a) *Eccentric (inferior) positioning*: provides a space between the glenosphere and the scapular neck that may decrease notching and creates additional distance between the greater tuberosity and coracoacromial arch allowing greater impingement-free range of motion during abduction with an increased adduction deficit (11° to 39° of additional adduction) [16].
(b) *Inferior inclination*: the advantages of inferior inclination are still debated. In a cadaveric study by Nyffeler et al., the glenoid components was implanted with an inferior inclination of 15°, and the results showed increased abduction and adduction impingement-free range of motion compared with a component placed in neutral position [17]. In a prospective randomized controlled trial of 42 patients, Edwards et al. compared cohorts with glenoid components implanted in either a neutral position or with a 10° inferior inclination, and they reported no benefit of inferior inclination [18].
(c) *Lateral offset*: lateralization relative to this new medialized center of rotation provides for a larger impingement-free range of motion but creates an additional destabilizing torque at the bone-implant interface. Grammont's Delta III glenosphere was designed with 19 mm of lateral offset. Harman et al. demonstrated in vitro that glenospheres with increased lateral offsets of 23 and 27 mm

generate 44% and 69% more torque, respectively, at the baseplate interface [19, 20]. Lateralization may improve shoulder range of motion after RTSA, but the medialization of the shoulder's center of rotation decreases the rotator cuff muscle tension with a reduction of their respective moment arms by as much as 36% [21]. Furthermore, limited shoulder rotation with RTSA may be, in part, related to the limited excursion of the cup around the medialized glenosphere as well as mechanical impingement of the tuberosities against the coracoid process in internal rotation and the scapular spine in external rotation. However, lateralization may be less important if the glenosphere is placed in an eccentric (inferior) position as demonstrated by De Wilde et al. [15].

(d) *Humeral component version*: the 155° prosthesis is certainly the most widely accepted inclination angle and has been essentially the only prosthesis used in Europe for more than 10 years [22]. With increasing neck-shaft angle, the polyethylene cup is positioned in a more horizontal orientation [15], resulting in progressive mechanical conflict between the cup and inferior scapular neck as demonstrated by Gutierrez [23]. To solve this problem, an increased humeral component could raise the amount of external rotation and decreases the amount of internal rotation before impingement [24]. Erickson et al. [25] reported in a systematic review that there is much more possibility of scapular notching with 155° inclination rather than 135° but no difference of instability. Boileau et al. [26] attempted to decrease the rate of scapular notching in patients with a 155° prosthesis by lateralizing the glenoid using cancellous humeral head autograft. The study concluded that the rate of notching decreased (reported in the study at 19%) with bony lateralization without increasing torque on the glenoid component as is seen with more lateralized glenoid system.

(e) *Inherent stability*: the normal shoulder stability is characterized by two important factors: the balance stability angle defined as the maximal angle that the limit joint reaction force can form with the concavity before a dislocation [27] and the stability ratio defined as the maximum allowable subluxation force/joint compression force (V.N. 0.5). Regarding the balance stability angle, a RTSA is able to tolerate a joint reaction force vector of up to 45° and has got a stability ratio > 2.0, four to five times more stable than a normal joint and two to three times more stable than a conventional total shoulder prosthesis [28]. Despite this, the semiconstrained design is susceptible to anterior instability in the fully adducted position, a complication reported in 1.5 to 31% of patients, [29] and this problem is likely due to inferior impingement that can generate distractive forces. Increasing the humeral cup's depth to radius ratio exponentially improves the inherent stability of the reverse prosthesis [30]. In contrast, varying glenosphere size has no notable effect on joint stability [23]. Stability also depends on glenosphere position that with a retroversion >20° has been shown to reduce anterior stability, while the arm is in the resting position [30]. In addition, placing the glenosphere in a position of inferior offset has been shown to increase stability by approximately 17% [31]. Humeral component version has little effect on stability. Although a noncadaveric shoulder simulator demonstrated that version of the humeral component had a significant effect on stability, a conflicting study using cadaveric shoulders, which provide an additional element of soft tissue constraint, showed that humeral component version did not significantly alter dislocation forces [28, 31].

(f) *Deltoid, teres minor, and rotator cuff function*: the function of RTSA involved the deltoid muscle because a medialized center of rotation increases the deltoid's function by 20–42% with additional anterior and posterior fibers as abductors [32], instead of flexor and extensor, respectively, as they work in a normal shoulder. In details the inferior-most portion of the anterior deltoid becomes a flexor-abductor and the posterior deltoid an extensor-abductor, and the middle deltoid increases its abductor function [33]. The maximum deltoid fluctuation is reached at 90° of abduction that can compensate the deficiency of the supraspinatus [13], and the distalized center of rotation shortened the fibers with an improved muscle function by 30% [34] and gives a less restricted range of motion. This "new" abductor muscle function is present from the start of movement due to a lower level of fibers from the RTSA with reduced forces of middle and anterior deltoid during the flexion [35]. Despite most patients' improvement in flexion and abduction, active internal rotation and external rotation often remain unchanged or reduced [36] due to an absence or detensioning of the subscapularis tendon and teres minor [21]. The outcome of RTSA is influenced by the integrity of the external rotators, specifically the teres minor (TM) [37]. According to Grammont [10] and Boileau [14], a potential solution to improve active external rotation is to increase humeral retroversion to improve the mechanical advantage of the TM, when it is present. Berton et al. [30] showed that RTSA increases TM external rotation moment arms compared with a normal shoulder. Such increase is less pronounced in high degrees of arm abduction. At the same time, because of humeral medialization, RTSA decreases TM length, especially in low degrees of humeral abduction. They concluded that the 0° to 20° retroversion was the optimum compromise between sufficient TM length and moment arm with minimum impingement. In case of teres minor absence with a full rotator cuff deficiency, it could indicate to restore the external rotation a latissimus dorsi transfer associated to RTSA [38].

(g) *Prosthesis design*: the planning of the reverse shoulder prosthesis is based on the idea of a fixed rotating center on the scapula and a cup on the humerus to create a fulcrum for the joint. This fixed fulcrum prevents the superior migration of the humeral head and allows the deltoid lift up the arm despite the absence of muscles of the rotating cuff. The planning has been tested to recreate the anatomical glenoidal face rotation center with a highly constrained design. There are two current design: The first one is based on the original Grammont-style prosthesis, with a medialized center of rotation at the baseplate-glenoid interface. The second design places the center of rotation more laterally within the glenosphere. Despite the differing biomechanics, both prostheses allow for a greater deltoid lever arm, which enables arm elevation in the absence of a functioning rotator cuff. The glenoid component can be a hemisphere with a diameter of 36 as in the original Grammont prosthesis, but in the last 10 years, many companies created different sizes of glenosphere from 36 to 42 mm, creating a greater potential arc of motion [39]. Reverse shoulder patients with severe deficiency in the rotator cuff often demonstrate a lack of external rotation strength, particularly with the arm abducted. The deficiency is not typically due to physical limitations of the implant as many patients have good passive external rotation. The result of external rotation deficiency is the hand falls into internal rotation as the arm is elevated and stays in front of the face in a motion resembling a person holding a horn to their mouth, termed "hornblower's sign." The 42 mm glenosphere, compared with the 36 mm glenosphere, has been shown to increase average abduction amplitude by approximately 5° and to provide an additional 22° of adduction before inferior impingement occurs [40] but can be difficult to demonstrate in the common practice because the mechanical effect is not constant for all patients treated with 42 glenospheres. The humeral component's neck-shaft angle is an important factor that affects the clinical range of motion. Grammont's humeral component is designed with a nonanatomic humeral neck inclination of 155°; the polyethylene cup is positioned in a more horizontal orientation, resulting in progressive mechanical conflict between the cup and inferior scapular neck [16]. A retrospective review of 65 patients after RTSA compared 2 cohorts with varying neck-shaft angles and glenoid offsets and showed that the group with a smaller neck-shaft angle (143° vs. 155°) and larger glenosphere offset (2.5 mm vs. 0 mm) had a significantly lower incidence of notching (16.2% vs. 60.7%) [23]. Stephenson et al., in a cadaveric study, showed that humeral retroversion between 20° and 40° most closely restores a functional range of motion [24]. Placing the humeral component in neutral version or anteversion results in greater than physiologic internal rotation while increasing the risk of posterior notching. As the shoulder is abducted in the scapular plane, mechanical limitations on internal and external rotation diminish. At 60° of abduction, the humeral bearing is able to rotate unimpeded around the glenosphere; and at 90° of abduction, supraphysiologic internal rotation and external rotation are possible [41]. In the last years, a new short humeral stem design has been introduced in order to avoid complications related to the normal accounted for 10 to 20% such as periprosthetic fracture, shaft perforation, disassembly, and loosening [42]. Levy et al. [43] reported midterm good results in 102 patients using this new stem with an improved rotational movements, low incidence of glenoid notching, and no implant loosening, subsidence, or stress shielding. The baseplate screw fixation is the most important factor leading to long-term fixation through osseous integration [44], and it depends on the anatomy of scapula (the three-column concept), the bone quality and screw type, and location [45]. Locking screws create a more stable construct and reduce baseplate micromotion in vitro compared with similar diameter nonlocking screws [46], and we can use four or two screws depending on a baseplate model with a central peg. In the screw placement, there is a risk of a soft tissue damage including the suprascapular nerve, the suprascapular artery, and the subscapularis muscle, and several studies have showed that the mean screw length should be 30 mm for the superior screw holes, 28 mm for the inferior screw holes, 13 mm for the anterior screw holes, and 15 mm for the posterior screw holes in order to avoid this problem [47]. About the screw position, it is important to keep in mind the safe zone of the glenoid during surgery that usually is identified with the vertical axis crossing the supraglenoid tubercle and the infraglenoid tubercle (Fig. 3.5). Screws placed anterior to this axis would be in the safe zone with a relatively low risk to the axillary nerve; screws placed posterior to this axis would enter the danger zone and pose a risk to the suprascapular nerve and artery [48]. Glenoid deficiency and erosion (excessive retroversion/inclination) must be corrected in reverse shoulder arthroplasty (RSA) to avoid prosthetic notching or instability and to maximize function, range of motion, and prosthesis longevity [40]. Historically, options to address glenoid bone defects combined eccentric reaming with glenoid bone grafting with an autograft iliac crest bone graft (ICBG) or allograft or augmented

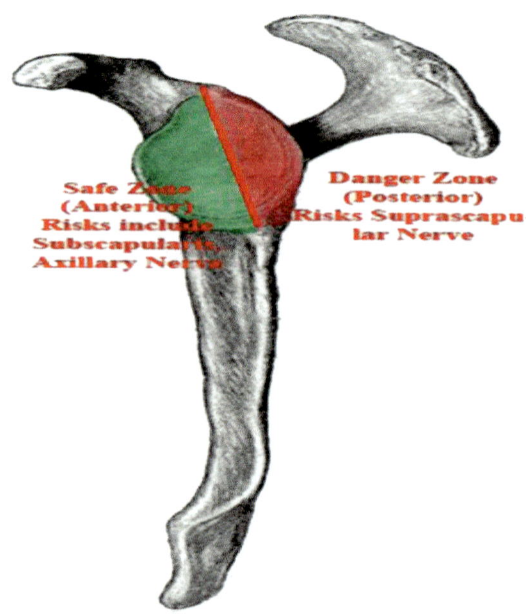

Fig. 3.5 Safe zone of glenoid. Hart ND, Clark JC, Wade Krause FR, Kissenberth MJ, Bragg WE, Hawkins RJ. Glenoid screw position in the encore reverse shoulder prosthesis: an anatomic dissection study of screw relationship to surrounding structures. J Shoulder Elbow Surg. 2013 Jun;22(6):814–20. doi: https://doi.org/10.1016/j.jse.2012.08.013. Epub 2012 Nov 14

glenoid baseplates [49]. Since 2006, a new technique was described by Neyton et al. [50] based on the use of an autologous bone graft harvested from the humeral head to restore the glenoid bone stock and obtain correct alignment of the implant with minimal morbidity (BIO-RSA). The humeral head autograft may be symmetrical (BIO-RSA) for the type A and B1 glenoid according to Walch classification [51] or asymmetrical (angled BIO-RSA) in the case of type B2/C glenoid. The results published by Jones et al. [52] on the BIO-RSA demonstrated a higher rate of graft incorporation in RSA for autografts compared with allografts (86% complete or partial incorporation for autografts vs. 66% for allografts); Boileau et al. [53] recently published their results on the angled BIO-RSA with 94% of complete radiographic incorporation of the graft, mild notching occurred in 25% of patients, and Constant-Murley and subjective shoulder value assessments increased from 31 to 68 and from 30% to 83%, respectively.

3.1 Reverse Shoulder Arthroplasty for Proximal Humeral Fractures

RSA has recently been applied to the treatment of acute four-part proximal humeral fractures [54]. This implant can provide reliable forward elevation, improve functional scores, and relieve pain in the carefully selected patient. Shoulder surgeons currently restrict its use to complex three- or four-part fractures in elderly patients because the longevity of this type of implant has yet to be determined. RSA has been used more frequently for these fractures because it is less reliant on a functioning rotator cuff and healing of the tuberosities. The management of the lesser and greater tuberosity for the RSA implant in these complex fracture is still debated, and few studies are present on this topic. In the first cases, the tuberosities were removed based on the mechanical concept of the isolated deltoid action to supply the cuff deficiency, and the results [55] demonstrated high numbers of complication especially relative to the frequent instability and lack of extrarotation. Tuberosity fixation and implant positioning remain important for the RSA when used for fracture. Recent evidence has shown that improved rotation may be obtained if the tuberosities are repaired anatomically to the RSA implant. Gallinet et al. [56] treated elderly patients with proximal humeral fractures with RSA and found that patients with anatomic healing of the tuberosities had improved forward elevation (127.2° vs. 96.5°), external rotation at the side (19.7° vs. 1.6°), and external rotation at 90° of abduction (49.4° vs. 10.3°) when compared with patients who had nonunion or malunion. Nonabsorbable sutures are placed through the bone-tendon junction of each fragment and can be placed before glenosphere placement because the implant may limit one's ability to suture the greater tuberosity. Vertical sutures are also placed to secure the shaft to the tuberosities [57]. The humeral implant should be done with 0°–20° of retroversion and its height in relation with humeral calcar; it is the most important factor in minimizing postoperative dislocation [58] and can be extremely challenging in cases of severe shaft comminution. About this topic, we have done a contribution by publishing a modified Brems' technique [59] with BCAT (bone collar and tie) technique [60] in order to improve the bone quantity around the humeral prosthesis, especially in the case of comminuted greater tuberosity fractures, the bone healing, and the tension of teres minor with a more lateral tendon insertion. The B-CAT technique is made with a part of fractured humeral head, shaped, and placed as a collar around the prosthesis and under the great tuberosity [61] with an improved elevation and external rotation as reported in our results. A recent study of Hermann [21] demonstrated that a moment arms for humeral rotation are significantly smaller for the cranial segments of subscapularis muscle and all segments of teres minor in abduction angles of 30° and above ($p \leq 0.05$). Abduction moment arms were significantly decreased for all segments ($p \leq 0.002$). Origin to insertion distance was significantly smaller for all muscles at the 15° position ($p \leq 0.005$), apart from the cranial SSC segment. This study could confirm some aspects on the improving function in external rotation due to the improved tension of teres minor using the bone augmentation.The baseplate and glenosphere position and fixation on the native glenoid are crucial to the success and longevity of the RSA, and several studies have been done on these aspects. The "three-column concept" of scapula fixation was introduced in 2008 [16], and based on this, shoulder surgeons have placed three to four screws in the glenoid baseplate to obtain good cortical fixation. Typically, one screw is aimed at the coracoid, one toward the scapular spine, and one down the lateral pillar. Recent studies have shown that the glenoid baseplate may only need two screws for adequate fixation. Parsons et al. [62] showed that longer screw fixation is obtained by aiming the inferior screw more parallel to the baseplate as opposed to aiming anteroinferiorly down the lateral pillar. There are a variety of RSA implants available today that limit the surgeon to two or four screws. Given this recent evidence, it is advisable to fix the baseplate with at least two locking screws and to aim the screws in such a manner as to obtain the largest amount of bone purchase. Proper tensioning of the RSA should be addressed to prevent postoperative instability. Shoulder surgeons often rely on the tension of the conjoined tendon and deltoid muscle to assist in the determination of the height of the implant. The implant should be stable before fixation of the tuberosities. Recently, Walch et al. [63] proposed that lengthening the humerus with the RSA was associated with improved active anterior elevation. They determined that when the humerus was shortened, all of the patients had poorer functional results. Although the optimum lengthening of the arm was not determined in this study, they advised that the humerus should not be lengthened more than 2.5 cm compared with the opposite side.

References

1. Boyle MJ, Youn SM, Frampton CM, Ball CM. Functional outcomes of reverse shoulder arthroplasty compared with hemiarthroplasty for acute proximal humeral fractures. J Shoulder Elb Surg. 2013;22:32–7.
2. Guery J, Favard L, Sirveaux F, Oudet D, Mole D, Walch G. Reverse total shoulder arthroplasty. Survivorship analysis of eighty replacements followed for five to ten years. J Bone Joint Surg Am. 2006;88:1742–7.
3. Hattrup SJ, Sanchez-Sotelo J, Sperling JW, Cofield RH. Reverse shoulder replacement for patients with inflammatory arthritis. J Hand Surg Am. 2012;37:1888–94.
4. Wall B, Nove-Josserand L, O'Connor DP, Edwards TB, Walch G. Reverse total shoulder arthroplasty: a review of results according to etiology. J Bone Joint Surg Am. 2007;89:1476–85.
5. Bodey WN, Yeoman PM. Prosthetic arthroplasty of the shoulder. Acta Orthop Scand. 1983;54:900–3.
6. Buechel FF, Pappas MJ, DePalma AF. 'Floating-socket' total shoulder replacement: anatomical, biomechanical, and surgical rationale. J Biomed Mater Res. 1978;12:89–114.
7. Fenlin JM Jr. Total glenohumeral joint replacement. Orthop Clin North Am. 1975;6:565–83.
8. Bayley J, Kessel L. The Kessel total shoulder replacement. In: Bayley I, Kessel L, editors. Shoulder surgery. New York: Springer-Verlag; 1982. p. 160–4.
9. Nyffeler RW, Werner CML, Simmen BR, Gerber C. Analysis of a retrieved Delta III total shoulder prosthesis. J Bone Joint Surg Br. 2004;86:1187–91.
10. Grammont PM, Baulot E. Delta shoulder prosthesis for rotator cuff rupture. Orthopedics. 1993;16:65–8.
11. Gerber C, Pennington SD, Lingenfelter EJ, Sukthankar A. Reverse Delta-III total shoulder replacement combined with latissimus dorsi transfer. A preliminary report. J Bone Joint Surg Am. 2007;89:940–7.
12. Fischer L, Carret J, Gonon G, Dimnet J. Etude cinematique des mouvements de l'articulation scapulohumerale. Rev Chir Orthop Reparatrice Appar Mot. 1977;63:108–15.
13. Kontaxis A, Johnson GR. The biomechanics of reverse anatomy shoulder replacement–a modelling study. Clin Biomech (Bristol, Avon). 2009;24:254–60.
14. Boileau P, Watkinson D, Hatzidakis AM, Hovorka I. Neer Award 2005: the Grammont reverse shoulder prosthesis: results in cuff tear arthritis, fracture sequelae, and revision arthroplasty. J Shoulder Elb Surg. 2006;15:527–40.
15. Levigne C, Boileau P, Favard L, Garaud P, Mole D, Sirveaux F, et al. Scapular notching in reverse shoulder arthroplasty. J Shoulder Elb Surg. 2008;17:925–35.
16. De Wilde LF, Poncet D, Middernacht B, Ekelund A. Prosthetic overhang is the most effective way to prevent scapular conflict in a reverse total shoulder prosthesis. Acta Orthop. 2010;81:719–26.
17. Nyffeler RW, Werner CM, Gerber C. Biomechanical relevance of glenoid component positioning in the reverse Delta III total shoulder prosthesis. J Shoulder Elb Surg. 2005;14:524–8.
18. Edwards TB, Trappey GJ, Riley C, O'Connor DP, Elkousy HA, Gartsman GM. Inferior tilt of the glenoid component does not decrease scapular notching in reverse shoulder arthroplasty: results of a prospective randomized study. J Shoulder Elb Surg. 2012;21:641–6.

19. Harman M, Frankle M, Vasey M, Banks S. Initial glenoid component fixation in "reverse" total shoulder arthroplasty: a biomechanical evaluation. J Shoulder Elb Surg. 2005;14(Suppl S):162S–7S.
20. Frankle M, Siegal S, Pupello D, Saleem A, Mighell M, Vasey M. The reverse shoulder prosthesis for glenohumeral arthritis associated with severe rotator cuff deficiency. A minimum two-year follow-up study of sixty patients. J Bone Joint Surg Am. 2005;87:1697–705.
21. Herrmann S, Konig C, Heller M, Perka C, Greiner S. Reverse shoulder arthroplasty leads to significant biomechanical changes in the remaining rotator cuff. J Orthop Surg Res. 2011;6:42.
22. De Biase CF, Delcogliano M, Borroni M, Castagna A. Reverse total shoulder arthroplasty: radiological and clinical result using an eccentric glenosphere. Musculoskelet Surg. 2012;96(Suppl 1):S27–34.
23. Gutierrez S, Levy JC, Frankle MA, Cuff D, Keller TS, Pupello DR, et al. Evaluation of abduction range of motion and avoidance of inferior scapular impingement in a reverse shoulder model. J Shoulder Elb Surg. 2008;17:608–15.
24. Stephenson DR, Oh JH, McGarry MH, Rick Hatch GF 3rd, Lee TQ. Effect of humeral component version on impingement in reverse total shoulder arthroplasty. J Shoulder Elb Surg. 2011;20:652–8.
25. Erickson BJ, Frank RM, Harris JD, Mall N, Romeo AA. The influence of humeral head inclination in reverse total shoulder arthroplasty: a systematic review. J Shoulder Elb Surg. 2015;24:988–93.
26. Boileau P, Moineau G, Roussanne Y, O'Shea K. Bony increased-offset reversed shoulder arthroplasty: minimizing scapular impingement while maximizing glenoid fixation. Clin Orthop Relat Res. 2011;469:2558–67.
27. Matsen FA 3rd, Boileau P, Walch G, Gerber C, Bicknell RT. The reverse total shoulder arthroplasty. J Bone Joint Surg Am. 2007;89:660–7.
28. Favre P, Sussmann PS, Gerber C. The effect of component positioning on intrinsic stability of the reverse shoulder arthroplasty. J Shoulder Elb Surg. 2010;19:550–6.
29. Gutierrez S, Keller TS, Levy JC, Lee WE 3rd, Luo ZP. Hierarchy of stability factors in reverse shoulder arthroplasty. Clin Orthop Relat Res. 2008;466:670–6.
30. Berton A, Gulotta LV, Petrillo S, Florio P, Longo UG, Denaro V, Kontaxis A. The effect of humeral version on teres minor muscle moment arm, length, and impingement in reverse shoulder arthroplasty during activities of daily living. J Shoulder Elb Surg. 2015;24:578–86.
31. Clouthier AL, Hetzler MA, Fedorak G, Bryant JT, Deluzio KJ, Bicknell RT. Factors affecting the stability of reverse shoulder arthroplasty: a biomechanical study. J Shoulder Elb Surg. 2013;22:439–44.
32. Terrier A, Reist A, Merlini F, Farron A. Simulated joint and muscle forces in reversed and anatomic shoulder prostheses. J Bone Joint Surg Br. 2008;90:751–6.
33. Ackland DC, Roshan-Zamir S, Richardson M, Pandy MG. Moment arms of the shoulder musculature after reverse total shoulder arthroplasty. J Bone Joint Surg Am. 2010;92:1221–30.
34. Henninger HB, Barg A, Anderson AE, Bachus KN, Tashjian RZ, Burks RT. Effect of deltoid tension and humeral version in reverse total shoulder arthroplasty: a biomechanical study. J Shoulder Elb Surg. 2012;21:483–90.
35. Ackland DC, Roshan-Zamir S, Richardson M, Pandy MG. Muscle and joint-contact loading at the glenohumeral joint after reverse total shoulder arthroplasty. J Orthop Res. 2011;29:1850–8.
36. Werner CM, Steinmann PA, Gilbart M, Gerber C. Treatment of painful pseudoparesis due to irreparable rotator cuff dysfunction with the Delta III reverse-ball-and-socket total shoulder prosthesis. J Bone Joint Surg Am. 2005;87:1476–86.
37. Sirveaux F, Favard L, Oudet D, Huquet D, Walch G, Mole D. Grammont inverted total shoulder arthroplasty in the treatment of glenohumeral osteoarthritis with massive rupture of the cuff. Results of a multicentre study of 80 shoulders. J Bone Joint Surg Br. 2004;86:388–95.
38. Favre P, Loeb MD, Helmy N, Gerber C. Latissimus dorsi transfer to restore external rotation with reverse shoulder arthroplasty: a biomechanical study. J Shoulder Elb Surg. 2008;17:650–8.
39. Chou J, Malak SF, Anderson IA, Astley T, Poon PC. Biomechanical evaluation of different designs of glenospheres in the SMR reverse total shoulder prosthesis: range of motion and risk of scapular notching. J Shoulder Elb Surg. 2009;18:354–9.
40. Berhouet J, Garaud P, Favard L. Evaluation of the role of glenosphere design and humeral component retroversion in avoiding scapular notching during reverse shoulder arthroplasty. J Shoulder Elb Surg. 2014;23:151–8.
41. Gulotta LV, Choi D, Marinello P, Knutson Z, Lipman J, Wright T, et al. Humeral component retroversion in reverse total shoulder arthroplasty: a biomechanical study. J Shoulder Elb Surg. 2012;21(9):1121–7.
42. Boyle S, Watts A, Trail I. Periprosthetic fractures around the shoulder. Shoulder Elbow. 2012;4(1):1–10.
43. Levy O, Narvani A, Hous N, Abraham R, Relwani J, Pradhan R, Bruguera J, Sforza G, Atoun E. Reverse shoulder arthroplasty with a cementless short metaphyseal humeral implant without a stem: clinical and radiologic outcomes in prospective 2- to 7-year follow-up study. J Shoulder Elb Surg. 2016;25(8):1362–70.
44. Hopkins AR, Hansen UN, Bull AM, Emery R, Amis AA. Fixation of the reversed shoulder prosthesis. J Shoulder Elb Surg. 2008;17:974–80.
45. Humphrey CS, Kelly JD 2nd, Norris TR. Optimizing glenosphere position and fixation in reverse shoulder arthroplasty, part two: the three-column concept. J Shoulder Elb Surg. 2008;17:595–601.
46. Chebli C, Huber P, Watling J, Bertelsen A, Bicknell RT, Matsen F 3rd. Factors affecting fixation of the glenoid component of a reverse total shoulder prothesis. J Shoulder Elb Surg. 2008;17:323–7.
47. Codsi MJ, Bennetts C, Powell K, Iannotti JP. Locations for screw fixation beyond the glenoid vault for fixation

of glenoid implants into the scapula: an anatomic study. J Shoulder Elb Surg. 2007;16:S84–9.
48. Hart ND, Clark JC, Wade Krause FR, Kissenberth MJ, Bragg WE, Hawkins RJ. Glenoid screw position in the encore reverse shoulder prosthesis: an anatomic dissection study of screw relationship to surrounding structures. J Shoulder Elb Surg. 2013;22:814–20.
49. Denard PJ, Walch G. Current concepts in the surgical management of primary glenohumeral arthritis with a biconcave glenoid. J Shoulder Elb Surg. 2013;22:1589–98.
50. Neyton L, Boileau P, Nové-Josserand L, Edwards TB, Walch G. Glenoid bone grafting with a reverse design prosthesis. J Shoulder Elb Surg. 2007;16(3 Suppl):S71–8.
51. Walch G, Badet R, Boulahia A, Khoury A. Morphologic study of the glenoid in primary glenohumeral osteoarthritis. J Arthroplast. 1999;14:756–60.
52. Jones RB, Wright TW, Zuckerman JD. Reverse total shoulder arthroplasty with structural bone grafting of large glenoid defects. J Shoulder Elb Surg. 2016;25:1425–32.
53. Boileau P, Morin-Salvo N, Gauci MO, Seeto BL, Chalmers PN, Holzer N, Walch G. Angled BIO-RSA (bony-increased offset–reverse shoulder arthroplasty): a solution for the management glenoid bone loss and erosion. J Shoulder Elbow Surg. 2017;26(12):2133–42.
54. Klein M, Juschka M, Hinkenjann B, Scherger B, Ostermann PA. Treatment of comminuted fractures of the proximal humerus in elderly patients with the Delta III reverse shoulder prosthesis. J Orthop Trauma. 2008;22:698–704.
55. Tischer T, Rose T, Imhoff AB. The reverse shoulder prosthesis for primary and secondary treatment of proximal humeral fractures: a case report. Arch Orthop Trauma Surg. 2008;128(9):973–8.
56. Gallinet D, Adam A, Gasse N, Rochet S, Obert L. Improvement in shoulder rotation in complex shoulder fractures treated by reverse shoulder arthroplasty. J Shoulder Elb Surg. 2012;22:38–44.
57. Boileau P, Walch G, Krishnan S. Tuberosity osteosynthesis and hemiarthroplasty for four-part fractures of the proximal humerus. Tech Shoulder Elbow Surg. 2000;1:96–109.
58. Ladermann A, Walch G, Lubbeke A, Drake GN, Melis B, Bacle G, et al. Influence of arm lengthening in reverse shoulder arthroplasty. J Shoulder Elb Surg. 2012;21:336–41.
59. Brems JJ. Shoulder arthroplasty in the face of acute fracture: puzzle pieces. J Arthroplast. 2002;17:32–5.
60. Russo R, Cautiero F, Fontanarosa A, Della Rotonda G, Valerio G. Reconstruction techniques in comparison for reverse shoulder trauma prosthesis in the elderly: a follow-up between 2 and 4 years. Arch Orthop Trauma Surg. 2015;135(7):905–12.
61. Bufquin T, Hersan A, Hubert L, Massin P. Reverse shoulder arthroplasty for the treatment of three- and four-part fractures of the proximal humerus in the elderly: a prospective review of 43 cases with a short-term follow-up. J Bone Joint Surg Br. 2007;89:516–20.
62. Parsons BO, Gruson KI, Accousti KJ, Klug RA, Flatow EL. Optimal rotation and screw positioning for initial glenosphere baseplate fixation in reverse shoulder arthroplasty. J Shoulder Elb Surg. 2009;18:886–91.
63. Werner BS, Ascione F, Bugelli G, Walch G. Does arm lengthening affect the functional outcome in onlay reverse shoulder arthroplasty? J Shoulder Elb Surg. 2017;26(12):2152–7. pii: S1058-2746(17)30307-5

4 Epidemiology and Demographics of Reverse Shoulder Arthroplasty

Luigi Murena, Bramir Hoxhaj, Roberto Fattori, and Gianluca Canton

4.1 Introduction

Since the first documented shoulder arthroplasty in 1893 [1], there have been many advances in shoulder implants, particularly within the last two decades. Shoulder arthroplasty has become the established treatment for severe glenohumeral disease from rheumatoid arthritis (RA) to osteoarthritis (OA), severe fracture, avascular necrosis (AVN), and cuff tear arthropathy. Various implant designs have been developed over the past 20 years resulting in a large number of available implants. Due to increased life expectancy and greater demand from the aging society for optimal quality of life into advanced old age, shoulder arthroplasty has become more popular worldwide [2, 3]. The widespread of shoulder arthroplasty is more recent than that of hip and knee arthroplasty, the incidence is 7.5-fold lower, and the range of disease indication is wider [4]. Hip and knee arthroplasty is more common (40% of patients) in non-elderly adult patients compared to shoulder arthroplasty, in which 30% of patients are non-elderly [5]. The occurrences of hip and knee arthroplasty are increasing faster among the middle-aged population (45–64 years) than in the elderly population, while shoulder arthroplasty is a phenomenon that primarily affects the elderly [2]. The introduction of reverse total shoulder arthroplasty (rTSA) is one of the factors responsible for the predominance of elderly patients among those who are managed with TSA. Currently, rTSA is recommended predominantly for patients over 70 years old with disabling rotator cuff arthropathy [6]. However, a wider range of pathologies and complications, such as revision of failed anatomic total shoulder arthroplasty (aTSA) or hemiarthroplasty (HA), are nowadays managed with rTSA. Therefore, the increase in rTSA cases may be due in part to broader emerging indications [2]. Identifying actual epidemiology and demographics of rTSA may be difficult because of the poor data available in literature studies. In fact, while hundreds of thousands of shoulder arthroplasties are performed each year around the world, data are available on very few of them. Most of the publications on shoulder arthroplasty procedure and outcomes are published by a relatively small number of medical centers, which may not be representative of the situation on national or global scale [7].

Registries may thus provide the most reliable evidence on rTSA epidemiology and demographics [7].

L. Murena · B. Hoxhaj · R. Fattori · G. Canton (✉)
Orthopaedics and Trumatology unit,
Cattinara Hospital-ASUITS, Trieste, Italy

S. Gumina et al. (eds.), *Reverse Shoulder Arthroplasty*,
https://doi.org/10.1007/978-3-319-97743-0_4

4.2 Shoulder Arthroplasty Epidemiology Before rTSA Separate Coding in National Shoulder Arthroplasty Registers

Until recently, rTSA was coded as aTSA in different national registers. In the USA, the option for separate coding of rTSA and aTSA was implemented only in 2011 despite rTSA approval by the Food and Drug Administration (FDA) in 2003. According to US data reported by Kim et al. [2], in 1993 the total number of shoulder arthroplasties was 13,873, of which 7,545 (54.4%) HA and 6292 (45.6%) TSA (rTSA + aTSA) [2]. In 2003 the total number of shoulder arthroplasties doubled to 25,948 cases, of which 15,290 (58.9%) HA and 10,658 (41.1%) TSA (rTSA and aTSA) [2]. In 2006, short after the approval of rTSA by the FDA (2003), the number of TSA cases in the USA (20,086) became higher than the HA cases (18,052) for the first time. In 2008, of 46,951 shoulder arthroplasties implanted in the USA, 57% were TSA (26,773 cases) and 43% were HA (20,178 cases).

The number of shoulder arthroplasties performed in the USA indicated a 2.5-fold increase over the decade between years 1998 (19,000 cases) and 2008 (nearly 47,000) [8]. During this time, the elderly population increased approximately by 11%, and the number of surgeons implanting shoulder arthroplasties increased by 24% [2]. However, the augmented number in shoulder arthroplasty cases was much steeper than the growth of the elderly population or the density of orthopedic surgeons in the USA, suggesting that multiple other factors were responsible for this result. Kim et al. [2] suggested that the abrupt increase in TSA but a steadily growing HA since 2003 was due to the FDA approval of rTSA in 2003 [2] (Fig. 4.1). The same trend can be noticed in the German experience [9]. In Germany, the option to code rTSA was introduced in 2008. In 2005 the number of shoulder arthroplasties implanted was 7781, of which 5460 (70.2%) were HA and 2321 (29.8%) were TSA (rTSA + aTSA). In 2007, of 10,268 shoulder arthroplasties, 6640 (64.7%) were HA, and 628 (35.3%) were TSA (rTSA and aTSA). Since 2008 the number of TSA cases exceeded that of the HA cases, reaching in 2012 a total number of HA of 5975 and TSA 21340. Moreover, in the period 2005–2012, HA number showed an increase until 2008 followed by a continuous decrease, while TSA number increased over the years [9].

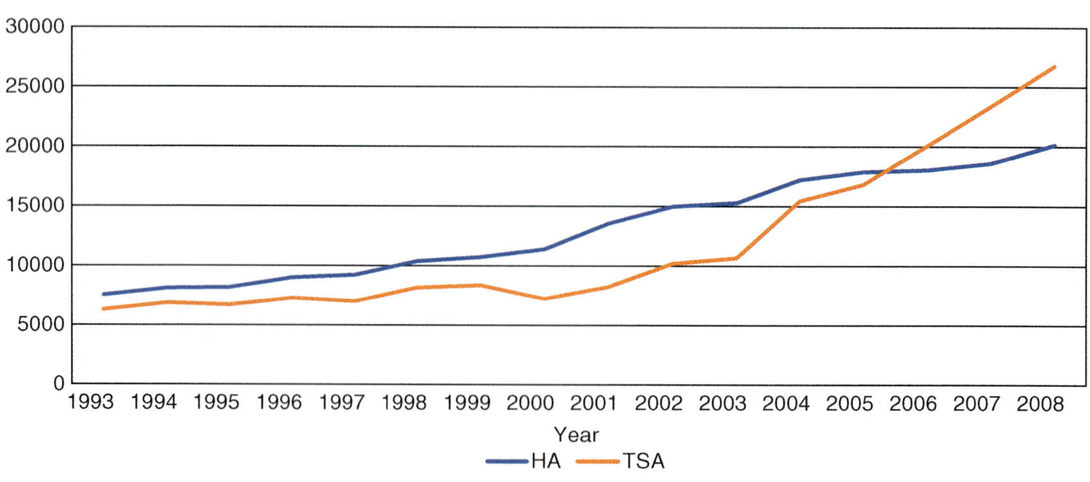

Fig. 4.1 Graphic illustrating annual implant rate for HA (hemiarthroplasty) and TSA (total shoulder arthroplasty) between 1993 and 2008 in the USA. Data from Kim et al. [2]

4.3 Epidemiology and Demographics of rTSA in National Shoulder Arthroplasty Registers

In the USA, the option to code rTSA was introduced in 2011 for the first time. Based on the Nationwide Inpatient Sample (NIS), 66,485 patients underwent shoulder arthroplasty in the USA in 2011, respectively, 21,692 (32.6%) rTSA, 29,359 (44%) aTSA, and 15,434 (23%) HA [10]. The incidence of shoulder arthroplasty nearly doubled in year 2011 ($54.4/10^5$ per year) compared to year 2002 ($24.5/10^5$ per year) [10]. The number of HA decreased from $14.5/10^5$ per year in 2002 to $12.6/10^5$ per year in 2011. The number of aTSA increased from $14.5/10^5$ per year in 2002 to $24/10^5$ per year in 2011 [10]. In 2011, the incidence of rTSA was $17.8/10^5$ per year [10].

The mean age of patients undergoing rTSA was 71 years, and females represented 63.68% of the patients [11]. The main pathologies leading to rTSA were osteoarthritis (43.67%), disorders of the bursae and tendons (14.03%), cuff tear arthropathy (11.83%), and fractures of the proximal humerus (9.36%).

The Australian national shoulder register started in 2004 but only in 2008 was widespread among all territories in Australia [12]. From 2008 to 2015, the total number of rTSA implanted was 12,362, with an increase of 2680 procedures in 2015 compared to 2014. Primary rTSA increased from 43.3% of all shoulder arthroplasties in 2008 to 64.1% in 2015. In 2012 there were more rTSA implanted than aTSA for the first time. Since 2008 gender distribution had a minor change, with 65.9% of cases in females and 34.1% in males. The mean age was 75.8 years for females and 73.4 years for males. The percentage of patients over 75 years old declined from 61.4% in 2010 to 51.9% in 2015. The main pathologies leading to rTSA were osteoarthritis (43.8%), rotator cuff arthropathy (34.1%), and fracture (14.6%). The diagnosis of osteoarthritis in rTSA declined from 57.8% in 2008 to 43.8% in 2015, while the diagnosis of rotator cuff arthropathy increased from 21% in 2008 to 34.1% in 2015. Regarding HA, the procedure had a drop from 30% to 10% between 2008 and 2014.

Norway is the first country in which the shoulder arthroplasty register was introduced in 1994 [11]. From 1994 to 2006, the total number of shoulder arthroplasties implanted was 2308, of which 301 (13%) were rTSA. In 2010, the percentage of rTSA (140/490; 28.57%) doubled with respect to the period between 1994 and 2001. Likely, in 2015 the percentage of rTSA reached 53.9% (377/700), reporting an increase in popularity of rTSA over the last 15 years. Conversely, HA number showed a significant decrease passing from 220 cases/year in 2006–2012 to 150 cases/year in 2013–2014 [11] (Fig. 4.2). Reverse TSA was implanted as a primary procedure in the majority of cases throughout the whole period considered. As far as surgical indication is concerned, from 1994 to 2015, the main pathologies leading to rTSA implantation were (1) proximal humerus fracture in 696 (33.6%) patients, (2) idiopathic osteoarthritis in 607 (29.3%) patients, (3) rheumatoid arthritis in 330 (15.9%) patients, and (4) rotator cuff arthropathy in 258 (12.4%) patients. There is no available data reported on the mean age and gender for rTSA on this registry (Fig. 4.3).

In the UK, data collection for the national shoulder arthroplasty registry began in 1 April 2012 [13]. Since then 9968 (42.2%) rTSA have been implanted. The mean age of patients who received rTSA was 76 years. The vast majority of patients were females. The number of rTSA implants has increased from 806 (31.7%) reported in 2012 to 3015 (50.7%) in 2016 [13]. The main pathologies leading to rTSA were (1) rotator cuff arthropathy (50.5%), (2) osteoarthritis (24.8%), (3) acute fractures of the proximal humerus (9.7%), (4) trauma sequelae (8%), and (5) inflammatory arthritis (3.4%) [13].

According to the New Zealand national shoulder arthroplasty registry, from January 2000 to December 2013 there were 5528 primary shoulder arthroplasties implanted, of which 1553 (28%)

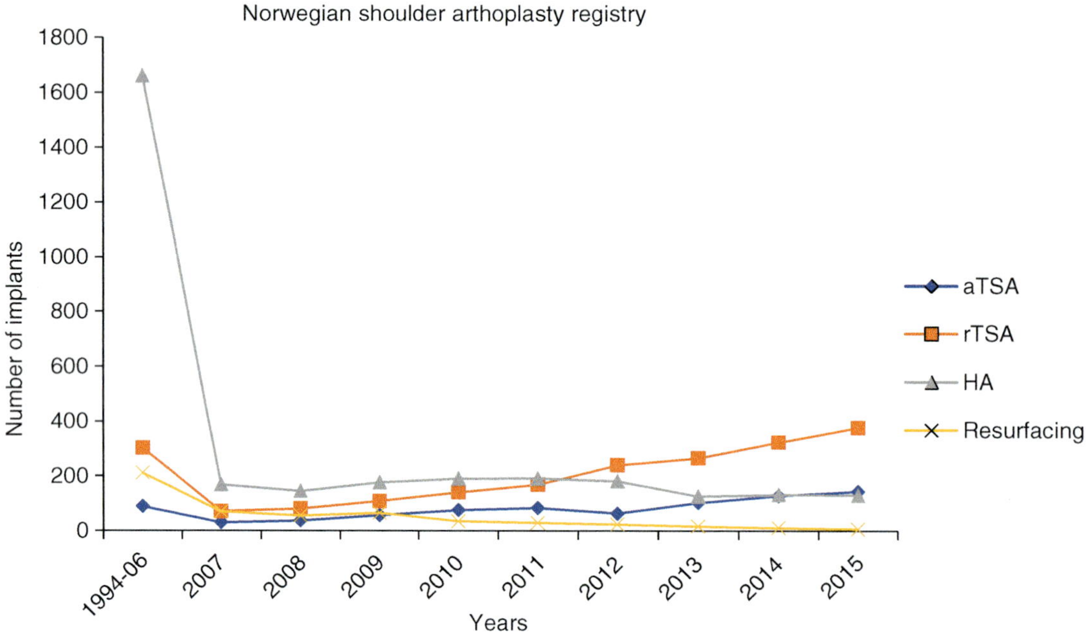

Fig 4.2 Graphic illustrating annual variation in shoulder arthroplasty implant between 1994 and 2015. Data from Norway national shoulder arthroplasty registry

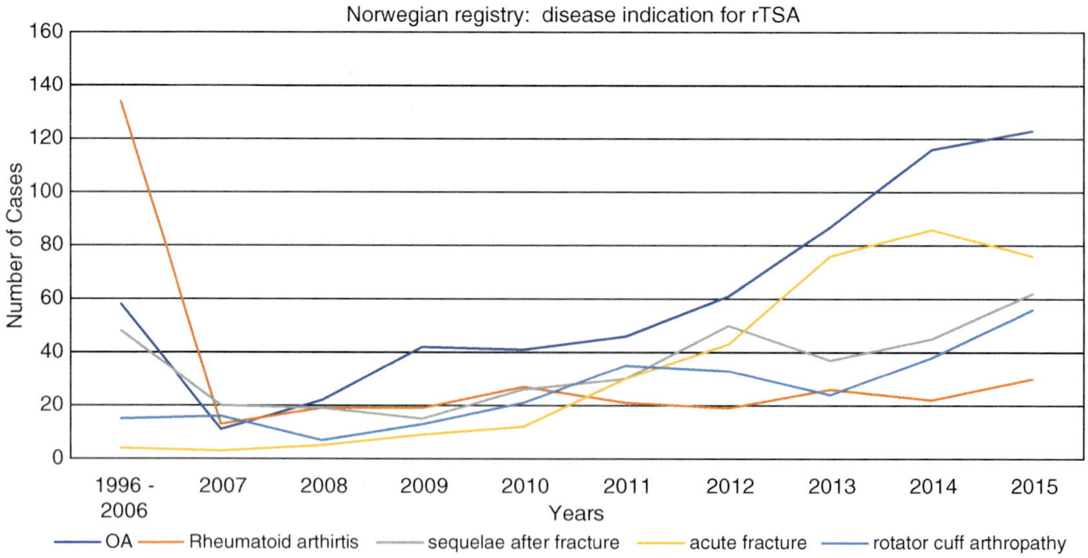

Fig 4.3 Graphic illustrating annual variation of disease indication for rTSA in Norway between 1996 and 2015. Data from Norway national shoulder arthroplasty registry

were rTSA (63.75% females and 36.25% males) [14]. Lübbeke et al. [15] recently reported in New Zealand an increase of rTSA from 2% in 2002 to 56% in 2012, although indications for surgery were not reported [15].

Germany has the highest incidence rate ($34/10^5$ per year) of shoulder arthroplasty among countries with available national data (mean incidence $13.3/10^5$ per year) [15]. The option to code rTSA was introduced in 2008. Between January 2008 and December 2012, the number of rTSA implanted was 27,011, with a tremendous increase in the number of cases over the years from 2008 to 2012. For example, in 2008 the number of rTSA implanted was 2935 while in 2012 was 8011, nearly a 273% increase. Women represented the vast majority of patients who underwent rTSA (75.5%). The main pathologies leading to rTSA were osteoarthritis (male 70.7%; female 58.97%), fracture of proximal humerus (male 18.5%; female 33.93%), and cuff tear arthropathy (male 9.21%; female 5.22%). Due to inconclusive information regarding causative pathology, 20% of the patients were not assigned to an indication group. Differently from previously considered registries, the ratio of aTSA/rTSA is in favor of anatomic implants (65/35). Anyway, since 2008 this ratio has become less divergent because of a relative increase of rTSA [16].

The study conducted by Bayona et al. [7] on national shoulder arthroplasty registers available concluded that shoulder arthroplasty indications have an important geographical variation that should be considered when comparing outcomes from different locations. Moreover, heterogeneity of information regarding diagnosis, age, gender, and procedure type in different registries, together with variable length of data collection, might lead to unease registries comparison [8].

Lübbeke et al. compared data within registries and from different registries regarding aTSA and rTSA as well as HA at different points in time. Considering all the national and regional registers available, rTSA was most commonly used in Norway, Australia, and the UK, HA in Scandinavia, and aTSA in New Zealand, California, and Germany [10–15]. The use of rTSA over the last 15 years in Norway and New Zealand increased from 12% to 52% and from 2% to 56%, respectively, whereas in Sweden its use remained stable (6–10%) over the examined period [11, 14, 15].

The distinction of different disease indications for each implant in national registers begun in recent years (from 2008 on, with the exception of California and Denmark). To quantify how much the different procedures varied across registries, Lübbeke et al. used meta-analysis techniques and evaluated the three most common disease-implant combinations, which were OA-aTSA, cuff tear arthropathy-rTSA, and fracture-HA. [15]. In the study conducted by Lübbeke et al. [15] for rTSA in patients with cuff tear arthropathy, the combined proportion was 77% (confidence interval 60–91). The variability between registers was relevant, and the prediction interval was from 13 to 100% [15]. A similar wide variability in indications was noted also for the other disease-implant combinations [15]. This large variation for different procedures could be related to the lack of long-term data and international guidelines.

4.4 Epidemiology and Demographics of TSA and rTSA in Italy

The national shoulder registry in Italy was introduced in 2001, with aTSA and rTSA codified as the same procedure since then. Since 2001 the total number of shoulder arthroplasties has increased, from 1539 in 2001 to 6588 in 2015 [17] (Fig. 4.4) (Table 4.1). During the last 15 years, the number of HA has increased until 2010 and has stabilized since then. The proportion of HA has rapidly decreased from 54.84% in 2001 to 19.44% in 2014, while the total number of shoulder arthroplasty and the number of TSA has proportionally increased (Table 4.1).

In the Italian scenario, a regional shoulder arthroplasty register with a different coding for aTSA and rTSA can be found. In fact, in Emilia-Romagna (a region of 4.5 million inhabitants in northeast Italy), separate coding was introduced in 2008 [17, 18] (Fig. 4.5). Between 2008 and 2015, 2855 shoulder arthroplasties out of 4653 (61.4%) were rTSA. Since 2008 the number of rTSA implanted has encountered a continuous increase, while HA is decreasing since 2011 (Table 4.1). For rTSA, female gender prevails with 2208 implants (77.3%) versus 647 (22.7%). The mean age of patients at surgery was 71.8 years for males and 74.1 for females.

The main disease indication for rTSA is eccentric osteoarthritis in 1495 cases (52.4%), proximal fracture management in 544 cases (19.1%), concentric osteoarthritis in 417 cases

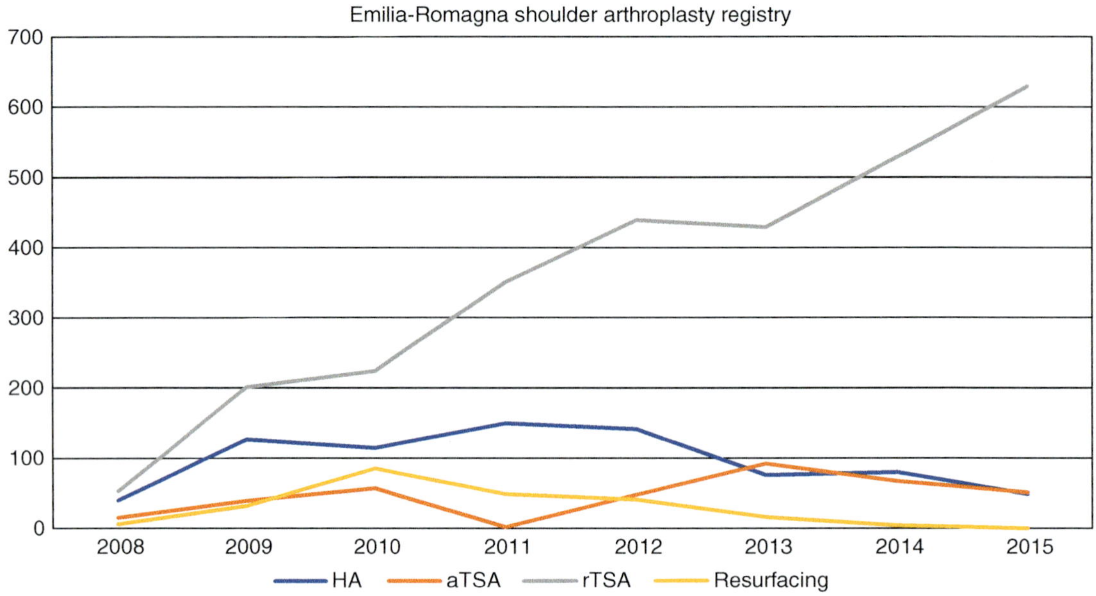

Fig 4.4 Graphic illustrating annual variation in shoulder arthroplasty implant between 2007 and 2014 in Italy. Data from Italian arthroplasty registry (RIAP)

(14.6%), cuff tear arthropathy in 82 cases (2.9%), sequelae of fractures in 78 cases (2.7%), and avascular necrosis of the humeral head in 67 cases (2.3%). The main indication for aTSA is concentric osteoarthritis, accounting for 80.9% of cases in the aTSA group. Conversely, the main indication for HA is fracture, accounting for 63.4% of cases in the HA group [15, 18].

4.5 Conclusions

Shoulder arthroplasty has seen a rapid acceleration in clinical application in the past two decades in the developed countries [2, 7, 15], although its incidence remains lower compared to hip and knee arthroplasty. The increase of rTSA implants seems to be at least partially responsible for this phenomenon [2, 7, 15]. Although reverse TSA has been primarily indicated in patients with rotator cuff arthropathy, a recent broadening of clinical indications has been documented. These factors coupled with the progressive aging of the population could be an acceptable explanation for the increase of rTSA implantation [2]. Several differences in indications for rTSA and relative use of rTSA compared to other implants emerge from different shoulder arthroplasty registers examinations. The steep increase in shoulder arthroplasty worldwide is not accompanied by a paired availability of published data. Outcomes published in the literature on shoulder arthroplasty are based on small series from a limited number of centers, nonreflecting the international practice. National shoulder registries can conversely provide important information on shoulder arthroplasty use in different countries, although they present some limitations especially regarding clinical indication for rTSA together with clinical and radiographic outcomes. Broadening of standardized and nationally founded shoulder arthroplasty registers could provide a better overview on today's practice and standardize shoulder arthroplasty indications in the future.

Table 4.1 Summary of data reported in the national shoulder arthroplasty registers of Italy, the UK, the USA, Germany, Australia, Norway, and Emilia-Romagna

		1993–2001	2002	2003	2004	2005	2006	2007	2008	2009	2010	2011	2012	2013	2014	2015	2016
Norway	HA	1660						168	145	176	190	191	181	126	132	130	
	aTSA	89						31	38	57	76	84	64	103	128	144	
	rTSA	301						71	81	108	140	168	239	265	323	377	
	Resurfacing	210						70	55	65	35	29	24	7	11	7	
USA	HA	77,443	14,988	15,298	17,231	17,883	18,052	18,601	20,178	/	/	15,434	/	/	/	/	
	aTSA	66,086	10,192	10,658	15,432	16,811	20,086	23,358	26,773	/	/	29,359	/	/	/	/	
	rTSA									/	/	21,692	/	/	/	/	
Germany	HA					5460	6130	6640	7512	7243	7055	6726	5975				
	aTSA					2321	2911	3628	6788	8426	10,190	11,928	13,329				
	rTSA								2935	3936	5326	6804	8011				
UK	HA												855	1261	1244	1204	927
	aTSA												827	1459	1786	1927	1939
	rTSA												806	1531	2100	2516	3015
Italy	HA	844	/	917	/	1051	/	1203	1234	1242	1333	1211	1352	1432	1281		
	aTSA + rTSA	695	/	934	/	1455	/	2036	2175	2515	2965	3444	3793	4421	5307		
	Total	1539	/	1851	/	2506	/	3239	3409	3757	4298	4655	5145	5853	6588		
Australia	HA												3627	4335	4956	5415	5810
	aTSA												5055	6347	7560	8906	10,230
	rTSA												4010	5530	7416	9682	12,362
	Resurfacing												85	120	157	181	198
Emilia-Romagna	HA								40	127	115	150	142	76	80	49	
	aTSA								15	39	57	2	48	92	67	51	
	rTSA								53	201	224	351	439	429	529	629	
	Resurfacing								6	32	85	49	41	16	4	/	

The number of different shoulder arthroplasty implants is reported for each disposable time interval

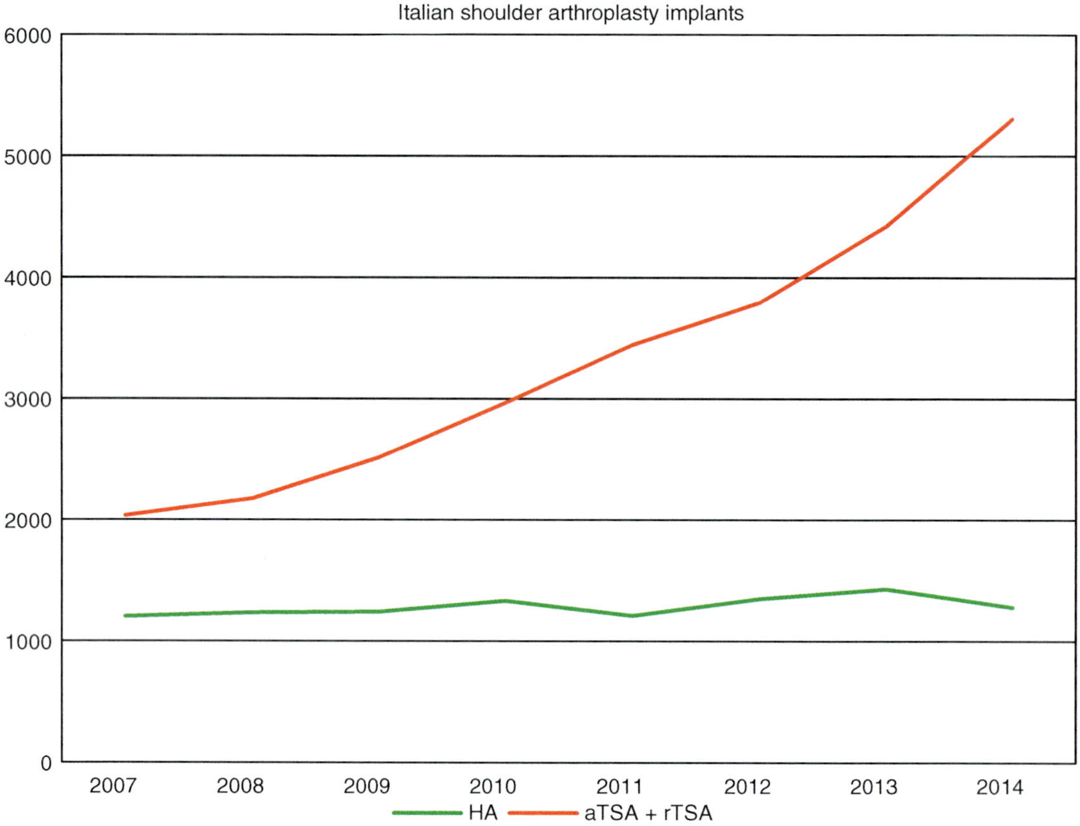

Fig 4.5 Graphic illustrating annual variation in shoulder arthroplasty implant between 2008 and 2015 in Emilia-Romagna (Italy). Data from Emilia-Romagna Register of the Orthopaedic Prosthetic Implants (RIPO)

References

1. Bankes MJ, Emery RJ. Pioneers of shoulder replacement: Themistocles Gluck and Jules Emile P'ean. J Shoulder Elbow Surg. 1995;4:259–62.
2. Kim SH, Wise BL, Zhang Y, Szabo RM. Increasing incidence of shoulder arthroplasty in the United States. J Bone Joint Surg Am. 2011;93:2249–54.
3. Glicklich R, Dreyer NA. Registries for evaluating patient outcomes: a user's guide. Rockville, MD: AHRQ; 2014.
4. Pabinger C, Geissler A. Utilization rates of hip arthroplasty in OECD countries. Osteoarthr Cartil. 2014;22(6):734–41.
5. Kim S. Changes in surgical loads and economic burden of hip and knee replacements in the US: 1997–2004. Arthritis Rheum. 2008;59:481–8.
6. Guery J, Favard L, Sirveaux F, Oudet D, Mole D, Walch G. Reverse total shoulder arthroplasty. Survivorship analysis of eighty replacements followed for five to ten years. J Bone Joint Surg Am. 2006;88:1742–7.
7. Bayona CEA, Somerson JS, Matsen FA. The utility of international shoulder joint replacement registries and databases: a comparative analytic review of two hundred and sixty one thousand, four hundred and eighty four cases. Int Orthop. 2017;42:351. https://doi.org/10.1007/s00264-017-3649-1.
8. Sharma S, Dreghorn CR. Registry of shoulder arthroplasty—the Scottish experience. Ann R Coll Surg Engl. 2006;88(2):122–6.
9. Oppermann J, Celik E, Bredow J, Beyer F, Hackl M, Spies CK, Muller LP, Burkhart KJ. Shoulder arthroplasty in Germany: 2005–2012. Arch Orthop Trauma Surg. 2016;136(5):723–9.
10. Westermann RW, Pugely AJ, Martin CT, Gao Y, Wolf BR, Hettrich CM. Reverse shoulder arthroplasty in the United States: a comparison of national volume, patient demographics, complications and surgical indications. Iowa Orthop. 2015;J35:1–7.

11. Norwegian National Advisory Unit on arthroplasty and hip fractures. http://nrlweb.ihelse.net/eng/. Accessed 20 Oct 2017.
12. Australian Orthopaedic Association. National Joint Replacement Registry. https://aoanjrr.sahmri.com/. Accessed 20 Oct 2017.
13. National Joint Registry for England, Wales Northern Ireland and the Isle of Man. http://www.njrcentre.org.uk/njrcentre/default.aspx. Accessed 20 Oct 2017.
14. New Zealand Orthopaedic Organisation. New Zealand Joint Registry. https://nzoa.org.nz/nz-joint-registry. Accessed 20 Oct 2017.
15. Lübbeke A, Rees JL, Barea C, Combescure C, Carr AJ, Silman AJ. International variation in shoulder arthroplasty. Acta Orthop. 2017;88:592. https://doi.org/10.1080/17453674.2017.1368884.
16. Hyun YS, Huri G, Garbis NG, McFarland EG. Uncommon indications for reverse total shoulder arthroplasty. Clin Orthop Surg. 2013;5:243–55.
17. Registro Italiano ArtroProtesi (RIAP). http://www.iss.it/riap/. Accessed 20 Oct 2017.
18. Registro dell'implantologia Protesica Ortopedica (Register of the Orthopaedic Prosthetic Implants). R.I.P.O. https://ripo.cineca.it/. Accessed 20 Oct 2017.

Part II

Cuff Tear Arthropathy

Etiopathogenesis of Rotator Cuff Arthropathy

5

Vittorio Candela, Daniele Passaretti, and Stefano Gumina

5.1 Definition and Historical Review

In the early 1980s, Neer et al. [1, 2] have coined the term "rotator cuff arthropathy" to indicate a nosological condition characterized by arthritic degeneration of the glenohumeral joint consequent to the massive posterosuperior rotator cuff tear. However, more than a century earlier, Adams [3], in his book on rheumatic gout, and Smith [4, 5] had described cases of shoulder arthropathy characterized by erosion of the upper portion of the humeral head, of the acromion, of the distal third of the clavicle, and of the rotator cuff tear. Codman [6], in his monograph published in 1934, had described the case of a woman, 51 years old, whose shoulder underwent rotator cuff tear, glenohumeral arthropathy, loose bodies, and swelling for the abundant articular synovial fluid.

Further papers have not been published until the end of the 1950s when Galmiche and Deshayes [7], Burman et al. [8], Banna and Hume [9], Shepard [10], and Snook [11] reported a total of 30 cases of shoulder arthropathies, some of them with the characteristics of cuff tear arthropathy.

In 1968, De Seze [12] described the hemorrhagic shoulder of three elderly women whose clinical (blood streaked recurrent effusion; rotator cuff tear) and radiographical (severe degenerative glenohumeral humeral arthritis) characteristics suggested a rotator cuff arthropathy. One year later, Bauduin and Famaey [13] described an analogous case.

Jensen et al. [14], in a prestigious publication of 1999, described the three main clinical and radiographical characteristics of the cuff arthropathy: (a) massive tear of the rotator cuff, associated with shoulder pain, supra and infraspinatus atrophy, and loss of motion (Fig. 5.1a–c); (b) degenerative changes of the glenohumeral joint (Fig. 5.2a, b); (c) upward migration of the humeral head observable on AP view (Fig. 5.3a). Humeral head collapse (Fig. 5.3b), erosive changes of superior glenoid or acromion, periarticular soft tissue calcifications, and subdeltoid effusion are other possible features that may be present [15].

5.2 Etiopathogenesis

Mechanical theory. Neer et al. [2] hypothesized that mechanical factors were at the origin of cuff arthropathy. According to this theory, loss of downward force performed by a healthy rotator

V. Candela (✉) · D. Passaretti (✉)
Department of Anatomy, Histology, Legal Medicine and Orthopedics, Sapienza, University of Rome, Rome, Italy

Istituto Chirurgico Ortopedico Traumatologico (ICOT), Latina, Italy

S. Gumina
Department of Orthopaedics and Traumatology, Sapienza University of Rome, Rome, Italy

S. Gumina et al. (eds.), *Reverse Shoulder Arthroplasty*, https://doi.org/10.1007/978-3-319-97743-0_5

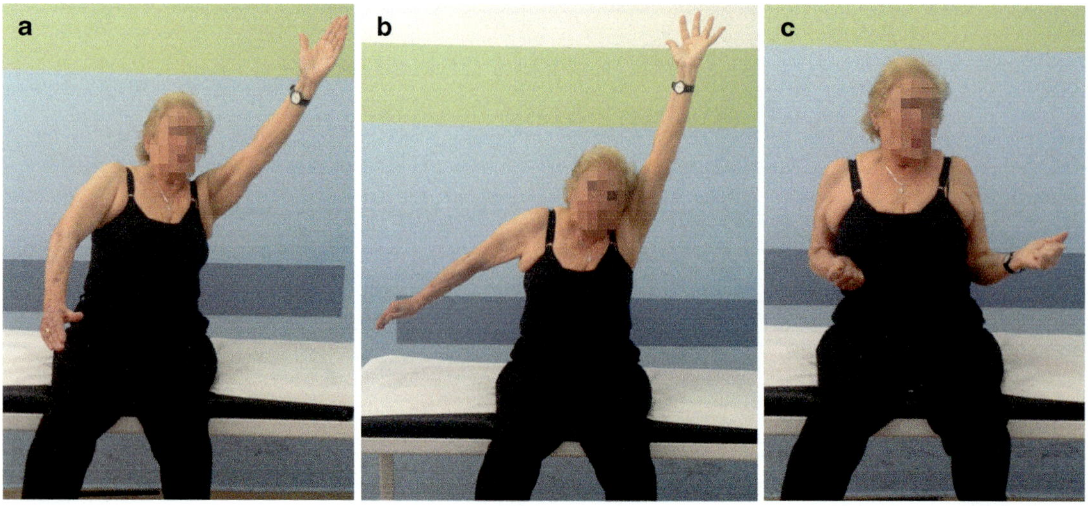

Fig. 5.1 (**a**–**c**) Decrease in range of motion in a 75-year-old female patient with cuff tear arthropathy

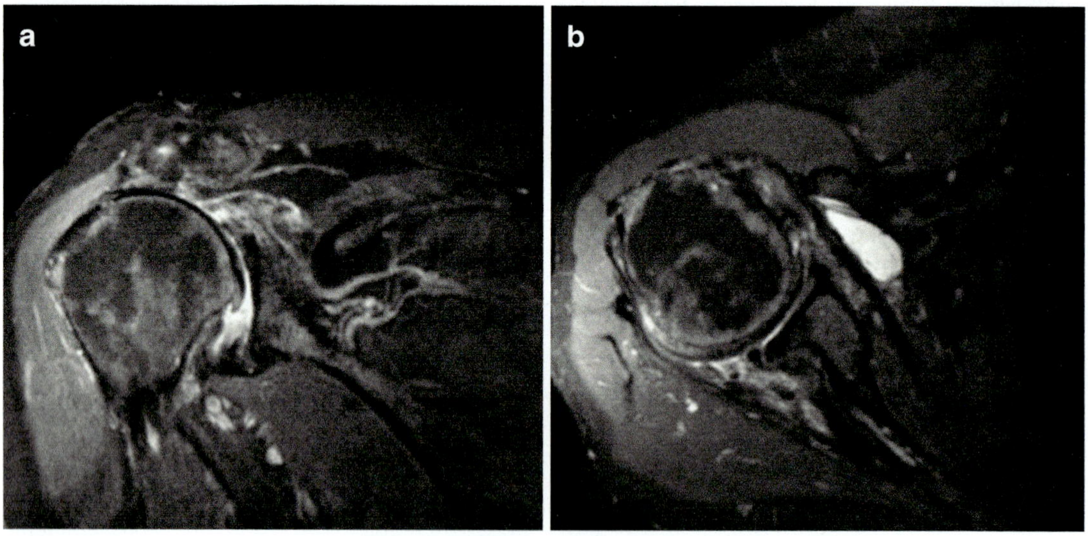

Fig. 5.2 MRI of a right shoulder of a 77-year-old male patient with Hamada 3 cuff tear arthropathy. (**a**) Coronal T2 fat suppressed FSE. Acromiohumeral distance <5 mm with acetabularization of acromion. (**b**) Axial PD fat suppressed FSE: Walch A1 glenoid morphology (humeral head centered with minimal erosion)

cuff on the humeral head would result in a superior migration of the humerus. This might facilitate an erosion of the superior surface of the glenoid and of the anteroinferior aspect of the acromion. In addition, the upward migration of the humeral head could cause a joint instability, an eccentric work of the humeral head, and, consequently, a premature wear of the articular cartilage in the areas of higher glenohumeral compression. Since 21 of the 26 patients cited in the paper had the rupture of the long head of the biceps tendon, Neer thought that this injury would help the upward migration of the humeral head.

Burkhart's hypothesis [16] seems to support the mechanical theory. The author believes that the healthy inferior portion of the rotator cuff (below the center of rotation) creates a moment that must balance the deltoid moment (force coupling). Furthermore, the subscapularis is anteriorly balanced against the infraspinatus and teres minor posteriorly. Uncoupling of the essential force couples results in anterior superior

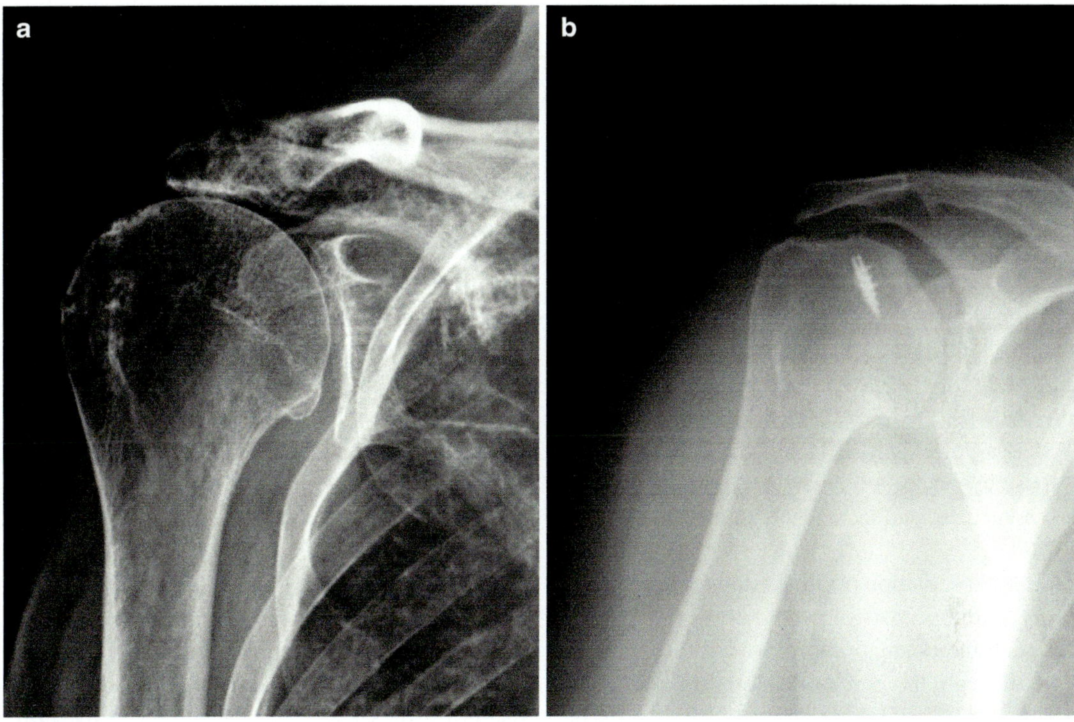

Fig. 5.3 (**a**) True AP X-ray view of a right shoulder: Hamada 3 cuff tear arthropathy. (**b**) AP X-ray view of a right shoulder: Hamada 5 cuff tear arthropathy bony destruction-humeral head collapse after a cuff repair failure

translation of the humeral head with attempted elevation of the shoulder.

In 1997, Collins and Harryman [17] hypothesized that cuff arthropathy was initially due to supraspinatus tear and later to the infraspinatus lesion; the complex tendon tear would cause the upward migration of the humeral head and, consequently, the contact of articular cartilage of the humeral head against the anteroinferior margin of the acromion. Cartilage fragmentation results in particulate debris, which causes synovial thickening and effusion as well as calcium phosphate crystal formation. The enzymatic response to the crystals furthers the damage of the articular surfaces.

Concavity-compression mechanism, suggested by Hurov [18], further corroborates the mechanical theory. According to the author, the healthy cuff compresses the convexity of the humeral head against the pseudo-concavity of the glenoid; therefore, the cuff, with other periscapular muscles, would act as an important dynamic stabilizer of the joint. This action may be even more important in the presence of severe laxity of the static stabilizers of the shoulder (capsule, labrum, and glenohumeral ligaments).

Oh et al. [19] identified that critical tear sizes responsible for disrupted joint kinematics are those with full-thickness supraspinatus tears and 50% detachment of the infraspinatus.

Nutritional theory. Neer et al. [1, 2] have also suggested that the osteoarthritis could depend on the loss of the "water tight" effect (loss of negative pressure normally existing inside the shoulder joint in normal conditions) due to the cuff tear.

This would cause dispersion of synovial fluid, normally contained in the joint, in the subacromial space. The dispersion would make the diffusion of synovial fluid into the joint cartilage difficult; consequently, the cartilage would be poorly nourished and would easily run into atrophy. Furthermore, diffusion of the fluid into the cartilage should be further hindered by the decrease in range of motion caused by the shoulder pain due to the cuff tear (loss of water and mucopolysaccharides content). In addition, decrease in mobility, resulting in pain, would lead the subchondral bone to be osteoporotic and more exposed to possible collapse.

It is known that cytokine and catabolic enzyme concentration increases in the early phases of osteoarthritis. Many studies have also proved that the rotator cuff tear leads to an increased production of interleukin 1β and TNF, which helps to explain the presence of pain and inflammation. It was also noted that the production of many cartilage matrix-specific matrix metalloproteinases (MMPs) increased, including MMP-1, MMP-2, MMP-3, MMP-8, and MMP-13 [20, 21]. The presence of MMP-3 is important because it is implicated in the proteolytic activation of the other MMPs. Yoshihara et al. [22] observed that there is a correlation between the concentration of these cytokines, collagenases, and aggrecanases and accelerated cartilage degeneration after a cuff tear.

These observations redimension the nutritional theory in the genesis of cuff tear arthropathy. In fact, with the evacuation of a part of the synovial fluid through the tendon lesion, inflammation factors and proteolytic enzymes should be removed, and, thus, health status of articular cartilage should be preserved.

In 2012, Reuter et al. [23] sonographically assessed the articular surface of the glenohumeral joint in rats with a rotator cuff tear and observed a thickness decrease in the cartilage. Kramer et al. [24] histologically studied the glenohumeral cartilage of rats, respectively, submitted to detachment of the posterosuperior rotator cuff and to suprascapular nerve root transection passing through the trapezoid (joint capsule was kept intact). The animals were killed 12 weeks after surgery. In the first case, if there had been degenerative changes of the cartilage, it would have been attributed, in accordance with Neer's hypotheses [1, 2], to the altered mechanical loading and to the nutritional theory, instead, in the second case, only to the mechanical hypothesis. Surprisingly, the amount of cartilage degeneration was similar between the groups. This result suggests that aberrant mechanical forces are the primary causes of articular cartilage degeneration in the setting of cuff tear arthropathy.

Crystalline-induced arthritis of the shoulder theory. In orthopedic literature, almost simultaneously to Neer's hypotheses, a nosologic entity similar to the cuff arthropathy has been described: the "Milwaukee syndrome" [25]. Although it is responsible for a clinical condition similar to that of the cuff arthropathy, this disease has been attributed to the presence in the synovial fluid of basic calcium phosphate crystals encapsulated into microspheroids without apparent inflammatory cell response. Indeed an altered capsular degenerated cartilage and synovium, possibly with a macrophage response and subsequent release of collagenase and neutral proteases, are associated with this condition, resulting in the attack and subsequent destruction of the joint.

In 1985, Dieppe and Watt [26] noted that basic calcium phosphate crystals could be found in arthritic and neuropathic joints and in apparently healthy joints of elderly subjects. In addition, the apatite crystals are found especially in the most destructive atrophic situations. Therefore, the authors hypothesized that the crystals are produced by the processes that are secondary to joint degeneration. This hypothesis redimensions the inflammatory theory and suggests that the syndrome is a form of cuff arthropathy.

Autoimmune rheumatic diseases. Cuff arthropathy could be considered an autoimmune rheumatic disease. As well as for scleroderma or systemic lupus erythematous, patients with cuff tear arthropathy are frequently females. No study has ever confirmed this hypothesis. We are conducting a study to verify the reliability of this hypothesis; however, available data do not allow us to formulate conclusions.

Idiopathic theory. It is possible that the cuff arthropathy is the result of a fortuitous coincidence between rotator cuff tear, which is frequently found in elderly patients [27, 28], and idiopathic glenohumeral arthropathy. In other words, arthropathy would occur regardless of cuff tear.

Upward migration of the humeral head consequent to the cuff tear would only be responsible for the fast evolution of the arthritic process, and it would only cause a more precocious wear of the upper portion of the glenoid surface. If this hypothesis is correct, the cuff arthropathy should not have a clear preference for sex, and patients should have an average age similar to that of patients with concentric arthropathy; instead, the cuff arthropathy is predominantly found in females and in older patients.

Theory related to joint laxity. Since cuff tear arthropathy and youth joint laxity are significantly more frequent in females, we hypothesized that these two conditions are associated with each other. If the rotator cuff tear occurs in patients who have/had joint laxity, it is possible that the involved shoulder could develop a severe static instability that might be responsible for a premature wear of the cartilage of the superior glenoid. This assumption justifies the evident difference in the prevalence of cuff arthropathy due to gender.

In order to verify this theory, 133 consecutive patients with glenohumeral osteoarthritis [(48M, 85F; mean age (SD): 72.32 (7.05)] were divided into 2 groups: Group I (patients with CTA) and Group II (patients with concentric shoulder arthropathy) composed of 71 (22M–49F) and 62 (26M–36F) patients, respectively. The presence of current or previous joints hypermobility in all participants was assessed by two standardized methodologies: the Beighton criteria/score and a 5-item self-report questionnaire [29, 30]. The questionnaire investigates, using major and minor criteria, patient's ability to perform uncommon activities, the presence of joint diseases, or the tendency to dislocation.

Beighton criteria led to a diagnosis of joint hypermobility in 16 patients (22.5%) in Group I and in 15 patients (24.2%) in Group II. According to the 5-item self-report questionnaire, juvenile joint laxity was diagnosed in 11 (15.5%) and 12 (19.4%) patients belonging to Groups I and II, respectively. No significant association between the two groups and both Beighton criteria [$\chi^2(1) = 0.051$, $p = 0.82$] and 5-item self-report questionnaire [$\chi^2(1) = 0.67$, $p = 0.41$] was found.

Our data excluded this possible correlation. In fact, surprisingly, in the two groups, percentage of patients who, in juvenile period, have been considered subjects with joint hyperlaxity was the same (Group I, 16 pts. on 71 = 22:53%; Group II, 14 pts. on 62 = 22:58%). Therefore, it is presumable that hyperlaxity condition runs out before the onset of tendon rupture and cannot enhance the joint instability consequent to cuff tear.

5.3 Clinical Presentation

Generally, patients with cuff tear arthropathy are older than 65. They refer shoulder pain; rarely pain intensity is marked. Patients typically are women with shoulder symptoms of long duration. The dominant side is most commonly affected. Usually, pain is distributed in the anterolateral region of the shoulder; rarely it is also at the neck base; it does not extend beyond the elbow; scapular region is not interested; pain is not accompanied by paresthesia. The pain characteristically interferes with sleep and intensifies with activity.

Many patients experience audible crepitus. When these are present, it is easy to evocate them during the Jobe or the Full can test maneuvers.

In thin patients, it is sometimes possible to observe shoulder profile deformity, because of the humeral head upward migration. Occasionally the shoulder is swollen by the presence of abundant synovial fluid that is spread in the subacromial space and glenohumeral and acromioclavicular joints.

Atrophy of infraspinatus and supraspinatus muscles is constantly observable. Weakness of the external rotators may be marked; generally Full can test and Patte test are positive. Very often, the lag signs are also positive.

In the vast majority of patients, the active and passive range of motion is severely limited because of soft tissue contractures or fixed glenohumeral subluxation [14]. Patients who maintain a stable core can keep mobility in flexion and abduction.

5.4 Differences Between Concentric and Eccentric Glenohumeral Arthritis

5.4.1 Histology

At our knowledge, no studies have been conducted regarding histological differences between shoulder arthropathies with or without cuff tear. Actually, the vast majority of the studies have considered histological and ultrastructural characteristics of the idiopathic arthritis, assuming that there were no differences between the two conditions. In both, articular cartilage layer is thinned or, as in the areas submitted to higher mechanical stress, has deep and broad splits or is completely absent, leaving wide exposition of the subchondral bone. In the most severe cases, cells are arranged in clusters in the deeper layer of the cartilage; sometimes chondrocyte lacunae are empty, surrounded by thickened collagen fibers [31]. The living cells are in intense activity and have well-developed cytoplasmic granules. They are enclosed in lacunae that contain numerous fibrils and mature collagen fibers. Matrix is represented by thickened collagen fibers, arranged in all directions, often perpendicularly disposed with respect to articular surface. Colloidal iron staining shows the presence of mucopolysaccharides around the living chondrocytes.

Neer [2] histologically described 26 shoulders with cuff arthropathy. Authors observed three consistent findings: areas with atrophic cartilage and osteoporotic subchondral bone in the humeral head; areas where cartilage is denuded and subchondral bone is sclerotic; and fragments of articular cartilage in the subsynovial layer. A histological study performed by Jensen et al. [14] on specimens of patients with cuff arthropathy revealed foci of calcific deposits in synovial microvilli.

Kramer et al. [24] performed an elegant study on rats whose cuff tendons were previously excised. The histological analysis was performed 12 months after surgery. Authors observed significant cartilage changes in the humeral head compared with the control side. Applying the modified Mankin score [32] (widely used for histologic evaluation of osteoarthritis), they obtained a value of 5.7 ± 1.9 in the involved shoulder and 2.0 ± 1.0 in the control side ($P < 0.001$). The score considers the structure, cellularity, safranin O staining, and tidemark integrity. Analogously, glenoid values were, respectively, 5.1 ± 1.9 and 2.4 ± 0.8 ($P < 0.001$).

CT studies [33–35] have demonstrated that bone density, below the superficial cartilaginous layer of the glenoid, varies with the different forms of arthropathy. In particular, the calcified cartilage layer, which is deeper than the noncalcified layer, is thicker in cuff arthropathy with respect to the concentric arthropathy; instead, the subchondral bone is thinner [35].

Kekatpure et al. [36] submitted to histopathologic analysis the humeral head of nine women who underwent total shoulder arthroplasty for a rapidly destructive arthrosis (rapid collapse of the humeral head with no evidence of other nonseptic articular arthropathy). Of the nine cases, seven had a rotator cuff tear (however fatty infiltration of the rotator cuff muscles were not indicative of a chronic condition), whereas tendinosis in the supraspinatus tendons was found in two cases. Analysis showed absence of articular cartilage. In the subchondral zone, both fragmentation and regeneration of bone matrix, which represented fracture healing, were observed. There was no evidence of inflammatory changes, microorganisms, or crystal-induced arthropathy. Authors did not observe typical AVN findings in the marrow, medullary bone, and cortex.

5.4.2 Age and Gender

It is known that patients with cuff tear arthropathy usually are older than those with concentric arthropathy and are very often females. To check the reliability of these data, we reviewed all the scientific papers published in English from 2000 to date, relative to shoulder arthropathy without rotator cuff tear. We excluded all the papers conducted on patients with rheumatologic diseases, traumas, infections, previous surgical treatments, and cohorts of less than 20 patients. We were able to have demographic information on about 2761 patients with concentric arthropathy [37–45]. Data obtained were compared with those of a meta-analysis conducted by Samitier et al. [46] in 2015 relative to patients with cuff tear arthropathy. This cohort consisted of 581 patients. Data were not statistically analyzed. The weighted average age of the 2761 patients was 66.7 years while that of patients with cuff arthropathy was 72.0 years. These differences reflect my personal experience. In fact, in my series, the mean age of cuff intact arthropathy patients was 70.1 years while that of patients with cuff tear arthropathy was 75.6 years. The different age justifies a different etiology.

Analyzing the 2761 patients with concentric shoulder arthropathy, the weighted percentage of females was 48.8%; that relative to cuff tear arthropathy was 74%. In my series, the percentages were 56% and 70.3%, respectively.

Literature data indicate that the prevalence of cuff tear does not vary between genders. These data reflect our experience. In our series of 586 patients with different sized cuff tear, males and females were, respectively, 280 and 306 [47]. Nevertheless, cuff tear arthropathy is much more common in females. Different hypotheses may be formulated to explain this sexual predisposition:

(1) The percentage of females with joint hyperlaxity is higher than that of males [48–54]; therefore, in absence of cuff tendons and with less effective static stabilizers, the shoulder could result excessively unstable.

(2) Muscle mass in females is less represented [55]; also in this case, the shoulder, in absence of cuff tendons, could be less stable.

(3) Cuff tear arthropathy might be an autoimmune disease and therefore belong to those diseases that notoriously are more frequent in females. In this case estrogens would play a primary role. In fact, estrogen receptors are present on cells of the immune system involved in the pathogenic mechanism of the autoimmune disease.

(4) Genetics.

(5) Environmental factors and lifestyle.

5.4.3 Functional Evaluation

Absolute values of ASES and SST scores are lower in patients with cuff arthropathy than those reported for patients with concentric arthropathy (Table 5.1). This is partly due to the fact that patients with cuff arthropathy are older. However, the marked difference between the mean values of flexion, abduction, and external rotation recorded in the two groups of patients (Table 5.2) indicates an actual functional difference. In addition, patients with cuff arthropathy have a decrease in external rotation strength that further compromises shoulder function. Surprisingly, it shows no significant differences between the two groups when the shoulder function is evaluated with the constant score.

Table 5.1 Functional evaluation in patients with shoulder arthropathy

	Concentric arthropathy	Cuff tear arthropathy Data relative to 581 patients [46]
	Weighted average	Weighted average
Constant score	27.9 (57 patients) [40, 44] 26.8 (210 patients) [56] 26.3 (41 patients) [57] 30.1 (41 patients) [57] 37.3 (62 patients) [58]	30.5
ASES score	39.3 (635 patients) [37, 42, 43, 45]	31.8
SST	3.3 (57 patients) [42, 45]	1.8

Comparison between concentric arthropathy and cuff tear arthropathy

Table 5.2 Range of motion in patients with shoulder arthropathy

	Concentric arthropathy	Cuff tear arthropathy Data relative to 581 patients [46]
	Weighted average	Weighted average
Forward flexion	90.1° (771 patients) [37, 38, 42–45]	63.7°
Abduction	76.2° (488 patients) [43–45]	51.2°
External rotation	21.8° (771 patients) [37, 38, 42–45]	12.5°

Comparison between concentric arthropathy and cuff tear arthropathy

References

1. Neer CS, Watson K, Stanton F. Recent experience in total shoulder replacement. J Bone Joint Surg Am. 1982;64:319–37.
2. Neer CS, Craig EV, Fukuda H. Cuff-tear arthropathy. J Bone Joint Surg Am. 1983;65:1232–1244J.
3. Adams R. A treatise on rheumatic gout or chronic rheumatic arthritis of all the joints. London: John Churcill & Sons; 1873. p. 91–175.
4. Smith RW. Observations upon chronic rheumatic arthritis of the shoulder (part I). Dublin Quart J Med Sci. 1853;15:1–16.
5. Smith RW. Observations upon chronic rheumatic arthritis of the shoulder (part II). Dublin Quart J Med Sci. 1853;15:343–58.
6. Codman E. Rupture of the supraspinatus tendon and others lesions in or about the subacromiale bursa. In: Codman E, editor. The shoulder. Boston: Thomas Todd; 1934. p. 478–80.
7. Galmiche P, Deshayes P. Hemarthrose essentielle récidivante. Rev Rhumat. 1958;25:57–9.
8. Burman M, Sutro C, Guariglia E. Spontaneous hemorrhage of bursae and joint in the elderly. Bull Hosp Joint Dis. 1964;25:217–39.
9. Banna A, Hume KP. Spontaneous hemarthrosis of the shoulder joint. Ann Phys Med. 1964;7:180–4.
10. Shephard E. Swelling of the subacromial bursa: a report on 16 cases. Proc R Soc Med. 1963;56:162–3.
11. Snook GA. Pigmented villonodular synovitis with bony invasion. A report of two cases. JAMA. 1963;184:424–5.
12. DeSeze S, Hubault A, Rampon S. L'épaule sénile hémorragique. L'actualité rhumatologique. Paris: Expansion Scientifique Francaise; 1967. p. 107–15.
13. Bauduin MP, Famaey JP. A propos d'un cas d'épaule sénile hémorragique. Belge Rhum Med Phys. 1969;24:135–40.
14. Jensen KL, Williams GR Jr, Russell IJ, Rockwood CA Jr. Rotator cuff tear arthropathy. J Bone Joint Surg Am. 1999;81:1312–24.
15. Ecklund KJ, Lee TQL, Tibone J, Gupta R. Rotator cuff tear arthropathy. J Am Acad Orthop Surg. 2007;15:340–9.
16. Burkhart SS. Fluoroscopic comparison of kinematic patterns in massive rotator cuff tears. A suspension bridge model. Clin Orthop Relat Res. 1992;284:144–52.
17. Collins DN, Harryman DT II. Arthroplasty for arthritis and rotator cuff deficiency. Orthop Clin North Am. 1997;28:225–39.
18. Hurov J. Anatomy and mechanics of the shoulder: review of current concepts. J Hand Ther. 2009;22:328–42.
19. Oh JH, Jun BJ, McGarry MH, Lee TQ. Does a critical rotator cuff tear stage exist?: a biomechanical study of rotator cuff tear progression in human cadaver shoulders. J Bone Joint Surg Am. 2011;93:2100–9.
20. Gotoh M, Hamada K, Yamakawa H, Nakamura M, Yamazaki H, Ueyama Y, Tamaoki N, Inoue A, Fukuda H. Perforation of rotator cuff increases interleukin 1beta production in the synovium of glenohumeral joint in rotator cuff diseases. J Rheumatol. 2000;27:2886–92.
21. Osawa T, Shinozaki T, Takagishi K. Multivariate analysis of biochemical markers in synovial fluid from the shoulder joint for diagnosis of rotator cuff tears. Rheumatol Int. 2005;25:436–41.
22. Yoshihara Y, Hamada K, Nakajima T, Fujikawa K, Fukuda H. Biochemical markers in the synovial fluid of glenohumeral joints from patients with rotator cuff tear. J Orthop Res. 2001;19:573–9.
23. Reuther KE, Sarver JJ, Schultz SM, Lee CS, Sehgal CM, Glaser DL, Soslowsky LJ. Glenoid cartilage mechanical properties decrease after rotator cuff tears in a rat model. J Orthop Res. 2012;30:1435–9.
24. Kramer EJ, Bodendorfer BM, Laron D, Wong J, Kim HT, Liu X, Feeley BT. Evaluation of cartilage degeneration in a rat model of rotator cuff tear arthropathy. J Shoulder Elb Surg. 2013;22:1702–9.
25. Halverson PB, Cheung HS, McCarty DJ, Garancis J, Mandel N. "Milwaukee shoulder"—association of microspheroids containing hydroxyapatite crystals, active collagenase, and neutral protease with rotator cuff defects. II. Synovial fluid studies. Arthritis Rheum. 1981;24:474–83.
26. Dieppe P, Watt I. Crystal deposition in osteoarthritis: an opportunistic event? Clin Rheum Dis. 1985;11:367–92.
27. Fukuda H, Mikasa M, Ogawa K, Yamanaka K, Hamada K. The partial thickness tear of the rotator cuff. Orthop Trans. 1983;11:237–8.
28. Minagawa H, Yamamoto N, Abe H, Fukuda M, Seki N, Kikuchi K, Kijima H, Itoi E. Prevalence of symptomatic and asymptomatic rotator cuff tears in the general population: from mass-screening in one village. J Orthop. 2013;10:8–12.

29. Hakim AJ, Grahame R. A simple questionnaire to detect hypermobility: an adjunct to the assessment of patients with diffuse musculoskeletal pain. Int J Clin Pract. 2003;57:163–6.
30. Hakim A, Grahame R. Joint hypermobility. Best Pract Res Clin Rheumatol. 2003;17:989–1004.
31. Postacchini F, Gumina S. Ultrastructural and histochemical aspects of osteoarthritic cartilage. In: Osteoarthritis. Florence: OIC Medical Press; 1992. p. 189–201.
32. Mankin HJ, Dorfman H, Lippiello L, Zarins A. A biochemical and metabolic abnormalities in articular cartilage from osteo-arthritic human hip II. Correlation of morphology with biochemical and metabolic data. J Bone Joint Surg Am. 1971;53:523–37.
33. von Eisenhart-Rothe R, Müller-Gerbl M, Wiedemann E, Englmeier KH, Graichen H. Functional malcentering of the humeral head and asymmetric long-term stress on the glenoid: potential reasons for glenoid loosening in total shoulder arthroplasty. J Shoulder Elb Surg. 2008;17:695–702.
34. Knowles NK, Athwal GS, Keener JD, Ferreira LM. Regional bone density variations in osteoarthritic glenoids: a comparison of symmetric to asymmetric (type B2) erosion patterns. J Shoulder Elb Surg. 2015;24:425–32.
35. Simon P, Gupta A, Pappou I, Hussey MM, Santoni BG, Inoue N, Frankle MA. Glenoid subchondral bone density distribution in male total shoulder arthroplasty subjects with eccentric and concentric wear. J Shoulder Elb Surg. 2015;24:416–24.
36. Kekatpure AL, Sun JH, Sim GB, Chun JM, Jeon IH. Rapidly destructive arthrosis of the shoulder joints: radiographic, magnetic resonance imaging, and histopathologic findings. J Shoulder Elb Surg. 2015;24:922–7.
37. Gartsman GM, Roddey TS, Hammerman SM. Shoulder arthroplasty with or without resurfacing of the glenoid in patients who have osteoarthritis. J Bone Joint Surg Am. 2000;82:26–34.
38. Bryant D, Litchfield R, Sandow M, Gartsman G, Guyatt G, Kirkley A. A comparison of pain, strength, range of motion, and functional outcomes after hemiarthroplasty and total shoulder arthroplasty in patients with osteoarthritis of the shoulder: a systematic review and meta-analysis. J Bone Joint Surg Am. 2005;87:1947–56.
39. Radnay CS, Setter KJ, Chambers L, Levine WN, Bigliani LU, Ahmad CS. Total shoulder replacement compared with humeral head replacement for the treatment of primary glenohumeral osteoarthritis: a systematic review. J Shoulder Elb Surg. 2007;16:396–402.
40. Sandow MJ, David H, Bentall SJ. Hemiarthroplasty vs total shoulder replacement for rotator cuff intact osteoarthritis: how do they fare after a decade? J Shoulder Elb Surg. 2013;22:877–85.
41. Smith T, Gettmann A, Wellmann M, Pastor F, Struck M. Humeral surface replacement for osteoarthritis. Acta Orthop. 2013;84:468–72.
42. Cvetanovich GL, Chalmers PN, Streit JJ, Romeo AA, Nicholson GP. Patients undergoing total shoulder arthroplasty on the dominant extremity attain greater postoperative ROM. Clin Orthop Relat Res. 2015;473(10):3221–5. [Epub ahead of print].
43. Hussey MM, Steen BM, Cusick MC, Cox JL, Marberry ST, Simon P, Cottrell BJ, Santoni BG, Frankle MA. The effects of glenoid wear patterns on patients with osteoarthritis in total shoulder arthroplasty: an assessment of outcomes and value. J Shoulder Elb Surg. 2015;24:682–90.
44. Maier MW, Lauer S, Wolf SI, Dreher T, Klotz MC, Zeifang F, Rickert M. Low preoperative constant score is a negative predictive factor for postoperative proprioception after total shoulder arthroplasty in osteoarthritis. Arch Orthop Trauma Surg. 2015;135:171–7.
45. Steen BM, Cabezas AF, Santoni BG, Hussey MM, Cusick MC, Kumar AG, Frankle MA. Outcome and value of reverse shoulder arthroplasty for treatment of glenohumeral osteoarthritis: a matched cohort. J Shoulder Elbow Surg. 2015;24(9):1433–41. pii: S1058-2746(15)00043-9.
46. Samitier G, Alentorn-Geli E, Torrens C, Wright TW. Reverse shoulder arthroplasty. Part 1: systematic review of clinical and functional outcomes. Int J Shoulder Surg. 2015;9:24–31.
47. Gumina S, Carbone S, Campagna V, Candela V, Sacchetti FM, Giannicola G. The impact of aging on rotator cuff tear size. Musculoskelet Surg. 2013;97(Suppl 1):69–72.
48. Al-Rawi ZS, Al-Aszawi AJ, Al-Chalabi T. Joint mobility among university students in Iraq. Br J Rheumatol. 1985;24:326–31.
49. Larsson LG, Baum J, Mudholkar GS. Hypermobility: features and differential incidence between the sexes. Arthritis Rheum. 1987;30:1426–30.
50. Didia BC, Dapper DV, Boboye SB. Joint hypermobility syndrome among undergraduate students. East Afr Med J. 2002;79:80–1.
51. Seçkin U, Tur BS, Yilmaz O, et al. The prevalence of joint hypermobility among high school students. Rheumatol Int. 2005;25:260–3.
52. Quatman CE, Ford KR, Myer GD, Paterno MV, Hewett TE. The effects of gender and pubertal status on generalized joint laxity in young athletes. J Sci Med Sport. 2008;11:257–63.
53. Cameron KL, Duffey ML, DeBerardino TM, Stoneman PD, Jones CJ, Owens BD. Association of generalized joint hypermobility with a history of glenohumeral joint instability. J Athl Train. 2010;45:253–8.
54. Wolf JM, Schreier S, Tomsick S, Williams A, Petersen B. Radiographic laxity of the trapeziometacarpal joint is correlated with generalized joint hypermobility. J Hand Surg Am. 2011;36:1165–9.
55. Kasper DL, Braunwald E, Fauci AS, Hauser SL, Longo DL, Jameson JL. Harrison's principles of internal medicine., 16th/e. Part 1: 33–38. ISBN: 978883863929-6. New York: McGraw Hill; 2005.

56. Young A, Walch G, Boileau P, Favard L, Gohlke F, Loew M, Molé D. A multicentre study of the long-term results of using a flat-back polyethylene glenoid component in shoulder replacement for primary osteoarthritis. J Bone Joint Surg Br. 2011;93:210–6.
57. Berth A, Pap G. Stemless shoulder prosthesis versus conventional anatomic shoulder prosthesis in patients with osteoarthritis: a comparison of the functional outcome after a minimum of two years follow-up. J Orthop Traumatol. 2013;14:31–7.
58. Montoya F, Magosch P, Scheiderer B, Lichtenberg S, Melean P, Habermeyer P. Midterm results of a total shoulder prosthesis fixed with a cementless glenoid component. J Shoulder Elb Surg. 2013;22:628–35.

Cuff Tear Arthropathy: Classifications

6

Vincenzo Campagna, Vittorio Candela, and Stefano Gumina

6.1 Introduction

Rotator cuff tear arthropathy is a term coined by Neer in 1983, and it encompasses a broad spectrum of pathology [1]. All patients with rotator cuff tear arthropathy possess at least three critical features: (1) rotator cuff insufficiency, (2) degenerative changes of the glenohumeral joint, and (3) superior migration of the humeral head [2].

The glenohumeral joint lacks substantial intrinsic osseous restraints, and thus the joint's stability relies heavily on the rotator cuff's ability to center the humeral head within the glenoid fossa [3, 4]. This key concept has been coined concavity-compression. Through this mechanism, the shoulder musculature—including the rotator cuff—becomes the primary stabilizer of the glenohumeral joint as the arm moves through positions in which the capsule ligamentous structures are lax [3, 5].

V. Campagna
Department of Shoulder and Elbow Surgery, Celio Military Hospital, Rome, Italy

V. Candela
Department of Anatomy, Istology, Forensic Medicine, Orthopaedics and Traumatology, Sapienza, University of Rome, Rome, Italy

Polo Pontino, Latina, Italy

S. Gumina (✉)
Department of Orthopaedics and Traumatology, Sapienza University of Rome, Rome, Italy

S. Gumina et al. (eds.), *Reverse Shoulder Arthroplasty*, https://doi.org/10.1007/978-3-319-97743-0_6

Patients with a massive rotator cuff tear may present with a clinical pattern of combined loss of active elevation and external rotation (CLEER) [6]. Their daily activities may be reversely limited due to a muscle imbalance in both the horizontal and vertical planes.

In particular, activities involving external rotation (eating, drinking, brushing teeth, etc.) may be impossible and lead to a severe handicap in daily life. In such situation, the absence of the rotator cuff causes the head of the humerus to ride upward.

The definition of an irreparable rotator cuff varies widely. At one extreme some surgeons argue that all rotator cuff tears are reparable. Others consider tears with a chronic acromiohumeral distance (AHD) less than 7 mm [7] or atrophy greater than grade 2 [8] irreparable. Fatty degeneration is irreversible even with repair and leads to reduced function of the rotator cuff musculature [9]. If associated with preoperative supraspinatus tendon length of less than 15 mm, MRCT (massive rotator cuff tear) with Goutallier Stages 2 to 3 MRCT fails to completely heal in up to 92% of cases [10]. Acetabularization of the acromion and femoralization of the humeral head are preoperative factors reflecting significant chronic static instability and are a contraindication for repair.

Once a MRCT is identified, it can be further classified according to Collin et al. [11]. In this classification, the rotator cuff is divided into five components: supraspinatus, superior subscapularis, inferior subscapularis, infraspinatus, and teres minor (Fig. 6.1).

Rotator cuff tear patterns can then be classified into five types: type A, supraspinatus and superior subscapularis tears; type B, supraspinatus and entire subscapularis tears; type C, supraspinatus, superior subscapularis, and infraspinatus tears; type D, supraspinatus and infraspinatus tears; and type E, supraspinatus, infraspinatus, and teres minor tears (Fig. 6.2) [11].

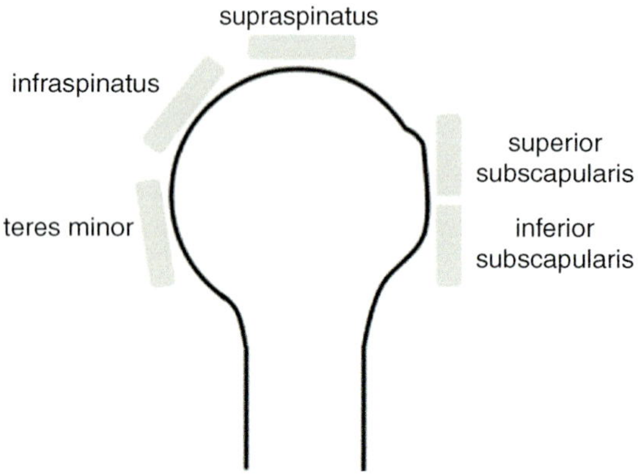

Fig. 6.1 The rotator cuff is divided into five components: supraspinatus, superior subscapularis, inferior subscapularis, infraspinatus, and teres minor (Reproduced from Collin P, Matsumura N, Lädermann A, Denard PJ, Walch G (2014). Relationship between massive chronic rotator cuff tear pattern and loss of active shoulder range of motion. J Shoulder Elbow Surg 23(8):1195–202. doi:https://doi.org/10.1016/j.jse.2013.11.019)

This classification not only subclassifies massive tears but has also been linked to function, particularly the maintenance of active elevation [11].

6.2 Cuff Tear Arthropathy Classification

A concise definition of cuff tear arthropathy would probably be glenohumeral osteoarthritis with a concomitant massive rotator cuff tear and rotator cuff dysfunction. The spectrum of cuff tear arthropathy ranges from superior migration of the humeral head with only regional chondromalacia to collapse of the humeral head with full-thickness cartilage defects. Numerous radiologic classification schemes have been proposed [12].

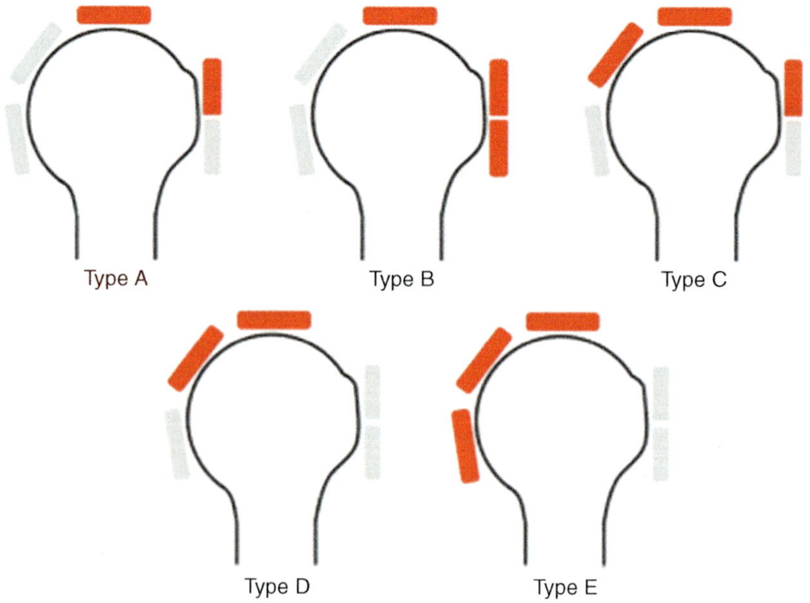

Fig. 6.2 Rotator cuff tears classified by the involved components: type A, supraspinatus and superior subscapularis tears; type B, supraspinatus and entire subscapularis tears; type C, supraspinatus, superior subscapularis, and infraspinatus tears; type D, supraspinatus and infraspinatus tears; and type E, supraspinatus, infraspinatus, and teres minor tears (Reproduced from: Collin P, Matsumura N, Lädermann A, Denard PJ, Walch G (2014). Relationship between massive chronic rotator cuff tear pattern and loss of active shoulder range of motion. J Shoulder Elbow Surg 23(8):1195–202. doi:https://doi.org/10.1016/j.jse.2013.11.019)

Classification systems applicable to rotator cuff tear arthropathy include the Hamada system [13] and the Seebauer system [14].

- The *Hamada classification* [13] grades the acromion humeral distance, morphologic alterations of the acromion and humeral head, and glenohumeral joint space narrowing. This system divides massive rotator cuff tears into five radiographic stages, with successive stages demonstrating findings consistent with progression of the rotator cuff tear arthropathy. In Stage 1, the acromiohumeral interval is >6 mm. In Stage 2, the acromiohumeral interval is <5 mm. In Stage 3, the acromiohumeral interval is <5 mm and acetabulization of the coracoacromial arch is present. In Stage 4, the glenohumeral joint is narrowed, either without acetabulization (Stage 4a) or with acetabulization (Stage 4b). In Stage 5, humeral head osteonecrosis results in collapse (Fig. 6.3).
- The *Seebauer classification* system [15] is a biomechanical description of rotator cuff tear arthropathy, in which each type is distinguished on the basis of the degree of superior migration from the center of rotation and the amount of instability. The amount of decentralization seen on radiographs is dependent on "the extent of the rotator cuff tear, the integrity of the coracoacromial arch, and the degree and direction of the glenoid bone erosion," and thus this classification system is intended to be a radiographic correlate of the underlying pathology seen in rotator cuff tear arthropathy (Fig. 6.4).
- The *Favard classification* of cuff tear arthropathy is shown in Fig. 6.5.
  - Group 1: this group is characterized by upward migration of the humeral head, superior glenohumeral joint space narrowing, an acromion changed in shape due to the imprint of the humeral head and subacromial arthritis.
  - Group 2: this group is characterized by central glenohumeral joint space narrowing and with little alteration in the shape of

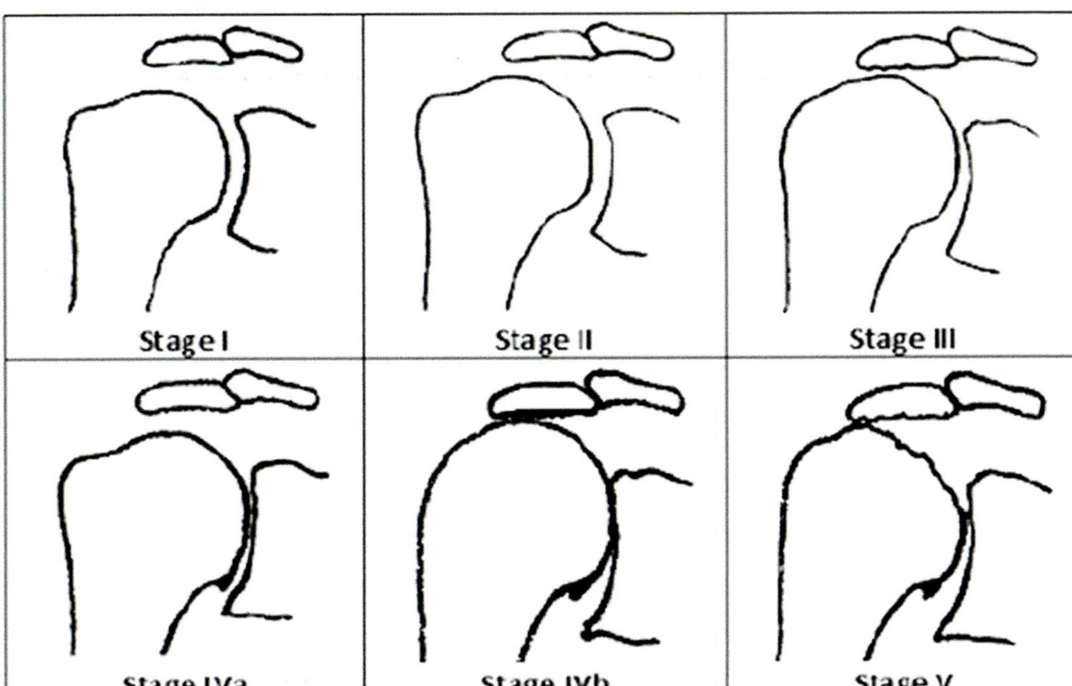

Fig. 6.3 Hamada classification system according to the acromiohumeral interval and progression of arthropathy (Reproduced from Hamada K, Fukuda H, Mikasa M, Kobayashi Y. Roentgenographic findings in massive rotator cuff tears. A long-term observation. Clin Orthop Relat Res. 1990; 254:92–6)

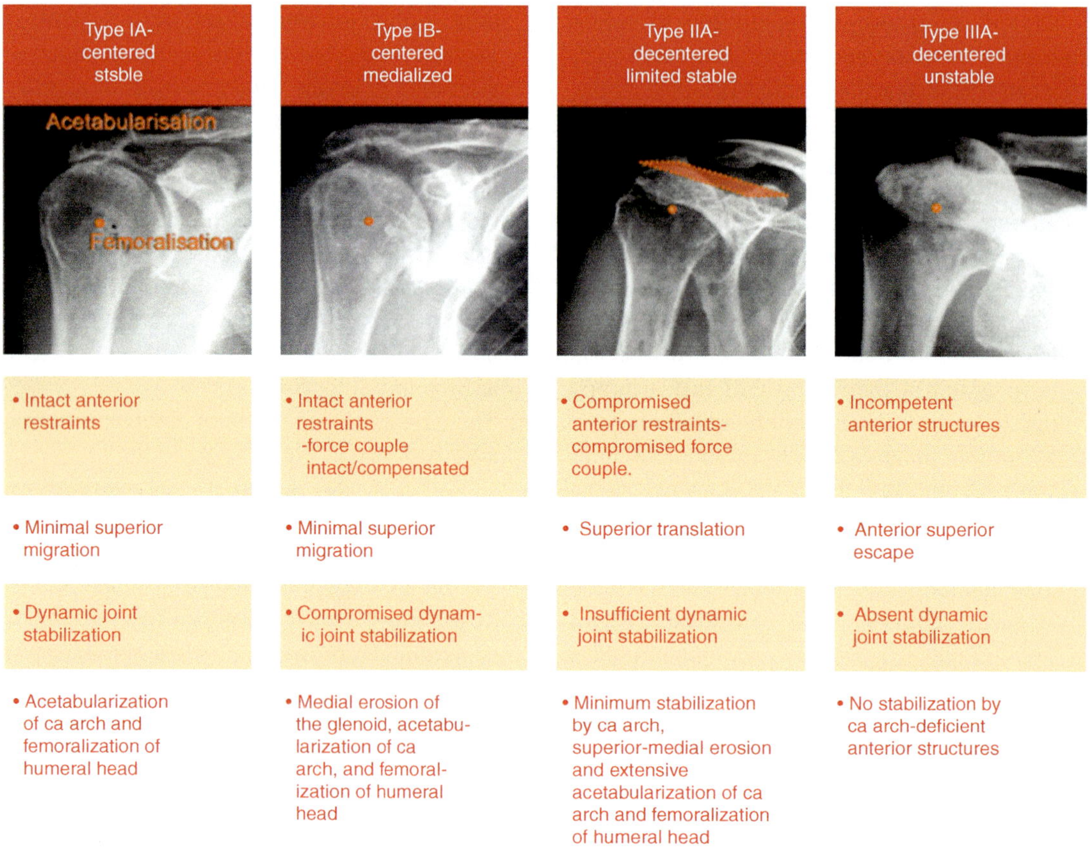

Fig. 6.4 The Seebauer classification system is a biomechanical description of rotator cuff tear arthropathy based on clinical and radiographic parameters (Reproduced from Visotsky JL, Basamania C, Seebauer L, Rockwood CA, Jensen KL. Cuff tear arthropathy: pathogenesis, classification, and algorithm for treatment. J Bone Joint Surg Am. 2004;86)

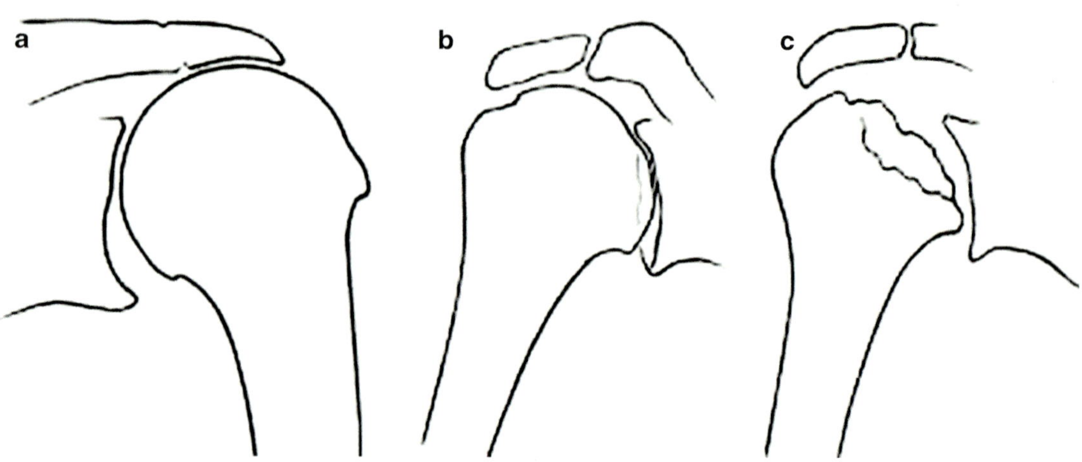

Fig. 6.5 Favard classification of cuff tear arthropathy (Reproduced from Favard et al., OA with massive RCT: the limitations of its current definitions. In: The Cuff, edited by Gazielly D, Elsevier, 1997)

the acromion which does not have a humeral head imprint.
- Group 3: this group is characterized by signs of bony destruction in the form of lysis of either the head or the acromion. The bony elements not affected by the lysis do not undergo any modification in their shape, for example, the greater tuberosity is not eroded and the acromion does not have a humeral head imprint. Glenohumeral joint space narrowing is either minimal or nonexistent.

Classification of glenoid erosion in glenohumeral osteoarthritis with massive rupture of the cuff according to *Sirveaux* [16]: the authors defined four types of glenoid erosion. In type E0, the head of the humerus migrated upward without erosion of the glenoid. Type E1 was defined by a concentric erosion of the glenoid. In type E2 there was an erosion of the superior part of the glenoid, and in type E3 the erosion extended to the inferior part of the glenoid (Fig. 6.6).

There is no general agreement as to which classification system should be used. No comparison of radiographic classification schemes of cuff tear arthropathy has been attempted yet, nor has their reliability been determined yet. A classification scheme specifically for cuff tear arthropathy has to display three core characteristics: it has to be valid and to preferably allow treatment strategies to be derived from the stage of disease determined by the classification. In addition, it has to possess at least comparable reliability to classification schemes that were not specifically designed for cuff tear arthropathy.

Moreover, an improved understanding of the risk factors for radiographic progression of cuff tears may improve treatment paradigms for patients with degenerative cuff tears. Keener et al. [14] performed an analysis of risk factors for proximal humeral migration. These authors found it to be significantly greater in tears with symptoms, tears with involvement of the infraspinatus, and tears with larger size. In multivariate analysis, tear size was the strongest predictor

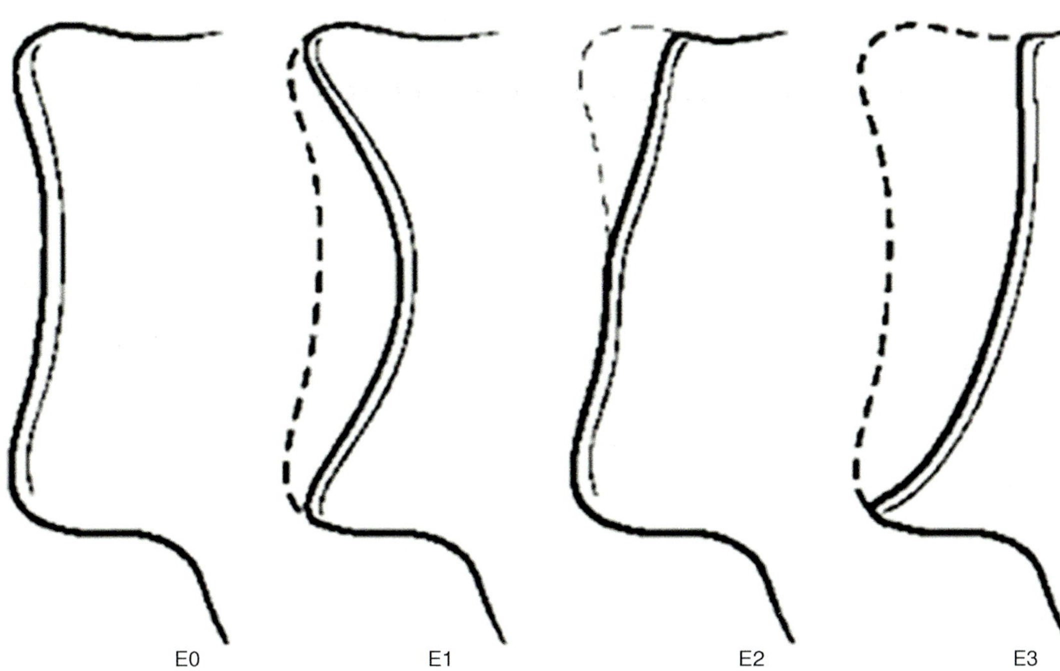

Fig. 6.6 Sirveaux classification of glenoid erosion in cuff tear arthropathy (Reproduced from Sirveaux F, Favard L, Oudet D, Huquet D, Walch G, Mole D. Grammont inverted total shoulder arthroplasty in the treatment of glenohumeral osteoarthritis with massive rupture of the cuff. Results of a multicentre study of 80 shoulders. J Bone Joint Surg Br 2004;86:388–95 (PMID 15125127))

of migration. Patients with small or medium size tears and minimal arthritic changes had low risk for arthritic progression. Those patients who present with larger tears and more advanced arthritic changes may have more accelerated progression.

Paxton et al. [17] reported no correlation between tear characteristics or clinical findings and the progression of rotator cuff tear arthropathy, although non-comparative series have suggested that large, irreparable recurrent tears have rapid progression rates.

References

1. Neer CS 2nd, Craig EV, Fukuda H. Cuff-tear arthropathy. J Bone Joint Surg Am. 1983;65:1232–44.
2. Jensen KL, Williams GR Jr, Russell IJ, Rockwood CA Jr. Rotator cuff tear arthropathy. J Bone Joint Surg Am. 1999;81:1312–24.
3. Hurov J. Anatomy and mechanics of the shoulder: review of current concepts. J Hand Ther. 2009;22:328–42.
4. Zeman CA, Arcand MA, Cantrell JS, Skedros JG, Burkhead WZ Jr. The rotator cuff-deficient arthritic shoulder: diagnosis and surgical management. J Am Acad Orthop Surg. 1998;6:337–48.
5. Lippitt S, Matsen F. Mechanisms of glenohumeral joint stability. Clin Orthop Relat Res. 1993;291:20–8.
6. Boileau P, Chuinard C, Roussanne Y, Neyton L, Troiani C. Modified latissimus dorsi and teres major transfer through a single delto pectoral approach for external rotation deficit of the shoulder: as an isolated procedure or with a reverse arthroplasty. J Shoulder Elb Surg. 2010;19:20–30.
7. Nove-Josserand L, Edwards TB, O'Connor DP, Walch G. The acromiohumeral and coracohumeral intervals are abnormal in rotator cuff tears with muscular fatty degeneration. Clin Orthop Relat Res. 2005;433:90–6.
8. Warner JJ, Higgins L, Parsons IM, Dowdy P. Diagnosis and treatment of anterosuperior rotator cuff tears. J Shoulder Elb Surg. 2001;10:37–46. https://doi.org/10.1067/mse.2001.112022.
9. Gladstone JN, Bishop JY, Lo IK, Flatow EL. Fatty infiltration and atrophy of the rotator cuff do not improve after rotator cuff repair and correlate with poor functional outcome. Am J Sports Med. 2007;35:719–28. https://doi.org/10.1177/0363546506297539.
10. Meyer DC, Farshad M, Amacker NA, Gerber C, Wieser K. Quantitative analysis of muscle and tendon retraction in chronic rotator cuff tears. Am J Sports Med. 2012;40:606–10. https://doi.org/10.1177/0363546511429778.
11. Collin P, Matsumura N, Lädermann A, Denard PJ, Walch G. Relationship between massive chronic rotator cuff tear pattern and loss of active shoulder range of motion. J Shoulder Elb Surg. 2014;23(8):1195–202. https://doi.org/10.1016/j.jse.2013.11.019.
12. Arkawi M, Cakir B, Reichel H, Kappe T. Reliability of radiologic glenohumeral osteoarthritis classification. J Shoulder Elb Surg. 2013;22:1063–7.
13. Hamada K, Fukuda H, Mikasa M, Kobayashi Y. Roentgenographic findings in massive rotator cuff tears. A long-term observation. Clin Orthop Relat Res. 1990;254:92–6.
14. Keener JD, Wei AS, Kim HM, Steger-May K, Yamaguchi K. Proximal humeral migration in shoulders with symptomatic and asymptomatic rotator cuff tears. J Bone Joint Surg Am. 2009;91:1405–13. https://doi.org/10.2106/JBJS.H.00854.
15. Visotsky JL, Basamania C, Seebauer L, Rockwood CA, Jensen KL. Cuff tear arthropathy: pathogenesis, classification, and algorithm for treatment. J Bone Joint Surg Am. 2004;86(Suppl 2):35–40.
16. Sirveaux F, Favard L, Oudet D, Huquet D, Walch G, Mole D. Grammont inverted total shoulder arthroplasty in the treatment of glenohumeral osteoarthritis with massive rupture of the cuff. Results of a multicentre study of 80 shoulders. J Bone Joint Surg Br. 2004;86:388–95. (PMID: 15125127).
17. Paxton ES, Teefey SA, Dahiya N, Keener JD, Yamaguchi K, Galatz LM. Clinical and radiographic outcomes of failed repairs of large or massive rotator cuff tears: minimum ten-year follow-up. J Bone Joint Surg Am. 2013;95:627–32. https://doi.org/10.2106/JBJS.L.00255.

7 Natural History

Eraclio Siuni

The anatomopathological aspects of the glenohumeral arthropathy associated with the massive rupture of the rotator cuff were already described in the nineteenth century.

R. W. Smith, a professor of surgery in the University of Dublin, in the original communications section published in the *Quarterly Journal of Medical Science* in Dublin in February 1853 [1, 2], described the case of a man of about 60 years of age where a chronic rheumatic arthritis had been established in the shoulder joint.

He wrote "Upon the right side, the head of the humerus, placed much farther back than natural, and elevated so as to be in contact with the under surface of the acromion process"...."it was found that no articular surface existed in the normal situation of the glenoid cavity, but upon the external aspect of the neck of the scapula, there had been formed a glenoid-shaped, concave surface, for the reception of the head of the humerus"...."The head of the humerus had lost completely the globular form which it possesses in the normal state; it was flattened from within outwards."

Adams, a Regius Professor of surgery at the University of Dublin, explained in his *A Treatise on Rheumatic Gout, or Chronic Rheumatic Arthritis of All the Joints* published in 1873 [3] a localized form of chronic rheumatoid arthritis involving the shoulder, characterized by biceps tendon rupture and rotator cuff tear, erosion of the upper portion of the humeral head, and erosion of the undersurface of the acromion process and of the distal third of the clavicle.

Codman, in his text *The Shoulder* published in 1934 [4], described the case of a 51-year-old woman suffering from a traumatic rotator cuff tear resulting from a fall. At the time of the intervention, 6 years after the traumatic event, he found a major defect in the rotator cuff associated with an atrophy of the surrounding muscle, a severe glenohumeral arthropathy, intra-articular loose bodies, a chronic synovitis, and effusion of the bursa or joint. He attributed the pathological changes to the mechanical forces acting on the shoulder joint as a result of the functional insufficiency of a chronically neglected large rotator cuff tear.

In the 1950s and 1960s of the last century, several authors, Galmiche and Deshayes [5] in 1958, Shephard [6] and Snook [7] in 1963, Burman [8] and Banna [9] in 1964, and Bauduin and Famaey [10] in 1969, have published numerous cases of elderly patients with supraspinatus tendon tears and shoulder arthropathy associated with recurrent spontaneous hemorrhage into the subdeltoid bursa and glenohumeral joint.

DeSeze [11] in 1968 exposed "l'épaule sénile hémorragique" characterized by a chronic rupture of the rotator cuff, associated with recurrent hemorrhage of the shoulder and severe

E. Siuni (✉)
Responsible "Shoulder Surgery Unit", SCOMR
Marino Hospital, Cagliari Ats Sardinia, Italy

S. Gumina et al. (eds.), *Reverse Shoulder Arthroplasty*,
https://doi.org/10.1007/978-3-319-97743-0_7

arthropathy. Also referring to previous reports in the literature, he then studied this clinical entity in three elderly women who did not have a history of trauma.

Lamboley [12] in 1977 presented a report of nine cases of elderly women who suffered from recurrent painful swelling on the shoulder and identified an association between rotator cuff tear and glenohumeral arthropathy and arthritis of the knee joint.

Charles S. Neer in 1977 [13] then introduced, for the first time, the term "cuff tear arthropathy" to describe degenerative changes in the glenohumeral joint associated with a chronic cuff tear, including erosion of the articular surfaces, restricted shoulder motion, osteopenia, and collapse of the humeral head.

Halverson et al. in 1981 [14–16] coined the term "Milwaukee shoulder" to describe the condition of elderly women who had chronic rotator cuff tear with recurrent bilateral shoulder effusions and radiographic destructive changes of the glenohumeral joints. They found out that basic calcium phosphate (BCP) crystals, such as hydroxyapatite, accumulate in elevated levels, in the synovial tissue and fluid of shoulders with rotator cuff deficiency and arthropathy.

They then suggested the so-called inflammatory-mediated theory to explain the arthropathy associated with the rotator cuff tear and hypothesized that the basic calcium phosphate crystals such as hydroxyapatite initiate a cascade of events. The resulting phagocytosis of these crystals by macrophages would induce the release of proteolytic enzymes such as collagenases and proteases that would cause degradation of cartilage matrix components and periarticular and articular structures [17–19].

Tissue damage involves an additional release of crystals in the synovial fluid by triggering a vicious circle and resulting in an accelerated degeneration of the rotator cuff and biceps tendon, leading to glenohumeral joint destruction [20, 21].

Dieppe et al. in 1984 [22] introduced the term "apatite-associated destructive arthritis," and in 1985 [23], after noticing that the basic calcium phosphate crystals were found in osteoarthritis, neuropathic joints, and joint tissue of healthy elderly patients, they argued that BCP crystals were actually the product of the wear and destruction of the articular surfaces and not the triggering cause. In 1988 [24] they later proposed the term "idiopathic destructive arthritis" to describe the arthropathy of the shoulder associated with rotator cuff tear.

In contrast, Neer et al. hypothesized in 1983 [25] that a massive rotator cuff tear was the inciting event in the development of rotator cuff tear arthropathy and that both mechanical and nutritional factors contributed to the subsequent progression of the arthropathy.

The scapulohumeral cingulum muscles, the rotator cuff, and the deltoid muscle act synergistically to maintain the balance of the shoulder joint on both the coronal and the transverse plane.

The mechanical theory suggests that the glenohumeral arthropathy was due to the deficient rotator cuff because without the superior stabilizing effect of the supraspinatus tendon, the humeral head for the action of the deltoid muscle tends to subluxate superiorly (Fig. 7.1a, b). The deterioration of the articular cartilage is a direct result of abnormal physical stresses imparted to the humeral head, leading to erosion of the upper portion of the humeral head (Fig. 7.2a, b, c), the superior glenoid fossa, and undersurface of the acromion (Fig. 7.3a, b) and erosion of the acromioclavicular joint and the coracoid (Fig. 7.4a, b).

The rotator cuff acts in the dynamic stability of the shoulder with balance between the subscapularis anteriorly and infraspinatus and teres minor posteriorly. A massive rotator cuff tear extends posteriorly with infraspinatus, and teres minor involvement entails an imbalance of this "force couples" (Burkhart 1992) resulting in further wear on the articular surfaces and acromion [26].

The concept of "concavity-compression" was coined by Hurov in 2009 [27], to explain the role of the rotator cuff in the dynamic stabilization of the shoulder by centering the convex humeral head on the concave glenoid fossa in all directions of movement.

A massive rotator cuff tear and rupture or dislocation of the long head of the biceps leads to unbalanced force coupling and loss of the

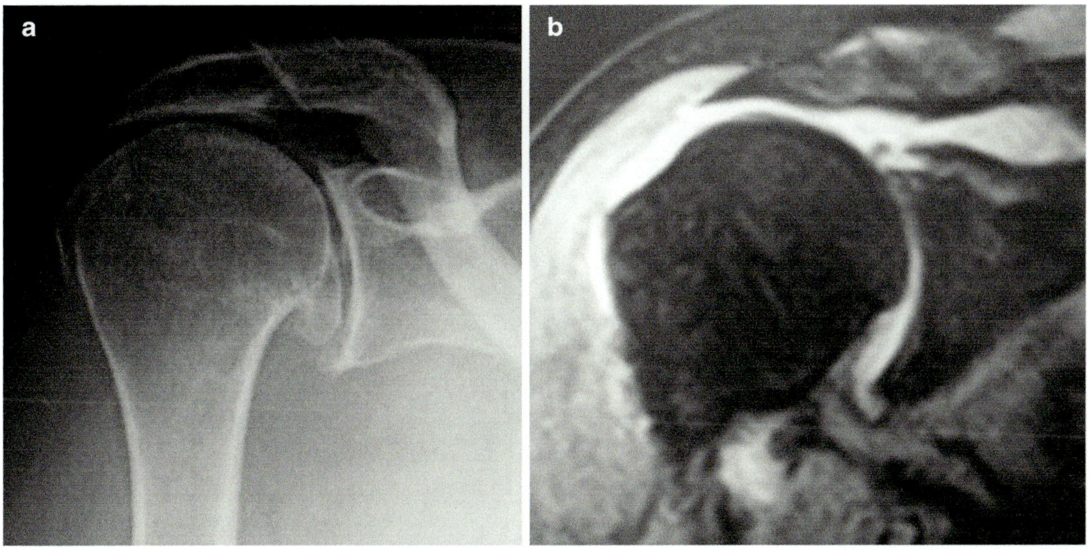

Fig. 7.1 (**a**, **b**) The humeral head, for the action of the deltoid muscle, tends to subluxate superiorly

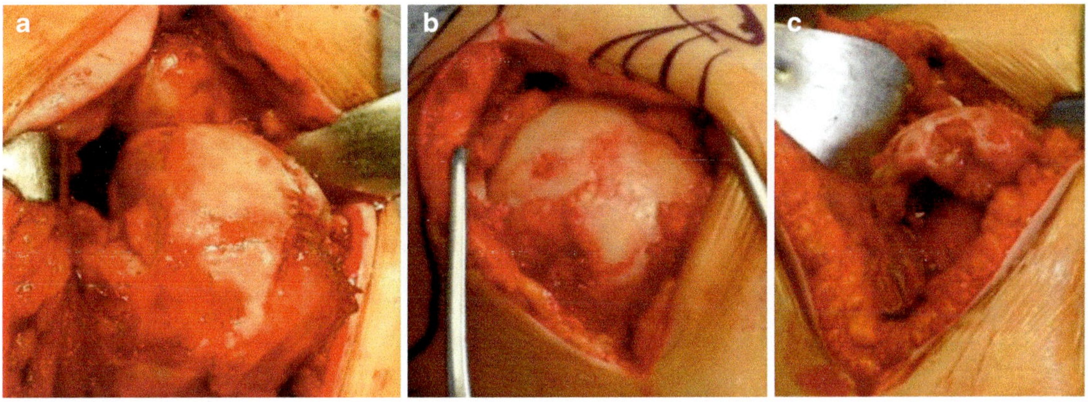

Fig. 7.2 (**a–c**) The deterioration of the articular cartilage is a direct result of abnormal physical stresses imparted to the humeral head, leading to erosion of the upper portion of the humeral head

concavity-compression mechanism which ultimately result in altered glenohumeral joint biomechanics [28–30]. In a study on eight cadaver shoulders performed by Ho et al. in 2011 [31], it was noted that biomechanical alterations in the shoulder develop after a full-thickness supraspinatus tear and at least 50% of the infraspinatus.

Neer, in 1983, also described the nutritional theory that, in association with alteration of the shoulder joint kinematic due to the massive full-thickness rotator cuff tear, leads to the development of the cuff tear arthropathy. The defect of the rotator cuff results in the loss of normal negative pressure within the joint space and the consequent spread of the synovial fluid in the surrounding tissues with loss of regular nutrition of articular cartilaginous surfaces. The defect of the rotator cuff also involves the reduction of joint movement and function, resulting in biochemical alteration of the synovial fluid and glycosaminoglycan content of cartilage, osteoporosis, cartilage atrophy and subchondral collapse (Fig. 7.5a, b), and the development of arthropathy cuff tear.

Collins and Harryman in 1997 [32] have suggested the combination of mechanical, nutritional, and biological concepts. The repeated

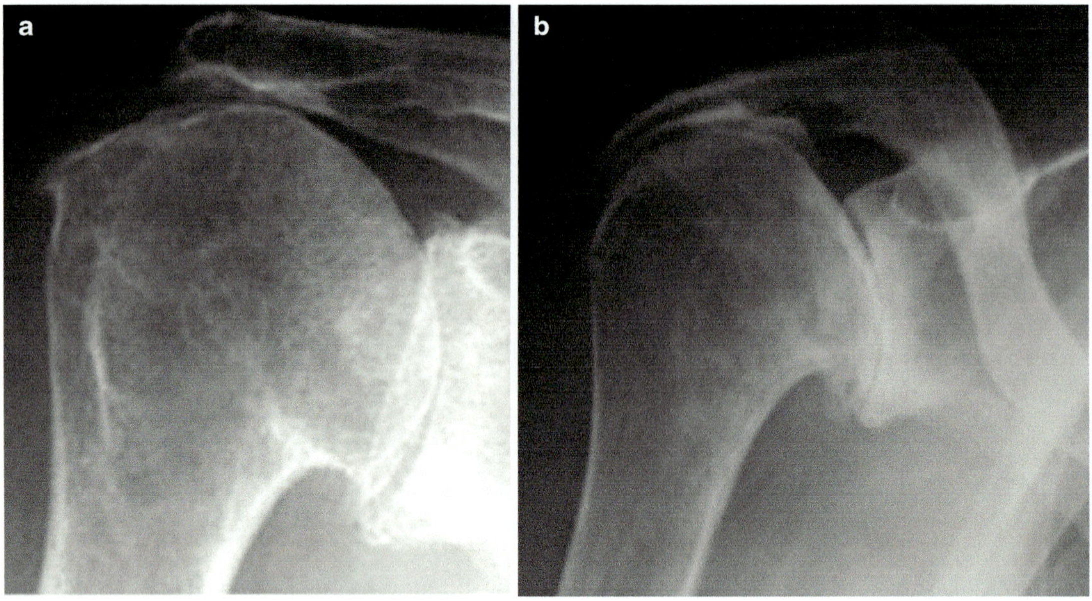

Fig. 7.3 (**a**, **b**) Erosion of the superior glenoid fossa and undersurface of the acromion

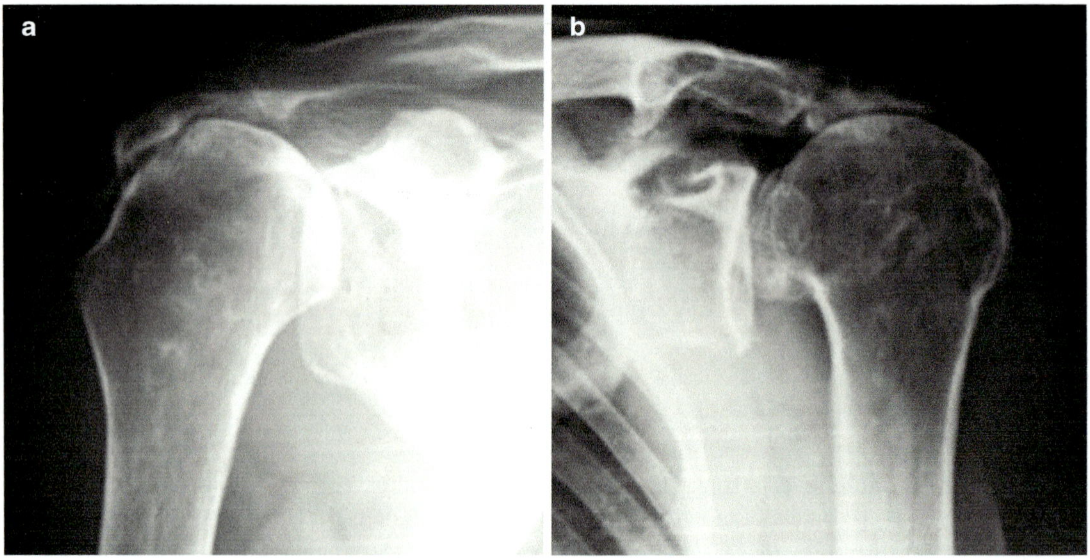

Fig. 7.4 (**a**, **b**) Erosion of the acromion and acromioclavicular joint

microtrauma created by the humeral head resting on the acromion leads to a fragmentation of the cartilage and particulate debris. Something that not only induces an enzymatic response, always associated with the pain and loss of movement, but also leads to further damage to the articular cartilage surface.

Nutrition theory has been questioned by some studies showing an increase in cartilage matrix metalloproteinase and both the correlation between the cytokine concentration and catabolic enzymes and the deterioration of articular cartilage after a massive rotator cuff tear [33–35].

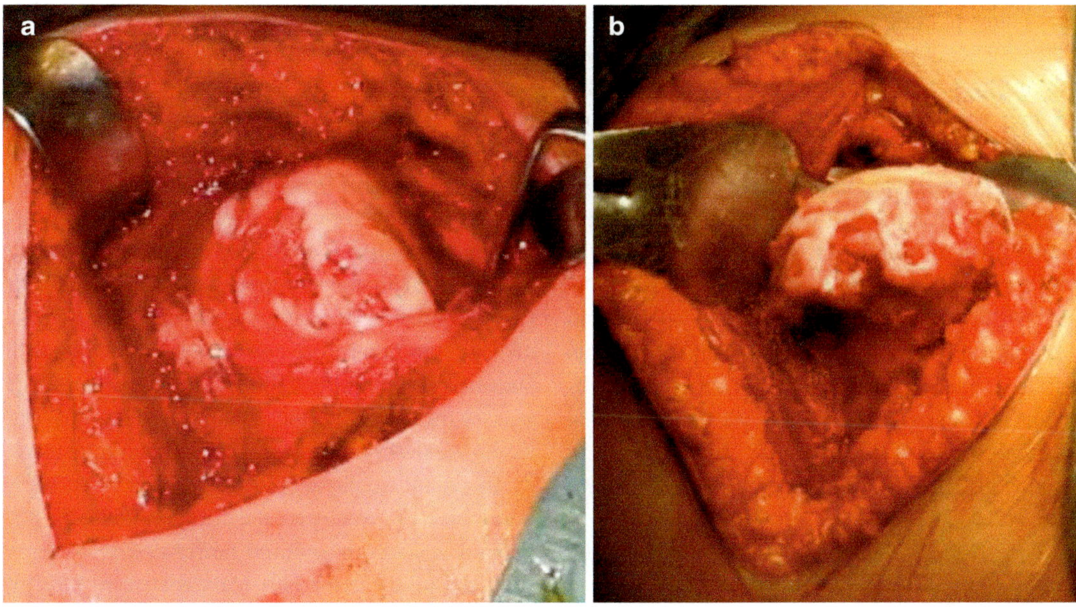

Fig. 7.5 (**a**, **b**) Cartilage atrophy and subchondral collapse of the humeral head

Kramer et al. in 2013 [36] performed a histological study on the shoulder joint cartilage of two rat groups, one with an induced rotator cuff tear and another with suprascapular nerve injury and intact rotator cuff. The results obtained over time have shown that cartilage deterioration was similar in the two groups. It must have been thought that perhaps the wear of the cartilage was due to the loss of balance of the mechanical forces acting on the glenohumeral joint.

Literature data [37, 38] indicates that rotator cuff injuries increase with age progression and that the percentage evolves from an average of 10.7% between the ages of 50 and 59 to 36.6% in the age from 80 to 89 years, with no significant differences between male and female subject [39]. Already Tempelhof et al. [40] in an ultrasound study published in 1999 highlighted the prevalence of 51% of full-thickness rotator cuff tears in asymptomatic patients over the age of 80 years.

However, a recent study published in 2016 [41] on the ultrasound examination of 486 volunteers showed contrasting results, with a prevalence of 11.1% of full-thickness rotator cuff tears in asymptomatic patients over the age of 70 years.

From the literature we gather that a rotator cuff tear, not subjected to surgical repair, though asymptomatic, can evolve toward a massive tear [42–45].

In a recent study published in 2017 [46], 69 patients were evaluated, of whom 45 with partial-thickness tears (PTT) and 24 with full-thickness tears (FTT), undergoing acromioplasty without tendon repair. It has been observed in a 22-year long-term evaluation that 74% of patients with FTT had developed X-ray cuff tear arthropathy >2° according to the Hamada classification and 87% had increased the tear size with ultrasonic examination. These authors stated that patients with full-thickness cuff tear and undergoing acromioplasty without cuff repair have, after 22 years, a high frequency of tear progression and cuff tear arthropathy. They concluded that only full thickness was a significant variable.

Several authors [29, 46, 47] also analyzed risk factors such as advanced age, sex, cuff tendon and biceps tendon status, trauma, high shoulder activity and manual labor, and their possible influence on the onset of cuff tear arthropathy for the progression of the tear rotator cuff. Nevertheless, other risk factors, such as hypercholesterolemia [48], hypertension [49, 50], and smoking [51, 52], only studied to evaluate the evolutionary rotator cuff tear on a degenerative basis could also be cited for possible influences on the arthropathy cuff tear.

Neer et al. [25] reported that the arthropathy cuff tear would only develop in 4% of patients suffering from a complete tear of the rotator cuff.

It can be therefore stated that the progressive worsening of rotator cuff tear toward arthropathy is quite difficult to predict.

In a recent study [53] of 138 subjects, evaluated with 8-year radiographic and ultrasound examination, 24% of whom were control patients and 28% had partial-thickness and 49% full-thickness rotator cuff tears, it was showed that the magnitude of radiographic progression in Hamada grade is not influenced by the tear severity or enlargement. The size of rotator cuff damage alone does not seem to be associated with the development of typical alterations of the cuff tear arthropathy. Other individual, biological, or genetic factors may interfere with the natural progression to this severe and disabling pathology of the shoulder [37].

Cuff tear arthropathy is more common in elderly women [19, 29, 54–56] and dominant shoulder [55].

To explain the reason as to why arthropathy cuff tear is more common in female patients, Gumina et al. in 2017 [56] hypothesized both an autoimmune theory and a theory related to joint hyperlaxity, as the two pathological conditions are more frequent in women. In the first hypothesis, estrogens may interfere with the autoimmune mechanism seen that estrogen receptors are also present in the immune system complex. In the second theory, static stabilizers may be less effective and therefore conditions for an unstable shoulder in patients with massive rotator cuff tear. Unfortunately the available data did not allow the authors to make any valid conclusions.

In recent years, numerous studies have been conducted to investigate the etiopathogenesis, but several aspects that would better define patients with massive rotator cuff tears that may face an arthropathy still remain unknown.

Being able to identify and fully understand the risk factors related to rotator cuff disease, but above all to progression to the cuff tear arthropathy, would be crucial to implement a prevention strategy aimed at avoiding this severe disabling disease (Fig. 7.6a–d).

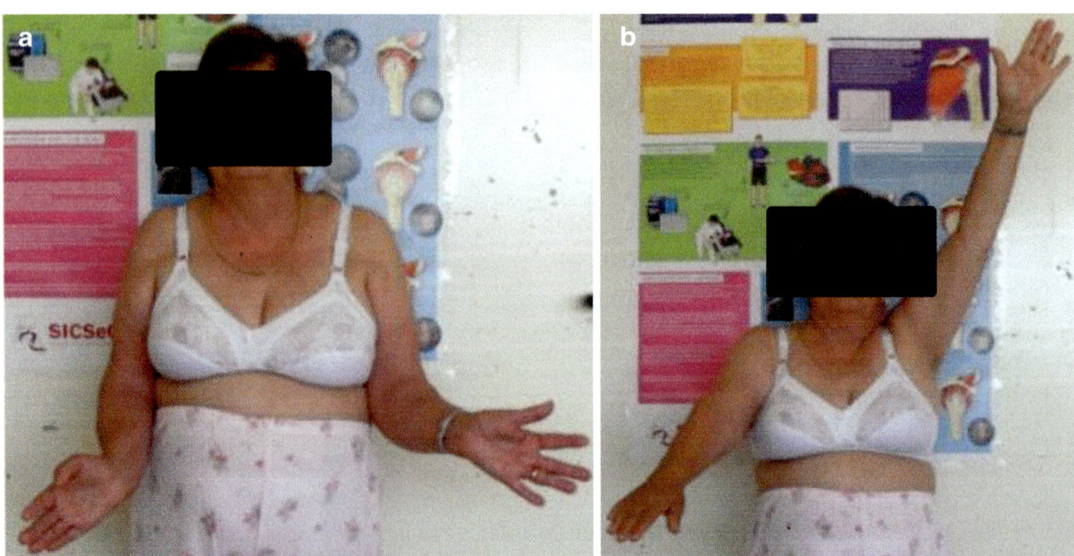

Fig. 7.6 (**a**–**d**) Active preoperative range of movement in woman patient with a cuff tear arthropathy: severe disabling disease

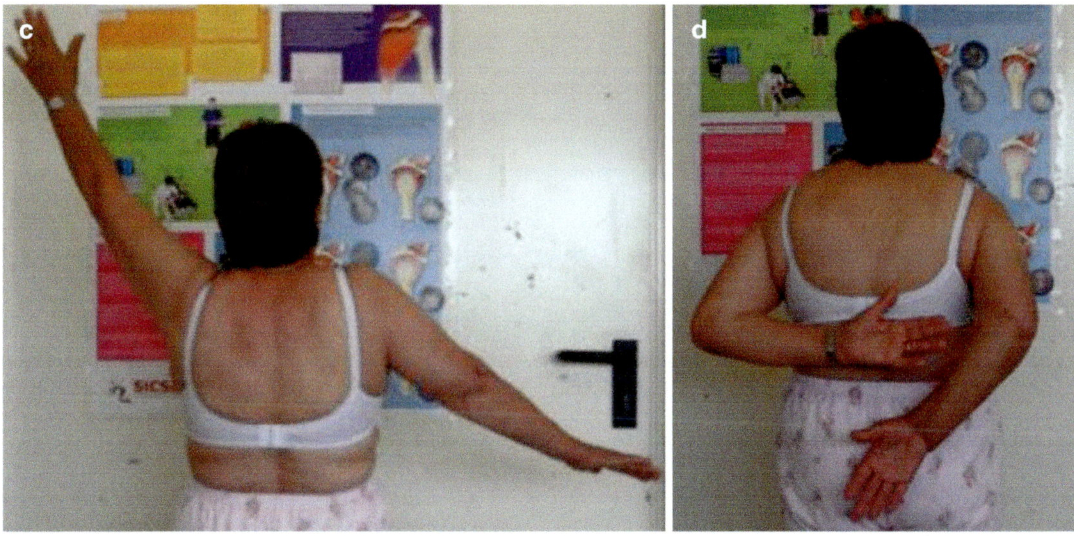

Fig. 7.6 (continued)

References

1. Smith RW. Observations upon chronic rheumatic arthritis of the shoulder (part I). Dublin Quart J Med Sci. 1853;15:1–16.
2. Smith RW. Observations upon chronic rheumatic arthritis of the shoulder (part II). Dublin Quart J Med Sci. 1853;15:343–58.
3. Adams R. A treatise on rheumatic gout or chronic rheumatic arthritis of all the joints. London: John Churchill & Sons; 1873. p. 91–175.
4. Codman E. Rupture of the supraspinatus tendon and others lesions in or about the subacromial bursa. In: Codman E, editor. The shoulder. Boston: Thomas Todd; 1934. p. 478–80.
5. Galmiche P, Deshayes P. Hemarthrose essentielle récidivante. Rev Rhumat. 1958;25:57–9.
6. Shephard E. Swelling of the subacromial bursa: a report on 16 cases. Proc R Soc Med. 1963;56:162–3.
7. Snook GA. Pigmented villonodular synovitis with bony invasion. A report of two cases. JAMA. 1963;184:424–5.
8. Burman M, Sutro C, Guariglia E. Spontaneous hemorrhage of bursae and joint in the elderly. Bull Hosp Joint Dis. 1964;25:217–39.
9. Banna A, Hume KP. Spontaneous hemarthrosis of the shoulder joint. Ann Phys Med. 1964;7:180–4.
10. Bauduin MP, Famaey JP. A propos d'un cas d'épaule sénile hémorragique. Belge Rhum Med Phys. 1969;24:135–40.
11. DeSeze S, Hubault A, Rampon S. L'épaule sénile hémorragique. L'actualité rhumatologique. Paris: Expansion Scientifique Francaise; 1967. p. 107–15.
12. Lamboley C, Bataille R, Rosenberg F, Sany J, Serre H. L'épaule sénile hémorragique. A propos de 9 observations. Rhumatologie. 1977;29:323–30.
13. Neer CS, Watson K, Stanton F. Recent experience in total shoulder replacement. J Bone Joint Surg Am. 1982;64:319–37.
14. Garancis JC, Cheung HS, Halverson PB, McCarty DJ. "Milwaukee shoulder"—association of microspheroids containing hydroxyapatite crystals, active collagenase, and neutral protease with rotator cuff defects. III. Morphologic and biochemical studies of an excised synovium showing chondromatosis. Arthritis Rheum. 1981;24:484–91.
15. Halverson PB, Cheung HS, McCarty DJ, Garancis J, Mandel N. "Milwaukee shoulder"—association of microspheroids containing hydroxyapatite crystals, active collagenase, and neutral protease with rotator cuff defects. II. Synovial fluid studies. Arthritis Rheum. 1981;24:474–83.
16. McCarty DJ, Halverson PB, Carrera GF, Brewer BJ, Kozin F. "Milwaukee shoulder"—association of microspheroids containing hydroxyapatite crystals, active collagenase, and neutral protease with rotator cuff defects. I. Clinical aspects. Arthritis Rheum. 1981;24:464–73.
17. Halverson PB, Garancis JC, McCarty DJ. Histopathological and ultrastructural studies of synovium in Milwaukee shoulder syndrome a basic

calcium phosphate crystal arthropathy. Ann Rheum Dis. 1984;43:734–41.
18. Halverson PB, Carrera GF, McCarty DJ. Milwaukee shoulder syndrome: fifteen additional cases and a description of contributing factors. Arch Intern Med. 1990;150:677–82.
19. McCarty DJ. Milwaukee shoulder syndrome. Trans Am Clin Climatol Assoc. 1991;102:271–84.
20. Cheung HS, Ryan LM. Role of crystal deposition in matrix degradation. In: Woessner FJ, Howell DS, editors. Joint cartilage degradation: basic and clinical aspects, vol. 209. New York: Marcel Dekker; 1995.
21. Zeman C, Arcand M, Cantrell J, et al. The rotator cuff deficient arthritic shoulder: diagnosis and surgical management. J Am Acad Orthop Surg. 1998;6:337–48.
22. Dieppe PA, Doherty M, Macfarlane DG, Hutton CW, Bradfield JW, Watt I. Apatite associated destructive arthritis. Br J Rheumatol. 1984;23:84–91.
23. Dieppe P, Watt I. Crystal deposition in osteoarthritis: an opportunistic event? Clin Rheum Dis. 1985;11:367–92.
24. Campion GV, McCrae F, Alwan W, Watt I, Bradfield J, Dieppe PA. Idiopathic destructive arthritis of the shoulder. Semin Arthritis Rheum. 1988;17:232–45.
25. Neer CS, Craig EV, Fukuda H. Cuff-tear arthropathy. J Bone Joint Surg Am. 1983;65:1232–44.
26. Burkhart SS. Fluoroscopic comparison of kinematic patterns in massive rotator cuff tears. A suspension bridge model. Clin Orthop Relat Res. 1992;284:144–52.
27. Hurov J. Anatomy and mechanics of the shoulder: review of current concepts. J Hand Ther. 2009;22:328–42.
28. Nam D, Maak TG, Raphael BS, et al. Rotator cuff tear arthropathy: evaluation, diagnosis, and treatment: AAOS exhibit selection. J Bone Joint Surg Am. 2012;94(6):e34.
29. Aumiller WD, Kleuser TM. Diagnosis and treatment of cuff tear arthropathy. JAAPA. 2015;28(8):33–8.
30. Eajazi A, Kussman S, LeBedis C, Guermazi A, Kompel A, Jawa A, Murakami AM. Rotator cuff tear arthropathy: pathophysiology, imaging characteristics, and treatment options. AJR. 2015;205:W502–11.
31. Oh JH, Jun BJ, McGarry MH, Lee TQ. Does a critical rotator cuff tear stage exist? A biomechanical study of rotator cuff tear progression in human cadaver shoulders. J Bone Joint Surg Am. 2011;93:2100–9.
32. Collins DN, Harryman DTI. Arthroplasty for arthritis and rotator cuff deficiency. Orthop Clin North Am. 1997;28:225–39.
33. Gotoh M, Hamada K, Yamakawa H, Nakamura M, Yamazaki H, Ueyama Y, Tamaoki N, Inoue A, Fukuda H. Perforation of rotator cuff increases interleukin 1beta production in the synovium of glenohumeral joint in rotator cuff diseases. J Rheumatol. 2000;27:2886–92.
34. Osawa T, Shinozaki T, Takagishi K. Multivariate analysis of biochemical markers in synovial fluid from the shoulder joint for diagnosis of rotator cuff tears. Rheumatol Int. 2005;25:436–41.
35. Yoshihara Y, Hamada K, Nakajima T, Fujikawa K, Fukuda H. Biochemical markers in the synovial fluid of glenohumeral joints from patients with rotator cuff tear. J Orthop Res. 2001;19:573–9.
36. Kramer EJ, Bodendorfer BM, Laron D, Wong J, Kim HT, Liu X, Feeley BT. Evaluation of cartilage degeneration in a rat model of rotator cuff tear arthropathy. J Shoulder Elbow Surg. 2013;22:1702–9.
37. Tashjian RZ. The natural history of rotator cuff disease: evidence in 2016. Tech Should Elb Surg. 2016;17(4):132–8.
38. Minagawa H, Yamamoto N, Abe H, et al. Prevalence of symptomatic and asymptomatic rotator cuff tears in the general population: from mass-screening in one village. J Orthop. 2013;10(1):8–12.
39. Gumina S, Carbone S, Campagna V, Candela V, Sacchetti FM, Giannicola G. The impact of aging on rotator cuff tear size. Musculoskelet Surg. 2013;97(Suppl 1):69–72.
40. Tempelhof S, Rupp S, Seil R. Age-related prevalence of rotator cuff tears in asymptomatic shoulders. J Shoulder Elbow Surg. 1999;8:296–9.
41. Jeong J, Shin DC, Kim TH, et al. Prevalence of asymptomatic rotator cuff tear and their related factors in the Korean population. J Shoulder Elbow Surg. 2017;26(1):30–5.
42. Ecklund KJ, Lee TQ, Tibone J, Gupta R. Rotator cuff tear arthropathy. J Am Acad Orthop Surg. 2007;15(6):340–9.
43. Lashgari C, Rediniaki D. Upper extremity. The natural history of RTC tears. Current Orthop Pract. 2012;1:10–3.
44. Moosmayer S, Tariq R, Stiris M, Smith HJ. The natural history of asymptomatic rotator cuff tears: a three-year follow-up of fifty cases. J Bone Joint Surg Am. 2013;95(14):1249–55.
45. Keener JD, Galatz LM, Teefey SA, Middleton WD, Steger-May K, Stobbs-Cucchi G, et al. A prospective evaluation of survivorship of asymptomatic degenerative rotator cuff tears. J Bone Joint Surg Am. 2015;97:89–98.
46. Ranebo MC, Björnsson Hallgren HB, Norlin R, Adolfsson LE. Clinical and structural outcome 22 years after acromioplasty without tendon repair in patients with subacromial pain and cuff tears. J Shoulder Elbow Surg. 2017;26:1262–70.
47. Schmidt CC, Jarrett CJ, Brown BT. Management of rotator cuff tears. J Hand Surg Am. 2015;40:399–408.
48. Abboud JA, Kim JS. The effect of hypercholesterolemia on rotator cuff disease. Clin Orthop Relat Res. 2010;468:1493–7.
49. Gumina S, Arceri V, Carbone S, Albino P, Passaretti D, Campagna V, et al. The association between arterial hypertension and rotator cuff tear: the influence on rotator cuff tear sizes. J Shoulder Elbow Surg. 2013;22:229–32.
50. Djerbi I, Chammas M, Mirous MP, Lazerges C, Coulet B. Impact of cardiovascular risk factor on the

prevalence and severity of symptomatic full-thickness rotator cuff tears. Orthop Traumatol Surg Res. 2015;101(6 Suppl):S269–73.
51. Kane SM, Dave A, Haque A, Langston K. The incidence of rotator cuff disease in smoking and non-smoking patients: a cadaveric study. Orthopedics. 2006;29(4):363–6.
52. Carbone S, Gumina S, Arceri V, Campagna V, Fagnani C, Postacchini F. The impact of preoperative smoking habit on rotator cuff tear: cigarette smoking influences rotator cuff tear sizes. J Shoulder Elbow Surg. 2012;21:56–60.
53. Chalmers PN, Salazar DH, Steger-May K, Chamberlain AM, Stobbs-Cucchi G, Yamaguchi K, Keener D, D J. Radiographic progression of arthritic changes in shoulders with degenerative rotator cuff tears. J Shoulder Elbow Surg. 2016;25(11):1749–55.
54. Samitier G, Alentorn-Geli E, Torrens C, Wright TW. Reverse shoulder arthroplasty. Part 1: systematic review of clinical and functional outcomes. Int J Shoulder Surg. 2015;9:24–31.
55. Jensen KL, Williams GR Jr, Russell IJ, Rockwood CA Jr. Rotator cuff tear arthropathy. J Bone Joint Surg Am. 1999;81(9):1312–24.
56. Gumina S, Candela V. Rotator cuff arthropathy. What is it? In: Gumina S, editor. Rotator cuff tear, pathogenesis, evaluation and treatment. New York: Springer; 2017. p. 383–90.

8 Rotator Cuff Tear Arthropathy: Clinical Evaluation

Alessandro Marinelli, Marco Cavallo, Alice Ritali, and Roberto Rotini

Rotator cuff tear arthropathy (RCTA) includes a wide spectrum of clinical signs and symptoms caused by the contemporary presence of three main features: rotator cuff insufficiency, degenerative changes of the glenohumeral joint, and superior migration of the humeral head. Consequently, the severity of the symptoms complained by the patients can be different, depending on the severity of the glenohumeral joint arthritis, the possible compensation of the residual rotator cuff tendons and deltoid muscle, the severity of the joint effusion, and finally the pain. In end-stage arthropathy, RCTA can be severely painful and debilitating, affecting the shoulder function and the patient's quality of life. Patients with rotator cuff tear arthropathy are typically elderly, usually in their 70s, more commonly female with the dominant side involved. Bilateral RCTA involvement is reported up to 60% of the cases [1].

Medical History: For a complete clinical examination, it is important to collect a complete record of the patient, investigating the past medical history and the current general conditions. Age, comorbidities, medical therapy, previous surgeries, occupation, activity level, and functional requests are essential for addressing the treatment. Regarding the shoulder, the past medical history must consider all the previous attempted treatments that most of the times include multiple corticosteroid injections and previous surgeries, like acromioplasty or rotator cuff repair.

Patients affected by RCTA typically complain a long-standing pain (often worse at night and increasing with shoulder activity), progressive loss of motion, and chronic joint effusion, with recurrent and painful swelling episodes.

- *Pain*: Typically, patients refer a history of progressively worsening pain, which is perceived over the lateral and posterior side of the shoulder, with arm irradiation. The pain usually worsens at night and with the use of the shoulder, improving with rest and, sometimes, with local ice application. The scale of pain can range from mild and tolerable ache, generated only by forced shoulder movement, to sharp and constant pain, severely affecting the patient's quality of life.
- *Loss of motion*: A progressive loss of motion, causing a significant limitation in activities, is typical in patients affected by RCTA. Different degrees of muscle weakness, pain, and stiffness can influence the shoulder functions. In presence of a relative stable fulcrum of motion, the deltoid is still able to elevate and abduct the arm even without the rotator cuff action, so that, thanks to the compensation performed by the deltoid muscle, some patients demonstrate

A. Marinelli (✉) · M. Cavallo · A. Ritali · R. Rotini
Shoulder and Elbow Unit, Istituto Ortopedico Rizzoli, IRCS, Bologna, Italy
e-mail: alessandro.marinelli@ior.it

S. Gumina et al. (eds.), *Reverse Shoulder Arthroplasty*,
https://doi.org/10.1007/978-3-319-97743-0_8

an acceptable range of active shoulder motion [2]. Others, the majority, will show a pseudoparalysis, consisting in a complete inability to actively move the shoulder: attempting to abduct and forward flex the shoulder, a superior migration of the humeral head is easily noticed. Deficiencies in the active range of motion are also evident in external rotation, where the deltoid compensation possibilities are even lower.

- *Joint effusion*: Most of the patients report chronic shoulder swelling, with episodes of recurrent worsening, often associated to pain increase and function decrease (Fig. 8.1).

Physical Examination: A comprehensive systemic examination, including bilateral entire upper extremities and cervical region evaluation, should be undertaken. It is mandatory to investigate associated cervical disorders on patient's complains.

Initially the patient should be visited in a sitting position over the examination table. Both shoulders, back, and neck, both front and back sides, should be undressed and accessible for clinician's inspection. Many preliminary information can be obtained by observing the patient taking off his/her clothes: difficulties, compensation movement, functionality of the contralateral shoulder, and pain.

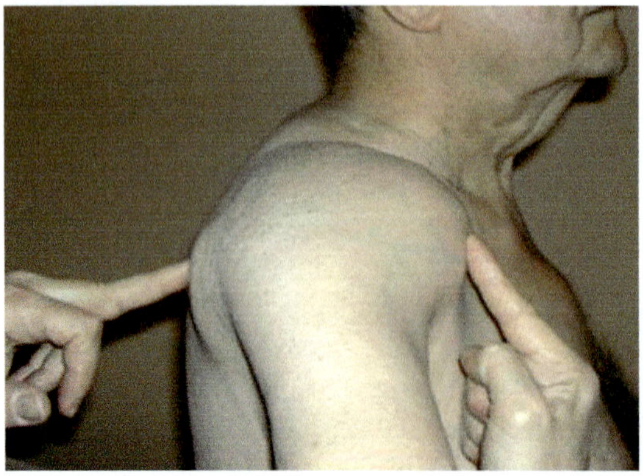

Fig. 8.1 Shoulder swelling, caused by synovial and/or hemorrhagic joint effusion

- *Inspection*: The initial physical examination starts with the inspection, focused on the shoulder and the scapular region. Typically, in patients affected by RCTA, it is possible to detect the following:
  - Shoulder swelling (Fig. 8.1).
  - Muscular atrophy of the supraspinatus and infraspinatus.
  - A "Popeye" biceps sign can be present, in cases when the long head of the biceps is already spontaneously ruptured. This sign is more evident in skinny patients where the biceps muscle is covered by a thin layer of subcutaneous fat.
  - A geyser sign: in case of a long-standing massive rotator cuff tear and advanced degenerative change of the shoulder, the glenohumeral joint fluid can herniate superiorly through the acromioclavicular (AC) interval, causing a subcutaneous pseudotumor, causing both symptoms and cosmetic impairment to the patient (Fig. 8.2).
- Palpation: By palpation, the perception of fluid collection around the shoulder joint can be easily confirmed (Fig. 8.1).
- During passive rotational movements of the shoulder, palpable crepitation is easily perceived. Tenderness and pain at the level of the long head of the biceps (if present and not already torn) are easily evoked, expression of a synovitis of the tendon sheet. Pain and contracture at the level of the trapezius muscle are frequently associated.
- *Motion*: Both active and passive glenohumeral range of motion should be assessed. A patient with cuff tear arthropathy may present varying degrees of active range of motion: if the glenohumeral fulcrum is compensated by a preserved deltoid muscle, a functional movement can be preserved. However, in the majority of severe cases, a pseudoparalysis, in abduction and forward flexion, is present. In these cases, the attempt of active shoulder abduction or elevation reveals the typical superior subluxation or escape [1, 3–7] of the humeral head (Fig. 8.3).

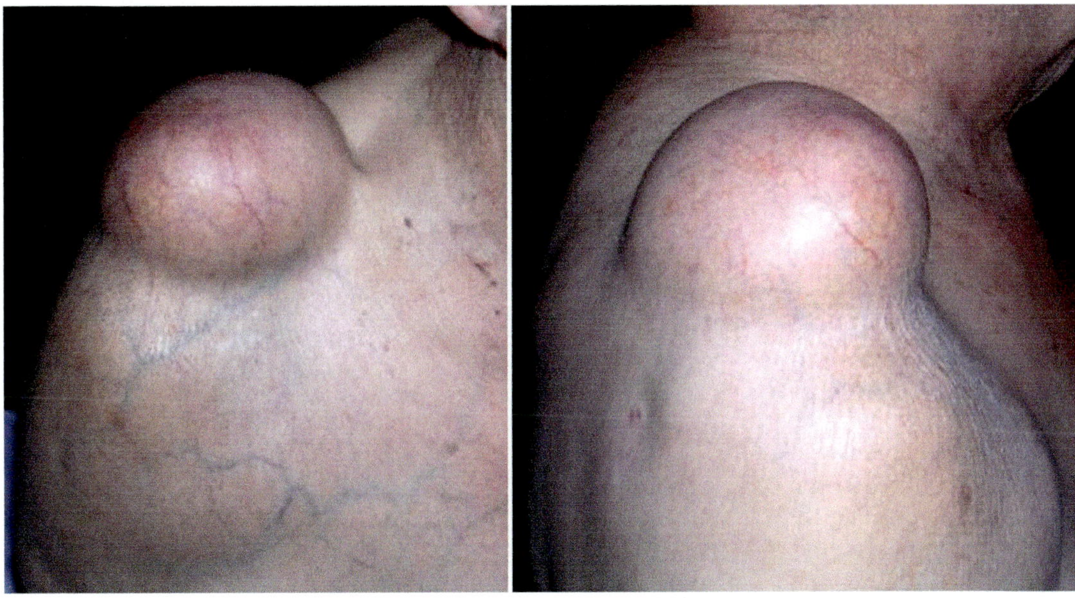

Fig. 8.2 Geyser sign above the AC joint. It is a pseudotumor caused by the synovial fluid passing from the glenohumeral to the AC joint that creates a one-way valve mechanism, entrapping the liquid in the soft tissues in the upper part of the shoulder

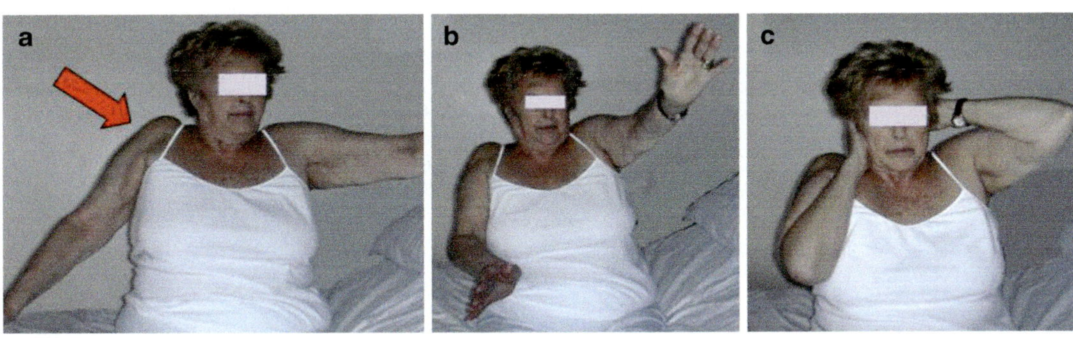

Fig. 8.3 A pseudoparalysis of the right shoulder is shown. (**a**, **b**) Typical anterior escape of the humeral head during active abduction and elevation attempt; (**c**) significant external rotation deficiency

- In case of concomitant severe subscapularis tendon, the escape of the humeral head from the glenoid fossa is frankly anterosuperior.
- After active shoulder movement evaluation, it is important to inspect the passive range of motion, to evaluate the severity of the shoulder stiffness. To reduce the possible spine compensation movements, the passive ROM examination can be better performed with the patient in a supine position.
- *Resistive movements*: After the evaluation of the active and passive motion of the shoulder, some tests should be performed on both shoulders, in order to carefully evaluate the residual presence of any rotator cuff muscle activity and to assess the validity of the other muscles around the shoulder.
- The Jobe test allows to evaluate the posterosuperior cuff strength. It was performed by applying downward force by 90° in shoulder

abduction, internal rotation, and elbow extension: this test usually cannot be performed, because of pain and stiffness, being the majority of the patients unable to reach the 90° of abduction required.

- The Patte test evaluates the external rotation strength. It can be measured with the 0° arm adduction and 90° elbow flexion.
- External rotation lag sign: the inability to maintain the externally rotated position with the elbow leaning to the chest is a sign of severe posterior and superior rotator cuff damage. If the lesion involves also the teres minor fibers, causing a complete active external rotation deficiency, the patient is forced to abduct the shoulder to bring the hand to the mouth: this pathognomonic sign has been called the "Hornblower sign" by Walch [8].
- The Napoleon test allows to evaluate the subscapularis muscle. The lift-off test, described by Gerber to analyze the subscapularis muscle, is usually too difficult and painful to be performed in patients affected by CTA.
- It is mandatory to assess the deltoid muscle function, in order to eventually consider the reverse prosthesis replacement as a possible surgical solution.

With an accurate clinical examination, completed by the medical history and a correct imaging (X-rays, MRI, and/or CT scan), it is possible to point out all the needed elements to address the patient to the more appropriate treatment.

References

1. Funk L, Haines J, Trail I. Rotator cuff arthropathy. Curr Orthop. 2007;21:415–21.
2. Visotsky JL, Basamania C, Seebauer L, Rockwood CA, Jensen KL. Cuff tear arthropathy: pathogenesis, classification, and algorithm for treatment. J Bone Joint Surg Am. 2004;86-A(Suppl 2):35–40.
3. Aumiller WD, Kleuser TM. Diagnosis and treatment of cuff tear arthropathy. JAAPA. 2015;28(8):33–8.
4. Jensen KL, Williams GR Jr, Russell IJ, Rockwood CA Jr. Rotator cuff tear arthropathy. J Bone Joint Surg Am. 1999;81:1312–24.
5. Ecklund KJ, Lee TQ, Tibone J, Gupta R. Rotator cuff tear arthropathy. J Am Acad Orthop Surg. 2007;15(6):340–9.
6. Feeley BT, Gallo RA, Craig EV. Cuff tear arthropathy: current trends in diagnosis and surgical management. J Shoulder Elb Surg. 2009;18(3):484–94.
7. Macaulay AA, Greiwe RM, Bigliani LU. Rotator cuff deficient arthritis of the glenohumeral joint. Clin Orthop Surg. 2010;2(4):196–202.
8. Walch G, Boulahia A, Calderone S, Robinson AH. The 'dropping' and 'hornblower's' signs in evaluation of rotator-cuff tears. J Bone Joint Surg Br. 1998;80(4):624–8.

CTA: Instrumental Evaluation

9

Domiziano Coppacchioli, Giacomo Ponte, and Tony Mangano

9.1 Standard Radiography and Ultrasound

The first cases of glenohumeral arthritis occurring with tears of the rotator cuff were described by Adams and Smith in the 1850s [1]. In 1983 Neer described a massive rotator cuff tear as the initial event in the development of degenerative arthritis, with a final spectrum of this condition ranging from superior migration of the humeral head with only regional chondromalacia to collapse of the humeral head with full-thickness cartilage defects. Neer defined this condition "cuff tear arthropathy" (CTA) and identified the diagnostic hallmarks in the superior humeral migration and diminished acromiohumeral distance, erosion of the great tuberosity ("femoralization") and of the inferior aspect of the acromion ("acetabularization"), joint space narrowing, and other arthritic changes at the glenohumeral joint [2]. All of these features have been variably considered by the historical works upon CTA, especially those dealing with the radiographic classifications, and have been widely accepted as the hallmarks not only of the diagnosis but also of the natural evolution itself of this pathology.

As the term itself suggests, however, cuff tear arthropathy is the final expression of a pathological mechanism that affects bone, cartilage, and soft tissues and therefore needs specific imaging methods for the study of such structures. All of these methods should not be exclusive but inclusive and complementary in order to give the orthopedic surgeon the few but essential structural informations he needs for a proper clinical framing.

Standard radiography (SR) still remains the most often performed imaging examination of the shoulder girdle anatomical region. The main advantages of SR are easy accessibility, low cost, panoramic view, and short time of examination. Further, the basic findings provided by radiography are well known and familiar both to radiologists and clinicians.

For these reasons, SR should always be the first technique to be used and especially if a CTA is suspected; a simple projection (if properly performed!) allows to obtain most of the necessary informations, through direct and indirect signs of pathology: the anteroposterior (AP) tangential view.

When obtaining an AP tangential view (Fig. 9.1), the X-ray beam is directed tangential to the glenohumeral joint and to the subacromial

D. Coppacchioli
Department of Orthopaedics and Traumatology, Ospedale San Giuseppe, Empoli, FI, Italy

G. Ponte
Unit of Radiodiagnostic, GruppoMed, Genoa, Italy

T. Mangano (✉)
Department of Orthopaedics and Traumatology, Casa di Cura Villa Igea, Acqui Terme, AL, Italy

Unit of Shoulder and Elbow Surgery, Ospedale Humanitas—San Pio X, Milan, Italy

S. Gumina et al. (eds.), *Reverse Shoulder Arthroplasty*, https://doi.org/10.1007/978-3-319-97743-0_9

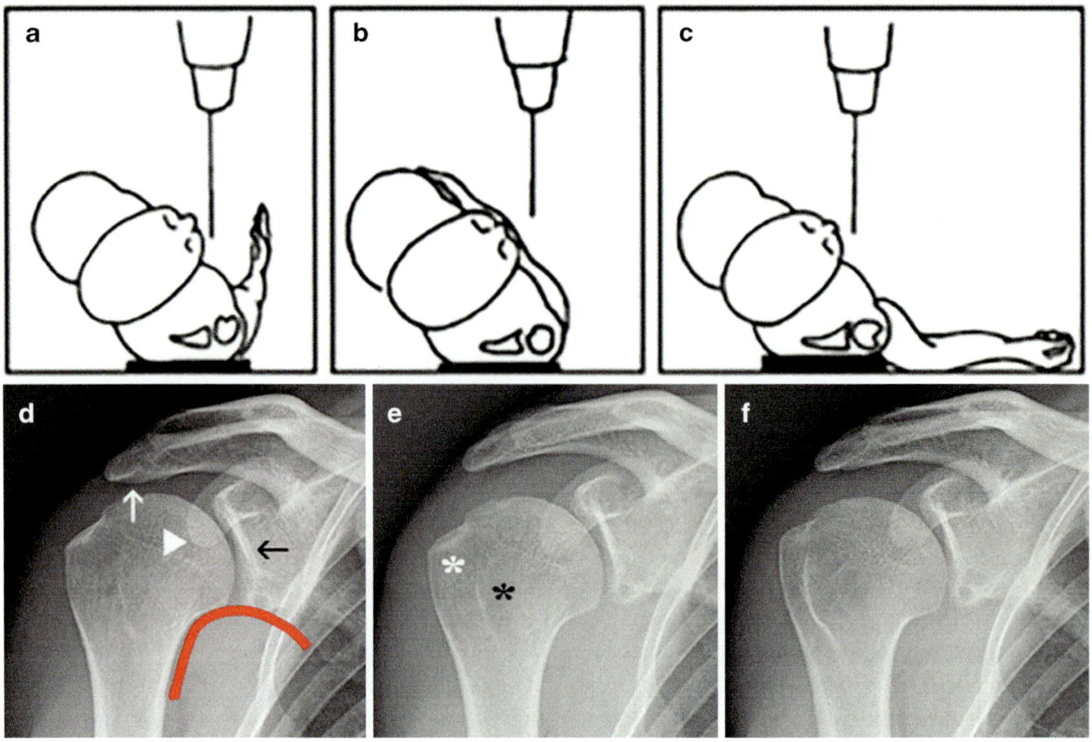

Fig. 9.1 AP tangential view and examination technique with corresponding radiographs. Radiographs obtained with (**a–d**) internal, (**b–e**) neutral, and (**c–f**) external rotation of the arm. The views allow optimal assessment of the glenohumeral joint and the subacromial space. Note superposition of the anterior and posterior glenoid rim (*black arrow*) and the sharply defined cortical line corresponding to the inferior surface of the acromion (*white arrow*). The *gothic arc* is indicated with the red line in d. The coracoid process overly the medial aspect of the humeral head (*arrowhead*). The different rotations of the arm lead to *en face* and *en profile* view of the greater tuberosity (*white asterisk*) and lesser tuberosity (*black asterisk*). (Modified from "Imaging of the Shoulder—Techniques and Applications," Springer Ed., Chap. 1: Shoulder Radiology, Bianchi S. et al. With permission from the authors)

space. The patient is standing in a 40° posterior oblique position with the shoulder to be examined in contact with the examining table. In this position the scapula lies parallel to the cassette and allows an optimal tangential view of the glenohumeral joint. The articular surface of the glenoid cavity is seen from a lateral sight and, in normal conditions, no overlap of the glenoid cavity and humeral head is observed. Additional craniocaudal angulation (10–20°) of the beam leads to excellent visualization of the subacromial space. Since the orientation of the scapula, as well as the obliquity of the acromial arch, can vary between patients, fluoroscopic control can be used to achieve accurate positioning of the patient and correct tilting of the X-ray beam. Three radiographs are obtained with the arm in different rotations (neutral, internal, and external). After each rotation of the humerus, the obliquity of the patient, as well as the correct visualization of the subacromial space, must be checked since changes in the rotation of the arm are frequently associated with changes in the position of the patient. The coracoid process overlies the medial aspect of the humeral head. Due to the tangential orientation of the beam, the inferior surface of the acromion appears as a regular cortical line, and the anterior and posterior rims of the glenoid fossa are superimposed. The glenohumeral joint space width can be accurately evaluated and reflects the thickness of both the humeral and glenoid cartilages (Fig. 9.1).

Finally, this radiological projection allows the evaluation of the glenohumeral joint congruency by measuring the distance between the limiters, inversely proportional to the cartilage wear condition, by analyzing the *gothic arch* continuity (Fig. 9.1d, red line), and by directly evaluating the state of the articular bony limiters (sclerosis, erosions, etc.). Through the careful study of this single X-ray projection, we can therefore define the arthropathy degree and severity.

Several classification systems based on standard radiography have been developed to define the bone changes that occur in CTA and its evolution as well. Although the main features of these systems often overlap, each system focuses on a different set of findings associated with the disorder. The classification schemes of Visotzky-Seebauer [3] and Hamada-Fukuda [4] respect both the glenoid and the humerus and have been recommended as highly reliable [5].

The Visotzky-Seebauer classification system separates CTA into four distinct types: IA, IB, IIA, and IIB. Each type is characterized by a massive rotator cuff tear, a distinctive level of joint instability, humeral head translation, and articular surface erosion. This classification system is a biomechanical description of CTA, in which each subtype is distinguished on the basis of the degree of superior migration of the humeral head from the center of rotation and the amount of instability. The extent of decentralization seen on radiographs depends on the size of the rotator cuff tear, the integrity of the coracoacromial arch, and the degree and direction of glenoid bone erosion (Fig. 9.2).

The Hamada classification system (Fig. 9.3) describes structural changes within the coracoacromial arch and changes in the acromiohumeral interval (AHI) on anteroposterior radiographs as the basis for classification. This system divides massive rotator cuff tears into five radiographic stages, with consecutive stages indicating disease progression. The following table shows the main features of each stage in this classification system:

Grade 1:	AHI > 6mm
Grade 2:	AHI 5 mm or less
Grade 3:	Grade 2 with acetabularization of acromion (concave deformity of acromion undersurface)
Grade 4A:	Glenohumeral arthritis with narrowing of glenohumeral joint, without acetabularization
Grade 4B:	Glenohumeral arthritis with narrowing of glenohumeral joint, with acetabularization
Grade 5:	Bony destruction—humeral head collapse

The AP tangential view also allows to quantify some more structural and biomechanical parameters, like the acromial index (AI) and the critical shoulder angle (CSA), useful in order to gain further predictive estimations around the shoulder [6]. The AI relies on the gleno-acromial and glenohumeral distances (Fig. 9.4) and shows a direct correlation to progression in large-to-massive rotator cuff tears. The CSA represents a morphological parameter that accounts for both glenoid inclination and lateral extension of the acromion (Fig. 9.5): larger CSA requires more rotator cuff activity to preserve joint stability. The intuitive biomechanical basis of this relationship is that the lateral extension of the acromion leads to a more vertical line of action of the deltoid and therefore promotes a trend toward a superior dislocation of the humeral head. Despite the speculative appeal of this hypothesis, however, recent studies seem to agree on noncorrelation of this parameter with tear size or tear progression [7]. On the contrary, an indirect correlation between CSA and glenohumeral osteoarthritis (OA) has been observed and confirmed [8]: the lower the value of the CSA, the greater the thickness of the rotator cuff tendons and their ability to maintain the humeral head centered in the glenoid, with relative facilitation in OA progression.

In the same way that an expert radiology technician is required to obtain, through a cost-effective and easily accessible method, a projection full of information for CTA diagnosis, similarly he must be experienced the radiologist that completes the diagnostic process through an equally inexpensive method like ultrasound (US) for the

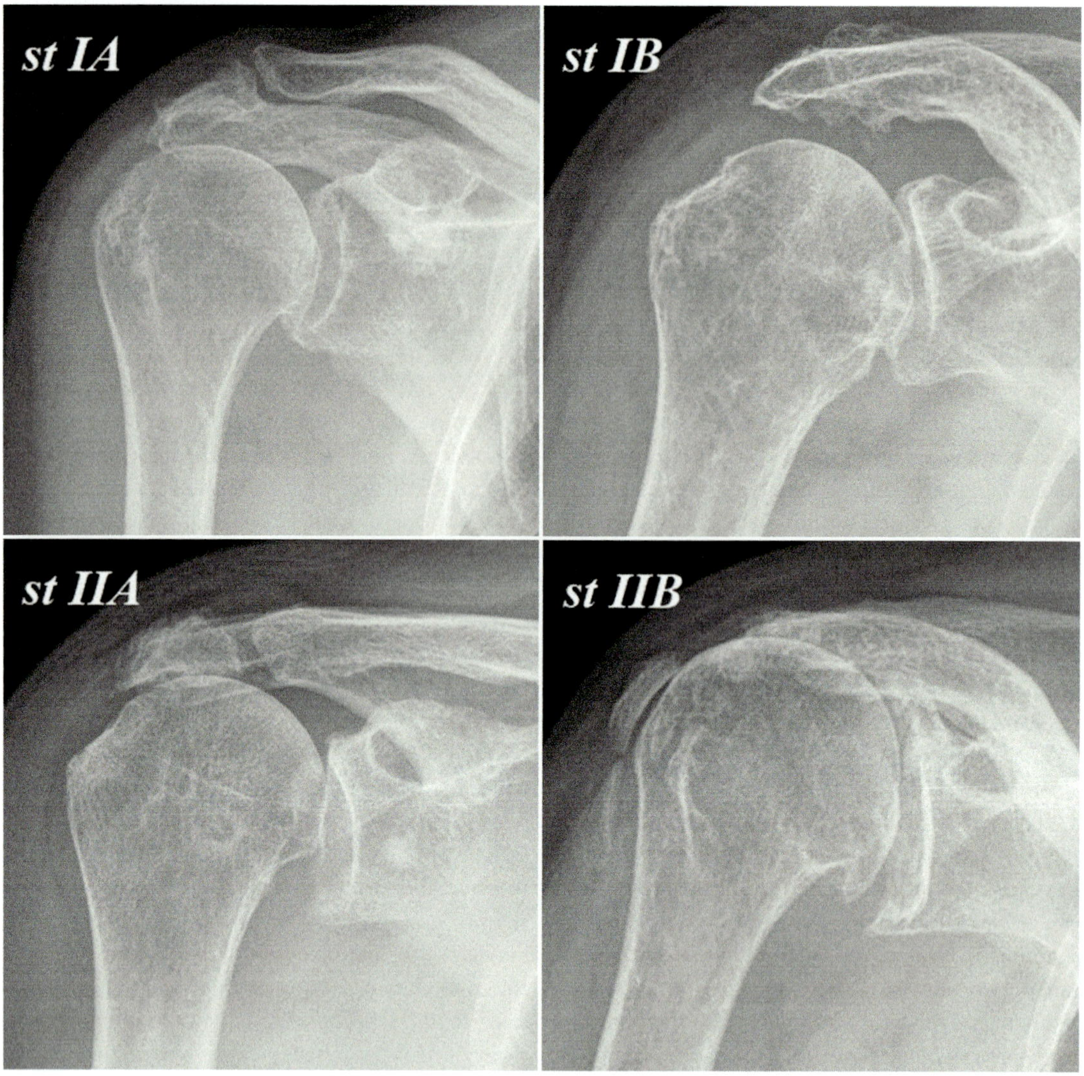

Fig. 9.2 Examples of types of rotator cuff tear arthropathy according to Visotzky-Seebauer classification system. Type IA is characterized as centered and stable. Imaging findings are intact anterior restraints, minimal superior migration, femoralization, and acetabularization. Type IB is characterized as centered and medialized. Imaging findings are intact anterior restraints, minimal superior migration, and medial erosion of glenoid bone. Type IIA is characterized as decentered, limited, and stable. Imaging findings are compromised anterior restraints, superior translation, minimal stabilization by coracoacromial arch, and superior and medial erosions of glenoid bone. Type IIB is characterized as decentered and unstable. Imaging findings are incompetent anterior structures, anterior-superior escape, and no stabilization by coracoacromial arch

study of soft tissues, always remembering that *"you look, what you know"*.

Ultrasound analysis is a cheap and easy accessibility study method, equally to SR but not involving exposure to X-rays; it allows an excellent full soft tissues study, while offering a further possibility for dynamic testing.

As shown in the images, the US method owns a high intrinsic resolution on tendon structures, allowing to accurately evaluate the fibrillary structure of the tendons of the rotator cuff (Fig. 9.6) and the acromion-humeral interval as well (Fig. 9.7). Further, it can show the eventual retraction of the myotendinous junction and the quality of the

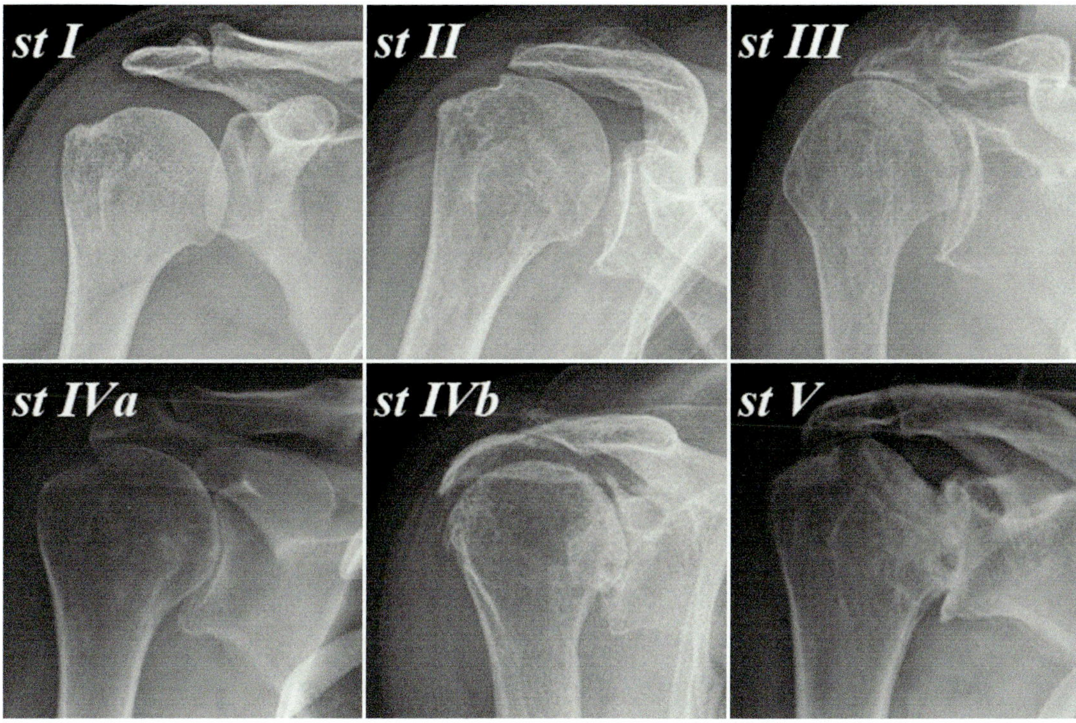

Fig. 9.3 The Hamada-Fukuda classification system. See text for description

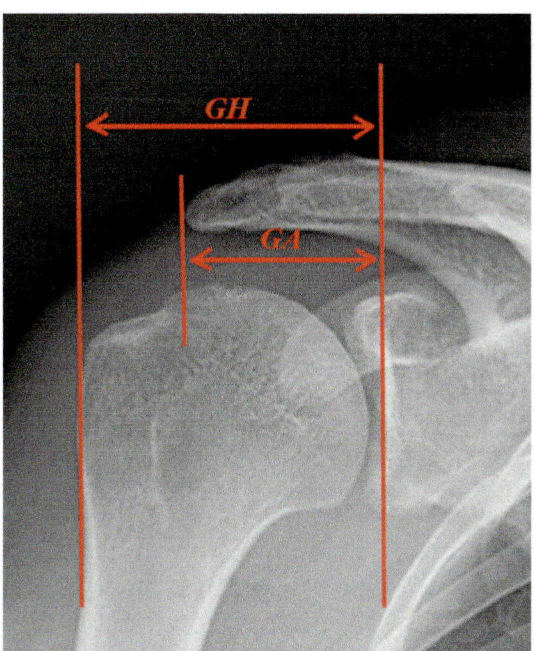

Fig. 9.4 The acromion index (AI) = GA/GH. *GA* is the gleno-acromial distance, *GH* is the glenohumeral distance. See text for description

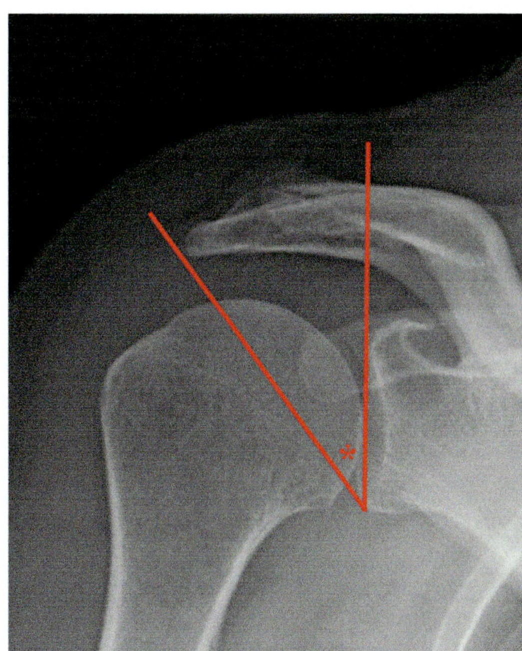

Fig. 9.5 Critical shoulder angle (CSA) (asterisk). It is a morphological parameter that accounts for both glenoid inclination and lateral extension of the acromion

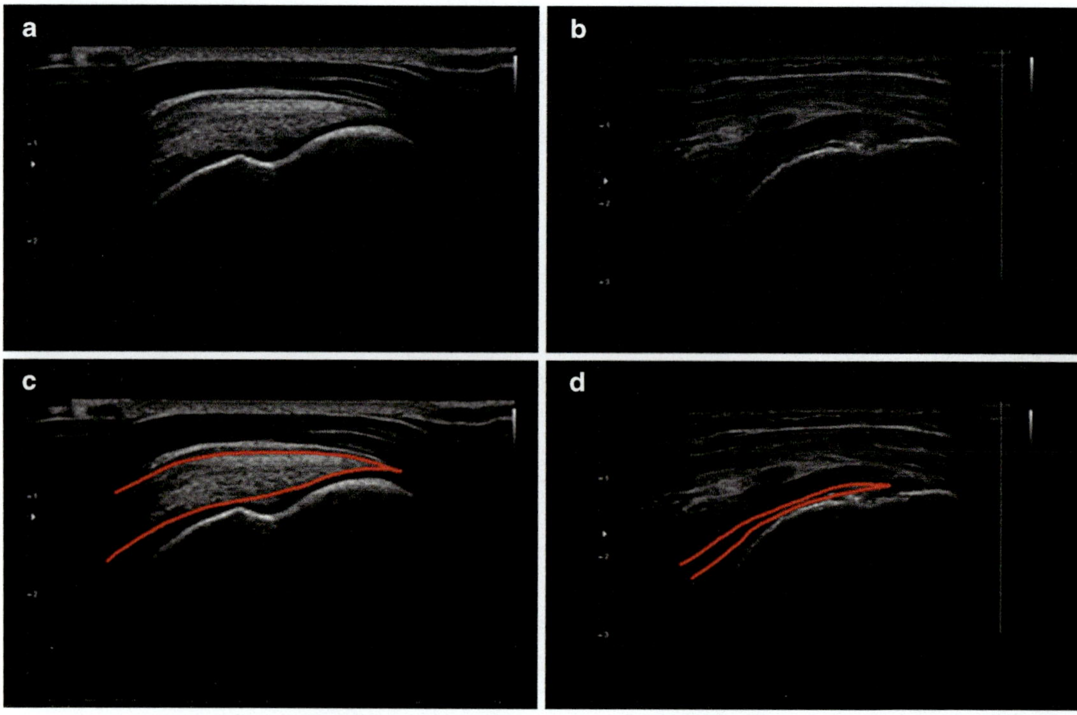

Fig. 9.6 Fibrillary structure and thickness of the supraspinatus tendon. On the left (**a**–**c**): preserved fibrillary structure and thickness of supraspinatus tendon. On the right (**b**–**d**): subtotal lesion of supraspinatus tendon with no more residual thickness

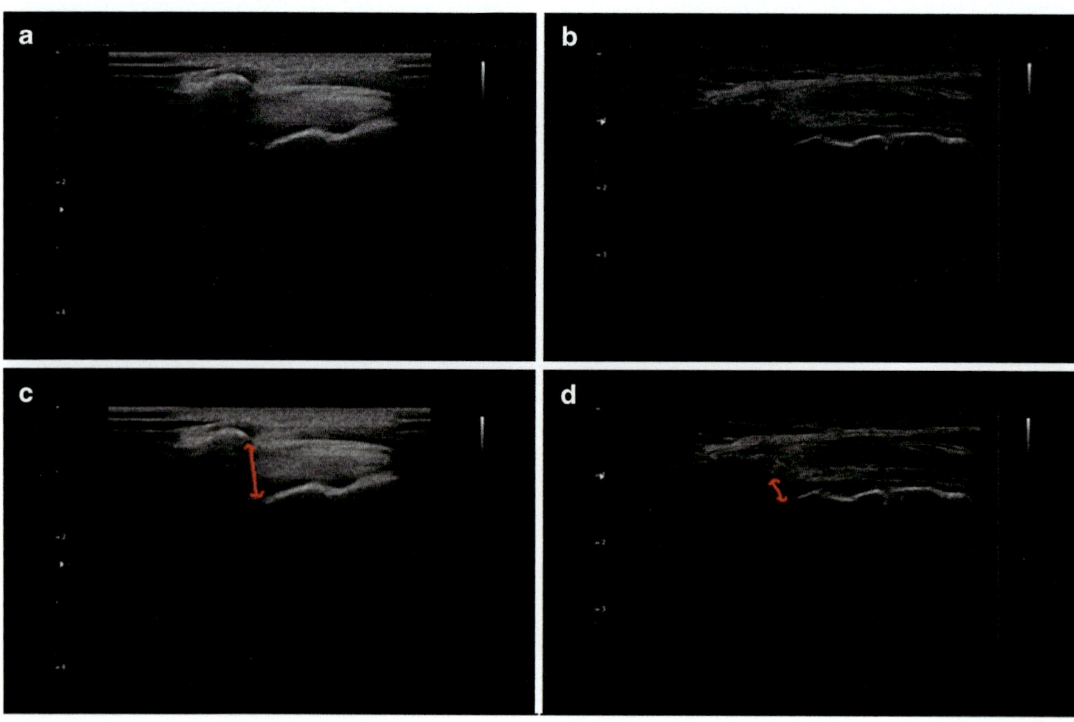

Fig. 9.7 The acromiohumeral interval as seen in US. On the left (**a**–**c**): preserved acromiohumeral interval. On the right (**b**–**d**): lower acromiohumeral interval in RCTA

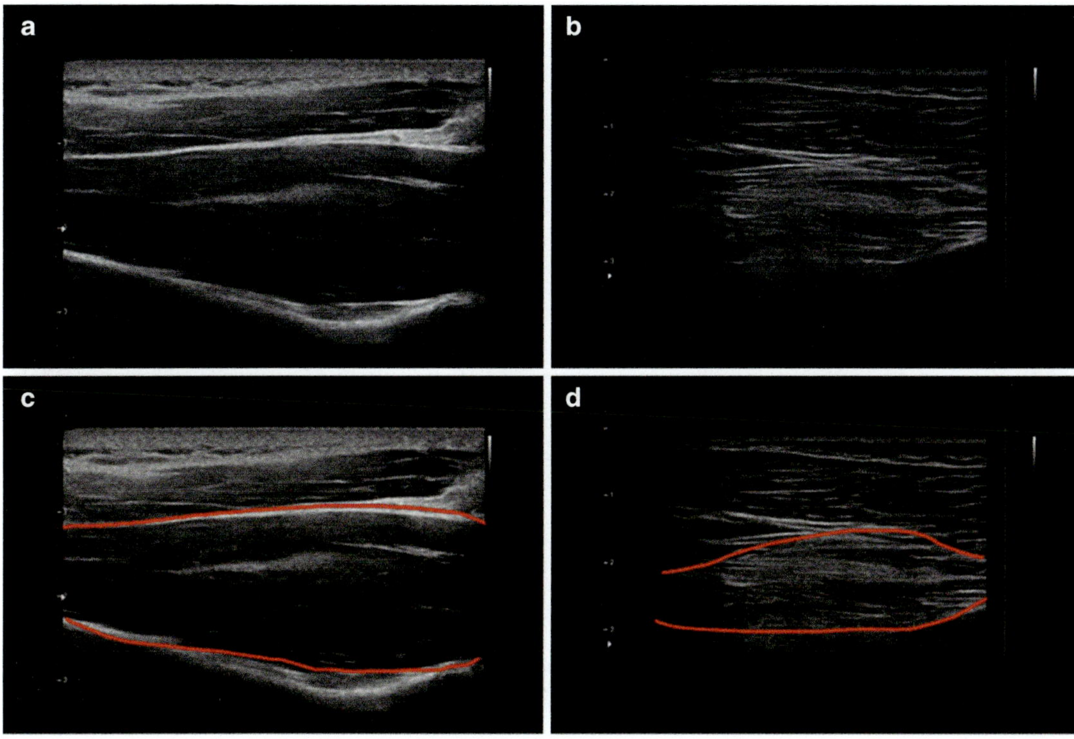

Fig. 9.8 Muscular trophism as seen in US. On the left (**a–c**): preserved muscular trophism and volume of supraspinatus. On the right (**b–d**): reduced muscular trophism with adipose infiltration (hyperechogenicity)

muscular trophic condition, with the final ability to calculate thickness and muscle volume and its eventual adipose infiltration, that progressively increases echogenicity (Figs. 9.8 and 9.9).

In the setting of the same examination, it is possible to make a dynamic study to evaluate the behavior under biomechanical stress of the same structure first examined under static conditions (the only possible study condition for other methods such as X-ray, CT, and MRI). The classic example is the long head of the biceps tendon (Fig. 9.10) [9, 10].

US can provide detailed accessory informations such as those regarding the status of the subacromial-subdeltoid (SASD) bursa and joint recesses. In particular, regarding the SASD bursa one can evaluate parietal thickness, synovial hyperplasia and hyperemia (thanks to the complementary color-Doppler module), and amount and type of contained fluid (Fig. 9.11).

US analysis combined with X-ray AP tangential view result in a perfect couple for CTA first-line diagnostic workup and framing, both for the quality/quantity of the information obtained and for the easy accessibility of these radiographic facilities, thanks to capillary territorial distribution.

9.2 Magnetic Resonance Imaging

As previously described, standard radiography and ultrasound examination should represent the first-line instrumental studies for a correct CTA diagnostic workup, together with accurate anamnestic interview and clinical examination. Despite widely diffused and often abused, *magnetic resonance imaging* (MRI) should be considered as a second-line analysis, being its true utility exerted in the surgical planning (i.e., after surgical treatment has been already identified as the next therapeutical step), and specially if a cuff tear reconstruction is hypothesized. MRI is extremely useful in soft tissue characterization and in the visualization and description of soft tissue traumatic and degenerative alterations [11]. It is then mostly indicated in

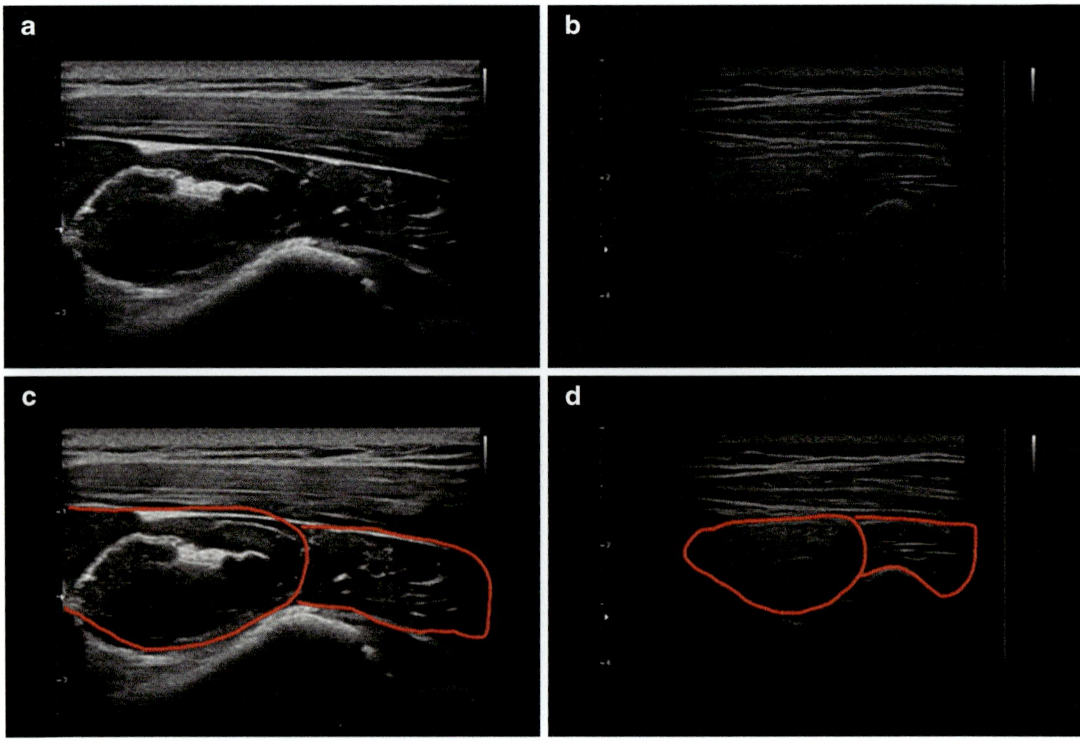

Fig. 9.9 Muscular trophism as seen in US. On the left (**a**–**c**): preserved muscular trophism and volume of infraspinatus and teres minor. On the right (**b**–**d**): reduced muscular trophism with adipose infiltration of infraspinatus, while the teres minor still shows trophic muscular features

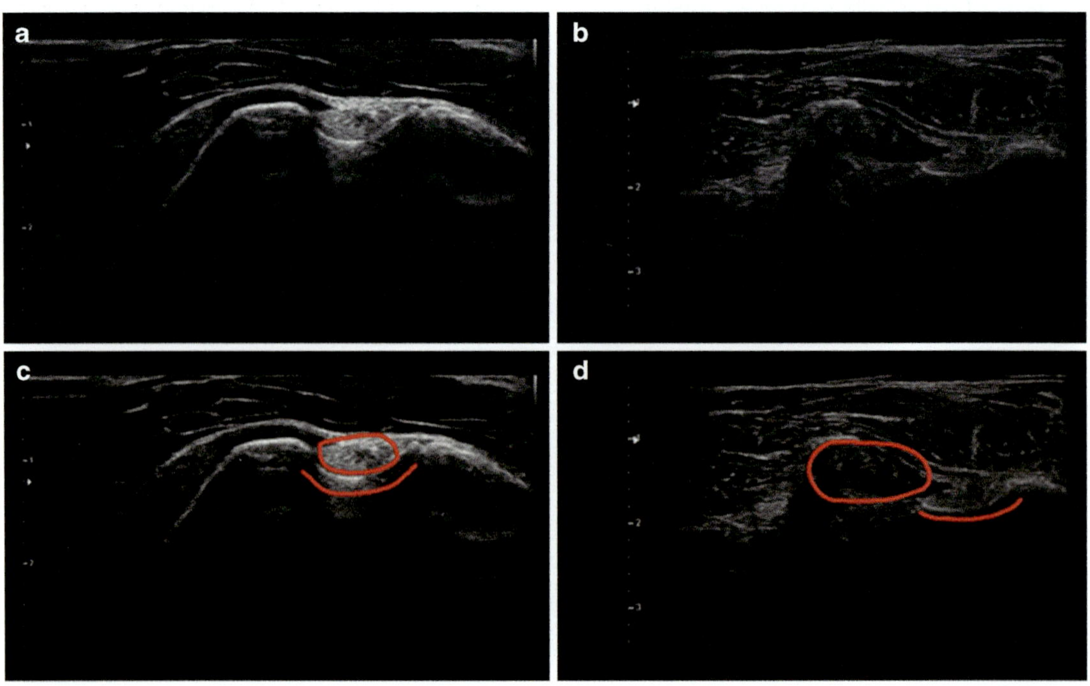

Fig. 9.10 Long head of the biceps brachii (LHBB) tendon position. On the left (**a**–**c**): LHBB maintains the physiological position and structure. On the right (**b**–**d**): LHBB presents increased volume by tendinosis and is medially dislocated behind the subscapularis tendon

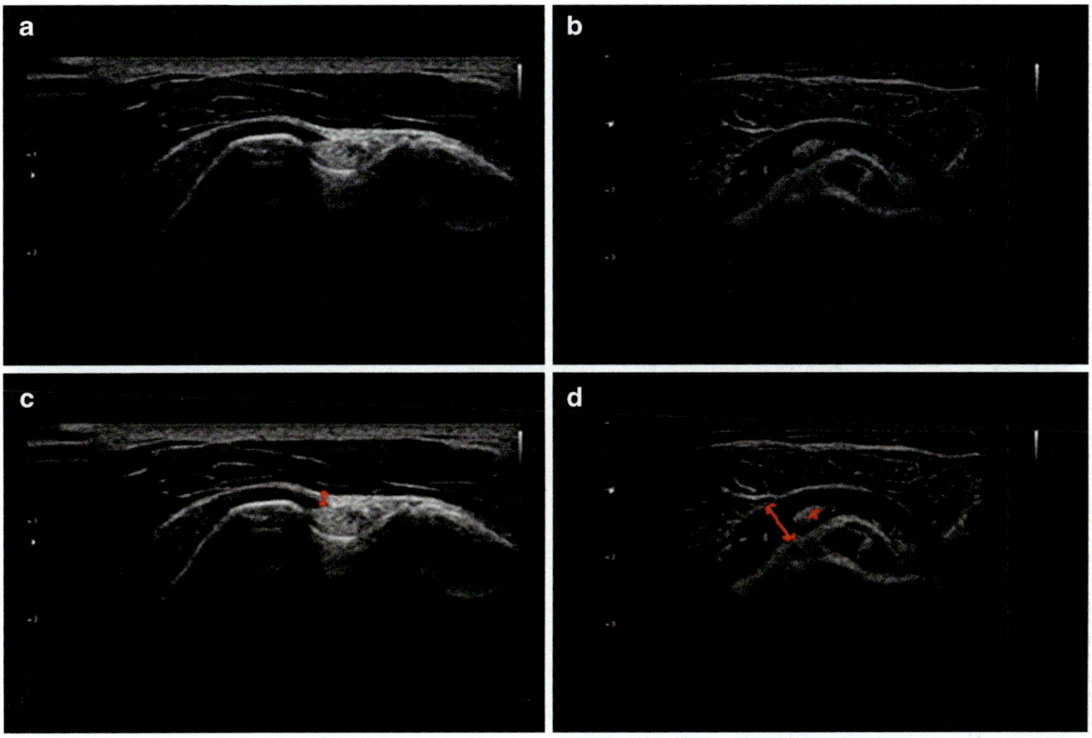

Fig. 9.11 SASD bursa status. On the left (**a–c**): no parietal thickening and no fluid content in the SASD bursa. On the right (**b–d**): parietal thickening with fluid content of SASD bursa; also visible are synovial hyperplasia nodules (*x*)

the setting of cuff tear severity definition, as well as in the pathology of the long head of the biceps brachii (LHBB), allowing a more adequate choice of the correct surgical treatment [12, 13]. On the contrary, magnetic resonance arthrography (MRA) represents a useful examination for partial thickness tears of the rotator cuff, and shoulder instability as well, very important pathologies in terms of incidence and prevalence in the general population, but not related to CTA and not included in the present work.

The shoulder MRI exam generally involves a three-spatial-planes study (Fig. 9.12). In the axial plane, perpendicular to the glenoid fossa, the tendons and the muscle bellies of the subscapularis, infraspinatus, and teres minor are studied, and LHBB and the acromioclavicular joint as well. In the coronal oblique plane it is possible to identify and study the supraspinatus tendon and the upper part of the infraspinatus tendon, the subacromial space and bursa, and the acromioclavicular joint. Finally, in the sagittal oblique plane, parallel to the glenoid fossa, the rotator cuff insertion and eventual muscle atrophy/degeneration are studied [13]. It is currently possible the choice between high (1.5–3T)- and low (0.3–0.5T)-field MRI. The high-field MRI is generally appreciated for the more precise spatial resolution and minor rate of movement artifacts, while the low-field MRI is someway more comfortable for the patient because of the open gantry, avoiding claustrophobic reactions. If the high-field MRI is then useful for a precise anatomical study before rotator cuff surgery, a low-field MRI could often be sufficient in order to define major cuff tear and muscle degeneration in the setting of CTA (Fig. 9.13), if the scan in the sagittal plane is correctly extended to include the scapular "Y." Depending on the specific used sequences (i.e., T1 or T2 weighted, fat suppression, etc.), different anatomical structures are highlighted, with eventual alterations due to inflammatory, traumatic, or degenerative processes. Particularly in the setting of rotator cuff pathology, a rotator cuff tear is easily identified as well as the specific tendon involved, the dimensions of the tear, the retraction of the tendon, and the fatty degeneration and atrophy of the relative muscle belly.

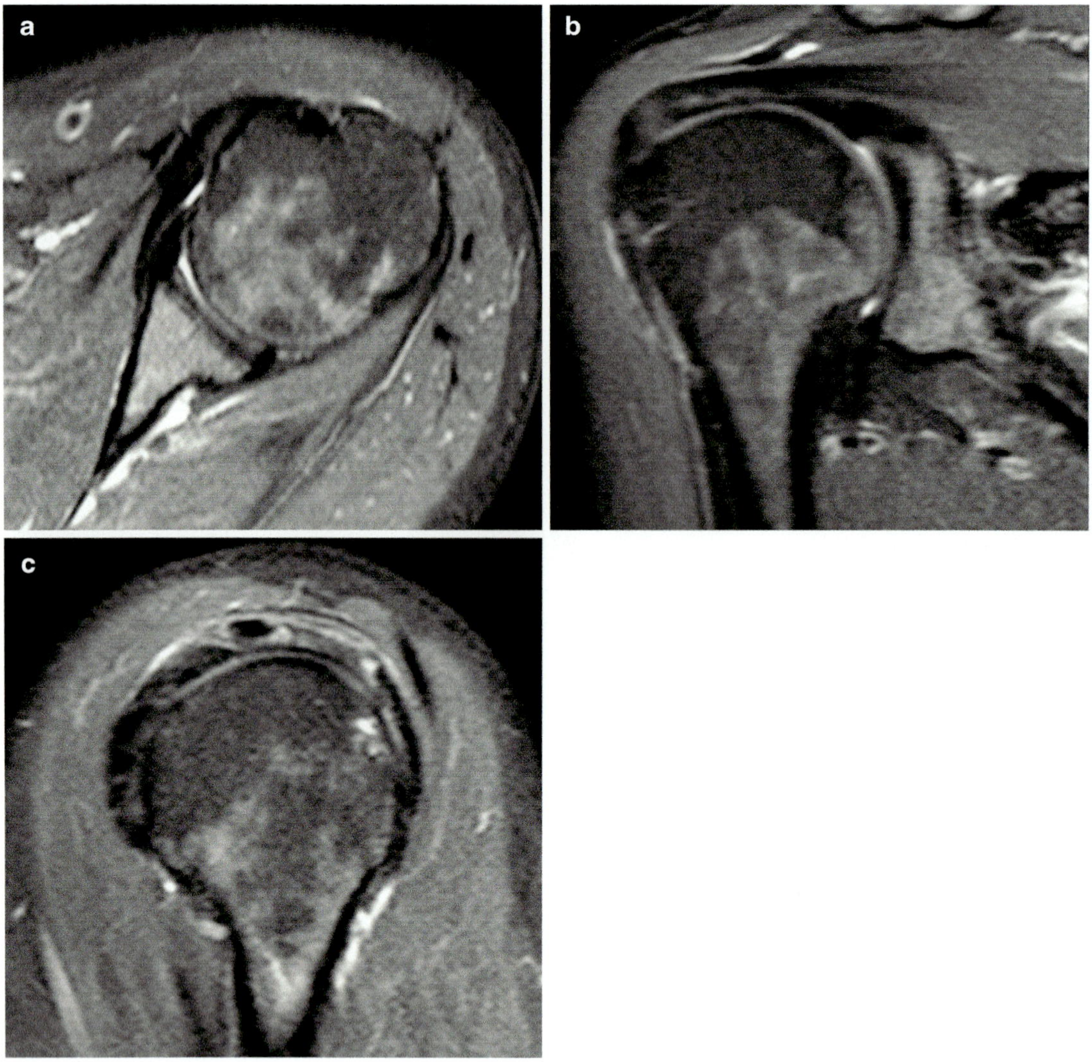

Fig. 9.12 Three spatial planes study with MRI. (**a**) Axial plane scan; (**b**) coronal plane scan; and (**c**) sagittal plane scan. See text for description

All of these are important structural features of the tear, first of all defining the reparability of the lesion and greatly influencing, then, the final surgical choice. In this sense, several classification systems have been developed, based on the morphostructural parameters of the muscles and tendons, allowing a plausible predictability on the clinical and biological results of a reconstructive surgery. Snyder developed and published in 2003 a comprehensive classification to describe the extent of the tear, the location, and the size [14]. The location of the tear is classified as *articular* (A), *bursal* (B), or *complete* (C) thickness tears. Full-thickness tears are classified as: C1, small complete tear, pinhole sized; C2, moderate tear < 2 cm of only one tendon without retraction; C3, large complete tear with an entire tendon with minimal retraction usually 3–4 cm; C4, massive rotator cuff tear involving two or more rotator cuff tendon with associated retraction and scarring of the remaining tendon. This classification system was originally described as based on arthroscopic findings; nevertheless, it can at least partially be utilized in preoperative MRI studies,

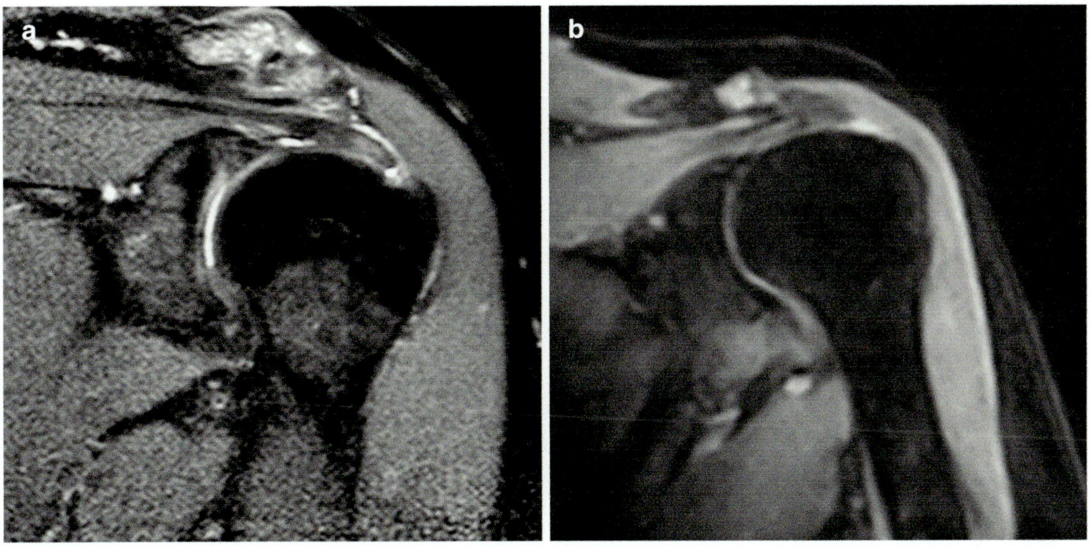

Fig. 9.13 High-field and low-field MRI. High-field MRI (**a**) and low-field MRI (**b**) coronal views of similar small tears of the supraspinatus tendon (T2-weighted sequences)

where T2-weighted sequences are mainly used, showing the bright liquid signal in substitution of the tendon signal in case of tendon tear. Despite a noncomplete interobserver agreement, this is a useful classification system giving solid information about type of surgery, technical difficulties, and prognosis [15]. Due to some intrinsic limitations of the Snyder classification, essentially involving the lack of consideration for tendon and muscle degeneration, however, a further classification system is commonly used by the authors. Goutallier introduced a classification of fatty infiltration of the supraspinatus based on the presence of fatty streaks within the muscle belly using CT images [16, 17]. Fuchs has subsequently published a similar classification using MRI, essentially based on T1-weighted sequences highlighting the fat signal [18]. In the Goutallier-Fuchs system, the grade 0 is normal muscle; grade I describes muscle with some fatty streaks; in grade II fatty infiltration is important, but there is still more muscle than fat; in grade III there is as much fat as muscle; and in grade IV more fat than muscle is present (Fig. 9.14).

If tendon retraction allows a confident evaluation of the reparability of the torn tendon itself, the muscle atrophy and fatty degeneration are equally important in order to allow some degree of predictability about the biologic healing of the repaired tendon and final functional results as well [19–21]. In summary, the higher the degree of fatty degeneration, the lower the probability of tendon healing after surgical repair. With a moderate to good interobserver agreement, the Goutallier-Fuchs score have shown a substantial prognostic utility and is often used to guide treatment. Indeed, despite a technically repairable tendon tear, the concomitance of grade II or superior Goutallier-Fuchs score represents a progressively poorer prognostic factor for surgical tendon suture. In such cases, alternative solutions should be considered, like tendon transfer or joint substitution with reverse shoulder arthroplasty, depending on patient-related factors and clinical and instrumental severity of the pathology.

9.3 Computed Tomography

With respect to MRI, the *computed tomography* (CT) analysis is generally preferred for the study of the bony component of a joint. In the shoulder district, CT reveals a great diagnostic utility in the traumatic and oncologic pathology, and in the shoulder instability chapter as well. Furthermore, in the setting of degenerative conditions such as

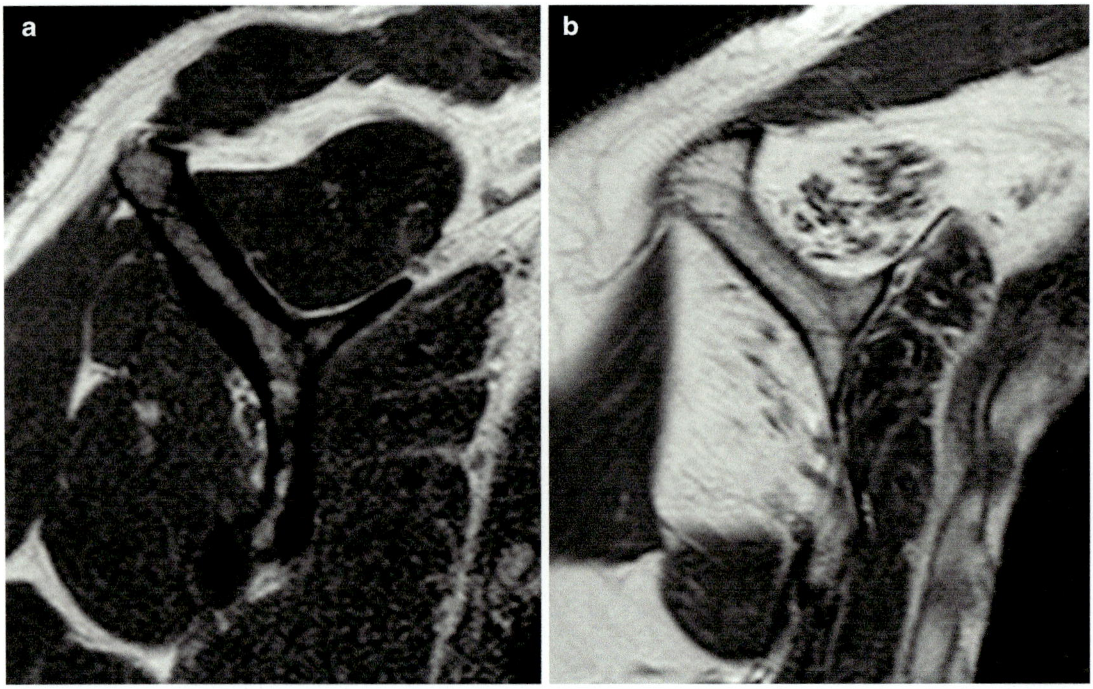

Fig. 9.14 Muscular trophism as seen in MRI. (**a**) Normal trophism of the rotator cuff muscle bellies as seen in T1-weighted sagittal view of the scapular "Y"; (**b**) severe fatty infiltration of the supraspinatus and infraspinatus bellies (Goutallier-Fuchs stage IV), with almost completely conserved trophism of subscapularis (stage I) and teres minor (stage 0)

primary osteoarthritis and CTA, CT represents a second-line exam, very useful for the precise definition of the glenoid morphology and version and for the study of the proximal humeral structure as well. Its importance is then widely accepted in the preoperative planning, essentially when a prosthetic substitution is already planned.

Despite the easy accessibility and the short time needed for the exam, CT presents some disadvantages, just like consistent exposure to ionizing radiations and low sensibility for soft tissue structures (i.e., rotator cuff, LHB).

The CT exam is conducted with the patient in supine position, with the arm at the side and shoulder in neutral rotation. A series of acquisitions is obtained from the superior margin of the clavicle down to the inferior margin of the glenoid fossa, with axial scanning perpendicular to the glenoid surface. Further image reconstructions are obtained in the coronal and sagittal planes and 3D reconstructions as well. CT scan has become the gold standard exam for studying traumatic lesions of the humerus and the glenoid, with particular importance in the setting of instability-related glenoid lesions [22]. The ability of precisely defining the glenoid bone defect drove up the CT scan to be the key examination in the decision process for shoulder surgical stabilization, allowing the correct choice between arthroscopic capsuloplasty and open or arthroscopic coracoid transposition or other bone-block procedures [23].

When dealing with degenerative shoulder disease, a prosthetic solution involving partial or total anatomic prosthesis or reverse total shoulder arthroplasty is often considered. In this particular setting, CT scan represents a fundamental step in the surgical planning, more than in the diagnostic workup. The glenoid surface shows a normal retroversion angle varying between 0 and 7 degrees. The bony wear generally linked to glenohumeral arthropathy could determine an increased retroversion angle, with eventual surface asymmetry (Fig. 9.15). Walch classified glenoid bone defects into three groups [24]. The A type glenoid is characterized by an equal balancing of the loads acting on the glenoid plane: the A1 subtype shows a moderate concentric wear, while the A2 subtype has a major glenoid wear, with concave glenoid surface. The B-type glenoid, on the contrary, is characterized by an asymmetric balancing of the loads acting on the glenoid plane: the B1 subtype shows a posterior joint space narrowing with subchondral sclerosis, while the B2 subtype shows a retroverted biconcave glenoid with posterior rim erosion. Finally, the C-type glenoid is a retroverted glenoid with more than 25° of retroversion, regardless of erosion, and normally related to a dysplastic condition. More recently, the B3 type, with posteriorly worn monoconcave morphology, and the D type or anteverted glenoid have been added to this classification (Fig. 9.16) [25]. Both the CT study of the glenoid and the humeral morphology are key steps in the surgical planning, allowing a correct choice and placing of the prosthetic components and eventually avoiding possible major complications (e.g., intraoperative fractures, post-operative component mobilization or implant instability).

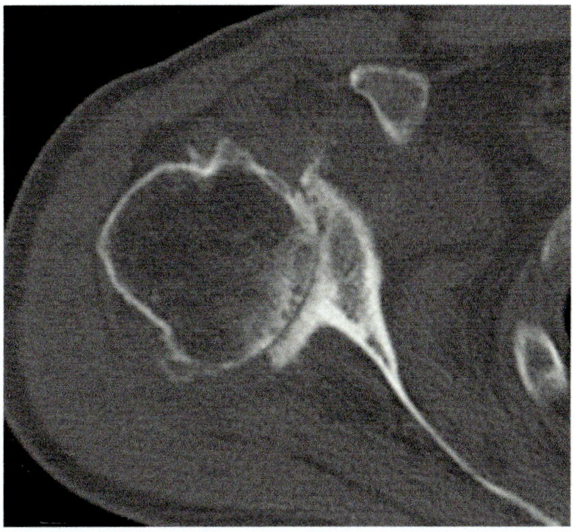

Fig. 9.15 Glenoid bone morphology. CT axial scan of a degenerated glenoid, with severe retroversion and prominent posterior osteophyte. Omitting this kind of analysis could easily lead to glenoid component malposition or glenoid intraoperative fracture in such a case

A limited role is currently reserved to the CT-arthrogram, with intra-articular contrastographic fluid. Despite the historical and current value in the study of instability-related lesions of the shoulder, no clear utility is actually recognized to this procedure in the setting of degenerative shoulder disease, with the exception for patients not analyzable with MRI or MRA (e.g., pacemaker owners, presence of metallic bodies of metallic vascular sutures, claustrophobic patients).

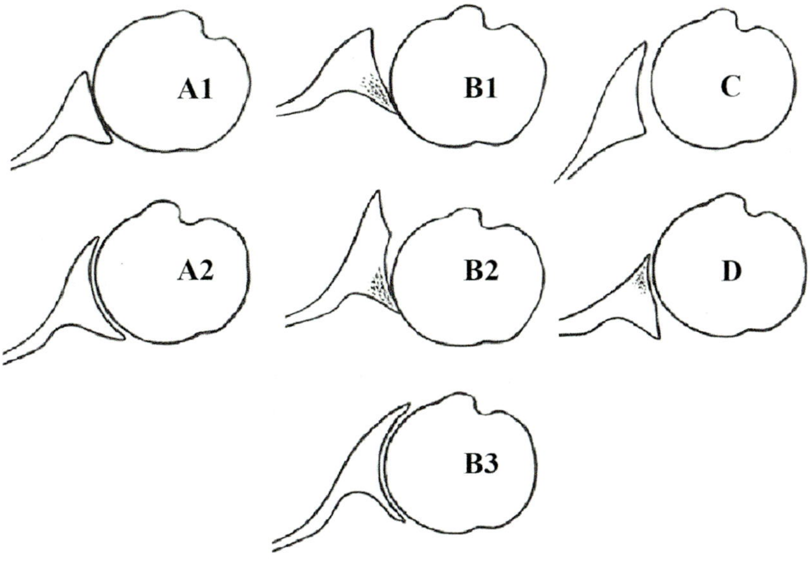

Fig. 9.16 The Walch classification system. See text for description. (Modified from Bercik et al., Ref. [25], with permission from the authors)

References

1. Smith JG. Pathologic appearance of seven cases of injury of the shoulder joint with remarks. London Medical Gazette. 1834;14:280.
2. Neer CS 2nd, Craig EV, Fukuda H. Cuff-tear arthropathy. J Bone Joint Surg Am. 1983;65:1232–44.
3. Visotsky JL, Bassamania C, Seebauer L, Rockwood CA, Jensen KL. Cuff tear arthropathy: pathogenesis, classification and algorithm for treatment. J Bone Joint Surg Am. 2004;86-A(2):35–40.
4. Hamada K, Fukuda H, Mikasa M, Kobayashi Y. Roentgenographic findings in massive rotator cuff tears. A long-term observation. Clin Orthop Relat Res. 1990;254:92–6.
5. Kappe T, Cakir B, Reichel H, Elsharkawi M. Reliability of radiologic classification for cuff tear arthropathy. J Shoulder Elb Surg. 2011;20(4):543–7.
6. Moor BK, Wieser K, Slankamenac K, Gerber C, Bouaicha S. Relationship of individual scapular anatomy and degenerative rotator cuff tears. J Shoulder Elb Surg. 2014;23(4):536–41.
7. Bjarnison AO, Sørensen TJ, Kallemose T, Barfod KW. The critical shoulder angle is associated with osteoarthritis in the shoulder but not rotator cuff tears: a retrospective case-control study. J Shoulder Elb Surg. 2017;26(12):2097–102.
8. Mantell MT, Nelson R, Lowe JT, Endrizzi DP, Jawa A. Critical shoulder angle associated with full-thickness rotator cuff tears in patients with glenohumeral osteoarthritis. J Shoulder Elb Surg. 2017;26(12):e376–81.
9. Bianchi S, Prato N, Martinoli C, Derchi LE. Shoulder radiography. In: Imaging of the shoulder, vol. 1. New York: Springer; 2004. p. 4–5.
10. Martinoli C, Bianchi S, Prato N, et al. US of the shoulder: non-rotator cuff disorders. Radiographics. 2003;23:381–401.
11. Huber DJ, Sauter R, Mueller E, et al. MR imaging of the normal shoulder. Radiology. 1986;158:405–8.
12. Iannotti JP, Zlatkin MB, Esterhai JL, et al. Magnetic resonance imaging of the shoulder. Sensitivity, specificity and predictive value. J Bone Joint Surg Am. 1991;73:17–29.
13. Seeger LL, Ruszkowski JT, Bassett LW, et al. MR imaging of the normal shoulder. Anatomic correlation. AJR Am J Roentgenol. 1987;148:83–91.
14. Snyder SJ. Arthroscopic classification of rotator cuff lesions and surgical decision making. In: Snyder SJ, editor. Shoulder arthroscopy. Philadelphia: Lippincott Williams & Wilkins; 2003. p. 201–7.
15. Choi S, Kim MK, Kim GM, Roh YH, Hwang IK, Kang H. Factors associated with clinical and structural outcomes after arthroscopic rotator cuff repair with a suture bridge technique in medium, large, and massive tears. J Shoulder Elb Surg. 2014;23:1675–81.
16. Goutallier D, Bernageau J, Patte D. Assessment of the trophicity of the muscles of the ruptured rotator cuff by CT scan. In: Post M, Morrey B, Hawkins R, editors. Surgery of the shoulder. St. Louis, MO: Mosby; 1990. p. 11–3.
17. Goutallier D, Postel JM, Bernageau J, Lavau L, Voisin MC. Fatty muscle degeneration in cuff ruptures: pre- and postoperative evaluation by CT scan. Clin Orthop Relat Res. 1994;304:78–83.
18. Fuchs B, Weishaupt D, Zanetti M, Hodler J, Gerber C. Fatty degeneration of the muscles of the rotator cuff: assessment by computed tomography versus magnetic resonance imaging. J Shoulder Elb Surg. 1999;8:599–605.
19. Goutallier D, Postel JM, Gleyze P, Leguilloux P, Van Driessche S. Influence of cuff muscle fatty degeneration on anatomic and functional outcomes after simple suture of full-thickness tears. J Shoulder Elb Surg. 2003;12:550–4.
20. Deniz G, Kose O, Tugay A, Guler F, Turan A. Fatty degeneration and atrophy of the rotator cuff muscles after arthroscopic repair: does it improve, halt or deteriorate? Arch Orthop Trauma Surg. 2014;134:985–90.
21. Gladstone JN, Bishop JY, Lo IK, Flatow EL. Fatty infiltration and atrophy of the rotator cuff do not improve after rotator cuff repair and correlate with poor functional outcome. Am J Sports Med. 2007;35:719–28.
22. Burkhart SS, De Beer JF. Traumatic glenohumeral bone defects and their relationship to failure of arthroscopic Bankart repairs: significance of the inverted-pear glenoid and the humeral engaging Hill-Sachs lesion. Arthroscopy. 2000;16(7):677–94.
23. Baudi P, Righi P, Bolognesi D, Rivetta S, Rossi Urtoler E, Giucciardi N, Carrara M. How to identify and calculate glenoid bone deficit. Chir Organi Mov. 2005;90(2):145–52.
24. Walch G, Badet R, Boulahia A, Khoury A. Morphologic study of the glenoid in primary glenohumeral osteoarthritis. J Arthroplast. 1999;14(6):756–60.
25. Bercik MJ, Kruse K II, Yalizis M, Gauci M-O, Chaoui J, Walch G. A modification to the Walch classification of the glenoid in primary glenohumeral osteoarthritis using three-dimensional imaging. J Shoulder Elb Surg. 2016;25:1601–6.

Part III

Proximal Humeral Fractures

10 Introduction and Classifications

Mario Borroni, Giacomo Delle Rose, and Alessandro Castagna

10.1 Introduction

Proximal humeral fractures are very common and incidence is very different considering the age.

In children, they are less than 1% of all the fractures, but as they never required a treatment with reverse shoulder arthroplasty, they will not be treated in this chapter.

Incidence rate of proximal humeral fracture in adults rates from 4 to 5% of all fractures, and in patients older than 40 years, they account for over 75% of humerus fractures [1, 2].

Women have a much higher incidence than men, probably because of postmenopausal osteoporosis, whereas in patients younger than 50 years, the main cause of this kind of fracture is a high-energy trauma [3, 4].

Classification should help orthopedic surgeons to characterize a problem, to suggest a prognosis, and to offer the optimal treatment for a particular pathology.

Understanding the particular fracture pattern in each case is complicated, especially when poorly positioned radiographs are the only available studies. Most well-accepted classification systems were developed based on radiographs complemented by intraoperative findings.

M. Borroni (✉) · G. Delle Rose · A. Castagna
Humanitas Research Hospital, Rozzano, Milan, Italy
e-mail: giacomo.delle_rose@humanitas.it; Alessandro.castagna@humanitas.it

S. Gumina et al. (eds.), *Reverse Shoulder Arthroplasty*,
https://doi.org/10.1007/978-3-319-97743-0_10

10.2 Historical Classifications

As in other districts, many different classifications have been proposed, starting with Kocher's classification based on different anatomic levels of fracture: anatomic neck, epiphyseal region, and surgical neck [5].

This classification is quite simple and reproducible, but do not consider the presence of fracture at multiple levels, the degree of fracture displacement, and the present of dislocations.

In 1934 Codman presented a modification of Kocher's classification, based on the epiphyseal region of the proximal humerus, and identified four possible fracture fragments: greater tuberosity, lesser tuberosity, anatomic head, and shaft [6].

10.3 Neer Classification

This classification was used till 1970, when Neer proposed his classification that is still the most used in clinical practice [7] (Fig. 10.1).

This system is based on the anatomic relationship of the four main anatomic parts (greater tuberosity, lesser tuberosity, proximal shaft, and humeral head) and on the grade of displacement of the fragments.

In this classification the main issue is the presence of displacement of one or more segments and not only the presence of a line of fractures.

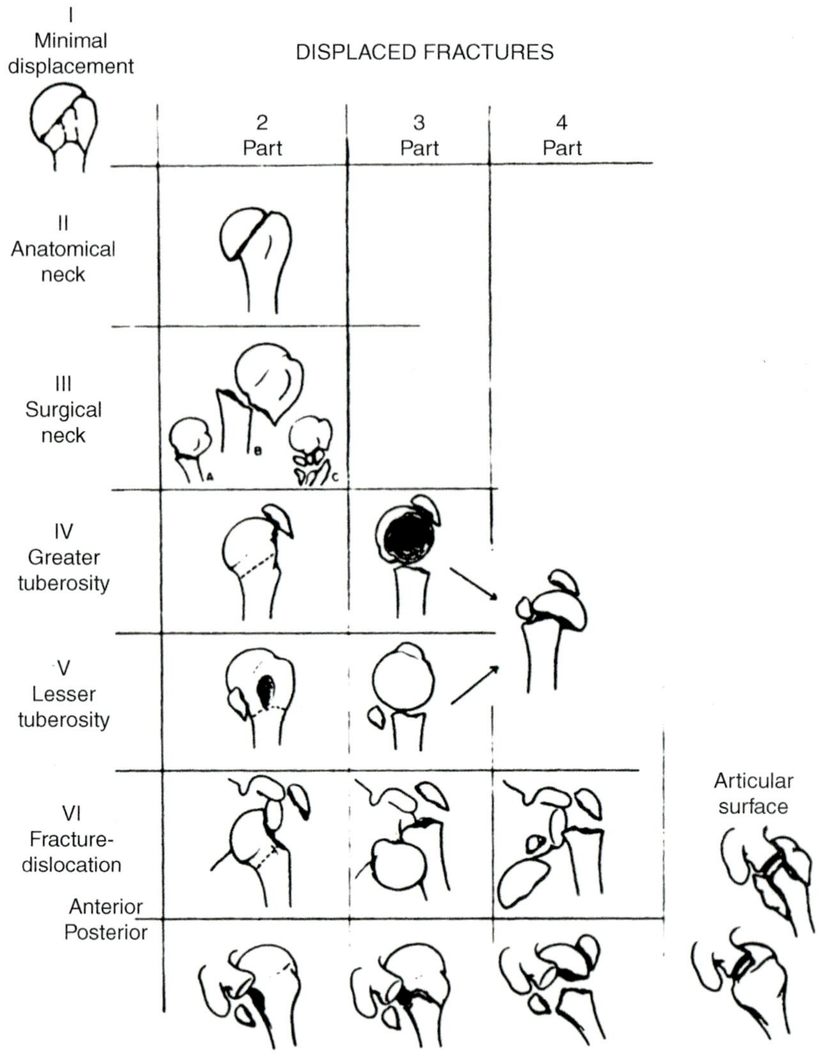

Fig. 10.1 The Neer classification of proximal humeral fractures [7]

A segment was considered displaced if it angulated more than 45 degrees from its anatomic position or if it's displaced more than 1 cm.

The most common fracture (85% of all proximal humeral fractures) is a one-part non-displaced or minimally displaced fracture even if these fractures have multiple fractures lines, because the fragments don't fulfill the criteria for displacement as stated by Neer [8].

Displaced fracture includes two-part fractures, characterized by displacement of one of the four-fragment, three-part fractures, in which there is a displacement of two fragments, and four-part fractures, where there is a displacement of all four segments.

So we could have four different two-fragment fractures (anatomic neck, surgical neck, greater tuberosity, or lesser tuberosity), two different three-fragment fractures (greater tuberosity and shaft or lesser tuberosity and shaft), and one four-fragment fracture.

Neer also introduced fracture dislocations which are displaced fractures (two-, three-, or four-part fractures) associated with anterior or posterior dislocations: so we could have six different types of fracture dislocations.

In the end Neer also introduced articular surface fractures dividing them into two types: impression fractures and head-splitting fractures.

Neer classification is the most widely used classification system for proximal humerus fractures [9]; however reliability of this classification has been discussed in many studies.

Radiographs of 50 proximal humerus fractures [10] were reviewed by an orthopedic shoulder specialist, an orthopedic traumatologist, a skeletal radiologist, an orthopedic resident in fifth year of training, and an orthopedic resident in second year of training.

These exams were reviewed two times at 6 months of interval, and the results showed a "moderate" level of reliability and the mean intra-observer reliability was 0.65.

This point is really important because a fracture could be classified as minimally displaced or as a three-part fracture by two different orthopedic surgeons leading to two different treatments [11].

10.4 AO Classification

The AO group proposed another classification based on risk of osteonecrosis due to modification of vascular supply (Fig. 10.2).

The fractures of the proximal humerus are divided in three types: extraarticular unifocal, extraarticular bifocal, and articular; each of these groups is further divided into three different groups based on presence of impaction and associated dislocation.

Type A fractures are extraarticular unifocal and A1 are the tuberosities fractures, A2 are impacted metaphyseal fractures, and A3 are nonimpacted metaphyseal fractures.

Type B group includes extraarticular bifocal fractures involving both tuberosities with a concomitant metaphyseal fracture or glenohumeral dislocations: B1 fractures are the fractures associated with an impacted metaphyseal fracture, B2 are nonimpacted metaphyseal fractures, and B3 are fractures associated to a glenohumeral dislocation.

Type C fractures are articular and involve vascular isolation: C1 are fractures with slight displacement, C2 are fractures impacted with marked displacement, and C3 are fractures associated with dislocation.

Each subgroup is divided in three different options according to alignment, degree, and direction of the displacement.

The risk of avascular necrosis is rare in type A, low in type B, and high in type C.

This classification seems to be more complex compared to the Neer classification, even if it should allow a more detailed guideline for treatment, but its interobserver reliability has not shown it to be better than Neer's classification [12].

10.5 LEGO System and HGLS Classification

Hertel [13] more recently developed a "binary system" (LEGO system). Emphasis was given to the location of fracture planes, rather than the nature of the fractured fragments. The system pictorially represented the four parts of the proximal

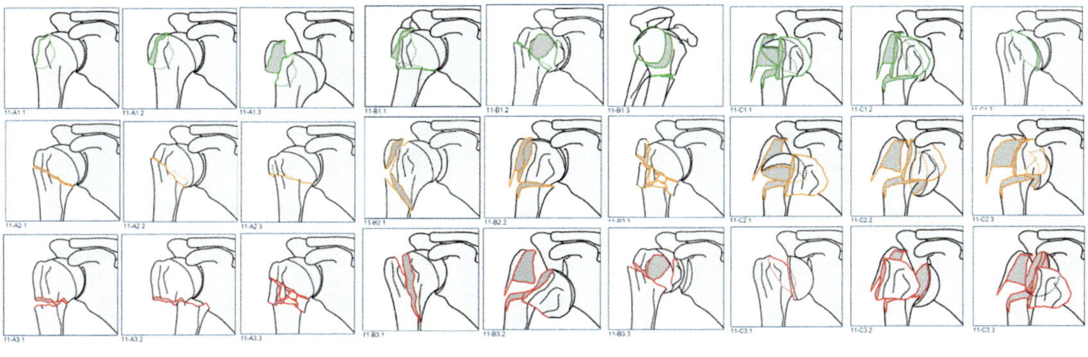

Fig. 10.2 The AO classification of proximal humeral fractures (https://www2.aofoundation.org)

humerus (head, greater and lesser tuberosities, and shaft) using LEGO blocks (Lego Group, Billund, Denmark). The absence of a bond between any of the four parts represents the location of a fracture plane. For a full fracture description, five yes-or-no questions had to be answered concerning the five basic fracture planes: (1) Is there a fracture plane between the head and greater tuberosity? (2) Is there a fracture plane between the greater tuberosity and shaft? (3) Is there a fracture plane between the head and lesser tuberosity? (4) Is there a fracture plane between the lesser tuberosity and shaft? (5) Is there a fracture plane between the greater tuberosity and lesser tuberosity? Thinking in fracture planes, not in fracture fragments, represented the change of paradigm. A number was then assigned to each fracture permutation (Fig. 10.3).

In addition, the following accessory criteria were determined (Figs. 10.2, 10.3, and 10.4): length of the posteromedial metaphyseal head extension; displacement of the shaft with respect to the head (the maximal displacement was measured between the posteromedial edge of the head and the posteromedial shaft fracture line); whether the shaft is displaced medially or laterally; displacement of the tuberosities (maximum displacement of either the greater or the lesser tuberosity); amount of angular displacement of the head, varus, or valgus; whether there is a glenohumeral dislocation (anterior or posterior); whether there is a head impression fracture (anterior or posterior); and whether there is a head-split component (>20% of head involvement) with one or two intraarticular fracture planes (Figs. 10.4 and 10.5).

The main purpose of this classification was to predict humeral head perfusion in proximal humeral fractures in order to identify the optimal treatment; the results were that specific fracture plane combinations (types 2, 7, 8, 9, 10, and 12) were associated with impaired head perfusion and that additional elements, such as the length of the posteromedial metaphyseal head extension and the integrity of the medial hinge, were the key elements for occurrence of vascular disruption.

However, despite validating this system well with intraoperative direct observation, the numerical coding of individual fracture patterns was considered difficult to remember and therefore likely to contribute to categorization error and poor reliability.

So, this classification was modified adopting an alphabetic-based "pictogram" that clearly

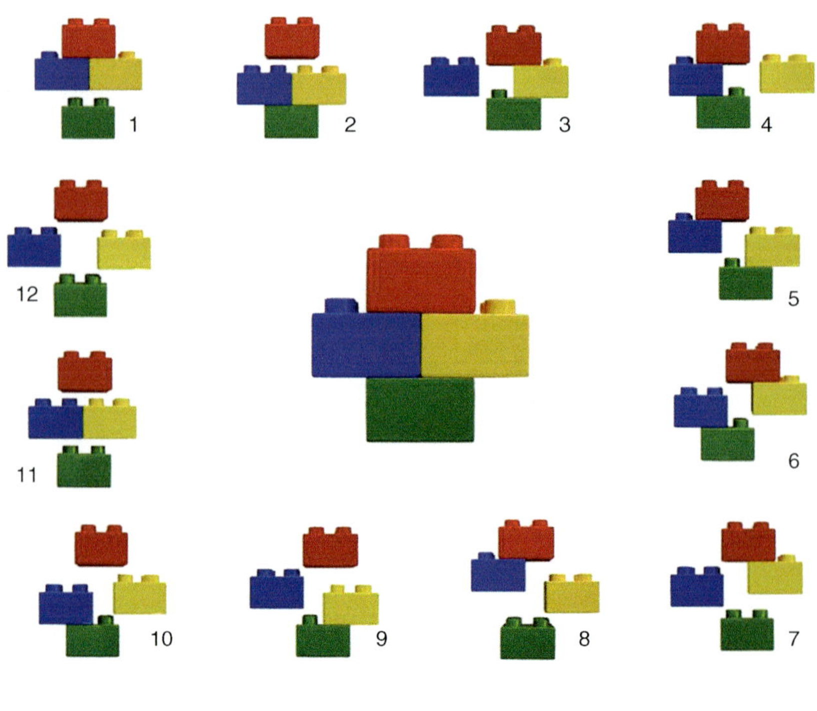

Fig. 10.3 The LEGO system classification of proximal humeral fractures (Ref. [13])

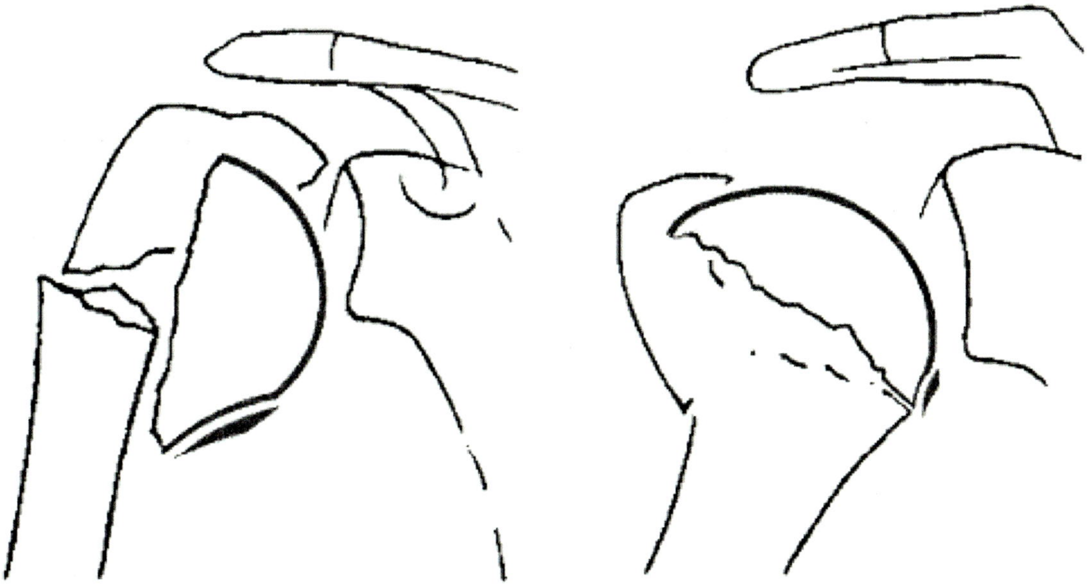

Fig. 10.4 First additional criterion: length of the medial metaphyseal head extension. The longer the extension, the more likely the head is perfused. Hertel, R., Hempfing, A., Stiehler, M., & Leunig, M. (2004). Predictors of humeral head ischemia after intracapsular fracture of the proximal humerus. *J Shoulder Elbow Surg, 13*, 427-33

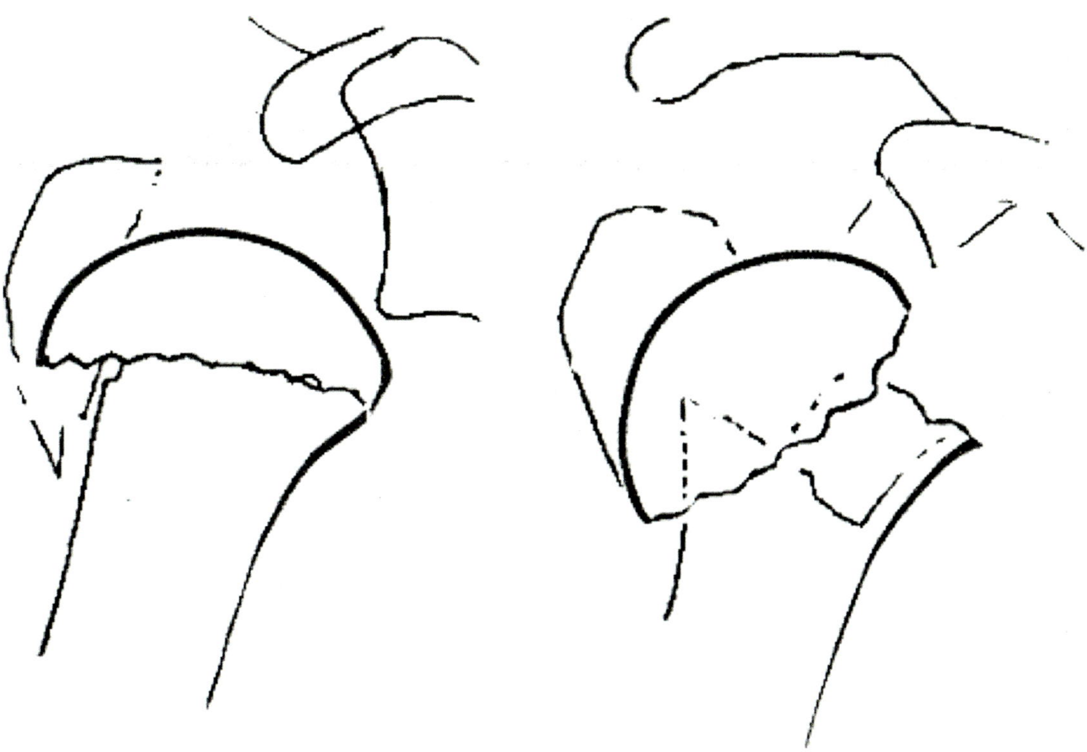

Fig. 10.5 Second additional criterion: integrity of the medial hinge. Integrity of the hinge is a predictor of both ischemia and practical feasibility of reduction. Hertel, R., Hempfing, A., Stiehler, M., & Leunig, M. (2004). Predictors of humeral head ischemia after intracapsular fracture of the proximal humerus. *J Shoulder Elbow Surg, 13*, 427-33

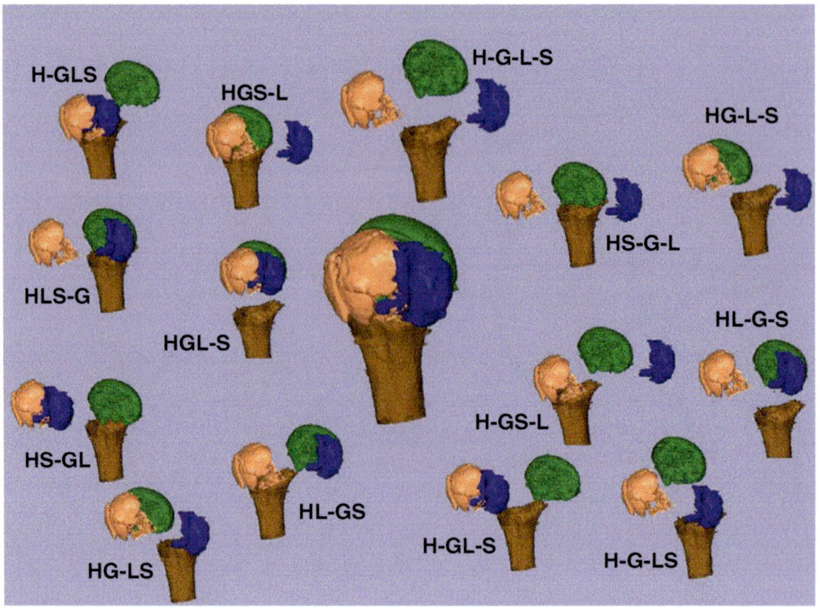

Fig. 10.6 HGLS classification. Sukthankar AV, Leonello DT, Hertel RW, Ding GS, Sandow MJ. J Shoulder Elbow Surg 2013, 22 e1–e6

defines the four anatomic parts of the proximal humerus and the location of a fracture plane(s) between these parts. This system is named the HGLS classification (Fig. 10.6).

In this classification, the proximal humerus is divided into four topographic parts: head (H), greater tuberosity (G), lesser tuberosity (L), and shaft (S). The line of fracture is symbolized by a hyphen (−) and represents a cortical interruption between two parts regardless of displacement and angulation. So a fracture of the greater tuberosity is documented as HLS-G and a fracture of the surgical neck (with tuberosities attached to the humeral head) is documented as HGL-S and so on.

In case of dislocation, a prefixed "d" must be inserted before H; furthermore, calcar length (so important for prediction of humeral head ischemia) is identified by bracketing the letter "c" followed by the length of the intact calcar segment in mm.

Comparing Neer, AO, and HGLS classifications, it seems that HGLS classification has a better intra- and interobserver reliability [14].

As previously stated, the aim of a classification should be to characterize the problem and offer the optimal treatment.

If the first issue has been satisfied by Neer and, more recently, by Hertel, the second one is still pending because even if the reliability of the classification system is quite high, there is not a unique treatment according to the classification itself.

In fact, whatever is the system used, the treatment may be different: analyzing 229 displaced humeral fractures classified with the most utilized system (Neer and AO), only 58.8% of the four-part Neer fractures and 67.7% type-C AO classified were surgically treated [15].

Maybe it could be due to the different cultures of each surgeon and/or the unpredictability of the outcome either of the conservative or surgical treatment [16].

References

1. Bigliani LU, E F. Fractures of the proximal humerus. In: Green RA, editor. Fractures in adults. Philadelphia: Lippincott-Raven; 1996.
2. Norris T. Fractures of the proximal humerus and dislocations of the shoulder. In: Jupiter J, Browner BD, editors. Skeletal trauma. Philadelphia: WB Saunders; 1992. p. 1201–90.
3. Baron J, Barret J, Malenka D. Racial difference in fracture risk. Epidemiology. 1994;5:42–7.
4. Kristiansen B, Barfod g, Bredesen J. Epidemiology of proximal humeral fractures. Acta Orthop Scand. 1987;68:75–7.

5. Kocher T. Bietrage zur Kenntnis einigir praktisch wichtiger Fracturen-formen. Basel: Carl Sallman Verlag; 1896.
6. Codman E. The shoulder: rupture of the supraspinatus tendon and other lesions in or about the subacromial bursa. Boston: Thomas Todd; 1934.
7. Neer C. Displaced proximal humeral fractures: part I Classification and evaluation. J Bone Joint Surg Am. 1970;52:1077–89.
8. Horak J, Nilsson B. Epidemiology of fractures of the upper end of the humerus. Clin Orthop. 1975;112:250–3.
9. Kristiansen B, Christansen S. Proximal humeral fractures. Late results in relation to classification and treatment. Acta Orthop Scand. 1987;58:124–7.
10. Sidor M, Zuckerman J, Lyon T, Koval K, Cuomo F, Schoenberg N. The Neer classification of proximal humeral fractures: an assessment of inter-observer reliability and intra-observer reproducibility. J Bone Joint Surg Am. 1993;75:1745–50.
11. Cowell H. Patient care and scientific freedom. J Bone Joint Surg. 1994;76:640–1.
12. Siebenrock K, Gerber C. The reproducibility of classification of fractures of the proximal end of the humerus. J Bone Joint Surg Am. 1993;75:1751–5.
13. Hertel R, Hempfing A, Stiehler M, Leunig M. Predictors of humeral head ischemia after intracapsular fracture of the proximal humerus. J Shoulder Elbow Surg. 2004;13:427–33.
14. Sukthankar A, Leonello D, Hertel R, Ding G, Sandow M. A comprehensive classification of proximal humeral fractures: HGLS system. J Shoulder Elbow. 2013;22:e1–6.
15. Okike K, Lee O, Makanji H, Harris M, Vrahas M. Factors associated with the decision for operative versus nonoperative treatment of displaced proximal humerus fractures in the elderly. Injury. 2013;44:448–55.
16. Tepass A, Rolauffs B, Weise K, Bahrs S, Dietz K, Bahrs C. Complication rates and outcomes stratified by treatment modalities in proximal humeral fractures: a systematic literature review from 1970–2009. Patient Saf Surg. 2013;7:34.

Instrumental Evaluation: X-Ray and CT

11

Rosario Lupo, Salvatore Morello,
Santo Alberto Rapisarda, and Riccardo Mandracchia

The first step in the evaluation of a fracture is represented by the exact definition deriving from the instrumental examinations that, allowing us to classify, represents a useful guide for the therapeutic decision [1].

In the proximal humerus, as in other anatomical districts, conventional radiology plays a major role as it is a readily available, fast and low-cost exam.

The simple radiographic examination (X-ray) is a useful tool in the diagnosis of the proximal humerus fractures, providing important information regarding the extent of the fracture, the number of fragments, their possible decomposition and the articular surface's involvement. Indirect signs such as the presence, in an anteroposterior radiogram performed in an upright position, of adipose tissue and blood in the articular capsule with the characteristic FBI (fat-blood interface) sign indicating an intra-articular extension of the fracture (Fig. 11.1) can help [2].

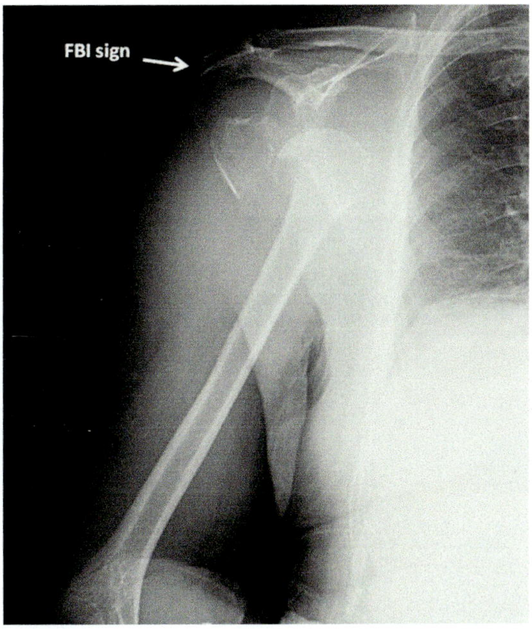

Fig. 11.1 An anteroposterior radiogram performed in an upright position with the characteristic *FBI* (fat-blood interface) *sign*, indicating an intra-articular extension of the fracture

However, there are several studies that highlight the difficulty in repeatability and reproducibility of a radiogram reading among different observers. Moreover, the quality of the slabs carried out under emergency conditions is often poor, both due to the poor collaboration of the patient suffering from the fractured event and to

R. Lupo (✉) · S. Morello
U.O.C. Ortopedia e Traumatologia Ospedale "San Giovanni di Dio", Agrigento, Italy

S. A. Rapisarda
U.O.C. Ortopedia e Traumatologia Ospedale "San Giacomo d'Altopasso", Licata, Italy

R. Mandracchia
U.O.C. Radiodiagnostica Ospedale "San Giovanni di Dio", Agrigento, Italy

S. Gumina et al. (eds.), *Reverse Shoulder Arthroplasty*,
https://doi.org/10.1007/978-3-319-97743-0_11

the difficulty in obtaining an accurate execution of standardized series of shoulder radiographs always under emergency conditions (trauma series). Furthermore, performing a correct radiographic examination cannot disregard an adequate knowledge of the shoulder's anatomy. It must be remembered that the scapula does not lie on the frontal plane of the chest but is inclined about 45° with respect to it; it follows that the anteroposterior radiographs on the frontal plane of the chest provide oblique images of the glenohumeral joint (Fig. 11.2a). An incomplete and inadequate X-ray examination because of the non-execution of some radiographic projections or a poor execution of the same can prevent a correct classification of the fracture and therefore induce to undertake a treatment, conservative or surgical, which is not the most suitable for that determined fracture or even, at worst, to make a fracture or a glenohumeral dislocation misunderstood [3]. Today, the trauma series remains the gold standard as a first-level examination when there is shoulder trauma [1]. It includes a true anteroposterior radiograph on the scapula plane which provides us with a real anteroposterior image of the glenohumeral joint, a lateral projection onto the scapula plane or a Y-projection of the scapula and an axial projection. The goal is to carry out an examination that altogether describes the fracture picture through the three floors of the space at best in order to obtain a description that is the most realistic and complete.

The two projections onto the scapula plane, anteroposterior and Y-lateral, can be performed keeping the traumatized limb in the bandage, thus avoiding its mobilization. This is a considerable advantage in particular for the patient, who avoids an accentuation of the algic

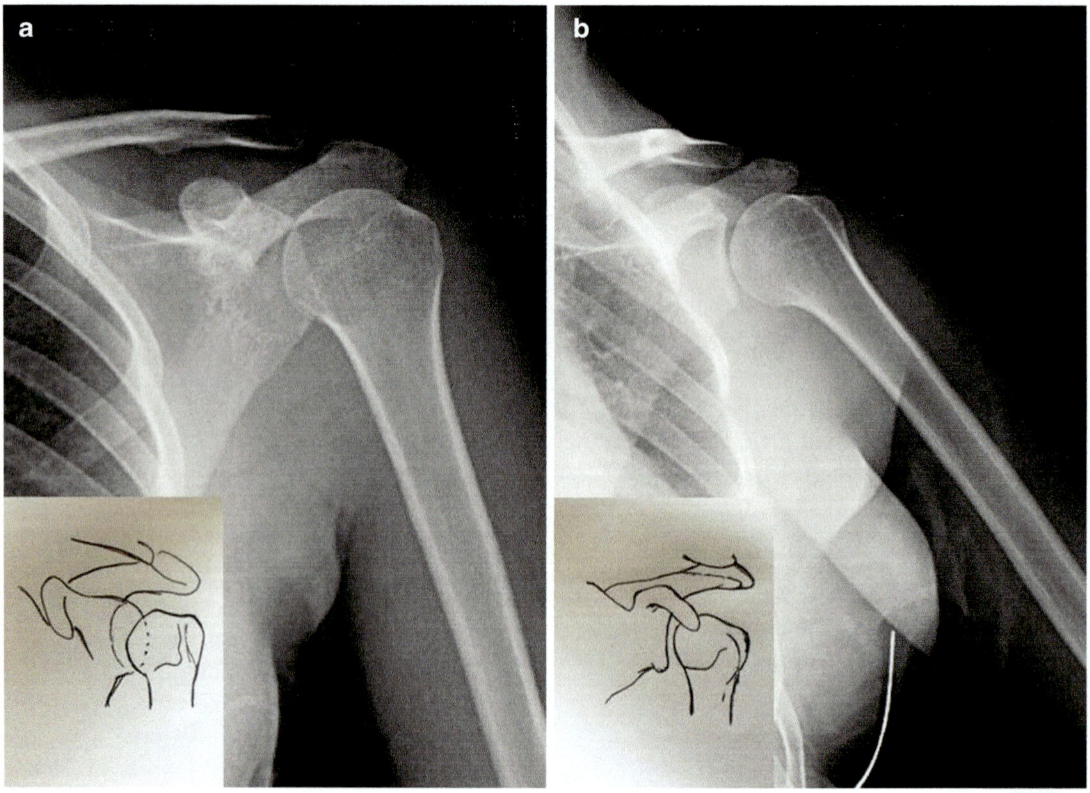

Fig. 11.2 (**a**) The anteroposterior radiograph on the frontal plane of the chest provides oblique images of the glenohumeral joint. (**b**) The anteroposterior projection on the scapula plane allows a visualization of the glenoid profile and thus allows the two articular components, the humeral head and the glenoid cavity, to be clearly seen at least in physiological conditions

symptomatology, and consequently also for the radiographic examination correct execution requiring a minor collaboration of the patient himself. The anteroposterior projection on the scapula plane can be performed in orthostatics or in supine position and in particular is carried out positioning the radiographic cassette posteriorly to the shoulder to be examined and inclining the contralateral shoulder with a forward angle of about 35°–45° so that the body of the scapula is positioned parallel to the sensitive plane. The radiating beam will thus be orthogonal to the sensitive plane and to the body of the scapula, inclined about 40° from the frontal plane in the mid-lateral direction and aimed at the centre of the scapula itself, approximately 5 cm below the coracoid process (Fig. 11.3). This allows a visualization of the glenoid profile and thus allows the two articular components, the humeral head and the glenoid cavity, to be clearly seen at least in physiological conditions (Fig. 11.2b).

On the contrary, if there is an anterior or posterior glenohumeral dislocation, the two structures will appear overlapped. However, the evaluation of the acromion, of the acromion-clavicular joint and of the clavicle's lateral portion appears more difficult with this projection rather than with the standard anteroposterior one.

The Y-lateral projection of the scapula [4] also known as projection of the defile of the supraspinatus, trans-scapular or lateral tangential can be performed with patient in orthostatics or sitting and, as the previous projection, can be performed without mobilizing the limb and maintaining it in the bandage or in the support. To perform the examination, the anterior region of the shoulder affected by the trauma lies on the X-ray cassette, while the contralateral shoulder is inclined forward approximately by 30°–45°. The radiating beam transits tangentially through the posterolateral chest wall and parallel with the spine of the scapula up to the radiographic cassette. The central ray's point of incidence must coincide with the centre of the median edge of the scapula. The radiological image must show the two median and lateral margins of the scapula perfectly overlapped to represent the stem of a "Y", whose arms are instead represented anteriorly by the

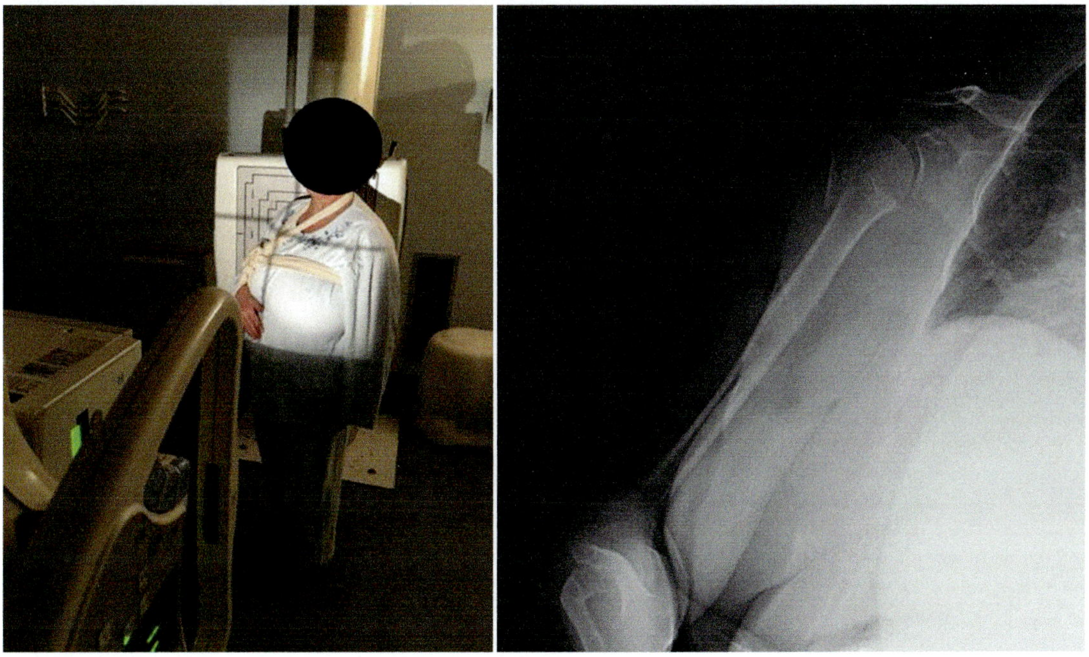

Fig. 11.3 The anteroposterior projection on the scapula plane is carried out, positioning the radiographic cassette posteriorly to the shoulder to be examined and inclining the contralateral shoulder with a forward angle of about 35°–45° so that the body of the scapula is positioned parallel to the sensitive plane

base of the coracoid process and posteriorly by the base of the acromial process. This projection is crucial to the study of the articular relationships between the humeral head and the glena. In physiological conditions, the head of the humerus is at the centre of the so-formed "Y", while it is forward or backward in the case of anterior or posterior dislocation, respectively. The Y-lateral projection is also particularly useful for the evaluation of the decomposition of the trochitis's possible fracture. It can help in the diagnosis of fractures of the coracoid process and of the acromial process and for the evaluation of the acromion's inferior margin, while it does not allow a careful study of the glena's anterior and posterior edges (Fig. 11.4).

The lateral axillary projection was first described by Lawrence [5], and it involves the 90° abduction, and it is a great method for the assessment of the anterior or posterior glenohumeral dislocation and for the detection of Bony Bankart involving the anterior glenoid fissure. The lateral axillary projection can be performed by the patient to a supine or upright position. The X-ray cassette is placed on the patient's shoulder and as close to the neck as possible, while the X-ray tube is placed slightly below the patient with the radiogenic beam directed inferior-superiorly and centred at the axillary cavity. Compared to the original projection, some variants in the literature have been described, providing a lower abduction angle so that this projection could be carried out even in traumatized patients, unable to reach that degree of abduction due to pain symptoms. In the technique described by Cleaves, the patient's limb, supine or seated, is abducted just enough to allow placement of the X-ray cassette below the shoulder [6]. If, because of the algic symptoms reported by the patient for the fracture, it's impossible to abduct the limb for correct execution of the axial, or in any case it is preferred not to remove the bandage to avoid any decomposition of the fracture, it is possible to make a Velpeau's axial [3, 7] (Fig. 11.5).

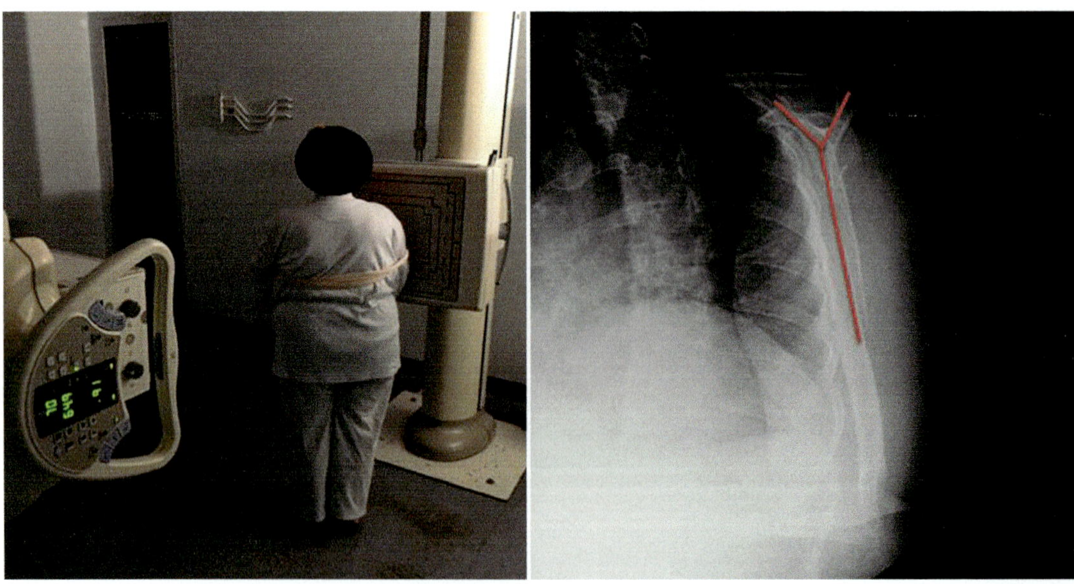

Fig. 11.4 In the Y-lateral projection of the scapula, the anterior region of the shoulder affected by the trauma lies on the X-ray cassette, while the contralateral shoulder is inclined forward approximately by 30°–45°. The radiating beam transits tangentially through the posterolateral chest wall and parallel with the spine of the scapula up to the radiographic cassette. The radiological image must show the two median and lateral margins of the scapula perfectly overlapped to represent the stem of a "Y", whose arms are instead represented anteriorly by the base of the coracoid process and posteriorly by the base of the acromial process. In physiological conditions, the head of the humerus is at the centre of the so-formed "Y", while it is forward or backward in the case of anterior or posterior dislocation, respectively

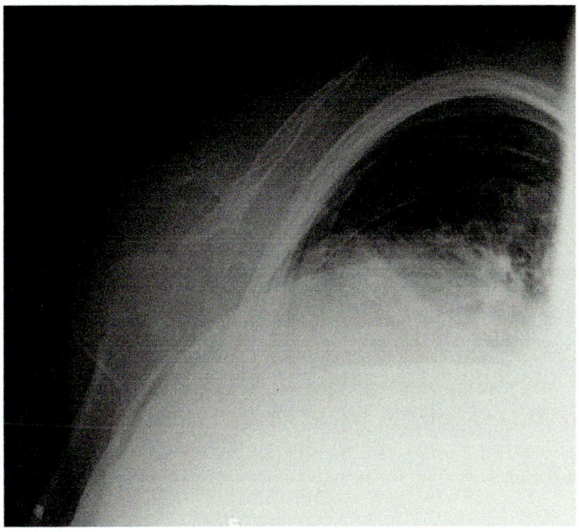

Fig. 11.5 In Velpeau's axial projection, the joint relationships can be assessed, although the glenohumeral joint appears enlarged and the humeral diaphysis shortened

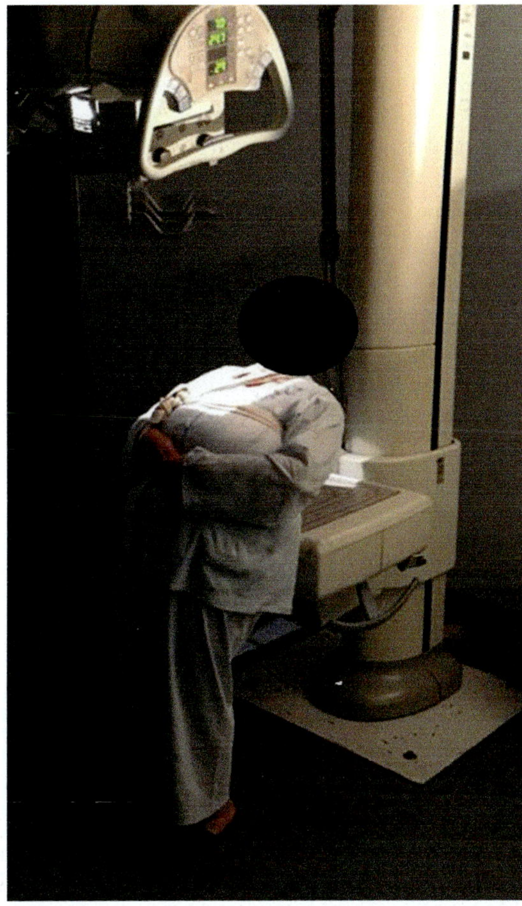

Fig. 11.6 Velpeau's axial projection allows maintaining the limb immobilized and adducted to the chest. The patient positions himself at the end of the radiological table by bending the thorax backwards by about 20°–30°. The X-ray cassette is placed directly below the shoulder, while the X-ray tube is placed above

This projection allows maintaining the limb immobilized and adducted to the chest and can be performed by the patient into an upright or sitting position. Specifically, the patient positions himself at the end of the radiological table by bending the thorax backwards by about 20–30°. The X-ray cassette is placed directly below the shoulder, while the X-ray tube is placed above. It follows that the X-ray beam is vertical and perpendicular to the table in the cranio-caudal sense, with incidence on the clavicle's lateral end (Fig. 11.6). Although the glenohumeral joint appears enlarged and the humeral diaphysis shortened, the joint relationships can be assessed. Further axillary projections have been described such as the trans-humeral axillary projection described by Tietge and Ciullo in 1982 [8], which can be carried out by keeping the immobilized arm in the bandage, like the previous ones, but it can be performed by the patient into a supine position.

The upper limb is anteriorly flexed by about 20° by placing a support below the elbow, and the radiological cassette is placed on the shoulder, perpendicular to the table. The X-ray beam will be horizontally directed following the cauda-cranial sense and incident towards the armpit. The axillary projections allow to evaluate the glenohumeral joint relationships, the glenoid's articular surface and the presence of potential Bony Bankart and glenoid fractures and allow an accurate study of the tuberosities and in particular of the decomposition degree of their potential fracture [9].

It is not always possible with simple radiographic examination to come to a correct classification of the fracture in order to plan the most suitable therapy. In recent years, thanks also to the technological development of diagnostic equipment, it is more and more frequent to resort to computed tomography (CT) for the assessment of proximal humerus fractures, especially when we decide to undertake the surgical treatment in such a way to carry out a pre-planning operation as accurately as possible and to have an idea as realistic as possible about what the intraoperative situation to be faced will be [10, 11]. As the common radiographic investigations, the CT is based upon the production by an X-ray tube of an X-ray beam whose attenuation is measured by some fixed detectors placed upon the stand at the machine that is named "gantry". During the rotation of the X-ray tube, the bed where the patient is placed moves along the horizontal axis, thus determining the reproduction by a software of the selected body volume, obtaining body sections of less than a millimetre (in modern equipment) which will allow us to have in addition to the traditional axial plane images some 2D multiplanar reconstructions (MPR, multiplanar reformation) on the coronal, sagittal and axial plane of the space and some 3D reconstructions (VR, volume rendering), thanks also to the contribution of modern equipment that allow us to obtain an isotropic voxel or an element characterized by the same dimensions on the three planes of the space with consequent, equal, spatial resolution in the

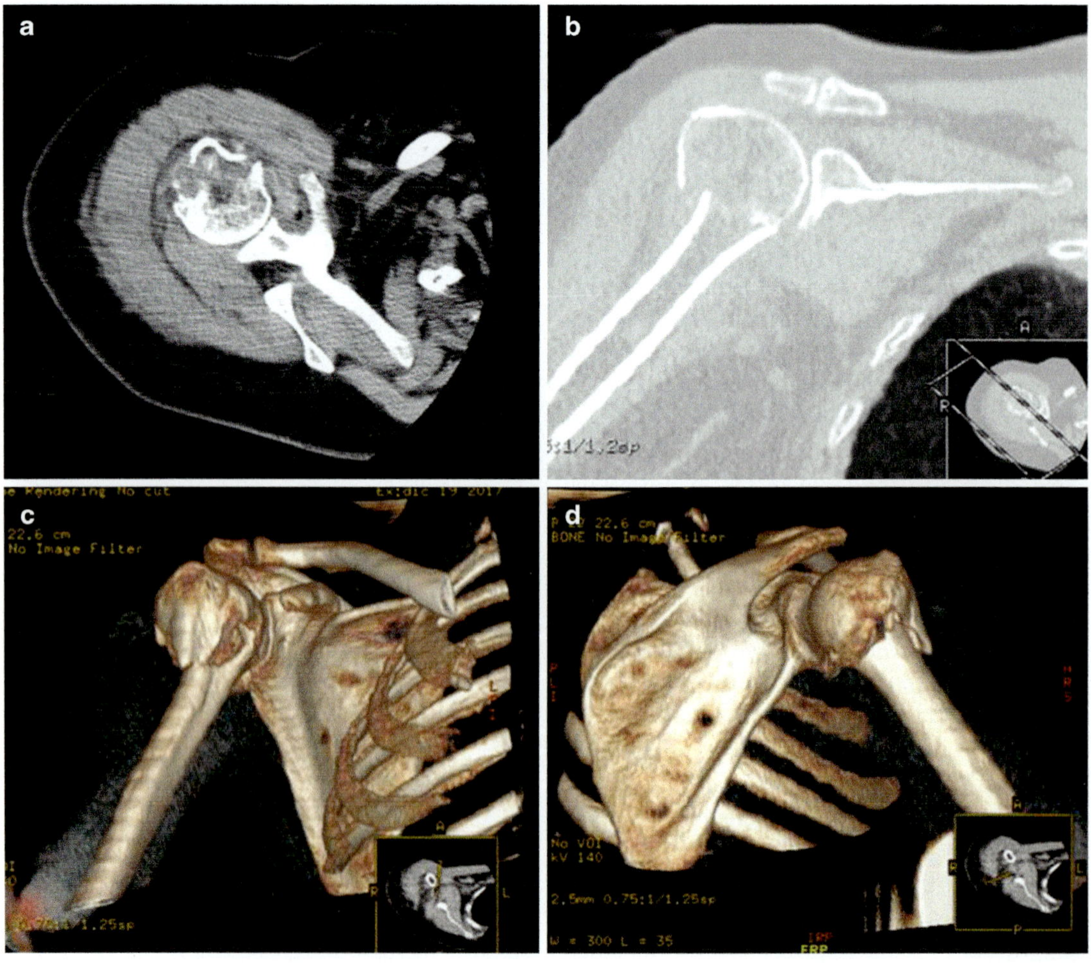

Fig. 11.7 CT scan: 2D multiplanar reconstructions (MPR, multiplanar reformation) on the axial (**a**) and coronal (**b**) plane of the space; 3D reconstructions (VR, volume rendering) (**c**–**d**)

reconstructions that we will carry out [12–14] (Fig.11.7).

The different X-rays' attenuation by the various anatomical structures will allow us to differentiate them within the images obtained [15]. The latest generation equipment (multidetector) allows us to acquire large body volumes in a few seconds, thus drastically reducing the time required to perform the examination and, therefore, any technical motion artefacts that affect it.

In the traumatic pathology of the proximal humerus, CT is extremely useful to define the presence and extent of the fracture or of a dislocation, to evaluate various intra-articular anomalies, to define the number and exact location of the fragments and to evaluate the adjacent soft tissues, in order to plan a conservative or, in alternative, a surgical treatment [16, 17].

CT is of particular importance in detecting small bone fragments located at the joint due to a trauma. The CT's advantage compared to conventional radiology is its ability to exceed the radiographic limits due to the overlap of several anatomical structures, providing great contrast resolution, to measure accurately the tissue attenuation coefficient and to obtain direct axial images. Multiplanar reconstructions (MPR) can be carried out on all floors of the space, thus offering greater diagnostic accuracy and adequate preoperative planning [18]. The three-dimensional images (VR) processed by the routinely used post-processing software allow the creation of a plastic model to the area in question, thus facilitating the operative planning and allowing a trial for complex reconstructive procedures' surgery [1, 19, 20]. The CT's disadvantages are related to the high radiant dose compared to common radiographic investigations and to a lower contrast resolution to the study of muscle-tendon structures compared with other imaging methods such as magnetic resonance, which, however, does not provide further information with respect to the TC for the bone study, and it is not usually indicated for patients with fracture of the proximal epiphysis of the humerus [21, 22].

References

1. Ney DR, Drebin RA, Fishman EK, Magid D. Volumetric rendering of computed tomographic data: principles and techniques. IEEE Comput Graph Appl. 1990;10:24–32.
2. Kilcoyne RF, Shuman WP, Matsen FA III, Morris M, Rockwood CA. The Neer classification of displaced proximal humeral fractures: spectrum of findings on plain radiographs and CT scans. AJR. 1990;154:1029–33.
3. Kontakis G, Koutras C, Tosounidis T, Giannoudis P. Early management of proximal humeral fractures with hemiarthroplasty: a systematic review. J Bone Joint Surg Br. 2008;90(11):1407–13.
4. Rubin SA, Gray RL, Wr G. The scapular Y: a diagnostic aid in shoulder trauma. Radiology. 1974;11:725–6.
5. Lawrence W. A new position in radiographing the shoulder joint. AJR Am J Roentgenol. 1915;2:728–30.
6. Cleaves EN. A new film holder for roentgen examinations of the shoulder. Am J Roentgenol. 1941;45(2):88–90.
7. Bloom MH, Obata WG. Diagnosis of posterior dislocation of the shoulder with use of Velpeau axillary and angle-up roentgenographic views. J Bone Joint Surg Am. 1967;49(5):943–9.
8. Tietge RA, Ciullo JV. The CAM axillary X-ray. Orthop Trns. 1982;6:451.
9. Jo MJ, Gardner MJ. Proximal humerus fractures. Curr Rev Musculoskelet Med. 2012;5(3):192–8.
10. Pretorius ES, Fishman EK. Volume-rendered three-dimensional spiral CT: musculoskeletal applications. Radiographics. 1999;19:1143–60.
11. Pretorius ES, Fishman EK. Helical (spiral) CT of the musculoskeletal system. Radiol Clin N Am. 1995;33:949–79.
12. Pretorius ES, Scott WW Jr, Fishman EK. Acute trauma of the shoulder: role of spiral CT imaging. Emerg Radiol. 1995;2:13–7.
13. Fishman EK. Protocols for helical CT of the musculoskeletal system. In: Silverman PM, editor. Helical (spiral) computed tomography: a practical approach to clinical protocols. New York, NY: Lippincott-Raven; 1998. p. 149–78.
14. Fishman EK. Spiral CT of the musculoskeletal system. In: Krestin GP, Glazer GM, editors. Advances in CT IV. Berlin: Springer-Verlag; 1998. p. 175–85.
15. Brink J. Technical aspects of helical (spiral) CT. Radiol Clin N Am. 1995;33:825–41.
16. Murray IR, Amin AK, White TO, Robinson CM. Proximal humeral fractures: current concepts in classification, treatment and outcomes. J Bone Joint Surg Br. 2011;93(1):1–11.
17. Fishman EK. Spiral CT evaluation of the musculoskeletal system. In: Fishman EK, Jeffrey RB, editors. Spiral CT: principles, techniques, and clinical

applications. New York, NY: Lippincott-Raven; 1998. p. 273–98.

18. Jurik AG, Albrechtsen J. The use of computed tomography with two- and three-dimensional reconstructions in the diagnosis of three- and four-part fractures of the proximal humerus. Clin Radiol. 1994;49:800–4.
19. Fishman EK, Magid D, Ney DR, et al. Three-dimensional imaging. Radiology. 1991;181:321–7.
20. Kuszyk BS, Heath DG, Bliss DF, Fishman EK. Skeletal 3D CT: advantages of volume rendering over surface rendering. Skelet Radiol. 1996;25:207–14.
21. Sandstrom CK, Kennedy SA, Gross JA. Acute shoulder trauma: what the surgeon wants to know. Radiographics. 2015;35:475–92.
22. Naeder H, Beat H. New trends in the treatment of proximal humeral fracture. Clin Orthop Relat Res. 2006;442:100–8.

Fix or Replace?

12

Paolo Paladini, Giovanni Merolla,
Carlo Alberto Augusti, and Giuseppe Porcellini

12.1 Introduction

Proximal humeral fractures account for about 10% of all fractures [1, 2], and the incidence is increasing [3]. The majority of minimally displaced fractures are successfully treated nonoperatively [4], but the optimal management of displaced or complex fracture remains controversial. Devascularization of the humeral head, associated injury to the rotator cuff, and the high prevalence of osteoporosis in elderly patients make the decision-making and the treatment very challenging. Current evidences are not able to give a useful guideline among prosthetic replacements, intramedullary nails, fixed angle locked plates, and conservative methods [5, 6]. Different classifications, based on fragment number and displacement, have been proposed for these difficult fractures [7–10]. This topic has been widely described in a previous chapter (2f—Borroni). However, no system can predict the ideal treatment option, and all ones have poor intra-and interobserver variability [11, 12]. Understanding the vascular supply of the humeral head is mandatory when planning surgical treatment. Arthroplasty surgery should be more useful in a fracture pattern in which the humeral head is at risk of avascular necrosis, while internal fixation should be better in a fracture pattern, whereby the risk of devascularization is low. The principal blood supply to the head has been shown to originate from the anterior humeral circumflex artery through the arcuate branch [13] with a helpful role by the posterior humeral circumflex [12]. Different fracture patterns have been associated with a higher risk of humeral head necrosis: medial metaphyseal head extension more than 8 millimeters, disruption of the posteromedial hinge, and any fracture disrupting the anatomical humeral head [12]. The presence of any of these features should prompt the clinician to consider arthroplasty surgery as a more reliable treatment option.

P. Paladini (✉) · G. Merolla · C. A. Augusti
Unit of Shoulder and Elbow Surgery, Cervesi Hospital, Cattolica, RN, Italy

G. Porcellini
Orthopaedic Department, Policlinico di Modena, University of Modena and Reggio Emilia, Modena, Italy
e-mail: Giuseppe.porcellini@unimore.it

12.2 Non-operative Treatment

The most part of patients with proximal humeral fractures can be managed nonoperatively [14] with a high union rate [15, 16]. The treatment would involve 2 or 3 weeks of immobilization followed by progressive mobility under the guidance of a physiotherapist. Retrospective studies have reported high rates of patients with good or excellent outcome [4, 14], with an average of 111–120° of forward flexion and 100–106° of

S. Gumina et al. (eds.), *Reverse Shoulder Arthroplasty*,
https://doi.org/10.1007/978-3-319-97743-0_12

abduction [15, 16]. The decision to proceed toward a surgical intervention is based on four factors: age, bone quality, fracture pattern, and timing of surgery [17]. The combination of a clinical history, examination findings, and radiographic investigations plays a critical role in decision-making process. Main elements of the history are patient age, date of injury, hand dominance, preinjury functional level, comorbidities, cognition, social status, and compliance to rehabilitation. Clinical examination should confirm the integrity of the axillary nerve, brachial plexus, and axillary artery.

12.3 Operative Treatment

Preoperative plain radiographs should include the complete shoulder series: anterior-posterior view of the glenohumeral joint and axillary and lateral views. Imaging studies should demonstrate the congruity of the glenohumeral joint, the number of fracture fragments, the degree of fracture displacement, and the presence of risk factors for a future humeral head necrosis. Computed tomography (CT) scanning with three-dimensional reconstructions is mandatory when planning internal fixation or prosthesis implant [12].

12.4 Plate Fixation

Surgical fixation should preserve articular surface congruency, alignment, and vascularity to the humeral head. It is mandatory to achieve an accurate reduction and to restore the medial calcar support [18, 19]. Screws should engage into the subchondral bone where the bone quality is greatest and should include inferior-medial screws [20]. The plate should be positioned at least 5 mm distal to the greater tuberosity to avoid impingement during abduction [21]. Reduction and fixation of the tuberosities can be done using screws but more commonly with sutures onto the plate. Intraoperative evaluation of the passive movement is necessary to check stability and to program the correct postoperative rehabilitation. Passive rehabilitation should start after few days from surgery. The surgical approach is performed through a deltopectoral or lateral deltoid splitting approach depending upon surgeon preference. The dissection may increase the risk of necrosis of the humeral head [22], and the plate use in three- and four-part fractures is uncertain especially in elderly patients. In young patients, where three- or four-part fractures can be reduced and the bone quality is adequate, a plate fixation can be performed. In elderly patients, when the bone is of poor quality, the articular surface damaged, and the blood supply compromised, then a prosthesis implant should be considered [23]. If the patient is under 60 years of age, open reduction and internal fixation should be considered even for complex cases. In these cases, a perfect tuberosity reduction should be searched, because, even if avascular necrosis occurs, the anatomic union of tuberosities will be advantageous for future arthroplasty surgery. In these cases, if plate fixation fails, salvage prosthesis implant is possible, but reported outcomes are poorer than in cases of primary hemiarthroplasty [24, 25].

12.5 Intramedullary Nailing

Usually intramedullary nailing has been used to treat humeral shaft fractures. To give more stability to the proximal part, nails with polyaxial screws were developed. This gives a valid option for the management of proximal humeral fractures. Two-part fractures are more eligible to be treated with intramedullary nails with respect to three- or four-part fractures. The advantage of the intramedullary devices is that less soft tissue disruption is required at the fracture site lessening the risk of humeral head necrosis. The entry point violates the rotator cuff often leading to residual shoulder pain [26, 27]. The complication rate is high with 10% developing impingement, 31% requiring removal of metal work, 12% developing AVN, and 4% requiring early revision [28, 29].

12.6 Hemiarthroplasty

The use of hemiarthroplasty for proximal humeral fractures was first described by Neer with 98% of satisfactory outcomes [30, 31]. At the present time, its ability to restore normal shoulder kinematics and function is still debated [32]. Indications for hemiarthroplasty are fracture dislocations and humeral head splitting fractures [33]. Hemiarthroplasty implant, in the management of these complex fractures, is difficult and still controversial depending on fracture features and patient's compliances. Elderly patients with low functional requirements, high comorbidities, and poor bone quality are more likely to benefit from hemiarthroplasty, but in these cases reverse shoulder prosthesis seems to be more effective in outcomes. Comminuted fractures, severely displaced, with features associated with avascular necrosis would be candidates to hemiarthroplasty. Tuberosity malunion or resorption returns to impaired functional outcome. A proper rehabilitation program is needed for achieving good outcomes [34]. Usually this will involve 4 weeks of shoulder support with pendulum and passive movement with active movement starting, in a pool, from 6 weeks. Complications as tuberosity non-union (11%), heterotopic ossification (9%), proximal migration of the prosthesis (6.8%), infection (2%), and nerve injury can affect the outcomes [32]. In addition, the glenoid can suffer for the pressure of the humeral head implant that can lead to glenoid wear causing pain and future revision surgery [35].

12.7 Reverse Arthroplasty

Reverse shoulder arthroplasty was dedicated and used for cuff tear arthropathy (CTA). The reverse arthroplasty medializes and lowers the center of rotation of the glenohumeral joint. This increases the torque force of the deltoid, by increasing tension and recruiting more muscle fibers, and allows greater shoulder elevation independent of the rotator cuff [36, 37]. The use of reverse shoulder athroplasty (RSA) was enlarged to treat complex proximal humerus fractures to restore function not taking into account the tuberosity healing which is extremely difficult in elderly patients with poor-quality tuberosities and with comminution of the bone fragment. It is mandatory to evaluate the right function of the axillary nerve because the denervation of the deltoid would result in a not recovered function. The use of RSA is recommended for patients over 75 years with complex fractures of the proximal humerus. This device usually provides similar pain relief to hemiarthroplasty and a better function in most of the cases even with tuberosity resorption in this elderly group [37]. Despite the good outcomes, there is a high complication rate with nerve palsy (11.6%), reflex sympathetic dystrophy (7%), prosthesis dislocation (2.3%), resorption and displacement of tuberosities (44.2%), and scapular notching (23.2%) [38]. Long-term follow-up showed radiographic evidence of glenoid loosening [39].

12.8 Discussion

The most part of proximal humeral fractures are minimally displaced and should be successfully managed conservatively. However, the treatment of displaced fractures remains controversial [5, 6], and it is still unclear when surgical intervention is necessary and with which surgical technique. The lack of adequately powered randomized controlled trials (RCT) precludes definitive conclusions over the optimal treatments.

Network meta-analysis (NMA) is a comparatively new evidence-based technique in medical disciplines which compares the relative benefits associated with multiple interventions and obtains hierarchies of these interventions for various treatment options. Chen et al. [40] evaluated the effectiveness and safety of open reduction and internal fixation (ORIF), hemiarthroplasty (HA), reverse shoulder arthroplasty (RSA), intramedullary nailing (IN), and nonoperative treatment (NOT) of displaced proximal humeral fractures in adults. RSA resulted in a lower incidence of additional surgery than ORIF and IN. The rank of treatments in terms of high constant score was RSA, ORIF, IN, NOT, and HA. The rank for reduction in total incidence of complications was RSA, NOT, HA, IN, and ORIF. For lowering the risk of additional surgery, the rank was RSA, NOT, HA, IN, and ORIF. RSA had the highest probability for improving functional outcome and reduction in the total incidence of complications and requiring additional surgery among the five interventions for treating adults with displaced proximal humeral fracture.

One RCT comparing hemiarthroplasty and locking plate fixation for four-part fractures has reported no significant difference in functional outcomes between the groups [41]. Systematic reviews have reported comparable functional results with reverse arthroplasty and hemiarthroplasty [37, 42]. The reverse arthroplasty is receiving increasing support due to its ability to restore function independent of tuberosity union. The problem of treatment of complex three- and four-part proximal humeral fractures with hemiarthroplasty in elderly patients has yielded mixed clinical results. Reverse shoulder arthroplasty has emerged as a treatment option for comminuted proximal humeral fractures for these patients. Reverse shoulder arthroplasty resulted in better clinical outcomes and a similar complication rate compared with hemiarthroplasty for the treatment of comminuted proximal humeral fractures in the elderly. The clinical outcomes and range of motion values of these elderly patients who were treated with a hemiarthroplasty for an acute comminuted proximal humeral fracture exhibited a bimodal distribution of good outcomes if tuberosity healing occurred or poor outcomes if their tuberosities underwent resorption. In comparison, the patients who underwent reverse shoulder arthroplasty had more consistent and superior results irrespective of tuberosity healing [43]. In a nationwide registry-based cohort study comparing patients undergoing primary RSA with patients undergoing primary hemiarthroplasty for acute proximal humeral fractures, RSA appeared to produce functionally superior results to hemiarthroplasty at 5 years postoperatively [44]. Theoretical advantages include relative independence from relying on a functioning supraspinatus for active elevation, potential rapid recovery, and reduced need for postoperative rehabilitation [45, 46]. Studies to date have demonstrated that RTSA provides predictable pain relief with reliable functional gains, especially with tuberosity healing. However, complication rates up to 50–68% have been

reported, including hematoma formation, scapular notching, loosening of the glenoid component, instability, and component dissociation [37, 38, 47, 48]. RTSA appears to provide range of motion superior to that of HA and ORIF. RTSA predictably restored active elevation over horizontal plane in all patients within 4 months. RTSA realized even significant cost savings compared with ORIF and HA [45].

12.9 Conclusion

Summarizing, the elderly patients treated with reverse shoulder arthroplasty had better clinical outcomes, better forward elevation, higher tuberosity healing rates, and a lower rate of revision surgery compared with those who had hemiarthroplasty and open reduction and internal fixation for the treatment of a comminuted proximal humeral fracture.

References

1. Jordan RW, Modi CS. A review of management options for proximal humeral fractures. Open Orthop J. 2014;8:148–56. https://doi.org/10.2174/1874325001408010148. eCollection 2014
2. Baron JA, Karagas M, Barrett J, et al. Basic epidemiology of fractures of the upper and lower limb among Americans over 65 years of age. Epidemiology. 1996;7:612–8.
3. Kannus P, Palvanen M, Niemi S, Parkkari J, Jarvinen M, Vuori I. Increasing number and incidence of osteoporotic fractures of the proximal humerus in elderly people. BMJ. 1996;313:1051–2.
4. Koval KJ, Gallagher MA, Marsicano JG, Cuomo F, McShinawy A, Zuckerman JD. Functional outcome after minimally displaced fractures of the proximal part of the humerus. J Bone Joint Surg Am. 1997;79(2):203–7.

5. Lanting B, MacDermid J, Drosdowech D, Faber KJ. Proximal humeral fractures: a systematic review of treatment modalities. J Shoulder Elb Surg. 2008;17:42–54.
6. Solberg BD, Moon CN, Franco DP, Paiement GD. Surgical treatment of three and four part proximal humeral fractures. J Bone Joint Surg Am. 2009;91:1689–97.
7. Neer CS II. Displaced proximal humerus fractures. Part I. Classification and evaluation. J Bone Joint Surg Am. 1970;52:1077–89.
8. Muller ME, Allgower M, Schneider R, Willeneger H. Manual of internal fixation: techniques recommended by the AO-Group. 2nd ed. Berlin, New York: Springer-Verlag; 1979.
9. Siebenrock KA, Gerber C. The reproducibility of classification of fractures of the proximal end of the humerus. J Bone Joint Surg. 1993;75:1751–5.
10. Sidor ML, Zuckerman JD, Lyon T, Koval K, Cuomo F, Schoenberg N. The Neer classification system for proximal humeral fractures. An assessment of interobserver reliability and intraobserver reproducibility. J Bone Joint Surg Am. 1993;75:1745–50.
11. Bernstein J, Adler LM, Blank JE, Dalsey RM, Williams GR, Iannotti JP. Evaluation of the Neer system of classification of proximal humeral fractures with computerized tomographic scans and plain radiographs. J Bone Joint Surg Am. 1996;78:1371–5.
12. Hertel R, Hempfing A, Stiehler M, Leunig M. Predictors of humeral head ischemia after intracapsular fracture of the proximal humerus. J Shoulder Elb Surg. 2004;13(4):427–33.
13. Hettrich CM, Boraiah S, Dyke JP, Neviaser A, Helfet DL, Lorich DG. Quantitative assessment of the vascularity of the proximal part of the humerus. J Bone Joint Surg Am. 2010;92:943–8.
14. Gaebler C, McQueen MM, Court-Brown CM. Minimally displaced proximal humeral fractures: epidemiology and outcome in 507 cases. Acta Orthop Scand. 2003;74:580–5.
15. Olerud P, Ahrengart L, Ponzer S, Saving J, Tidermark H. Internal fixation *versus* nonoperative treatment of displaced 3-part proximal humeral fractures in elderly patients: a randomised controlled trial. J Shoulder Elb Surg. 2011;20:747–55.
16. Zyto K. Non-operative treatment of comminuted fractures of the proximal humerus in elderly patients. Injury. 1998;29:349–52.
17. Krishnan SH, Bennion PW, Reineck JR, Burkhead WZ. Hemiarthroplasty for proximal humeral fracture: restoration of the Gothic arch. Orthop Clin North Am. 2008;39:441–50.
18. Gardner MJ, Boraiah S, Helfet DL, Lorich DG. Indirect medial reduction and strut support of proximal humerus fractures using an endosteal implant. J Orthop Trauma. 2008;22(3):195–200.
19. Gardner MJ, Weil Y, Barker JU, Kelly BT, Helfet DL, Lorich DG. The importance of medial support in locked plating of proximal humerus fractures. J Orthop Trauma. 2007;21(3):185–91.
20. Owsley K, Gorczyca JT. Fracture displacement and screw cutout after open reduction and locked plate fixation of proximal humeral fractures. J Bone Joint Surg Am. 2008;90:233–40.
21. Agudelo J, Schurmann M, Stahel P, et al. Analysis of efficacy and failure in proximal humerus fractures treated with locking plates. J Orthop Trauma. 2007;21:676–81.
22. Liew AS, Johnson JA, Patterson SD, King GJ, Chess DG. Effect of screw placement on fixation in the humeral head. J Shoulder Elb Surg. 2000;9:423–46.
23. Hagg O, Lundberg BJ. Aspects of prognostic factors in comminuted and dislocated proximal humerus fractures. In: Bateman JE, Welsh RP, editors. Surgery of the shoulder. Philadelphia: Decker; 1984.
24. Besch L, Daniels-Wredenhagen M, Mueller M, Varoga D, Hilgert RE, Seekamp A. Hemiarthroplasty of the shoulder after four part fracture of the humeral head: a long term analysis of 34 cases. J Trauma. 2009;66(1):211–4.
25. Mansat P, Guity MR, Bellumore Y, Mansat M. Shoulder arthroplasty for late sequelae of proximal humeral fractures. J Shoulder Elb Surg. 2004;13:305–12.
26. Agel J, Jones CB, Sanzone AG, Camuso M, Henley MB. Treatment of proximal humeral fractures with Polarus nail fixation. J Shoulder Elb Surg. 2004;13:191–5.
27. Rajasekhar C, Ray PS, Bhamra MS. Fixation of proximal humeral fractures with the Polarus nail. J Shoulder Elb Surg. 2001;10:7–10.
28. Cuny C, Scarlat MM, Irrazi M, et al. The telegraph nail for proximal humeral fractures: a prospective four year study. J Shoulder Elb Surg. 2008;17(4):539–45.
29. Giannoudis PV, Xypnitos FN, Dimitriou R, Manidakis N, Hackney R. Internal fixation of proximal humeral fractures using the Polarus intramedullary nail: our institutional experience and review of the literature. J Orthop Surg Res. 2012;19(7):1749–99.
30. Neer CSII. Displaced proximal humeral fractures. Part II. Treatment of three part and four part displacement. J Bone Joint Surg Am. 1970;52A:1090–103.
31. Neer CS. Indications for replacement of the proximal humeral articulation. Am J Surg. 1955;89:901–7.
32. Kontakis G, Koutras C, Tosounidis T, Giannoudis P. Early management of proximal humeral fractures with hemiarthroplasty: a systematic review. J Bone Joint Surg Br. 2008;90(11):1407–13.
33. Gerber C, Werner CM, Vienne P. Internal fixation of complex fractures of the proximal humerus. J Bone Joint Surg Br. 2004;86:848–55.
34. Dines DM, Warren RF. Modular shoulder hemiarthroplasty for acute fractures. Surgical considerations. Clin Orthop Relat Res. 1994;307:18–26.
35. Gronhagen CM, Abbaszadegan H, Revay SA, Adolphson PY. Medium-term results after primary hemiarthroplasty for comminute proximal humerus fractures: a study of 46 patients followed up for an average of 4.4 years. J Shoulder Elb Surg. 2007;16:766–73.

36. Sirveauz F, Favard L, Oudet D, Huguet D, Walch G, Mole D. Grammont inverted total shoulder arthroplasty in the treatment of glenohumeral osteoarthritis with massive rupture of the cuff. Results of a multicenter study of 80 shoulders. J Bone Joint Surg Br. 2004;86:388–95.
37. Bufquin T, Hersan A, Hubert L, Massin P. Reverse shoulder arthroplasty for the treatment of three and four part fractures of the proximal humerus in the elderly: a prospective review of 43 cases with a short-term follow up. J Bone Joint Surg Br. 2007;89:516–20.
38. Cazeneuve JF, Cristofari DJ. The reverse shoulder prosthesis in the treatment of fractures of the proximal humerus in the elderly. J Bone Joint Surg Br. 2010;92:535–9.
39. Klein M, Juschka M, Hinkenjann B, Scherger B, Ostermann PA. Treatment of comminuted fractures of the proximal humerus in elderly patients with the delta III reverse shoulder prosthesis. J Orthop Trauma. 2008;22(10):698–704.
40. Chen L, Xing F, Effectiveness XZ. Safety of interventions for treating adults with displaced proximal humeral fracture: a network meta-analysis and systematic review. PLoS One. 2016;11(11):e0166801. https://doi.org/10.1371/journal.pone.0166801. eCollection 2016. Review
41. Zyto K, Ahrengart L, Sperber A, Törnkvist H. Treatment of displaced proximal humeral fractures in elderly patients. J Bone Joint Surg Br. 1997;79(3):412–7.
42. Namdari S, Horneff JG, Baldwin K. Comparison of hemiarthroplasty and reverse arthroplasty for treatment of proximal humeral fractures: a systematic review. J Bone Joint Surg Am. 2013;95(18):1701–8.
43. Cuff DJ, Pupello DR. Comparison of hemiarthroplasty and reverse shoulder arthroplasty for the treatment of proximal humeral fractures in elderly patients. J Bone Joint Surg Am. 2013;95(22):2050–5. https://doi.org/10.2106/JBJS.L.01637.
44. Boyle MJ, Youn SM, Frampton CM, Ball CM. Functional outcomes of reverse shoulder arthroplasty compared with hemiarthroplasty for acute proximal humeral fractures. J Shoulder Elb Surg. 2013;22(1):32–7. https://doi.org/10.1016/j.jse.2012.03.006. Epub 2012 May 29
45. Chalmers PN, Slikker W 3rd, Mall NA, Gupta AK, Rahman Z, Enriquez D, Nicholson GP. Reverse total shoulder arthroplasty for acute proximal humeral fracture: comparison to open reduction-internal fixation and hemiarthroplasty. J Shoulder Elb Surg. 2014;23(2):197–204. https://doi.org/10.1016/j.jse.2013.07.044. Epub 2013 Sep 27
46. Gerber C, Pennington SD, Nyffeler RW. Reverse total shoulder arthroplasty. J Am Acad Orthop Surg. 2009;17:284–95.
47. Affonso J, Nicholson GP, Frankle MA, Walch G, Gerber C, Garzon- Muvdi J, et al. Complications of the reverse prosthesis: prevention and treatment. Instr Course Lect. 2012;61:157–68.
48. Cazeneuve JF, Cristofari D-J. Delta III reverse shoulder arthroplasty: radiological outcome for acute complex fractures of the proximal humerus in elderly patients. Orthop Traumatol Surg Res. 2009;95:325–9. https://doi.org/10.1016/j.otsr.2009.03.018.

Irreparable Rotator Cuff Tears

13

Fabrizio Campi, Raffaele Garofalo, and Alessandro Castagna

13.1 Introduction

Rotator cuff tears (RCT) are one of the most commonly treated orthopaedic pathologies. It is present in 20.7% of the general population, and the prevalence increases with age [1, 2]. The rate of patients with symptoms related to the shoulder affected by a cuff lesion is 36% in the general population, whereas 16.9% of the subjects without symptoms also had RCT. RCTs in the general population occur most commonly in elderly patients, male patients, the dominant arm, patients engaged in heavy labour, or patients having a history of trauma [2]. When conservative treatment fails, operative treatment is an option to improve patient condition [3, 4]. Most surgeons agree that an acute painful tear in young people should be treated operatively in order to decrease pain and provide satisfactory long-term function. However, great controversy exists with regard to tears that are large, chronic in nature, and not tractable to repair by standard means. These tears, considered "irreparable" or "massive", provide an ongoing challenge for the orthopaedic surgeon. Authors have attempted to classify these tears based on their size and location [5]. Others consider a massive rotator cuff tear to be one involving two or more tendons. A massive tear is not necessarily irreparable, and an irreparable tear does not mean it is massive in size. However, an irreparable tear can be defined surgically as a tear in which direct tendon-to-bone repair and healing are not possible. An irreparable tear was described by Warner and Parsons [6] as "the inability to achieve a direct repair of the native tendon to the humerus despite mobilizing the soft tissues". Small chronic tears in contradistinction to massive tears may be small and friable and unable to be repaired primarily to bone. Irreparable rotator cuff tears are usually large and retracted with nonfunctional muscle bellies and severe fatty degeneration. The true determination of an irreparable cuff tear, however, is definitively performed under direct visualization under the surgery.

Irreparable RCTs may occur through different mechanisms including acute (i.e. traumatic), acute on chronic, and chronic (i.e. degenerative) tears. Generally, acute massive tears greater than 5 cm are reparable, assuming fatty degeneration is minimal. Gerber et al. [7] showed that fatty infiltration in a sheep model of rotator cuff tears is a necessary consequence following macro-architectural change rather than degenerative process. As the tendon tears and the muscle

F. Campi (✉)
Orthosport Group, Private Hospital Villa Igea, Forlì, Italy

R. Garofalo
Unit of Shoulder Surgery, Miulli Hospital, Bari, Italy

A. Castagna
Shoulder and Elbow Unit, Humanitas Institute IRCCS, Milan, Italy

S. Gumina et al. (eds.), *Reverse Shoulder Arthroplasty*,
https://doi.org/10.1007/978-3-319-97743-0_13

retracts, the pennation angle of the muscle decreases, enabling the space between individual muscle fibres to become replaced with fat. As the muscle retracts and becomes filled with fat, it becomes stiffer and less compliant and has less strength.

The muscles of the rotator cuff provide dynamic stability to the shoulder. Burkhart described the force-couple concept of the rotator cuff after performing fluoroscopic evaluations of patients with massive rotator cuff tears. He stated that normal shoulder function is possible as long as there are balanced forces between the two force couples, i.e. the first force couple in the transverse plane and the second force couple in the coronal plane [8]. When this force couple is intact (or reparable), the shoulder moves perfectly without pain.

13.2 Clinical Evaluation and Imaging

We know that irreparable rotator cuff tears are unpredictable with respect to their clinical presentation. The spectrum of pain and functional disability varies widely. A shoulder may function well in the setting of a painless tear, whereas a small painful tear may result in substantial shoulder dysfunction and disability.

The physical examination should begin with inspection of both upper extremities with the shoulders exposed. The supraspinatus and infraspinatus fosse should be closely examined for signs of atrophy. Massive tears involving the infraspinatus will typically present with increases in passive internal rotation as well as an external rotation lag sign. Similarly, massive tears involving the subscapularis will often present with an increase in passive external rotation and an internal rotation lag sign. Further, supraspinatus tears may demonstrate a drop-arm sign.

Palpation of the long head of the biceps (LHB) tendon within the bicipital groove is essential during the examination, as lesions to the LHB are strongly associated with rotator cuff tears. The surgeon must also assess for concomitant symptomatic acromioclavicular joint arthritis through palpation as well as by assessing for pain with cross-body adduction.

Strength testing of all rotator cuff muscles is imperative. Posterosuperior cuff tears are associated with a positive lag sign when the patient is unable to maintain the shoulder externally rotated at 90° of abduction and adducted to the side.

Furthermore, special attention should be paid to the subscapularis, of which lesions to the upper part of the tendon are often correlated with biceps tendon lesions and LHBT instability. Tests for the subscapularis include the belly press test, the lift-off test, and the bear-hug test [9–11].

The imaging of the shoulder should include a standard set of three X-rays: true anteroposterior, axillary lateral, and outlet (scapular Y). Although plain radiographs will not clearly identify soft tissue, they are highly valuable in elucidating the chronicity of massive tears as well as identifying the presence of glenohumeral arthritis or rotator cuff arthropathy. The outlet view is used to assess the acromial morphology.

The magnetic resonance imaging is the preferred method to evaluate the structural integrity of the rotator cuff. Magnetic resonance imaging can be used to assess the size and location of the tear, the quality of the tendon, and the chronicity of the tear. The sagittal T2 image may show atrophy or fatty infiltration of the involved musculature, which can highlight the chronicity of the tear and also provide prognostic information (Fig. 13.1) [12]. Axial views can evaluate the integrity of the subscapularis as well as associated LHBT tendinosis, tears, or static instability.

13.3 Management Options

13.3.1 Nonsurgical Treatment

Nonsurgical treatment for patients with an irreparable RCT is generally reserved for low-demand patients who are not experiencing significant pain. The mainstay of nonoperative management is physical therapy, subacromial injections, and non-steroidal anti-inflammatory drug (NSAIDs).

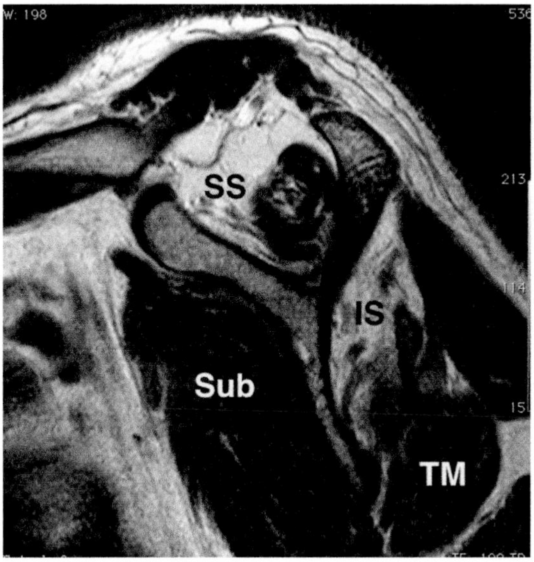

Fig. 13.1 Sagittal magnetic resonance image T2 weighted of a shoulder demonstrating a fatty infiltration of the supraspinatus and infraspinatus muscles. *IS* infraspinatus muscle, *SS* supraspinatus muscle, *Sub* subscapularis muscle, *TM* teres minor

Physical therapy focuses to strengthen the intact portion of the rotator cuff and deltoid as well as the periscapular musculature. Strengthening the intact rotator cuff and scapular stabilizers, in theory, should offload the tear edges and provide a strong foundation for maintenance of a strong force couple to prevent progressive rotator cuff arthropathy [13–15].

13.3.2 Surgical Treatment

This chapter does not describe the use of reverse shoulder arthroplasty in the treatment of irreparable rotator cuff tears.

When patients have failed nonsurgical management, surgical treatment should be considered. According to the AAOS guidelines, the only recommendation regarding irreparable rotator cuff tears was for partial repair when possible, debridement, or tendon transfers which all earned a weak recommendation [16].

Many operative techniques have been described for the treatment of massive RCTs with severe retraction where anatomic repair is not possible, such as arthroscopic debridement and/or biceps tenotomy, tendon transfers and grafting, partial repair of the remaining rotator cuff tendons, and a superior capsular reconstruction (SCR) [17].

13.4 Partial Repair, Margin Convergence

Burkhart et al. [18] first introduced the concept of functional repair of the cuff to restore the force couple of the humeral head and to increase the acromion-humeral distance (AHD). In these arthroscopic procedures, complete closure of the defect was not considered to be essential to restore the normal cuff and shoulder biomechanics [19]. In margin convergence technique, the free margin of the tear converges towards the greater tuberosity as side-to-side repair progresses (Fig. 13.2).

As the margin converges, the strain at the free edge of the cuff is reduced significantly, leaving an almost tension-free converged cuff margin overlying the humeral bone bed for partial or anatomic repair. Side-to-side closure of two-thirds of a U- or V-shaped tear reduces the strain at the cuff margin to one-sixth of the strain that existed at the pre-converged cuff margin. This strategy gives a lower probability of failure of fixation to bone. If the supraspinatus tendon retraction made direct reinsertion of tendon to bone not possible, the infraspinatus can be sutured to the bone in an attempt to cover its anatomic footprint. The technique allows repair of the peripheral margins of the tear to restore the force couples, anterior and posterior, and the "suspension bridge" system of force transmission in the shoulder. Clinical outcomes are obviously lesser than after complete rotator cuff repair [18–20] but remain stable for AHD even at medium-term follow-up [21].

Previous authors have introduced the radiographic evaluation of the AHD as a standard technique in routine orthopaedic treatment. A decreased AHD is the most reliable radiographic finding for RCTs [22–25], and in particular an AHD < 6 mm is a sign of rotator cuff rupture

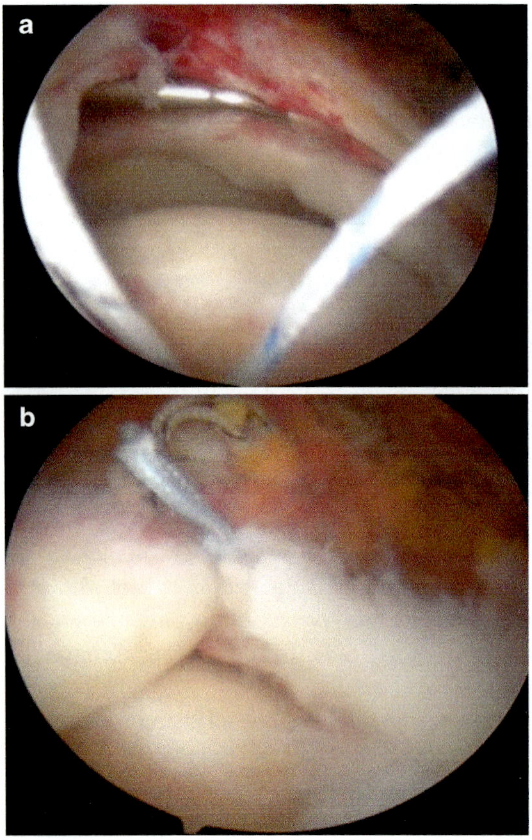

Fig. 13.2 (**a**) Massive superior and posterior RCT in a right shoulder observed with the scope through the lateral portal. A lateral anchor is placed on the greater tuberosity and is used after a margin convergence. (**b**) Same shoulder after that two latero-lateral nonabsorbable sutures are passed (margin convergence technique)

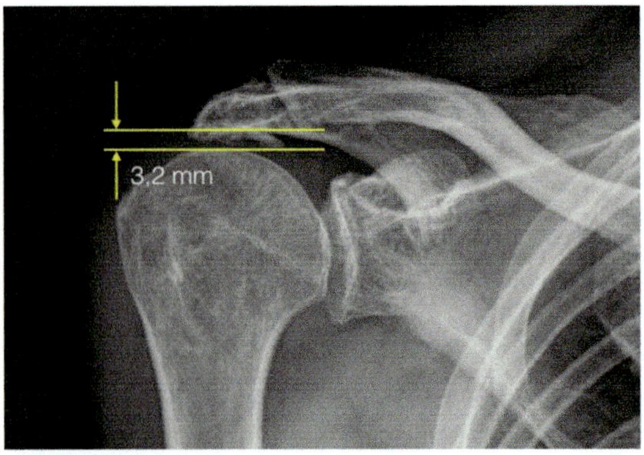

Fig. 13.3 X-ray in AP view of a right shoulder in a 67-year-old male patient with a degenerative massive rotator cuff tear. The measured AHD in this case in less than 6 mm indicating a not completely reparable RCT

almost systematically involving long-standing total infraspinatus tear, not always amenable to suture repair due to advanced fatty degeneration [26, 27]. AHD equal to or greater than 6 mm is of no diagnostic relevance and in no way indicates whether there is subscapularis tear and, if so, whether suture repair is feasible (Fig. 13.3).

Porcellini et al. [28] support the assumption that partial repair of a massive RCT may improve the biomechanics of the shoulder while re-establishing the shoulder's essential force couples, thus converting a "dysfunctional symptomatic" RCT into a "functional tear". This study indicates that, in cases of massive RCT with no subscapularis tear test, long-term results of partial repair of the posterior cuff with covering of the infraspinatus footprint showed improved outcome scores. In addition, AHD increased minimally and was stable at final follow-up. These results are superior to those of arthroscopic debridement alone in active patients. The ideal patient for partial repair of the cuff has good cuff balancing without signs of complete disruption of the posterior cuff (automatic internal recall), with no drop-arm or Hornblower sign, and with good function of the subscapularis. Postoperative outcomes of this investigation are comparable with those of the available literature. In a study on 24 patients with massive rotator cuff tear undergoing partial repair, Duralde et al. reported that 67% of patients showed good to excellent results at ASES score and 92% of patients were subjectively satisfied after this surgery [17].

Berth et al. reported good or satisfactory outcomes after partial rotator cuff repair, and regardless of the high rates of structural failure, the results of arthroscopic partial rotator cuff repair showed slightly better functional outcome than debridement [29]. In a study by Franceschi et al., patients with massive rotator cuff tear received either debridement or a partial repair. Postoperatively, both groups demonstrated highly significant improvements compared with preoperative values, and all scores in the partial repair group were superior to the outcome of the debridement group. These differences may be due to the ability of the partial repair to restore the functional anatomy of the shoulder, allowing a near-to-normal arc of movement, strength, and function [30]. Kim et al. in a recent report comparing pre- to postoperative results in a case series of 27 patients undergoing partial repair showed that all shoulder scores (simple shoulder test, Constant, and UCLA) had a significant improvement [31]. Arrigoni et al., recently, also showed similar clinical results in their case series [32].

In a cadaver laboratory study, Lee et al. [33] confirmed that if complete repair of massive cuff tear is not possible, posterior cuff (infraspinatus) repair is necessary to restore abnormal glenohumeral kinematics, and margin convergence anteriorly is recommended to decrease gap formation of the repaired tendon edge, which may provide a better biomechanical environment for healing. In 2012 Burkhart et al. demonstrated that repair of massive rotator cuff tears with advanced mobilization techniques can lead to reversal of preoperative pseudoparalysis in 90% of patients who have not had previous surgery. In these patients functional improvement can be obtained with a low rate of complications. However, in the setting of a revision and pseudoparalysis, only 43% of patients regained FF above 90° [34].

13.5 Debridement and LHB Tenotomy/Tenodesis

When partial repair is not possible because of the size, retraction, or fatty infiltration of the cuff, one can perform other palliative treatments for RCTs such as arthroscopic debridement or tenotomy/tenodesis of the LHB [35, 36]. There exists some strong evidence that the satisfactory results with debridement deteriorate during long-term follow-up [37]. For instance, Zvijac et al. [38] found a significant decrease in pain assessment and shoulder function at 3–6 years' follow-up in patients treated with arthroscopic subacromial decompression for irreparable RCT. Lee et al. [39] reported on 32 patients treated with arthroscopic decompression and tuberoplasty showing significant improvement in postoperative Constant and UCLA shoulder scores. The advantages of arthroscopic subacromial decompression and rotator cuff debridement include a short operative time, an accelerated rehabilitation program, and lower reported complication rates compared with the more extensive reconstructive procedures [37].

Lesions of the biceps tendon are frequently associated with RCT and have been identified as a source of persistent pain that can resolve with spontaneous rupture. This has led to the introduction of biceps tenotomy as a treatment option for patients with massive and/or irreparable RCTs. So far, discussions concerning this procedure have noted longevity of pain relief and a possible progression of arthritic changes in the glenohumeral joint. In addition, function of the biceps tendon in terms of generating elbow flexion strength is often a concern for patients who are presented with the option of cutting the LHB. After spontaneous rupture, loss of elbow flexion strength is found to be up to 16%. Arthroscopic biceps tenotomy in the treatment of RCTs in selected patients yields good objective improvement and a high degree of patient satisfaction. Despite these improvements, arthroscopic tenotomy or tenodesis can increase superior translation of the humeral head during active abduction of the shoulder in the scapular plane [40] and does not appear to alter the progressive radiographic changes that occur with long-standing RCT [41]. Walch et al. [42] reported the long-term results of 307 biceps tenotomies, 110 of which were performed with a concomitant acromioplasty, as palliative treatment for RCTs. At a mean of 57 months postoperatively, 87% of the patients were satisfied or very satisfied, and the mean Constant score had improved to 67.6 points, compared with 48 points preoperatively. As expected, active external rotation was not improved after the surgery.

Boileau et al. [43] evaluated the clinical and radiographic outcomes of isolated arthroscopic biceps tenotomy or tenodesis as treatment for irreparable RCT associated with a biceps lesion. They found a significant decrease in AHD by 1.1 mm, but only one patient progressed to a full RCT arthropathy, and they concluded that pseudoparalysis of the shoulder and severe rotator cuff arthropathy are contraindications to this procedure. Klinger et al. [44] compared the results of arthroscopic debridement in massive, irreparable RCTs with and without tenotomy of the LHB in 41 cases. They concluded that additional LHB tenotomy did not significantly influence the postoperative results at the latest follow-up, and they did not note significant humeral head migration or developing rotator cuff arthropathy after surgery. Recently, Su et al. [45] in a cadaveric study investigated the biomechanical effects of posterosuperior RCT size and loading the LHB tendon in the presence of various sized RCTs. They showed that if the inferior infraspinatus remained intact, there was no significant difference in glenohumeral translation for any different load studied. Once the supraspinatus and the entire infraspinatus were released, 50 N of load led to significantly increased translation in both directions: superior and anterosuperior. For intact specimens and for all sizes of RCTs, biceps loading led to a significant decrease in glenohumeral translation.

We postulate that these biomechanical data can justify the preventive role of partial repair on CTA development in cases of a good functional repair of the infraspinatus tendon on the original footprint, as recently demonstrated [46]. The good results of infraspinatus tendon repair can be indirectly shown by maintenance of the AHD at long-term follow-up for the well-known decrease in AHD with widening of the size of the cuff tear [28].

Some authors proposed the use of biodegradable spacer in case of massive irreparable RCT [47]. This spacer can be utilized alone or associated with a partial rotator cuff repair. The rationale using this device is to create a space between the acromion and humeral head by lowering and recentring the humeral head itself. In this manner the remaining rotator cuff can work in a better angle so to improve shoulder function.

13.6 Augmentation

All open and arthroscopic techniques have their limitations in treating this problem, and a number of different treatment options depending on patient age, activity level, and degree of disability have been proposed. The biceps tendon interposition technique for massive RCT offers a possible improvement in clinical outcomes and is comparable to that of conventional repair. In addition, the augmentation technique using the biceps as a potential graft for RCT is particularly useful in bridging the gap in immobile massive RCTs with posterior defects and retraction. In an effort to augment the deficient rotator cuff tissue while maintaining the anatomic integrity of the shoulder, some surgeons are incorporating biologic tissue scaffolds into the cuff deficiency [48–51].

Graft augmentation provides stability for torn tendons and increases the rate of healing. Tissue autografts and tendon transfers are subject to donor-site morbidity. Tendon augmentation grafts are derived from allografts, xenografts, or synthetic materials. Selection of augmentation grafts depends on the tissue of origin, graft processing, cross-linking of the material, surgeon experience, and physical properties of the tissue.

Augmentation grafts can provide strength by acting as conductive scaffolding for tissue ingrowth and provide a collagen reservoir for fibroblasts. Compared to tendon alone, augmentation grafts provide higher resistance to failure and minimize stress shielding [52]. Biomechanically, the stress-strain curve of each augmentation graft varies, depending on its origin and production process [53]. Further variation depends on the surgical method (e.g. whether the graft is interpositional or an on-lay device). Augmentation grafts increase stiffness [54] with strength approaching that of native tendons [55]. Some loss of mechanical properties is expected, as the augmentation graft integrates and remodels with the native tissue. One concern with using allografts or xenografts is the host-tissue morphological response. Cellular response depends on both the origin of the graft and the processing techniques and the host-tissue medium. Enhancing mechanical properties through over-chemical cross-linking may result in a foreign body response by the host tissue. Therefore, a balance of the biomechanical and biocompatibility properties of the grafts is needed. Chemical and physical properties of synthetic grafts can be controlled, but the trade-off is

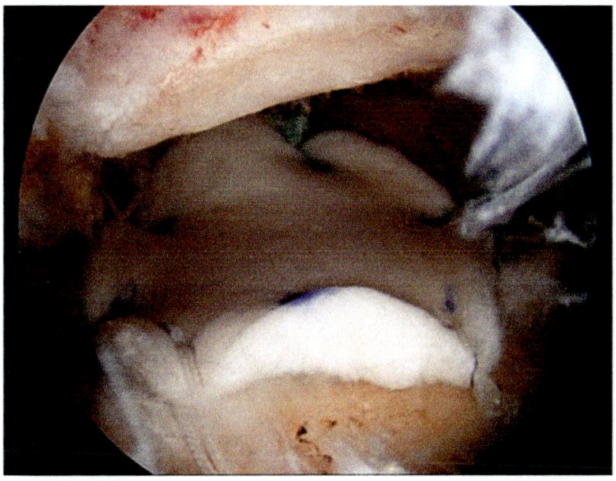

Fig. 13.4 Right shoulder observed through a lateral portal. A graft jacket patch is used to bridge the cuff defect in this massive RCT (Courtesy by SJ Snyder MD)

a lack of biocompatibility, which is usually being nonabsorbable by the tissue. A high rate of immune and inflammatory response has been reported [56]. A porcine submucosa subintestinal graft named Restore (DePuy, USA) was found to increase pain and lead to poorer tendon healing. Its clinical outcome was in contrast to the outcome of many preclinical animal studies. This suggests that Restore may not be suitable for human rotator cuff repair [57]. GraftJacket (Wright Medical Group, USA) is derived from human dermis and has been studied as interpositional graft in case of massive and not reparable RCT (Fig. 13.4). An improvement in UCLA shoulder scores at the 2-year follow-up has been demonstrated. Furthermore, magnetic resonance imaging demonstrated tissue incorporation into the graft [58].

Augmentation grafts can deliver cells and bioactive molecules. Repairing the supraspinatus of rabbits with mesenchymal stem cell-impregnated alginate beads enabled production of more well-organized tendon fibres and a higher ultimate failure load after 12 weeks [59]. Augmenting the infraspinatus of sheep with bovine type I collagen containing rhPDG-BB improved biomechanical strength and anatomic appearance, compared to controls [60]. Using a platelet-rich fibrin matrix suture construct in patients with rotator cuff tears enabled a lower retear rate (despite not being clinically significant) [61].

Mori et al. compared the arthroscopic patch graft procedure and partial repair for irreparable large or massive rotator cuff tears (RCTs) in shoulders with low-grade fatty degeneration of the infraspinatus (stage 1 or 2 according to Goutallier et al.) in terms of the functional and structural outcomes. The patch graft procedure showed an 8.3% retear rate for the repaired ISP with both improved clinical scores and recovery of muscle strength, whereas the partial repair had a retear rate of 41.7% [62].

13.7 Tendon Transfer

Tendon transfers of the latissimus dorsi [63–65], pectoralis major [66], and the pectoralis minor [67] have also been described to improve pain and function, usually in young and active patients with irreparable RCTs [68, 69]. Patients without glenohumeral arthritis but with marked weakness and pain in the setting of a massive, irreparable rotator cuff tear can benefit from a tendon transfer [70].

Latissimus dorsi transfer to reconstruct a massive posterosuperior rotator cuff tear was originally developed by Gerber et al. [71]. Patients with functional impairment who may also have loss of external rotation strength can be considered for this procedure if they do not have pseudoparalysis. The transferred latissimus dorsi was postulated to act as an effective depressor in restricting cranial migration of the humeral head. However, postoperative radiographs showed minimal or no depression, especially in the neutral or externally rotated position. With internal rotation, 9 of 14 treated patients showed slightly improved positioning of the humeral head in relation to the glenoid [68, 69]. Iannotti et al. [72] found that preoperative shoulder function and general strength influence the outcome after latissimus dorsi transfer. In their study of 14 patients undergoing latissimus dorsi transfer for massive rotator cuff tear, women with poor shoulder function had a greater probability of a poor result. The investigators reported that the most significant predictors of outcome were preoperative active range of motion and strength in forward flexion and external rotation. The transfer does not overcome pseudoparalysis.

Recently a systematic review of the literature was performed via a search of electronic databases. Ten studies that fulfilled all inclusion and exclusion criteria were included. The frequency-weighted mean age was 58.7 years. Patients were followed for a frequency-weighted mean of 45.5 months (range, 24–126 months). Patients had a frequency-weighted mean adjusted Constant score of 45.9 preoperatively compared with 73.2 postoperatively ($p < 0.001$). The frequency-weighted mean active forward elevation improved from 101.9° preoperatively to 137.4° postoperatively ($p < 0.001$), and the frequency-weighted mean active external rotation improved from 16.8° to 26.7° ($p < 0.001$). Subscapularis muscle insufficiency, advanced teres minor muscle atrophy, and the need for revision surgery were correlated with poor functional outcomes in some studies [73]. Recently transfer of the latissimus dorsi tendon has been reported to yield good-to-excellent long-term results in well-selected patients, with substantial and durable improvements in shoulder function and pain relief. Shoulders with fatty infiltration of the teres minor muscle and insufficiency of the subscapularis muscle tended to have inferior results, as did those with a large critical shoulder angle [71]. It remains unclear whether the clinical results of this technique are achieved either by active muscle contractions or by a passive tenodesis effect of the transfer. Henseler et al. evaluated the muscle activity with surface electromyography (EMG) and the clinical outcome of the latissimus dorsi transfer in selected patients. They demonstrated that latissimus dorsi has synergistic muscle activity after transfer. Apart from a tenodesis effect, directional muscle activity seems relevant for improved clinical outcome and pain relief. A specific gain was observed for external rotation in elevated arm positions, a motion essential for daily living tasks. The transfer remained active in all cases, as reflected by increased latissimus dorsi EMG activity and shifted from preoperative antagonistic co-activation in adduction to synergistic activation in abduction [74, 75]. In conclusion a majority of authors found less favourable results for revision cases besides detachment and/or atrophy of the anterior deltoid which seemed to be a major risk factor for postoperative lower results, whereas less aggressive previous surgery like arthroscopic debridement, acromioplasty, or LHB tenotomy might be more favourable. Those results may suggest that preserving deltoid muscle is important for success in a LD tendon transfer surgery [76–78]. A thorough examination of the literature on LD tendon transfer for irreparable posterosuperior tears and our own clinical experience showed that with correct indications this surgical procedure gives significant improvement in terms of pain, active elevation, active external rotation, and function of the shoulder. Strength is usually improved but not always in a statistically significant manner. LD tendon transfer does not seem to stop osteoarthritis progression or superior humeral head migration although those two issues have had no influence on postoperative subjective and objective results of the procedure so far. EMG analysis of the LD muscle after the transfer shows muscle activity mostly in active external rotation suggesting an active effect and not only a tenodesis effect to explain the new balance of the shoulder. In our opinion, this technique is the only solution in non-pseudoparalytic young patients who have no osteoarthritis after failure of a previous treatment for massive posterosuperior cuff tears to allow restoration of active external rotation. Recent advances in the technique with assistance of arthroscopy and tubularization are clearly a benefit as there are less danger for the deltoid muscle and stronger resistance of the transferred tendon to traction. Longer follow-up will be needed to determinate in which clinical situations LD tendon transfer will be the best surgical option [79, 80].

13.8 Superior Capsular Reconstruction

Mihata et al. [81] described a novel technique termed arthroscopic superior capsule reconstruction (ASCR) to restore stability of the glenohumeral joint after irreparable RCT [81]. A patch graft was used to reconstruct the superior capsule of the glenohumeral joint (Fig. 13.5); medially the graft is attached to the superior glenoid (Fig. 13.6) and laterally attached to the greater tuberosity. The graft demonstrated biomechanical evidence to decrease subacromial contact pressures [82]. In a clinical study of 24 patients with large or massive irreparable RCT, ASES scores improved from 23.5 to 92.9 postoperatively, and 84% of patients were free from graft tear at a mean of 34 month follow-up [82], even though Burkhart (et al.) concludes in a recent publication: "arthroscopic SCR using dermal allograft provides a successful outcome in approximately 70% of cases in an initial experience. The preliminary results are encouraging in this difficult to manage patient population, but precise indications are important and graft healing is low in our initial experience" [83].

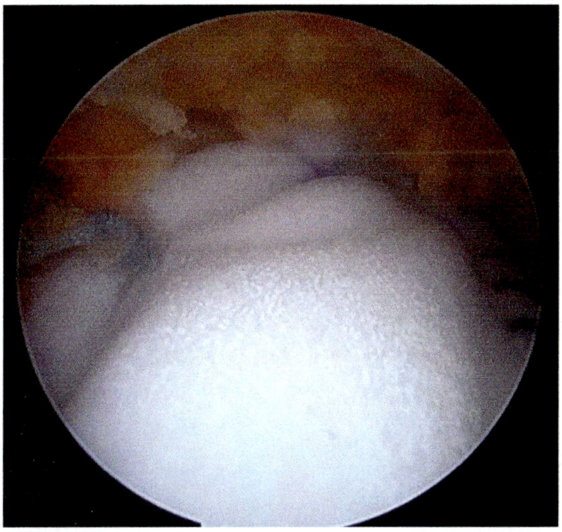

Fig. 13.5 Right shoulder observed through a lateral portal. Superior capsular reconstruction (note, on the left side, one of the two posterior sutures between the dermal matrix and the infraspinatus used to avoid the superior-posterior migration of the humeral head)

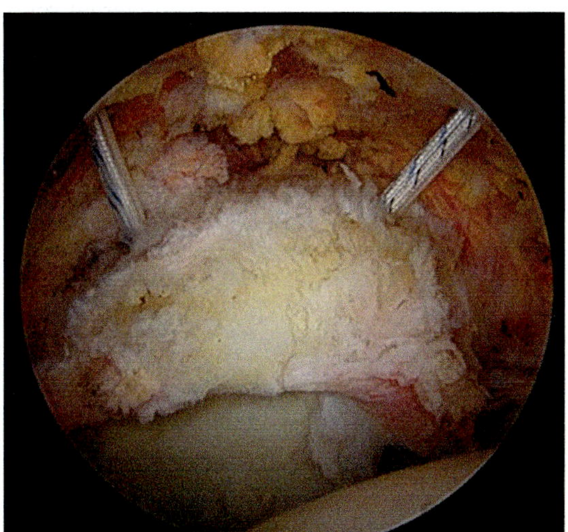

Fig. 13.6 Right shoulder observed through a lateral portal. Two anchors placed over the glenoid in the superior capsular reconstruction

13.9 Conclusion

Irreparable rotator cuff tears can be a challenging task for the orthopaedic surgeon. Treatment depends on patient functional status as well as the skill of the surgeon. Tendon transfer has become more recently popularized, with lower trapezius tendon transfer on the horizon. Salvage options for continued pain and decreased function include reverse total shoulder arthroplasty and hemiarthroplasty. Dermal allograft augmentation has shown some promise in small clinical and biomechanical series; however, larger long-term studies need to be done before definitive conclusions can be made.

References

1. Cofield RH. Current concepts review: rotator cuff disease of the shoulder. J Bone Joint Surg Am. 1985;67:974–9.
2. Yamamoto A, Takagishi K, Osawa T, Yanagawa T, Nakajima D, Shitara H, et al. Prevalence and risk factors of a rotator cuff tear in the general population. J Shoulder Elb Surg. 2010;19:116–20.
3. Iannotti JP. Full-thickness rotator cuff tears: factors affecting surgical outcome. J Am Acad Orthop Surg. 1994;2:87–95.
4. Williams GR Jr, Rockwood CA Jr, Bigliani LU, Iannotti JP, Stanwood W. Rotator cuff tears: why do we repair them? J Bone Joint Surg Am. 2004;86:2764–76.
5. Patte D. Classification of rotator cuff lesions. Clin Orthop Relat Res. 1990;(254):81–6.
6. Warner JJ, Parsons IM. Latissimus dorsi tendon transfer: a comparative analysis of primary and salvage reconstruction of massive, irreparable rotator cuff tears. J Shoulder Elb Surg. 2001;10(6):514–21.

7. Gerber C, Meyer DC, Schneeberger AG, Hoppeler H, von Rechenberg B. Effect of tendon release and delayed repair on the structure of the muscles of the rotator cuff: an experimental study in sheep. J Bone Joint Surg Am. 2004;86A(9):1973–82.
8. Burkhart SS. Arthroscopic treatment of massive rotator cuff tears. Clinical results and biomechanical rationale. Clin Orthop Relat Res. 1991;(267):45–56.
9. Barth JR, Burkhart SS, De Beer JF. The bear-hug test: a new and sensitive test for diagnosing a subscapularis tear. Arthroscopy. 2006;22:1076–84.
10. Bartsch M, Greiner S, Haas NP, Scheibel M. Diagnostic values of clinical tests for subscapularis lesions. Knee Surg Sports Traumatol Arthrosc. 2010;18:1712–7.
11. Gerber C, Hersche O, Farron A. Isolated rupture of the subscapularis tendon. J Bone Joint Surg Am. 1996;78:1015–23.
12. Thomazeau H, Boukobza E, Morcet N, Chaperon J, Langlais F. Prediction of rotator cuff repair results by magnetic resonance imaging. Clin Orthop Relat Res. 1997;344:275–83.
13. Ainsworth R. Physiotherapy rehabilitation in patients with massive, irreparable rotator cuff tears. Musculoskeletal Care. 2006;4(3):140–51.
14. Ainsworth R, Lewis JS. Exercise therapy for the conservative management of full thickness tears of the rotator cuff: a systematic review. Br J Sports Med. 2007;41(4):200–10.
15. Merolla G, Paladini P, Saporito M, Porcellini G. Conservative management of rotator cuff tears: literature review and proposal for a prognostic. Prediction Score. Muscles Ligaments Tendons J. 2011;1(1):12–9.
16. Tashjian RZ. AAOS clinical practice guideline: optimizing the management of rotator cuff problems. J Am Acad Orthop Surg. 2011;19(6):380–3.
17. Duralde XA, Bair B. Massive rotator cuff tears: the result of partial rotator cuff repair. J Shoulder Elb Surg. 2005;14:121–7.
18. Burkhart SS, Nottage WM, Ogilvie-Harris DJ, Kohn HS, Pachelli A. Partial repair of irreparable rotator cuff tears. Arthroscopy. 1994;10:363–70.
19. Nove-Josserand L, L_evigne C, No€el E, Walch G. The acromiohumeral interval. A study of the factors influencing its height (in French). Rev Chir Orthop Reparatrice Appar Mot. 1996;82:379–85.
20. Burkhart SS. Arthroscopic treatment of massive rotator cuff tears. Clin Orthop Relat Res. 2001;(390):107–18.
21. Yoo JC, Koh KH, Woo KJ, Shon MS, Koo KH. Clinical and radiographic results of partial repairs in irreparable rotator cuff tears: preliminary report (SS-05) [abstract]. Arthroscopy. 2010;26(Suppl):e3.
22. Golding FC. The shoulder-the forgotten joint. Brit J Radiol. 1962;35:149–58.
23. Gruber G, Bernhardt GA, Clar H, Zacherl M, Glehr M, Wurnig C. Measurement of the acromiohumeral interval on standardized anteroposterior radiographs: a prospective study of observer variability. J Shoulder Elb Surg. 2010;19:10–3.
24. Lehtinen JT, Lehto MU, Kaarela K, Kautiainen HJ, Belt EA, Kauppi MJ. Radiographic joint space in rheumatoid glenohumeral joints. A 15-year prospective follow-up study in 74 patients. Rheumatology (Oxford). 2000;39:288–92.
25. Saupe N, Pfirrmann CW, Schmid MR, Jost B, Werner CM, Zanetti M. Association between rotator cuff abnormalities and reduced acromiohumeral distance. Am J Roentgenol. 2006;187:376–82.
26. Liem D, Lengers N, Dedy N, Poetzl W, Steinbeck J, Marquardt B. Arthroscopic debridement of massive irreparable rotator cuff tears. Arthroscopy. 2008;24:743–8.
27. Keener JD, Wei AS, Kim HM, Steger-May K, Yamaguchi K. Proximal humeral migration in shoulders with symptomatic and asymptomatic rotator cuff tears. J Bone Joint Surg Am. 2009;91:1405–13.
28. Porcellini G, Castagna A, Cesari E, Merolla G, Pellegrini A, Paladini P. Partial repair of irreparable supraspinatus tendon tears: clinical and radiographic evaluations at long-term follow-up. J Shoulder Elb Surg. 2011;20(7):1170–7.
29. Berth A, Neumann W, Awiszus F, Pap G. Massive rotato cuff tears: functional outcome after debridement or arthroscopic partial repair. J Orthop Traumatol. 2010;11(1):13–20.
30. Franceschi F, Papalia R, Vasta S, Leonardi F, Maffulli N, Denaro V. Surgical management of irreparable rotator cuff tears. Knee Surg Sports Traumatol Arthrosc. 2012;23(2):494–501.
31. Kim SJ, Lee IS, Kim SH, Lee WY, Chun YM. Arthroscopic partial repair of irreparable large to massive rotator cuff tears. Arthroscopy. 2012;28(6):761–8.
32. Arrigoni P, Fossati C, Zottarelli L, Ragone V, Randelli P. Functional repair in massive immobile rotator cuff tears leads to satisfactory quality of living: results at 3-year follow-up. Musculoskelet Surg. 2013;97(Suppl 1):73–7.
33. Oh JH, McGarry MH, Jun BJ, Gupta A, Chung KC, Hwang J, Lee TQ. Restoration of shoulder biomechanics according to degree of repair completion in a cadaveric model of massive rotator cuff tear: importance of margin convergence and posterior cuff fixation. Am J Sports Med. 2012;40(11):2448–53.
34. Denard PJ, Lädermann A, Jiwani AZ, Burkhart SS. Functional outcome after arthroscopic repair of massive rotator cuff tears in individuals with pseudoparalysis. Arthroscopy. 2012;28(9):1214–9.
35. Gartsman GM. Massive, irreparable tears of the rotator cuff. Results of operative debridement and sub-acromial decompression. J Bone Joint Surg Am. 1997;79:715–21.
36. Rockwood CA Jr, Williams GR Jr, Burkhead WZ. Debridement of degenerative irreparable lesions of the rotator cuff. J Bone Joint Surg Am. 1995;77:857–66.
37. Mellio AS, Savoie FH, Field LD. Massive rotator cuff tears: debridement versus repair. Orthop Clin North Am. 1997;28:117–24.

38. Zvijac JE, Levy HJ, Lemak LJ. Arthroscopic subacromial decompression in the treatment of full thickness rotator cuff tears: a 3- to 6-year follow-up. Arthroscopy. 1994;10:518–23.
39. Lee BG, Cho NS, Rhee YG. Results of arthroscopic decompression and tuberoplasty for irreparable massive rotator cuff tears. Arthroscopy. 2011;27(10):1341–50.
40. Warner JJ, McMahon PJ. The role of the long head of the biceps brachii in superior stability of the glenohumeral joint. J Bone Joint Surg Am. 1995;77:366–72.
41. Szabo I, Boileau P, Walch G. The proximal biceps as a pain generator and results of tenotomy. Sports Med Arthrosc Rev. 2008;16:180–6.
42. Walch G, Edwards TB, Boulahia A, Nove-Josserand L, Neyton L, Szabo I. Arthroscopic tenotomy of the long head of the biceps in the treatment of rotator cuff tears: clinical and radiographic results of 307 cases. J Shoulder Elb Surg. 2005;14:238.
43. Boileau P, Baque F, Valerio L, Ahrens P, Chuinard C, Trojani C. Isolated arthroscopic biceps tenotomy or tenodesis improves symptom in patients with massive irreparable rotator cuff tears. J Bone Joint Surg Am. 2007;89:747–57.
44. Klinger HM, Spahn G, Baums MH, Steckel H. Arthroscopic debridement of irreparable massive rotator cuff tears comparison of debridement alone and combined procedure with biceps tenotomy. Acta Chir Belg. 2005;105:297–301.
45. Su WR, Budoff JE, Luo ZP. The effect of posterosuperior rotator cuff ears and biceps loading on glenohumeral translation. Arthroscopy. 2010;26:578–86.
46. Mochizuki T, Sugaya H, Uomizu M, Maeda K, Matsuki K, Sekiya I, et al. Humeral insertion of the supraspinatus and infraspinatus. New anatomical findings regarding the footprint of the rotator cuff. Surgical technique. J Bone Joint Surg Am. 2009;91(Suppl 2 Pt 1):1–7.
47. Savarese E, Romeo R. New solution for massive, irreparable rotator cuff tears: the subacromial "biodegradable spacer". Arthrosc Tech. 2012;1(1):e69–74.
48. Ahmad Z, Henson F, Wardale J, Noorani A, Tytherleigh-Strong G, Rushton N. Regenerative techniques for repair of rotator cuff tears. J Orthop Surg. 2013;21(2):226–31.
49. Bond JL, Dopirak RM, Higgins J, Burns J, Snyder SJ. Arthroscopic replacement of massive, irreparable rotator cuff tears using a Graft-Jacket allograft: technique and preliminary results. Arthroscopy. 2008;24:403–9.
50. Cho NS, Yi JW, Rhee YG. Arthroscopic biceps augmentation for avoiding undue tension in repair of massive rotator cuff tears. Arthroscopy. 2009;25:183–91.
51. Rhee YG, Cho NS, Lim CT, Yi JW, Vishvanathan T. Bridging the gap in immobile massive rotator cuff tears: augmentation using the tenotomized biceps. Am J Sports Med. 2008;36:1511–8.
52. Barber FA, Herbert MA, Boothby MH. Ultimate tensile failure loads of a human dermal allograft rotator cuff augmentation. Arthroscopy. 2008;24:20–4.
53. Derwin KA, Baker AR, Spragg RK, Leigh DR, Iannotti JP. Commercial extracellular matrix scaffolds for rotator cuff tendon repair. Biomechanical, biochemical, and cellular properties. J Bone Joint Surg Am. 2006;88:2665–72.
54. Schlegel TF, Hawkins RJ, Lewis CW, Motta T, Turner AS. The effects of augmentation with Swine small intestine submucosa on tendon healing under tension: histologic and mechanical evaluations in sheep. Am J Sports Med. 2006;34:275–80.
55. Nicholson GP, Breur GJ, Van Sickle D, Yao JQ, Kim J, Blanchard CR. Evaluation of a cross-linked acellular porcine dermal patch for rotator cuff repair augmentation in an ovine model. J Shoulder Elb Surg. 2007;16(5 Suppl):S184–90.
56. Chen J, Xu J, Wang A, Zheng M. Scaffolds for tendon and ligament repair: review of the efficacy of commercial products. Expert Rev Med Devices. 2009;6:61–73.
57. Iannotti JP, Codsi MJ, Kwon YW, Derwin K, Ciccone J, Brems JJ. Porcine small intestine submucosa augmentation of surgical repair of chronic two-tendon rotator cuff tears. A randomized, controlled trial. J Bone Joint Surg Am. 2006;88:1238–44.
58. Wong I, Burns J, Snyder SJ. Arthroscopic GraftJacket repair of rotator cuff tears. J Shoulder Elb Surg. 2010;19(2 Suppl):104–9.
59. Chen CH, Chang CH, Wang KC, Su CI, Liu HT, Yu CM, et al. Enhancement of rotator cuff tendon-bone healing with injectable periosteum progenitor cells-BMP-2 hydrogel in vivo. Knee Surg Sports Traumatol Arthrosc. 2011;19:1597–607.
60. Hee CK, Dines JS, Dines DM, Roden CM, Wisner-Lynch LA, Turner AS, et al. Augmentation of a rotator cuff suture repair using rhPDGF-BB and a type I bovine collagen matrix in an ovine model. Am J Sports Med. 2011;39:1630–9.
61. Barber FA, Hrnack SA, Snyder SJ, Hapa O. Rotator cuff repair healing influenced by platelet-rich plasma construct augmentation. Arthroscopy. 2011;27:1029–35.
62. Mori D, Funakoshi N, Yamashita F. Arthroscopic surgery of irreparable large or massive rotator cuff tears with low-grade fatty degeneration of the infraspinatus: patch autograft procedure versus partial repair procedure. Arthroscopy. 2013;29(12):1911–21.
63. Gerber C, Maquieira G, Espinosa N. Latissimus dorsi transfer for the treatment of irreparable rotator cuff tears. J Bone Joint Surg Am. 2006;88:113–20.
64. Habermeyer P, Magosch P, Rudolph T, Lichtenberg S, Liem D. Transfer of the tendon of latissimus dorsi for the treatment of massive tears of the rotator cuff: a new single-incision technique. J Bone Joint Surg Br. 2006;88:208–12.

65. Warner JJ. Management of massive irreparable rotator cuff tears: the role of tendon transfer. Instr Course Lect. 2001;50:63–71.
66. Resch H, Povacz P, Ritter E, Matschi W. Transfer of the pectoralis major muscle for the treatment of irreparable rupture of the subscapularis tendon. J Bone Joint Surg Am. 2000;82:372–82.
67. Paladini P, Campi F, Merolla G, Pellegrini A, Porcellini G. Pectoralis minor tendon transfer for irreparable anterosuperior cuff tears. J Shoulder Elb Surg. 2013;22(6):e1–5.
68. Weening A, Willems J. Latissimus dorsi transfer for treatment of irreparable rotator cuff tears. Int Orthop. 2010;16:1239–44.
69. Nove-Josserand L, Costa P, Liotard JP, Safar JF, Walch G, Zilber S. Results of latissimus dorsi tendon transfer for irreparable cuff tears. Orthop Traumatol Surg Res. 2009;95:108–13.
70. Omid R, Lee B. Tendon transfers for irreparable rotator cuff tears. J Am Acad Orthop Surg. 2013;21(8):492–501.
71. Gerber C, Rahm SA, Catanzaro S, Farshad M, Moor BK. Latissimus dorsi tendon transfer for treatment of irreparable posterosuperior rotator cuff tears: long-term results at a minimum follow-up of ten years. J Bone Joint Surg Am. 2013;95(21):1920–6.
72. Iannotti JP, Hennigan S, Herzog R, et al. Latissimus dorsi tendon transfer for irreparable posterosuperior rotator cuff tears. Factors affecting outcome. J Bone Joint Surg Am. 2006;88(2):342–8.
73. Namdari S, Voleti P, Baldwin K, Glaser D, Huffman GR. Latissimus dorsi tendon transfer for irreparable rotator cuff tears: a systematic review. J Bone Joint Surg Am. 2012;94(10):891–8.
74. Henseler JF, Nagels J, van der Zwaal P, Nelissen RG. Teres major tendon transfer for patients with massive irreparable posterosuperior rotator cuff tears: short-term clinical results. Bone Joint J. 2013;95-B(4):523–9.
75. Henseler JF, Nagels J, Nelissen RG, de Groot JH. Does the latissimus dorsi tendon transfer for massive rotator cuff tears remain active postoperatively and restore active external rotation? J Shoulder Elbow Surg. 2014;23:553–60.
76. Pearsall AW, Madanagopal S, Karas SG. Transfer of the latissimus dorsi as a salvage procedure for failed debridement and attempted repair of massive rotator cuff tears. Orthopedics. 2007;30:943–9.
77. Debeer P, De Smet L. Outcome of latissimus dorsi transfer for irreparable rotator cuff tears. Acta Orthop Belg. 2010;76:449–55.
78. Irlenbusch U, Bracht M, Gansen HK, Lorenz U, Thiel J. Latissimus dorsi transfer for irreparable rotator cuff tears: a longitudinal study. J Shoulder Elbow Surg. 2008;17:527–34.
79. Delaney RA, Lin A, Warner JJ. Nonarthroplasty options for the management of massive and irreparable rotator cuff tears. Clin Sports Med. 2012;31(4):727–48.
80. Grimberg J, Kany J. Latissimus dorsi tendon transfer for irreparable postero-superior cuff tears: current concepts, indications, and recent advances. Curr Rev Musculoskelet Med. 2014;7:22–32.
81. Mihata T, Lee TQ, Watanabe C, Fukunishi K, Ohue M, et al. Clinical results of arthroscopic superior capsule reconstruction for irreparable rotator cuff tears. Arthroscopy. 2013;29(3):459–70.
82. Mihata T, McGarry MH, Pirolo JM, Kinoshita M, Lee TQ. Superior capsule reconstruction to restore superior stability in irreparable rotator cuff tears: a biomechanical cadaveric study. Am J Sports Med. 2012;40(10):2248–55.
83. Denard PJ, Brady PC, Adams CR, Tokish JM, Burkhart SS. Preliminary results of arthroscopic superior capsule reconstruction with dermal allograft. Arthroscopy. 2018;34:93–9.

Glenohumeral Arthropathy in Patients with Healthy Rotator Cuff

14

Angelo De Carli, Antonio Vadalà, and Lorenzo Proietti

Sequelae of fractures of the proximal humerus, as first described by Neer, represent some of the most difficult situations to treat in shoulder reconstruction. Historically, a good functional result has been difficult to achieve [1].

As a consequence, a complex management decision is often due to the frequent bone loss, deformity, and periarticular soft tissue damages that come along with these types of fractures; moreover the affected patients are frequently elderly (mean age 75.5 years) with significant medical comorbidities. At this age, patients usually present a severe deficiency of the rotator cuff (RC) due to fatty degeneration or muscle atrophy [2]. Despite they have been traditionally treated with hemiarthroplasty (HA), the use of reverse shoulder arthroplasty (RSA) has been recently introduced [3].

In the last decade, the use of RSA, initially developed to manage massive and irreparable RC tears in old patients with or without glenohumeral arthritis and failed hemiarthroplasty, has been extended to trauma (acute proximal humeral fractures and management of fracture sequelae).

Patients who develop nonunion or malunion typically report pain, stiffness, and disability associated with shoulder dysfunction. The decision to perform unconstrained arthroplasty (hemiarthroplasty, total shoulder arthroplasty) is dependent on the degree of osteopenia, the viability of the humeral head, tuberosity integrity, and the functional status of the rotator cuff [4]. Total shoulder replacement is considered in the setting of concomitant glenohumeral arthritis with a functional rotator cuff. RSA is a treatment option in proximal humerus, nonunion or malunion with humeral head collapse, and/or a nonfunctioning RC [5]. However, experience with treating proximal humerus fracture sequelae with reverse total shoulder arthroplasty is limited, and its benefit has not been clearly established yet.

Because of the lack of a precedent valid classification, in 2006 Boileau et al. proposed a new classification for late sequelae of proximal humeral fractures [6]. They have classified these fracture sequelae in two categories and four types.

Fracture sequelae of Category I are related to intracapsular impacted fracture: usually there is no important distortion between tuberosities and humeral head. In this Category I, there are impacted fractures with humeral head collapse or necrosis (type 1) and locked dislocations or fracture-dislocations (type 2).

Fracture sequelae of Category II are related to extracapsular dis-impacted fracture with gross distortion between the tuberosities and the humeral head. In this Category II, there are nonunions of the surgical neck (type 3) and

The authors have acquired permission for any previously published material included in your chapter.

A. De Carli (✉) · A. Vadalà · L. Proietti
Orthopaedic Unit, Kirk Kilgour Sports Injury Center, La Sapienza, Rome, Italy

S. Gumina et al. (eds.), *Reverse Shoulder Arthroplasty*,
https://doi.org/10.1007/978-3-319-97743-0_14

severe tuberosity malunions or nonunions (type 4) (Fig. 14.1).

About surgical indication, in the same paper the author proposed different treatments for every type of sequelae. Fundamental criteria to take into consideration are (1) distortion of the proximal humeral anatomy, (2) tuberosity-diaphysis continuity, (3) potential need of a greater tuberosity osteotomy, and (4) quality of bone stock, status of the rotator cuff, and muscle trophicity. In case of moderate distortion of the anatomy and tuberosity-diaphysis continuity (types 1 and 2 sequelae), non-constrained shoulder prosthesis can be performed without greater tuberosity osteotomy, with good functional results expected. The prosthesis and technique should be modified to accommodate the distorted anatomy. If the rotator cuff has been involved with muscle atrophy, a RSA can be discussed in older patients. If there is tuberosity-diaphysis discontinuity (type 3 sequelae) and/or a severe distortion of the anatomy (type 4 sequelae), a greater tuberosity osteotomy is needed, with predictably poor functional results with a non-constrained shoulder replacement. Therefore, for type 3 sequelae, intramedullary bone graft with osteosynthesis can also be performed. Fracture prosthesis can also be indicated if the head cavitation is severe or if there is severe osteoarthritis. A reverse prosthesis is recommended for type 4 sequelae.

Results of shoulder arthroplasties (NCA) for old trauma are much less favourable than those of primary osteoarthritis or hemiarthroplasties performed for acute fractures. On the basis of a literature review, satisfactory results may be

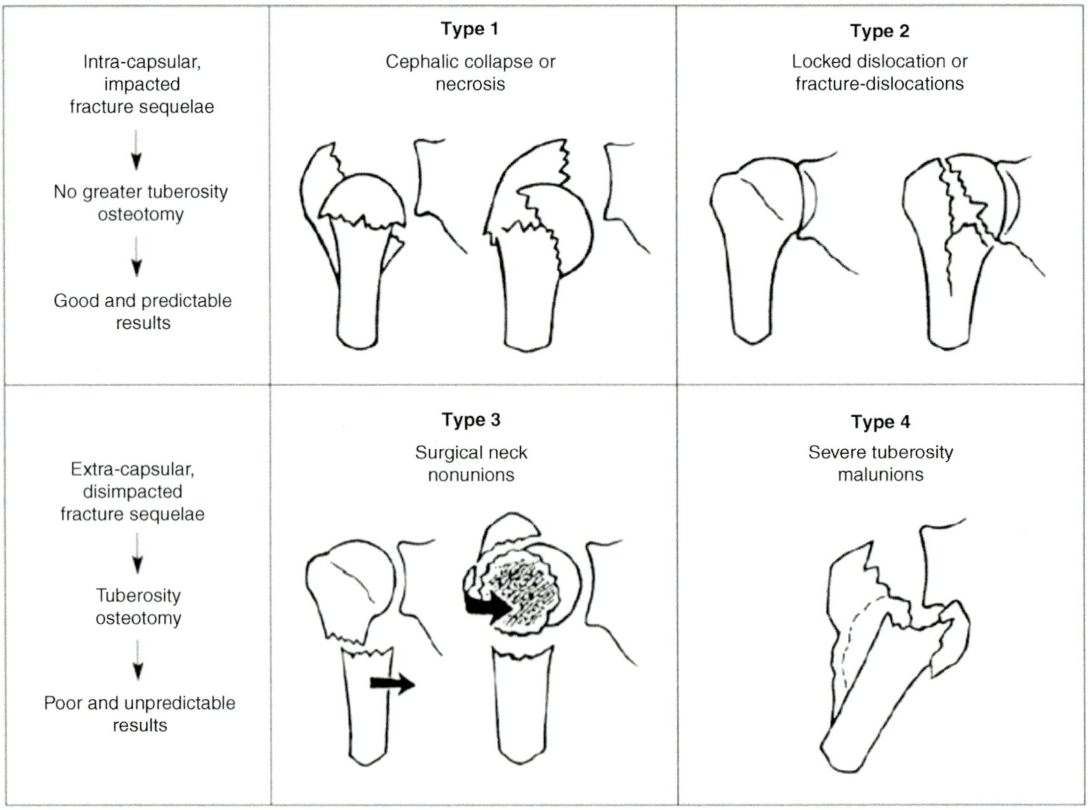

Fig. 14.1 Surgical classification of late sequelae of proximal humeral fractures described by Boileau in 2006 [6]

expected in 15–72% of the cases, with pain relief in more than 85% [7].

Poor results have been reported in 33–50% of patients with sequelae of the proximal humerus treated by hemiarthroplasty or total shoulder arthroplasty.

However, the use of RSA may be a better option than hemiarthroplasty for fracture sequelae given the trend towards a significantly better total Constant score and a significantly lower number of complications requiring revision of prosthesis [3].

Greater tuberosity osteotomy was the most important reason for poor and unpredictable results because of the high incidence of tuberosity nonunion or resorption. It is clear that RSA can improve range of movement and function following proximal humerus fracture sequelae. However, there is a risk of significant complications including dislocation (16.7%), infection (6.7%), intraoperative fracture (3%), and neurological injury (2.6%) [8].

Dislocation is widely considered the most important complication in this type of surgery: there are several factors that increase the risk for postoperative dislocation. The amount of soft tissues released and needed to implant the prosthesis is very important. In some cases there are paucities of tendons such as the subscapularis or infraspinatus and bone loss of the glenoid or proximal humerus: this makes the procedure more complicated because in these cases an allograft might be needed and the correct position and appropriate height of the prosthesis is difficult of calculate. This can result in poor muscular control and instability of the prosthesis [9].

Further additional issue in the sequelae setting is the biologic environment for bone healing. In the setting of secondary RSA for failed hemiarthroplasty, nonoperative treatment, or ORIF, the greater tuberosity is often malunited, non-united, and/or migrated or has undergone resorption making reduction and repair difficult or even impossible. Recent studies have also shown how RSA, hemiarthroplasty, and anatomic shoulder arthroplasty performed with unsatisfactory reduction or a malunion of the greater tuberosity leads to poor results [10, 11]. While both acute and secondary RSA for the treatment of proximal humerus fractures can yield successful clinical outcomes, acute RSA results in improved external rotation motion and decreased rate of complications in regard to scapular notching. The improved external rotation is likely related to the easiness of reducing and repairing the greater tuberosity when RSA is performed in the acute setting.

Comparing HA to RSA in the sequelae setting scenario, Kilic et al. [12] in 2010 reviewed the results of 55 patients with secondary fracture prostheses due to sequelae of fractures of the humeral head, 36 cases with unconstrained arthroplasty (NCA), and 19 with a RSA. In the NCA group, 32 had type 1 or 2 sequelae and 4 a type 3 or 4. In the RSA group, 2 patients had type 1 or 2 sequelae and 17 a type 3 or 4. After NCA the mean Constant scores improved from 19 to 68 points for fracture sequelae types 1 and 2 and from 9 to 47.5 points after RSA for fracture sequelae types 3 and 4. The authors confirmed the results and indications proposed by Boileau and Neyton. In fracture sequelae types 1 and 2, the NCA is the best choice; however, in fracture sequelae types 3 and 4 with severe deformities, the RSA is clearly superior to NCA.

Alentorn-Geli et al. [3] in their paper published in 2014 reported no significant differences in any of the preoperative parameters of the Constant score between the HA and RSA groups but a significantly different number of postoperative complications and reoperations between the two groups: in fact, while there were no complications in the RSA group requiring further surgery, in their cases there were three complications in the HA which required revision of the HA.

In conclusion despite the limitations and complications reported in literature, RSA seems to improve range of movement and functional outcome following proximal humerus fracture sequelae compared to unconstrained arthroplasty and also seems the best surgical treatment in patients with healthy rotator cuff. With this technique, it is possible to reduce the worsening effects of tuberosity malunions or nonunions succeeding cuff deficiency.

References

1. Neer CS II. Old trauma in glenohumeral arthroplasty In: Shoulder reconstruction. 3rd ed. Philadelphia: Saunders 222–234, 1990.
2. Goutallier D, Postel JM, Bernageau J, Lavau L, Voisin MC. Fatty muscle degeneration in cuff ruptures. Pre- and postoperative evaluation by CT scan. Clin Orthop Relat Res. 1994;304:78–83.
3. Alentorn-Geli E, Guirro P, Santana F, Torrens C. Treatment of fracture sequelae of the proximal humerus: comparison of hemiarthroplasty and reverse total shoulder arthroplasty. Arch Orthop Trauma Surg. 2014;134(11):1545–50. https://doi.org/10.1007/s00402-014-2074-9. Epub 2014 Aug 20
4. Ferrel JR, Trinh TQ, Fischer RA. Reverse total shoulder arthroplasty versus hemiarthroplasty for proximal humeral fractures: a systematic review. J Orthop Trauma. 2015;29:60–8.
5. Wang J, Zhu Y, Zhang F, et al. Metaanalysis suggests that reverse shoulder arthroplasty in proximal humerus fractures is a better option than hemiarthroplasty in the elderly. Int Orthop. 2016;40:531–9.
6. Boileau P, Chuinard C, Le Huec JC, Walch G, Trojani C. Proximal humerus fracture sequelae: impact of a new radiographic classification on arthroplasty. Clin Orthop Relat Res. 2006;442:121–30.
7. Mansat P. Les séquelles traumatiques ostéo-articulaires de l'articulation gléno-humérale. Montpellier: Sauramps Médical; 2006.
8. Holton J, Yousri T, Arealis G, Levy O. The role of reverse shoulder arthroplasty in management of proximal humerus fractures with fracture sequelae: a systematic review of the literature. Orthop Rev (Pavia). 2017;9(1):6977. https://doi.org/10.4081/or.2017.6977. eCollection 2017 Feb 20. Review
9. Martinez AA, Calvo A, Bejarano C, Carbonel I, Herrera A. The use of the Lima reverse shoulder arthroplasty for the treatment of fracture sequelae of the proximal humerus. J Orthop Sci. 2012;17(2):141–7. https://doi.org/10.1007/s00776-011-0185-5. Epub 2012 Jan 19
10. Boileau P, Krishnan SG, Tinsi L, Walch G, Coste JS, Mole D. Tuberosity malposition and migration: reasons for poor outcomes after hemiarthroplasty for displaced fractures of the proximal humerus. J Shoulder Elb Surg. 2002;11(5):401–12.
11. Boileau P, Trojani C, Walch G, Krishnan SG, Romeo A, Sinnerton R. Shoulder arthroplasty for the treatment of the sequelae of fractures of the proximal humerus. J Shoulder Elb Surg. 2001;10(4):299–308.
12. Kilic M, Berth A, Blatter G, Fuhrmann U, Gebhardt K, Rott O, Zenz P, Irlenbusch U. Anatomic and reverse shoulder prostheses in fracture sequelae of the humeral head. Acta Orthop Traumatol Turc. 2010;44:417–25. https://doi.org/10.3944/AOTT.2010.2272.

Proximal Humerus Neoplasia: Revision of the Literature

15

Silvana De Giorgi, Francesco Maruccia, Vito Belviso, and Biagio Moretti

The shoulder girdle, consisting of the proximal humerus, scapula, 1/3 lateral clavicle, and the surrounding soft tissue, is the third most common site of predilection for bone tumors [1]. In the shoulder girdle, the proximal humerus is the most common site, followed in descending order by scapula and clavicle.

15.1 Benign Humeral Neoplasms

The classification of bone tumors follows the histological findings. Benign bone tumors are *osteoid osteoma* which classically presents with night pain that disappears with salicylates. It is generally located in the cortical bone of diaphysis [2].

Osteoid osteoma generally occurs between 5 and 25 years old. In the upper limb, the elbow is generally interested. If the humerus is affected, the distal third of the bone is generally interested. Radiologically it presents with a radiotransparent nidus surrounded by a sclerotic ridge of bone. Osteoid osteoma requires a symptomatological therapy, but it often spontaneously regresses.

Tumors resulting from cartilaginous tissue are called *chondroid osteoma* or *osteocartilaginous exostosis* if benign and *chondrosarcoma* if malign.

Chondroid osteoma is the most frequent benign lesion. Generally it affects the knee, but it can be observed in the proximal humeral epiphysis, too. Radiologically a peduncle can be observed. If it is a single lesion, the chance to a malign conversion is less than 1%. A CT scan or an IRM may be fundamental for defining the features and dimensions of the cartilaginous coats [3].

Enchondroma is a lesion formed by well-differentiated cartilage, which affects the proximal humeral epiphysis in 7% of cases. It is often asymptomatic and, generally, it is casually diagnosed. In long bones it generally affects the metaphysis with calcific spots [4].

Chondroblastoma in contrast with enchondroma is a benign lesion of immature cartilaginous cells which generally affects the epiphysis of long bones in a not-mature skeleton. The most involved area is the distal femur and the proximal tibia but also the proximal epiphysis of the femur. It is a rare lesion and represents <1% of bone tumors. At the X-rays, it appears as a lytic lesion with sharp and well-defined sclerotic edges. Microscopically, chondroblasts are fused with thin calcific deposits [5].

Non-osseous fibroma is the commonest fibrous tumor, but it rarely involves the proximal humerus. The commonest area is the humeral shaft in young subjects with not-fused physis.

S. De Giorgi (✉) · F. Maruccia · V. Belviso
B. Moretti
Department of Basic Medical Sciences, Neurosciences and Sensory Organs, University of Bari, Bari, Italy
e-mail: silvanadegiorgi@virgilio.it

S. Gumina et al. (eds.), *Reverse Shoulder Arthroplasty*,
https://doi.org/10.1007/978-3-319-97743-0_15

Similarly, *fibrous dysplasia* in the humeral diaphysis is very rare, but it is more common in the tibia or femur.

In the proximal humerus, a *solitary bone cyst* is very common. It is generally observed between 3 and 14 years old, with a double involvement of male sex [6]. The cyst is filled with liquid. Generally, there are no particular symptoms, but a certain deformity of the bone profile can appear. At the X-rays, a radiotransparent area with a thin profile can be observed. If diagnosed in a mature bone, the solitary bone cyst can remain inside the physis of the bone. This lesion has to be differentiated from the fibrous dysplasia and aneurysmal bone cyst. The latter is multilobated, filled with blood, and locally destruent. It rearly interests the humerus and generally appears in the tibia, femur, or spine in the second decade of life. Solitary bone cysts (SBC) are benign, tumorlike lesions, which most frequently occur in the proximal metaphyseal-diaphyseal region of the humerus and femur of children and adolescents [7]. The lack of a clear pathoetiology has impeded the development of treatment strategies. Up to date, there is no consensus or official guideline for when and how to treat SBC [8]. Different techniques have been used dependent of the site of lesion, dimension, medical history, and activity status. Steroid injection remains a reliable method for treating solitary bone cysts owing to its low invasiveness [8]. To prevent fractures and allow a full weight bearing, internal fixation in combination with methylprednisolone acetate injections seems to be the most favorable in weight bearing bones [9]. Traub et al. reported no significant difference between the treatment groups with respect to secondary fractures, function, pain, or complications. In the individual groups, the failure rate after initial treatment was 36.6% with steroids, 50% with intramedullary nailing, 21.4% with intramedullary nailing plus steroids, and none in the remaining group [8].

15.2 Malign Humeral Tumors

Primitive malignant bone tumors are rare, while metastasis is much more frequent.

Bone tumors are classified by the following:

- Clinical features
- Histology
- Genetics
- Diagnosis
- Therapy
- Prognosis

The most used classification is the histological one, proposed by Schajowicz in 1972, which divides the tumors following the biological features (benign, low and high degree of malignity) and the histological one (fibrous and histiocytic, cartilaginous, bone, vascular, nervous, hemopoietic, epithelial, embryonal deriving from the notochord). Low-grade malignant neoplasms do not have a rapid growth, but it is more accelerated than benign lesions. They are classified as grade 1 or 2 following the histological classification by Broder. They can acquire a more aggressive behavior with time, thus becoming high malignant tumors, grade 3 or 4 in Broder's classification. In these cases the tumor has a very rapid growth and a sprouting development. It is really fundamental to study and well define a neoplasm. The most used system was proposed by Enneking in 1980. Its aim is to describe a bone lesion, following its extension and the natural frontiers it has to pass during its growth. The invasion of the cortical bone, the articular cartilage, fascia and tendons, the capsule, interstitial and fat tissues, and nervous and vascular structures has to be well described. In this classification three parameters are considered:

1. **G**: histological grade
2. **T**: local anatomical extension
3. **M**: presence of metastasis

The commonest primitive bone malign tumor is the *plasmacytoma*, but it is a bone marrow disease which affects the whole skeleton. Therefore, the commonest bone malign tumors are *osteosarcoma*, *Ewing's sarcoma*, and *chondrosarcoma*.

Sarcomas are classified according to:

Stage I (low grade of malignity): G1, M0
Stage II (high grade of malignity): G2, M0
Stage III (with metastasis): all kind of G, M1

Tumors can also be divided in A and B considering if it is intracompartmental (T1) or extracompartmental (T2).

Classical *osteosarcoma* is one of the most common primary malignant bone tumors in children and adolescents [10]. It more frequently occurs in the area of the highest growth plate proliferation: limb long bones particularly in the distal femur (30%), proximal tibia (15%), and proximal humerus (15%). In the long bones, the tumor is located usually in the metaphysis (90%), less frequently in the diaphysis (9%), and very rarely in the epiphysis. Osteosarcomas arising in the proximal femur, humerus, and tibia appear to have poorer outcomes than those arising in distal long bones [11]. However, the strength of this association is uncertain, particularly in light of other prognostic factors. Osteosarcoma is a malignant tumor formed by mesenchymal cells producing not-mature bone and osteoid matrix. It can be distinguished in classic- high degree, periosteal, and intramedullary low degree. Classic osteosarcoma is very rare. Its incidence is of two to three cases/million each year. The most involved areas are distal femur, humerus, and proximal tibia. It is related to the more rapid growing area. Generally at the diagnosis, the tumor is at IIB stage; only in 5% of cases, it is IIA stage.

X-ray is fundamental for diagnosis. The neoplasm initially is inside the bone canal, and then it reaches the cortical bones and surrounding soft tissues. The lesion can appear in a dense way or in a transparent one, while invasion of soft tissue is characterized by irregular radiodensity areas. Therapy is based on neoadjuvant chemotherapy, surgical exeresis, and adjuvant chemotherapy. The periosteal form rarely interests the humerus, while it is more frequently diagnosed in the femoral or tibial diaphysis. Parosteal sarcoma interests the metaphysis area of long bones, producing anaplastic dense bone. A typical area is the posterior side of the distal femur but also the humerus can be involved. On the X-rays a dense lobulated mass can appear, with a wide base of implant near to the cortical bone [12].

Ewing's sarcoma is one of the most common primary bone tumors of childhood. The tumor is almost always metaphyseal or diaphyseal, within long bones. In children, lesions of the epiphysis are often benign, with the most common diagnosis being chondroblastoma. Rarely, 1–2% of Ewing's sarcomas may involve epiphysis [13]. Therefore, the diagnosis should be considered for pediatric epiphyseal lesions. It has been genetically correlated to the peripheral neuroectodermal tumor and to Askin's tumor. It is formed by small and round cells with a low grade of differentiation. Its growth is fast and aggressive, and it can easily cause pulmonary, bone, or lymph nodal metastasis. It can affect the whole skeleton between 5 and 25 years old. In long bones, the diaphysis is often interested. Pain, swelling, and fever can be present. At the X-rays, it appears as an osteolytic lesion with a periosteal reaction. Patients are treated with systemic chemotherapy and eventually surgery or pharmacotherapy. There are no studies showing the superiority of each choice, so far.

Chondrosarcoma is a lesion producing cartilage with a mesenchymal origin. There are different subgroups:

- Peripheral chondrosarcomas: they start from the bone surface.
- Central chondrosarcomas: they are in the marrow canal.
- Extraosseous chondrosarcomas: they appear in soft tissues.

Central *chondrosarcoma* is generally located in the proximal part of the femur and pelvis, even if humeral cases are described. Males are generally interested between 20 and 50 years old. The lesion derives from exostosis with a malignant evolution. At the X-rays a wide cartilaginous coat often appears, suggesting the high malignant grade. It can rarely form metastasis, and surgery is the definitive therapy, even if recurrences can later appear.

Central *chondrosarcoma* generally interests adult population (between 30 and 70 years old) and is located in the proximal femur, proximal humerus, pelvis, and scapula. The main symptom is pain. The histological diagnosis is difficult, because different grades can be present; thus therapy and prognosis could be difficult to describe, too. Low malignant forms do not generally produce metastasis. The target organ for metastasis is the lung, with bone lesions that can occur even after several years. The therapy of the primitive lesion is surgery.

Zheng et al. reported a case with *chondrosarcoma* of the proximal humerus secondary to Ollier disease with treatment of wide resection of the tumor and a prosthetic replacement of the proximal humerus. So far an 8-year follow-up has been done for the patient, and the patient remains well with normal daily living and occupational activities [14].

Between intramedullary sarcomas, *malignant fibrous histiocytoma* generally interests the metaphysis of femur, humerus, or tibia. It can involve all ages, but not childhood. It is an osteolytic tumor, which generally does not have specific symptoms; therefore the diagnosis can be often made after a pathological fracture.

15.3 Treatment of Proximal Humerus Tumors

The treatment of malignant or invasive benign bone tumors of the shoulder girdle is a great challenge to orthopedic oncologists. As a result, before the 1970s, the forequarter amputation and shoulder disarticulation were the main treatment for malignant bone tumors of the shoulder girdle. With better understanding of the biological behavior of musculoskeletal tumors, application of effective adjuvant therapy, and the development of bone defect reconstruction, 80–90% of malignant tumors of the shoulder girdle can be safely resected through some limb-salvage procedures.

It is really important to describe the extension of the tumor mass and the behavior of the surrounding soft tissues. In massive lesions a resection of the whole humeral head is recommended with a later chemotherapy. During surgery, the features of rotator cuff and axillary nerve must be observed.

In this area, the most frequent neoplasia is a metastatic lesion. If the surgical neck of the humerus or the diaphysis is interested, rush or locked nails could be used. They can be inserted in a retrograde way (trans-tricipital), or in an anterograde way, with a deltopectoral approach.

In the anterograde approach, there is the risk of a cuff lesion and, in case of a prospicient nail, the risk of an axillary nerve lesion, during this approach.

Nails are rigid devices and can support bending forces, while proximal and distal screws can avoid torsion stresses.

This procedure of osteosynthesis can guarantee a high resistance and stability; it is tissue sparing with low invasiveness. Plates and screws, with PMMA, can be a solid construct after the curettage of the tumor. The disadvantage of this technique is the risk of fractures above and under the plate. To prevent it, an accurate evaluation of the tumor extension by an IRM (fast spin-echo inversion recovery sequences) is mandatory [15].

Bone tumors of the shoulder girdle can be treated mainly with various limb-salvage procedures, including prosthetic replacement, osteoarticular auto- or allograft, devitalization and replantation, and the Tikhoff-Linberg procedure that is safe and reliable. Meticulous evaluation and planning of the extent of resection and mode of reconstruction are mandatory. Local tumor control, stable and painless shoulder reconstruction, and good function of elbow and hand can be achieved in the majority of patients.

The treatment of proximal humerus tumors with reverse shoulder arthroplasty with allograft augmentation is still controversial. A tumor prosthesis represents a proven solution for such osseous defects [16]. Functionally satisfying results and a stable shoulder can be achieved by reverse shoulder arthroplasty without the need for an allograft. An intact abductor mechanism with a shorter resection humerus length produced good results. The treatment of malignant proximal humerus tumors with RSTP is an alternative that minimizes surgery time and complexity.

Reverse shoulder arthroplasty (RSA) provides an alternative for shoulder girdle reconstruction after wide transarticular resection of the proximal humerus for malignant tumors.

Use of RSA after resection of a malignant tumor of the proximal humerus seems to be an acceptable option to preserve function. However, radiographic evolution is worrisome, and long-term study remains necessary to validate this therapeutic option with follow-up [17].

Proximal humerus reconstructions after resection of tumors are challenging. Early success of the reverse shoulder arthroplasty for reconstructions has recently been reported. The reverse allograft-prosthetic composite offers the advantage of improved glenohumeral stability compared with hemiarthroplasty for proximal humeral reconstructions as it uses the deltoid for stability. Reverse allograft-prosthetic composites are a promising option for proximal humeral reconstructions, although nonunion of the allograft-host bone junction continues to be a challenge for this technique [18].

Scapula and proximal humerus are the most frequent site of primary bone tumors of upper limb. Surgical reconstruction after resection aimed to obtain a stable painful limb and active motion of the shoulder. Three major key points can affect functional results: intra- or extra-articular resection, ability to offer a strength fixation of rotator cuff tendons, and remaining function of the deltoid muscle after resection. When most of the deltoid muscle is active and there is an intra-articular resection, recent results of reversed prosthesis are very promising in terms of active motion. For other cases, conventional or tumor prosthesis can be proposed, but failure of rotator cuff tendons fixation on a prosthesis leads to very poor restoration of active motion.

Arthrodesis is an attractive option in this situation for young patients. In all cases, impairment of the shoulder function is the rule after resection, complication rate is high, and long-term deterioration of the reconstruction is frequent. Moreover, cosmetic results are always poor [19].

Patients with intra-articular resection and endoprosthetic replacement of the proximal humerus who have a preserved axillary nerve, rotator cuff, and deltoid and who chose synthetic mesh for reconstruction have better shoulder function, greater active shoulder ROM, and more joint stability than patients who did not choose to have synthetic mesh reconstructions [20]. The difference in outcome may be attributable to better soft tissue ingrowth in the synthetic mesh, patient motivation, surgical technique, or some combination of these factors. Therefore, a mesh reconstruction for these patients who have a preserved glenoid, axillary nerve, deltoid muscle, and rotator cuff is routinely used.

The optimal method for reconstructing the proximal humerus in patients with tumors is controversial. To determine functional outcomes and complication rates after different types of reconstructions, Potter et al. reviewed a consecutive series of 49 patients who underwent proximal humerus resection and osteoarticular allograft (17 patients), allograft-prosthetic composite (16), or endoprosthetic (16) reconstruction [21]. Operative indications included primary malignancies (24 patients), metastatic disease (19), and benign aggressive disease (6). Implant revision was more common after osteoarticular reconstruction (five of 17) than after allograft-prosthetic composite (one of 16) or endoprosthetic (zero of 16) reconstructions. At a minimum follow-up of 24 months (median, 98 months; range, 24–214 months) in surviving patients, Musculoskeletal Tumor Society functional scores averaged 79% for the allograft-prosthetic composite, 71% for the osteoarticular allograft, and 69% for the endoprosthetic reconstruction cohorts. Shoulder instability was associated with abductor mechanism compromise and was more common after endoprosthetic reconstruction. Allograft fractures occurred in 53% of patients receiving osteoarticular allografts. The authors recommend allograft-prosthetic composite reconstruction for younger patients with primary tumors of bone and endoprosthetic reconstruction for older patients with metastatic disease. Because of the unacceptable complication rate, they do not recommend osteoarticular allograft reconstruction for routine use in the proximal humerus [21].

Shoulder function is often limited after tumor resection and endoprosthetic replacement of the proximal humerus. This is partly attributable to the inability to reliably reattach rotator cuff tendons to the prosthesis and achieve adequate shoulder capsule repair with a metallic prosthesis. An option to attain these goals is to use synthetic mesh for the reconstruction, although the value of this method has not been well documented in the literature.

Patients with intra-articular resection and endoprosthetic replacement of the proximal humerus with reconstruction that included synthetic mesh had better shoulder function and ROM and more stable joints than patients who had reconstruction without synthetic mesh [20]. This result supports prior observations by others, and it remains to be shown whether use of the ligament advanced reconstruction system is superior to other types of mesh or other types of reconstructions. Using mesh should therefore be considered for patients with tumor resection and endoprosthetic replacement of the proximal humerus.

Tumors of the appendicular skeleton commonly affect the proximal humerus, but there is no consensus regarding the best reconstructive technique after proximal humerus resection for tumors of the shoulder. Several studies reported on reconstruction with prosthesis, osteoarticular allografts, and allograft-prosthesis composites.

They observed a higher fracture rate for osteoarticular allografts, but other specific complication rates were similar. The authors stated that allograft-prosthesis composites and prosthesis seem to have similar functional outcome and survival rates, and both seem to avoid fractures that are observed with osteoarticular allografts [22].

A patient with a malignant tumor of the proximal end of the humerus or glenoid may be treated with limb-sparing resection or with amputation. Although the oncologic and functional characteristics of shoulder amputations have been documented, little has been written comparing reconstructive options following limb salvage and amputation about the shoulder [23].

Resection of malignant tumors of the proximal humerus often requires dissection of the rotator cuffs and the deltoid muscle. There is no consensus on the ideal method for shoulder reconstruction. Viehweger et al. reported the functional outcome in a homogeneous series of eight patients treated by arthrodesis, using a vascularized free fibular flap [24]. All had an aggressive tumor of the upper humerus. Tumor resection was associated with a rotator cuff and deltoid muscle resection, in all patients. All patients then underwent shoulder arthrodesis, using a free vascularized fibular flap, fixed with a plate. The cosmetic outcome was considered poor by all patients. Radiographically, bone healing was achieved at last follow-up in all patients, but there was one case of failed fusion between the fibular graft and the scapula, which required secondary iliac grafting. Mean fibular graft hypertrophy was 32.8% at last follow-up. Two reconstruction methods have been described for patients, who require tumor resection of the upper humerus: reconstruction with preservation of glenohumeral joint function and shoulder arthrodesis. Many techniques have been described for each method. It is however difficult to compare the different series reported in the literature, because rotator cuff and deltoid muscle resection was not systematically performed and reconstruction methods varied between patients. An analysis of the literature shows that preservation of motion of the scapular glenoid joint can give good functional results, when the rotator cuff and deltoid muscle can be preserved. If they cannot, results favor shoulder arthrodesis, which provides the patient with very satisfactory upper limb function. Use of a vascularized fibular flap has provided very good arthrodesis results. The patient must however be informed of the probable poor final cosmetic result.

Techniques available for shoulder reconstruction after resection of a tumor of the proximal humerus include scapulohumeral arthrodesis, humerus prosthesis with or without an allograft, inverted prostheses, and massive allografts.

Resection of the upper portion of the humerus should be performed to achieve cancerologically satisfactory tumor resection and enable shoulder resection, if possible, with preservation of a viable and functional abductor system. The functional outcome after such reconstruction depends on the type of bony resection but also on the sacrifice of the rotator cuff and the deltoid muscle [25]. In light of their experience and results in the literature, the authors advocate, for the different reconstructions, the following decision-making algorithm after resection of the proximal humerus without joint invasion: when the resection removes the rotator cuff and the deltoid (or the axillary nerve), there are two options – scapulohumeral arthrodesis or massive humerus prosthesis for patients who do not desire a complex therapy with a long postoperative period. When the resection preserves the rotator cuff and/or the deltoid muscle, reconstruction can be achieved with a composite (inverted or not) prosthesis with suture of the cuff tendons. The authors prefer the inverted composite prosthesis; if the deltoid muscle can be preserved but not the rotator cuff, the composite inverted prosthesis appears to be the most logical solution, but scapulohumeral arthrodesis can be proposed in selected cases.

Limb salvage following resection of a tumor in the proximal part of the humerus poses many challenges. Reconstructive options are limited, because of the loss of periarticular soft tissue stabilizers of the glenohumeral joint, in addition to the loss of bone and articular cartilage. Abdeen et al. stated that extra-articular resections were associated with lower Musculoskeletal Tumor Society scores [26]. All patients had either mild or no pain and normal hand function at the time of final follow-up. The overall estimated rate of survival of the construct, with revision as the end point, was 88% at 10 years. There were three failures due to progressive prosthetic loosening that necessitated removal of the construct. Four patients required an additional bone-grafting procedure to treat a delayed union of the osteosynthesis site. An allograft-prosthesis composite used for limb salvage following tumor resection in the proximal part of the humerus is a durable construct, associated with an acceptable complication rate. Deltoid preservation and intra-articular resection are associated with a greater range of shoulder motion and a superior functional outcome, respectively.

Getty et al. evaluated the functional outcome and the complications of reconstruction with an osteoarticular allograft in patients who had intra-articular resection of the proximal aspect of the humerus [27]. At a median of 47 months (range, 14–130 months) after the operation, 14 of the patients in the study group were free of disease, and 2 had died of disease. No patient had local recurrence or nonunion. Late complications included four fractures of the allograft and one infection of the graft. A Kaplan-Meier survival curve demonstrated a 68% rate of survival of the allograft at 5 years. Instability of the glenohumeral joint in the form of ptosis and anterior subluxation was noted in three patients, and dislocation of the glenohumeral joint was seen in eight patients. On the basis of the modified Musculoskeletal Tumor Society functional evaluation, the mean score at the most recent follow-up evaluation (at a mean of 34 months) was 70%. This score was lower than the mean score of 81% at a mean of 14 months. All patients had normal manual dexterity and had mild or no pain at the most recent follow-up evaluation. However, all had restriction of recreational activities or partial disability in addition to limitations with regard to placement of the hand and the ability to lift. Reconstruction of the proximal aspect of the humerus with an osteoarticular allograft is an option that provides good relief of pain and preserves manual dexterity. There was an extremely high rate of complications, including joint instability, fracture of the allograft, and infection of the allograft. The authors no longer routinely perform this reconstruction at their institution [27].

References

1. Yang Q, Li J, Yang Z, Li X, Li Z. Limb sparing surgery for bone tumours of the shoulder girdle: the oncological and functional results. Int Orthop. 2010;34(6):869–75.
2. O'Connell JX, Nanthakumar SS, Nielsen GP, et al. Osteoid osteoma: the uniquely innervated bone tumor. Mod Pathol. 1998;11:175.
3. Sekiguchi K, Tsutsumi S, Arai S, Nonaka S, Suzuki T, Ishii H, Izumi H, Yasumoto Y. Osteochondroma presenting as a calcified mass in the sellar region and review of the literature. J Neurol Surg A Cent Eur Neurosurg. 2017;78:380–5.
4. Deckers C, Schreuder BH, Hannink G, de Rooy JW, van der Geest IC. Radiologic follow-up of untreated enchondroma and atypical cartilaginous tumors in the long bones. J Surg Oncol. 2016;114:987–91.
5. Karkhur Y, Tiwari A, Verma T, Maini L. Unusual presentation of chondroblastoma mimicking Trevor's disease. J Postgrad Med. 2017;63:197–9.
6. Geibel MA, Schreiber E, Bracher AK, Hell E, Ulrici J, Sailer LK, Rasche V. Characterisation of apical bone lesions: comparison of MRI and CBCT with histological findings—a case series. Eur J Oral Implantol. 2017;10:197–211.
7. Elsayad K, Kriz J, et al. Radiotherapy for aneurysmal bone cysts: a rare indication. Strahlenther Onkol. 2017;193:332–40.
8. Traub F, Eberhardt O, Fernandez FF, Wirth T. Solitary bone cyst: a comparison of treatment options with special reference to their long-term outcome. BMC Musculoskelet Disord. 2016;14(17):162.
9. Choi ES, Han I, Cho HS, Park IW, Park JW, Kim HS. Intramedullary nailing for pathological fractures of the proximal humerus. Clin Orthop Surg. 2016;8:458–64.
10. Rogozhin DV, Bulycheva IV, Konovalov DM, Talalaev AG, Roshchin VY, Ektova AP, Bogoroditsky YU, Strykov VA, Kazakova AN, Olshanskaya YU, Kachanov DY, Tereshchenko GV. Classical osteosarcoma in children and adolescent. Arkh Patol. 2015;77(5):68–74.
11. Cates JM, Schoenecker JG. Proximal location in extremity long bones is a poor prognostic factor for osteosarcoma: a retrospective cohort study of 153 patients. Acta Oncol. 2016;55(8):1036–9.
12. Simon MA. Diagnostic strategies. Surgery for bone and soft tissue tumors. Philadelphia: Lippincott-Raven; 1998. p. 21.
13. Esmaili HA, Niknejad MT. Mohajeri Ewing's sarcoma of proximal humeral epiphysis. Arch Iran Med. 2015;18(2):133–4.
14. Zheng K, Peng ZX, Zheng PP. Chondrosarcoma of the proximal humerus secondary to ollier disease: an 8-year follow-up of successful resection of the tumor with endoprosthetic replacement of the proximal humerus. J Clin Med Res. 2014;6(3):218–22.
15. Redmond BJ, Biermann JS, Blasier RB. Interlocking intramedullary nailing of pathologic fractures of the shaft of the humerus. J Bone Joint Surg. 1996;78:891–6.
16. Guven MF, Aslan L, Botanlioglu H, Kaynak G, Kesmezacar H, Babacan M. Functional outcome of reverse shoulder tumor prosthesis in the treatment of proximal humerus tumors. J Shoulder Elb Surg. 2016;25(1):e1–6.
17. Bonnevialle N, Mansat P, Lebon J, Lafosse JM, Bonnevialle P. Reverse shoulder arthroplasty for malignant tumors of proximal humerus. J Shoulder Elb Surg. 2015;24(1):36–44.
18. King JJ, Nystrom LM, Reimer NB, Gibbs CP Jr, Scarborough MT, Wright TW. Allograft-prosthetic composite reverse total shoulder arthroplasty for reconstruction of proximal humerus tumor resections. J Shoulder Elb Surg. 2016;25(1):45–54.
19. Gouin F, Creen V. Reconstruction following shoulder resection for bone tumor. Bull Cancer. 2014;101(10):951–7.
20. Tang X, Guo W, Yang R, Tang S, Ji T. Synthetic mesh improves shoulder function after intraarticular resection and prosthetic replacement of proximal humerus. Clin Orthop Relat Res. 2015;473(4):1464–71.
21. Potter BK, Adams SC, Pitcher JD Jr, Malinin TI, Temple HT. Proximal humerus reconstructions for tumors. Clin Orthop Relat Res. 2009;467(4):1035–41.
22. Teunis T, Nota SP, Hornicek FJ, Schwab JH, Lozano-Calderón SA. Outcome after reconstruction of the proximal humerus for tumor resection: a systematic review. Clin Orthop Relat Res. 2014;472(7):2245–53.
23. Kneisl JS. Function after amputation, arthrodesis, or arthroplasty for tumors about the shoulder. J South Orthop Assoc. 1995;4(3):228–36.
24. Viehweger E, Gonzalez JF, Launay F, Legre R, Jouve JL, Bollini G. Shoulder arthrodesis with vascularized fibular graft after tumor resection of the proximal humerus. Rev Chir Orthop Reparatrice Appar Mot. 2005;91(6):523–9.
25. Kassab M, Dumaine V, Babinet A, Ouaknine M, Tomeno B, Anract P. Twenty nine shoulder reconstructions after resection of the proximal humerus for neoplasm with mean 7-year follow-up. Rev Chir Orthop Reparatrice Appar Mot. 2005;91(1):15–23.
26. Abdeen A, Hoang BH, Athanasian EA, Morris CD, Boland PJ, Healey JH. Allograft-prosthesis composite reconstruction of the proximal part of the humerus: functional outcome and survivorship. J Bone Joint Surg. 2009;91(10):2406–15.
27. Getty PJ, Peabody TD. Complications and functional outcomes of reconstruction with an osteoarticular allograft after intra-articular resection of the proximal aspect of the humerus. J Bone Joint Surg Am. 1999;81(8):1138–46.

16 Humeral Head Nonunion

Stefano Di Fabio and Corrado D'Antimo

16.1 Introduction

Proximal humerus fractures are common injuries, accounting for about 5% of all fractures of the appendicular skeleton. The majority of these fractures (approximately 85%) occur as the result of a low-energy injury and are non-displaced or minimally displaced fractures. Such fractures heal without surgical intervention, but those that progress to nonunion have a negative effect on overall glenohumeral function and the ability to perform activities of daily living [1–6].

The incidence of nonunion of the proximal humerus fracture is quite rare ranging from 1 to 10%.

A large single-center clinical study performed by Court-Brown and McQueen [7] reported a nonunion rate of 1.1% in their prospective study of patients treated nonsurgically for proximal humerus fractures.

Hanson et al. [8] prospectively followed 124 patients with proximal humerus fractures that were managed nonsurgically. At 1-year follow-up, only 3% required surgery for fracture nonunion.

Iyengar et al. [9] performed a meta-analysis of 12 studies with a total of 650 patients who underwent non-operative treatment of their proximal humerus fracture and found a 2% incidence of nonunion (range 0–7%).

The etiology of a proximal humerus nonunion is multifactorial. There is an interaction between fracture-related issues, the medical conditions, and habits of the patients.

Fracture characteristics including translation and metaphyseal comminution can increase the risk of nonunion.

Several studies have identified two-part surgical neck fracture as the most common fracture pattern associated with fracture nonunion [10–12] probably due to the disruption of the medial soft tissues and blood supply that are important for fracture healing.

Court-Brown and McQueen [7] found an 8% rate of nonunion in patients with metaphyseal comminution and a 10% rate in patients with surgical neck translation between 33 and 100%. It is unclear if greater amount of comminution and translation increase the risk of nonunion because of decreased bone contact area or disruption of blood supply.

The authors of the largest prospective review of proximal humerus nonunion were not able to define predictive criteria for the development of nonunion due to the very low incidence of this pathology that should require studies with unrealistically large number of patients.

Interposed soft tissues between fracture fragments may also represent a crucial factor in nonunion development. Nayak et al. [13] in their

S. Di Fabio (✉) · C. D'Antimo
Orthopaedics Department, San Martino Hospital, Belluno, Italy

S. Gumina et al. (eds.), *Reverse Shoulder Arthroplasty*, https://doi.org/10.1007/978-3-319-97743-0_16

retrospective analysis found that interposed structures (especially the long head of biceps) blocked healing in 8 of 17 cases of nonunion (47%). Duralde et al. [14] reviewed 20 patients surgically treated for proximal humerus nonunion and found soft tissue interposition in 8 of 12 cases (67%) initially treated non-operatively.

Inadequate initial immobilization of humerus fracture after surgical operation or in patients treated conservatively may also compromise the bone healing process.

Nutritional deficiencies and metabolic bone disease (e.g., diabetes, osteopenia, obesity) are recognized as contributors to delayed unions or nonunions and should be identified with appropriate laboratory markers [10]. Persons who smoke are at 5.5 times higher risk than nonsmokers for developing nonunion [8].

16.2 Patient Evaluation

Patients with proximal humerus nonunion typically report pain, stiffness, and disability associated with shoulder dysfunction. The pain is usually absent or moderate at rest and increases during shoulder activities. Physical examination usually reveals diminished shoulder range of motion due to soft tissue contracture, with or without disuse atrophy of the deltoid and periscapular muscles. Axillary nerve function must be assessed, and electromyography is mandatory if neurologic injury is suspected. Integrity of rotator cuff should also be evaluated with a MRI scan.

Court-Brown and McQueen [7] measured the shoulder range of motion of patients following proximal humerus fractures that achieved union comparing to patients who developed nonunions at 6, 13, 26, and 52 weeks. They found that, instead of linear increasing of shoulder motion, patients with proximal humerus nonunion had less mobility with lost motion in all directions except external rotation after 26 weeks.

Radiographic evaluation of proximal humerus nonunion includes true AP view taken in the scapular plane with the shoulder in neutral, internal rotation, and external rotation. Outlet and axillary radiographs should also be made in the radiographic series.

The type of nonunion (e.g., hypertrophic versus atrophic) should be defined. Radiographically, hypertrophic nonunions are characterized by hypertrophic and sclerotic bone ends with fracture callus that failed to bridge the fracture site having the appearance of an "elephant's foot," whereas atrophic nonunions appear osteopenic with the absence of callus. In general, hypertrophic nonunions develop when insufficient mechanical stability and/or axial alignment exists and the vascularity and biologic environment for fracture healing are preserved. With atrophic nonunion, vascularity and the biologic environment are often compromised, which causes an inadequate fracture healing response. Lytic or mixed lytic and blastic lesions can be signs of underlying pathologic or metastatic processes. Signs of a sequestrum or involucrum are pathognomonic for infection.

Radiographs also should be evaluated for evidence of osteonecrosis of the humeral head and extent of bone loss. Comparison views of the contralateral shoulder may be helpful. In case of unclear diagnosis of nonunion, a CT scan should be performed with two- and three-dimensional reconstructions allowing better evaluation of tuberosity malunions, head cavitation, intra-articular extensions, and glenohumeral arthritic changes.

Nuclear imaging exams may offer additional information by evaluating callus vascularity and metabolic activity and presence of acute or chronic infection at nonunion sites.

Laboratory analysis in patients affected by proximal humerus nonunion can help to determine the cause of failure and the factors that should be corrected to allow bone healing. If infection is suspected, preoperative laboratory exams should include an erythrocyte sedimentation rate and C-reactive protein level, which are nonspecific markers of systemic inflammatory response. A white blood cell count may show leukocytosis with increased percentages of polymorphonuclear cells. However the gold standard for diagnosing infection is cultures taken from the nonunion fracture site.

Other endocrine markers should be assessed in patients affected by nonunion. Brinker et al. [15] founded that thyroid function, vitamin D, and calcium levels were altered in 37 patients with unexplained nonunion despite adequate reduction and stabilization or in case of history of multiple low-energy fractures with at least one progressing to nonunion or in non-displaced fracture of the pubic rami or sacral ala not healed, demonstrating that metabolic and endocrine abnormalities may be associated with nonunion.

When proximal humerus fracture nonunion is established, a descriptive classification should be used in order to compare the results from different studies and try to underline prognostic elements.

Checchia et al. [16] proposed a descriptive classification system based on their retrospective review of 21 cases.

They divided nonunions in four groups. High two-part nonunions include nonunions secondary to two-part fractures of the surgical neck of the humerus with very small proximal fragment and three-part fractures where the greater and lesser tuberosity is consolidated. Low two-part nonunions are also related to two-part fractures of the surgical neck, but nonunion occurs between the lesser tuberosity and the insertion of the pectoralis major tendon, and the proximal fragment is larger than in the previous group. Complex nonunions describe three-part, four-part, or head-splitting fractures where the surgical neck nonunion is associated with tuberosity nonunion that is displaced more than 5 mm. Finally lost fragment nonunion includes a scenario with a large degree of bone loss after open fractures and/or post-traumatic osteomyelitis.

Checchia classification has not widely been utilized in other studies, and therefore no treatment algorithms were performed basing on this system.

16.3 Timing of Surgery

Nonunion is typically diagnosed 6–9 months following injury [10]. The median time to union or bridging callus of nonsurgically managed proximal humerus fractures is 13–14 weeks, and an appropriate workup should be performed at that time in the absence of healing [7, 8]. The diagnosis of nonunion in the proximal humerus can be made when there is lack of callus formation on two consecutive radiographs taken 6 to 8–10 weeks after injury. Moreover, poor shoulder function and increasing pain should alert the physician about a nonunion risk.

Surgical management is recommended at approximately 3–6 months following injury if an impending nonunion is suspected, because wasting time increases soft tissue contractures at glenohumeral joint with predictable poor results after revision surgery.

Beredjiklian et al. [17] reviewed the results of 39 patients and noted significant difference in outcomes among patients who underwent late surgical management (after 1 year) of proximal humerus malunion. This was ascribed to more capsular contractures, muscle atrophy, and irreparable rotator cuff tear.

Intervening at this time (within 6 months) may help to prevent disabling glenohumeral dysfunction that is always associated with chronic proximal humerus nonunions in order to optimize the outcome.

16.4 Nonsurgical Management

Patients affected by symptomatic proximal humerus nonunion are commonly elderly with medical comorbidities. Moreover, surgical management of this pathology is technically challenging, and the postoperative course requires compliance and family assistance networks. Therefore surgical option is reserved for highly motivated patients with low medical comorbidities that place them at an acceptable risk for surgical management. Patients with minimal pain and mild shoulder function disability may be appropriate candidates for nonsurgical management [18]. Some authors consider a nonfunctional deltoid muscle a contraindication for operative treatment [16].

A few studies [13, 19] reported that up to 50% of patients affected by proximal humerus nonunion are minimally symptomatic with acceptable shoulder function.

A comprehensive conversation should be undertaken with patients in order to assess their pain and shoulder impairment and to elucidate them about the risks of surgical treatment and the duration of post-op rehabilitation program.

16.5 Surgical Management

16.5.1 ORIF

Many techniques have been described for surgical management of proximal humerus nonunion. Regardless of the implant used, the critical step is the preparation of the nonunion site with meticulously resection of scar, fibrous tissue, and avascular bone.

The aim of the therapy consists of an optimized combination of biological and biomechanical factors [10, 20–22].

Osteosynthesis using locking plate fixation techniques is preferred in the presence of good bone quality without significant medial calcar comminution or osteopenia that may compromise adequate fixation [23–28]. Clinical and radiographic assessment of function and integrity of tuberosity is mandatory in deciding whether or not osteosynthesis is the appropriate treatment. In case of surgical neck nonunion, rigid fixation can be achieved with a variety of plates, including 3.5- and 4.5-mm plates made for the proximal humerus, blade plates, and 4.5-mm T-plates. Fixed-angle locking or blade plates provide a biomechanically stable construct in the setting of osteoporotic bone [29, 30].

Isolated greater and lesser tuberosity nonunions are less common than surgical neck nonunions. The bone quality of the tuberosity fragment and rotator cuff function are critical components in determining the most appropriate surgical option. In patients with large tuberosity fragments and a viable and functional rotator cuff, osteosynthesis may be achieved with buttress plating with autogenous bone graft. Tension band techniques, transosseous suture fixation, or current suture anchor configurations used in modern rotator cuff repair techniques that provide compression across the fracture site with autogenous bone grafting augmentation can be used for comminuted tuberosity fragments, only if rotator cuff is intact without fatty degeneration. A deltoid-splitting or deltopectoral approach can be used for greater tuberosity osteosynthesis. A deltopectoral approach is suggested for lesser tuberosity nonunions. Arthroscopic techniques have also been described for managing greater tuberosity nonunions [31].

Autogenous or allograft bone augmentation is recommended to facilitate osteosynthesis. Large amounts of cancellous bone allograft can be obtained from the iliac crest, but the patient must be advised of the possibility of donor site pain. The alternative choice is using allograft if donor site morbidity is unacceptable [10].

Free vascularized fibular allograft may be considered for patients who need significant biologic augmentation along with mechanical support.

Healy et al. [32] retrospectively reviewed their experience and reported union in 12 of 13 patients following ORIF with bone graft in patients affected by proximal humerus nonunions. Ring et al. [33] reviewed 25 patients with proximal humerus fracture nonunion treated with blade plate and autogenous iliac crest cancellous bone graft. Fracture union was achieved in 23 patients (92%), and functional results were classified as good to excellent in 20 (80%). Two patients had complications due to iliac crest harvest. Allende and Allende [30] reported union in all seven patients treated with a locking 90° blade plate (average follow-up, 22 months). The average time to union was 5.9 months. At latest follow-up average DASH score was 25 points, and Constant score was 72.7 points.

The use of intramedullary peg graft with fixed-angle locked plating was first described by Walch et al. [34] that treated 20 patients with pseudarthrosis of the proximal humerus with 6–10 cm corticocancellous autogenous bone graft (11 iliac crest, 6 anterior tibial crest, and 3 middle-third of the fibula). The stability of the fracture site was obtained by T-plate osteosynthesis. Although a 96% union rate was achieved, donor site morbidity was high with 50% of patients developing a pathological fracture after harvesting from the anterior tibial crest. Other authors have strictly used iliac crest bone graft; however incidence of persistent pain postoperatively remains substantial.

Badman et al. [18] described the technique of using fibular strut allograft as an intramedullary implant that allows to maintain the humeral head in the correct position and to improve the stability of the implant (fixed-angle plate), without the morbidity of graft donor site. Badman and Mighell [35] reported 94% rate of union at an average of 5.4 months. Complications involved two posterior cord brachial plexus palsies that improved within 3 months and two cases of adhesive capsulitis treated with arthroscopic capsular release.

Fibular strut allograft has several advantages. It provides additional biologic and structural support to the poor-quality bone found at the proximal humerus, it is mechanically stronger than cancellous bone allograft or allograft, and it avoids the donor site morbidity. This technique is useful in both the acute proximal humerus fracture scenario and chronic nonunion scenario when medial calcar support is compromised secondary to significant medial calcar comminution or osteopenia (Figs. 16.1, 16.2a, b, and 16.3a, b).

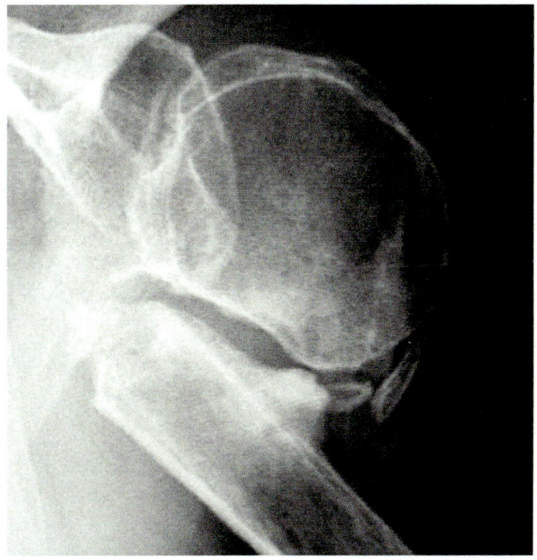

Fig. 16.1 Proximal humerus nonunion of surgical neck in 54-year-old patient (With permission of M. Fontana)

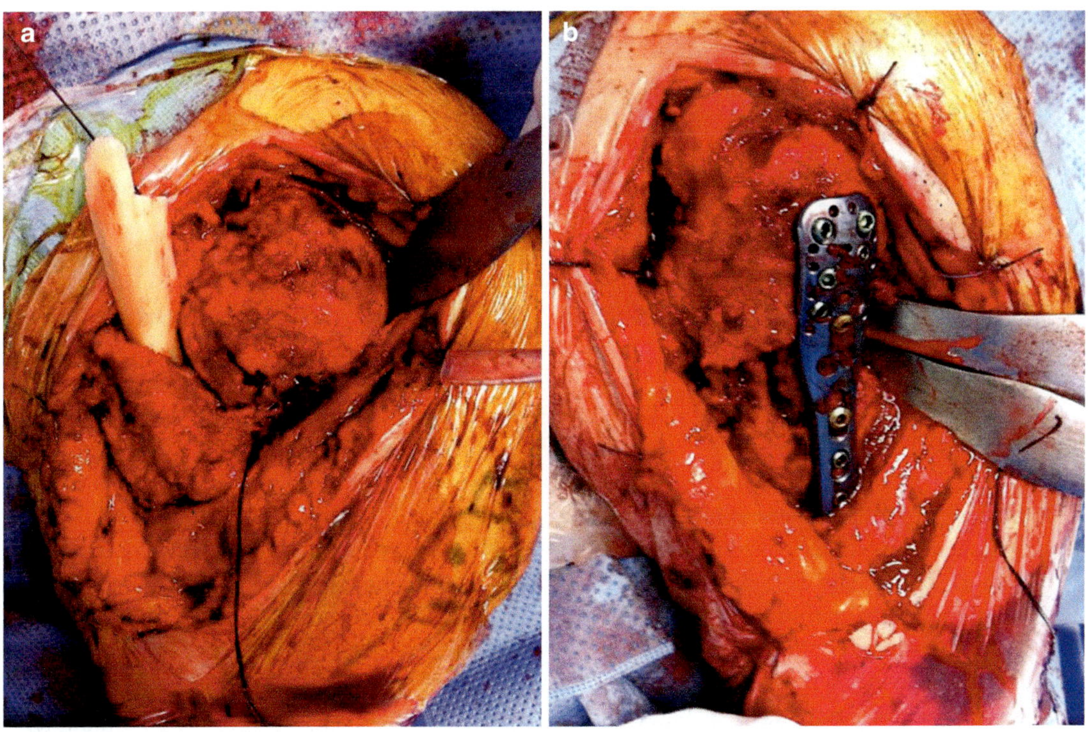

Fig. 16.2 (**a**) Intraoperative view of fibular allograft locked into humerus diaphysis with humeral head translated (With permission of M. Fontana). (**b**) Intraoperative view of reduced fracture with fixed-angled locked plate in place (With permission of M. Fontana)

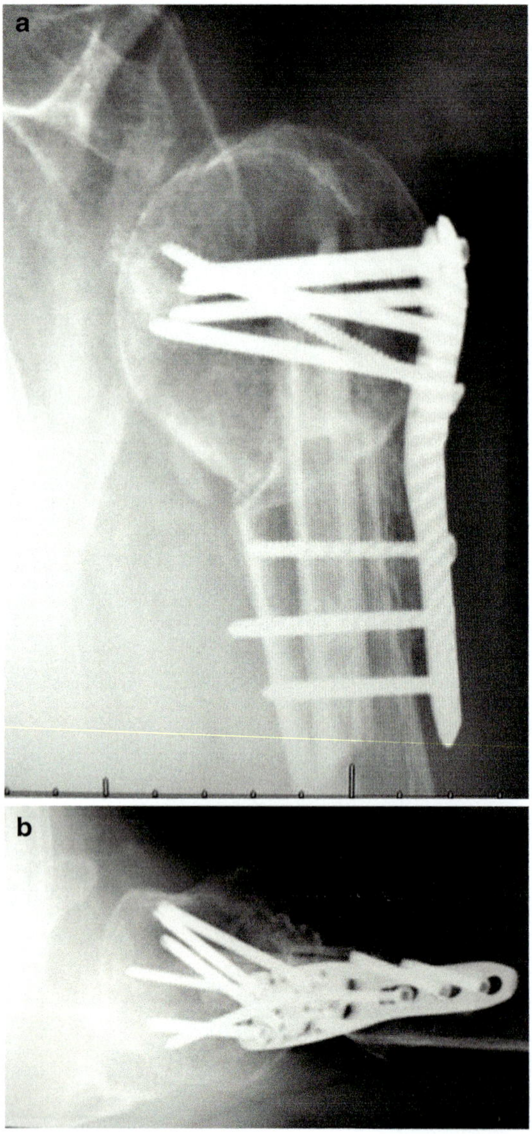

Fig. 16.3 (**a**, **b**) AP and axial view of healed proximal humerus nonunion treated with fibular allograft and fixed-angled locked plate (With permission of M. Fontana)

Another option of treatment is represented by the third generation of interlocked intramedullary nails. Historically, results were disappointing following intramedullary nailing to manage proximal humerus nonunion. Early mobilization of intramedullary devices with subsequent subacromial impingement necessitated a second surgery following union for nail removal. Most patients, however, progressed to union and regained good shoulder function [10].

Recently, Yamane et al. [11] published encouraging results with the use of interlocking intramedullary nails to manage proximal humerus fracture nonunion in 13 patients. The average follow-up was 37.8 months. All patients achieved union. All patients were satisfied with the results and had improved shoulder range of motion postoperatively. It is important to know that 11 of 13 patients treated in this study had no previous surgical operation and the other two were treated with percutaneous pinning or intramedullary nailing.

In addition to bone graft and hardware fixation, in case of proximal humerus nonunion, the human bone morphogenetic proteins (i.e., rhBMP-2) could be used combined with bone graft due to their important role in physiological fracture healing and bone regeneration [36].

The current literature supports the use of BMP only for tibial nonunion [37] and in general for long bone nonunion, but no studies were performed on its use in proximal humerus nonunion. A Cochrane review of BMP use for fracture nonunion in adults concluded that there is a paucity of data available and its role remains unclear. Therefore, the use of biologic augments such as rhBMP-2 has to be considered "off label" for the treatment of proximal humerus nonunion and is not approved by FDA.

16.6 Surgical Management

16.6.1 Shoulder Replacement

Proximal humerus nonunion with severe head cavitation, poor bone stock inadequate to achieve solid internal fixation, and glenohumeral osteoarthritis should be treated with an arthroplasty.

The decision to perform unconstrained arthroplasty (i.e., hemiarthroplasty, total shoulder arthroplasty) to manage proximal humerus nonunion depends in part on the quality of bone stock, the viability of the humeral head, and, most important, tuberosity integrity and position as well as rotator cuff functional status. Total shoulder replacement is considered in the setting of concomitant glenohumeral osteoarthritis with a functional and intact rotator cuff.

In case of tuberosity diaphysis discontinuity and/or severe distortion of the anatomy, a greater tuberosity osteotomy is needed, with predictable poor functional results of an unconstrained shoulder replacement.

When rotator cuff has been involved with muscle atrophy and/or tuberosity is absent, a reverse shoulder arthroplasty can be considered in older patients.

Boileau et al. [38] investigated factors important to successful patient selection for unconstrained arthroplasty (i.e., hemiarthroplasty, total shoulder arthroplasty) in the setting of proximal humerus malunion or nonunion. They retrospectively reviewed 203 consecutive patients with sequelae of proximal humerus fractures that had been managed with unconstrained glenohumeral arthroplasty. Of the unconstrained arthroplasties performed, 59% were hemiarthroplasty. Total shoulder arthroplasty was indicated for patients with preexisting pain secondary to glenohumeral osteoarthrosis or glenoid erosions noted at the time of surgery. The authors suggested that tuberosity integrity and anatomic position are critical for a good functional outcome following unconstrained arthroplasty. Furthermore, they recommended reverse total shoulder arthroplasty in cases of tuberosity osteotomy. Although arthroplasty has been shown to reliably relieve pain in patients with proximal humerus nonunion, return to preinjury function is less predictable [11, 14]. Nayak et al. [13] retrospectively reviewed seven patients who underwent hemiarthroplasty for proximal humerus nonunion. All patients were able to perform activities of daily living and had less pain as well as increased function and range of motion. However, no patients returned to their preinjury level of activity. Antuña et al. [12] published the results of 25 shoulders managed with unconstrained arthroplasty (mean follow-up, 6 years). Twenty-one patients underwent hemiarthroplasty and four total shoulder replacement. Twenty of 25 patients considered themselves better than preoperatively with variable Neer functional score (13 unsatisfactory results). Anatomic or near anatomic union of the tuberosity was a significant factor in achieving greater active forward elevation ($P = 0.02$). The authors pointed out the importance of using heavy no absorbable sutures, bone graft to fill gaps between the tuberosities and the diaphysis, and restricting post-op rehabilitation program to minimize the risk of complications.

Dunquin and all [39] reviewed the Mayo Clinic experience treating 67 proximal humerus nonunion with unconstrained shoulder replacement. Their results were similar to those published by Antuna: patient satisfaction in terms of pain was high, but motion was less predictable, with average elevation of 104° and external rotation of 50°. Active elevation was significantly decreased in patients with tuberosity nonunions, but this did not influence the pain level. Bone grafting did not prevent tuberosity nonunions. Other complications included 11 severe subluxations or dislocations, 2 deep infections, and 1 late periprosthetic fracture.

The strong relationship between postoperative range of motion and tuberosity healing has led some authors to suggest reverse total shoulder replacement as a viable alternative to unconstrained arthroplasty.

Reverse total shoulder arthroplasty is a viable option in the setting of proximal humerus nonunion with humeral head collapse, nonfunctional rotator cuff, and muscle atrophy and/or radiographic evidence of severe tuberosity malunion or resorption (Fig. 16.4a, b). Reverse implant relies on the deltoid muscle to achieve elevation and abduction, so it is crucial to perform electromyography in case of concerns about deltoid function. Otherwise reverse shoulder replacement requires tuberosity healing for optimum function especially to regain rotational movement and decrease post-op complications.

In a study of 18 patients treated with reverse total shoulder arthroplasty for proximal humerus nonunion, Martinez et al. [27] reported significant improvements in average active forward elevation (35–90°; $P < 0.0001$), external rotation (15–30°; $P < 0.0001$), and internal rotation (25–55°;

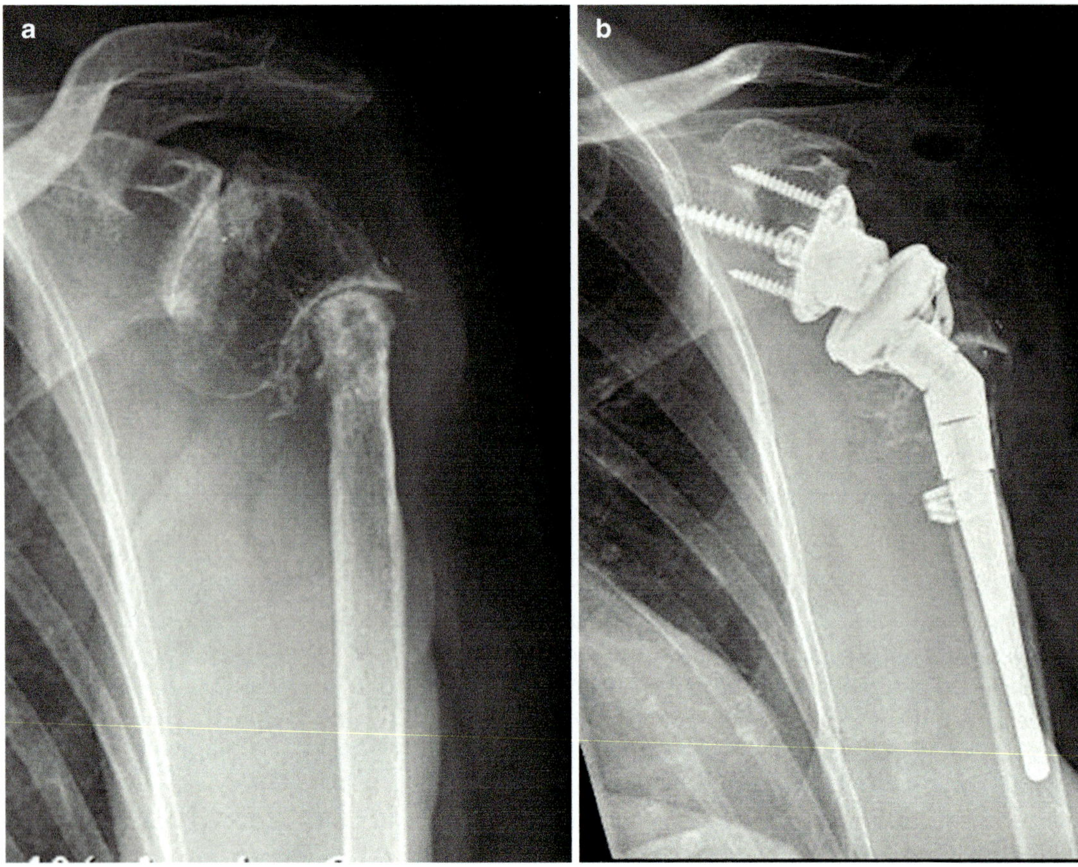

Fig. 16.4 (**a**) Long-lasting proximal humerus nonunion of surgical neck with resorption of tuberosity, relevant osteopenia, and glenohumeral osteoarthritis in 79-year-old patient (**b**) treated with reverse shoulder arthroplasty (With permission of H.R. Block)

$P < 0.0001$) at an average follow-up of 28 months. Fourteen patients were either satisfied or very satisfied with the result of the operation. Complications included one transient axillary nerve palsy, two deep infections, and two dislocations. Zafra et al. [40] published a prospective, multicentre study of 35 patients (mean follow-up of 51 months) who underwent a reverse total shoulder replacement for the treatment of proximal humerus nonunion. They reported a significant decrease of pain and significant improvement of range of motion and Costant score but a total of nine complications in seven patients: six dislocations, one glenoid loosening in a patient who had previously suffered dislocation, one transitory paresis of the axillary nerve and one infection.

16.7 Conclusions

Proximal humerus fractures are common, and the majority of them healed without any surgical procedure. A small percentage develop into nonunion, but the small study size available in the literature causes difficulty in determining the true rate. Nonunion of proximal humerus represents a big challenge due to biological problems from the initial injury and previous surgeries, poor bone stock, humeral head cavitation, soft tissue contracture, and infection.

Patients developing nonunions present restricted range of motion, pain, and greater problems to perform activities of daily living. Once nonunion has been identified, every effort should be made to treat the problem before 6 months after the initial injury in order to prevent the formation of soft tissue contractures.

Treatment options include nonsurgical management for minimally symptomatic patients with medical comorbidities. Surgical options range from osteosynthesis with standard, fixed-angle, or locked plate and interlocked intramedullary implants to arthroplasty using hemi-, total, or reverse shoulder replacement.

Surgery may provide for the use of augments such as cancellous allograft and allograft or structural grafts to increase rate of bone healing. When union is achieved with internal fixation, the results in terms of range of motion and Constant scores are significantly higher compared to arthroplasty options. Positive prognostic factors include simpler fracture patterns, better bone stock, and intact vascularity. Younger age and less medical comorbidity may also play a role in improving functional outcome. Moreover technological advances in locking plate and interlocking design had enlarged the indication for osteosynthesis in proximal humerus nonunion.

In case of head cavitation, poor bone quality, and glenohumeral osteoarthritis, shoulder arthroplasty offers favorable results in terms of pain control but less predictable functional outcome, which seems to be correlated with tuberosity healing.

Reverse shoulder replacement offers the theoretical advantage of decreased dependence on tuberosity union, but only one small study reviewed the results of this implant in treating proximal humerus nonunion. Therefore more studies are needed to better understand the role of inverse implant in treating this challenging pathology.

References

1. Lind T, Kroner K, Jensen J. The epidemiology of fractures of the proximal humerus. Arch Orthop Trauma Surg. 1989;108(5):285–7.
2. Court-Brown CM, Caesar B. Epidemiology of adult fractures: a review. Injury. 2006;37(8):691–7.
3. Court-Brown CM, Garg A, McQueen MM. The epidemiology of proximal humerus fractures. Acta Orthop Scand. 2001;72(4):365–71.
4. Palvenen M, Kannus P, Niemi S, Parkkari J. Update in the epidemiology of proximal humerus fractures. Clin Orthop Relat Res. 2006;442:87–92.
5. Green A, Norris TR. Proximal humeral fractures and glenohumeral dislocation. In: Browner BD, Levine AM, Jupiter JB, Trafton PG, Krettek C, editors. Skeletal trauma: basic science, management, and reconstruction. 4th ed. Philadelphia, PA: Saunders Elsevier; 2009. p. 1623–754.
6. Warner JP, Costouros JG, Gerber C. Fractures of the proximal humerus. In: Buchholz RW, Heckman JD, Court-Brown C, editors. Rockwood and Green's fractures in adults. 6th ed. Philadelphia: Lippincott, Williams & Wilkins; 2006. p. 1039–105.
7. Court-Brown CM, McQueen MM. Nonunions of the proximal humerus: their prevalence and functional outcome. J Trauma. 2008;64(6):1517–21.
8. Hanson B, Neidenbach P, de Boer P, Stengel D. Functional outcomes after nonoperative management of fractures of the proximal humerus. J Shoulder Elb Surg. 2009;18(4):612–21.
9. Iyengar JJ, Devcic Z, Sproul RC, Feley BT. Nonoperative treatment of proximal humerus fractures: a systematic review. J Orthop Trauma. 2011;25(10):612–7.
10. Galatz LM, Iannotti JP. Management of surgical neck nonunions. Orthop Clin North Am. 2000;31(1):51–61.
11. Yamane S, Suenaga N, Oizumi N, Minami A. Interlocking intramedullary nailing for nonunion of the proximal humerus with the straight nail system. J Shoulder Elb Surg. 2008;17(5):755–9.
12. Antuña SA, Sperling JW, Sánchez-Sotelo J, Cofield RH. Shoulder arthroplasty for proximal humeral non unions. J Shoulder Elb Surg. 2002;11(2):114–21.
13. Nayak NK, Schickendantz MS, Regan WD, Hawkins RJ. Operative treatment of nonunion of surgical neck fractures of the humerus. Clin Orthop Relat Res. 1995;(313):200–5.
14. Duralde XA, Flatow EL, Pollock RG, Nicholson GP, Self EB, Bigliani LU. Operative treatment of nonunions of the surgical neck of the humerus. J Shoulder Elb Surg. 1996;5(3):169–80.
15. Brinker MR, O'Connor DP, Monla YT, Earthman TP. Metabolic and endocrine abnormalities in patients with nonunions. J Orthop Trauma. 2007;21(8):557–70.
16. Checchia SL, Doneux P, Miyazaki AN, Sir IA, Bringel R, Ramos CH. Classification of non-unions of the proximal humerus. Int Orthop. 2000;24(4):217–20.
17. Beredjiklian PK, Iannotti JP, Norris TR, Williams GR. Operative treatment of malunion of a fracture of the proximal aspect of the humerus. J Bone Joint Surg Am. 1998;80(10):1484–97.
18. Badman B, Mighell M, Drake G. Proximal humeral nonunions: surgical technique with fibular strut allograft and fixed-angle locked plating. Tech Shoulder Elbow Surg. 2006;7(2):95–101.
19. Rockwood CA, Pearce JC. Management of proximal humerus nonunions. Orthop Trans. 1989;13:644.

20. Cadet ER, Yin B, Schulz B, Ahmad CS, Rosenwasser MP. Proximal humerus and humeral shaft nonunions. J Am Acad Orthop Surg. 2013;21(9):538–47.
21. Healy WL, White GM, Mick CA, Brooker AF Jr, Weiland AJ. Nonunion of the humeral shaft. Clin Orthop Relat Res. 1987;(219):206–13.
22. Rubel IF, Kloen P, Campbell D, et al. Open reduction and internal fixation of humeral nonunions: a biomechanical and clinical study. J Bone Joint Surg Am. 2002;84(8):1315–22.
23. Volgas DA, Stannard JP, Alonso JE. Nonunions of the humerus. Clin Orthop Relat Res. 2004;419:46–50.
24. Thanasas C, Kontakis G, Angoules A, Limb D, Giannoudis P. Treatment of proximal humerus fractures with locking plates: a systematic review. J Shoulder Elb Surg. 2009;18(6):837–44.
25. Wijgman AJ, Roolker W, Patt TW, Raaymakers EL, Matti RK. Open reduction and internal fixation of three and four-part fractures of the proximal part of the humerus. J Bone Joint Surg Am. 2002;84-A(11):1919–25.
26. Cadet ER, Ahmad CS. Hemiarthroplasty for three- and four-part proximal humerus fractures. J Am Acad Orthop Surg. 2012;20(1):17–27.
27. Martinez AA, Bejarano C, Carbonel I, Iglesias D, Gil-Albarova J, Herrera A. The treatment of proximal humerus nonunions in older patients with the reverse shoulder arthroplasty. Injury. 2012;43(Suppl 2):S3–6.
28. Clavert P, Adam P, Bevort A, Bonnomet F, Kempf JF. Pitfalls and complications with locking plate for proximal humerus fracture. J Shoulder Elb Surg. 2010;19(4):489–94.
29. Tauber M, Brugger A, Povacz P, Resch H. Reconstructive surgical treatment without bone grafting in nonunions of humeral surgical neck fractures. J Orthop Trauma. 2011;25(7):392–8.
30. Allende C, Allende BT. The use of a new locking 90 degree blade plate in the treatment of atrophic proximal humerus nonunions. Int Orthop. 2009;33(6):1649–54.
31. Gartsman GM, Taverna E. Arthroscopic treatment of rotator cuff tear and greater tuberosity fracture nonunion. Arthroscopy. 1996;12(2):242–4.
32. Healy WL, Jupiter JB, Kristiansen TK, White RR. Nonunion of the proximal humerus: a review of 25 cases. J Orthop Trauma. 1990;4(4):424–31.
33. Ring D, McKee MD, Perey BH, Jupiter JB. The use of a blade plate and autogenous cancellous bone graft in the treatment of ununited fractures of the proximal humerus. J Shoulder Elb Surg. 2001;10(6):501–7.
34. Walch G, Badet R, Nove Josserand L, Levigne C. Nonunions of the surgical neck of the humerus: surgical treatment with an intramedullary bone peg, internal fixation, and cancellous bone grafting. J Shoulder Elb Surg. 1996;5(3):161–8.
35. Badman BL, Mighell M, Kalandiak SP, Prasarn M. Proximal humeral nonunions treated with fixed-angle locked plating and an intramedullary strut allograft. J Orthop Trauma. 2009;23(3):173–9.
36. Garrison KR, Shemilt I, Donell S, et al. Bone morphogenetic protein (BMP) for fracture healing in adults. Cochrane Database Syst Rev. 2010;(6):CD006950.
37. Friedlaender GE, Perry CR, Cole JD, et al. Osteogenic protein-1 (bone morphogenetic protein-7) in the treatment of tibial nonunions. J Bone Joint Surg Am. 2001;83(Suppl 1 Pt 2):S151–8.
38. Boileau P, Chuinard C, Le Huec JC, Walch G, Trojani C. Proximal humerus fracture sequelae: impact of a new radiographic classification on arthroplasty. Clin Orthop Relat Res. 2006;442:121–30.
39. Duquin TR, Jacobson JA, Sanchez-Sotelo J, Sperling JW, Cofield RH. Unconstrained shoulder arthroplasty for treatment of proximal humeral nonunions. J Bone Joint Surg Am. 2012;94(17):1610–7.
40. Zafra M, Udeca P, Flores M, Carpintero P. Reverse total shoulder replacement for nonunion of a fracture of the proximal humerus. J Bone Joint Surg Br. 2014;96-B:1239–43.

Part IV

Surgical Treatment

17 Operating Room Setting

Eugenio Savarese

The chapter describes operating room setup for shoulder arthroplasty.

17.1 Patient Position and Preparation

The operating suite has one main entrance for the patient and a secondary door for sterilization area; during the surgery, the main door should be closed to minimize the staff traffic. Anesthesia equipment is located at the head of the patient; power source, cautery generator, and tubing for suction are located at the foot of the patient. Two Mayo stands, which contain the most commonly used instrument, and other one table, for the specific prosthetic equipment, are positioned on the operative side (Fig. 17.1). The main light is positioned above the left shoulder of the surgeon and the secondary light on the right shoulder of the surgeon but more on the head of patient.

17.2 Operating Room

Is placed in the modified beach chair position, with the knees of patient flexed at 80–90° (Fig. 17.2) and the back of the patient at 45–60° relative to the floor. The head of patient should be in neutral alignment and secured on the table. The patient is positioned laterally on the operating table to increase adduction helping humeral preparation (Fig. 17.3). Generally, we used the hydraulic arm assistant (Fig. 17.4). The epilation is recommended a day before surgery to avoid skin irritation; after patient positioning on operating table, precleaning is performed with povidone-iodine (Betadine); if patient is allergic to Betadine, the scrub is performed with 4% chlorhexidine gluconate solution. Draping is initiated from the hand of patient with an impermeable tubular knitted to over the elbow joint secured with an elastic wrap. An impermeable reinforced "U" drape is

E. Savarese (✉)
Casa di Cura Bernardini, Taranto, Italy

S. Gumina et al. (eds.), *Reverse Shoulder Arthroplasty*,
https://doi.org/10.1007/978-3-319-97743-0_17

Fig. 17.1 Operating room setting

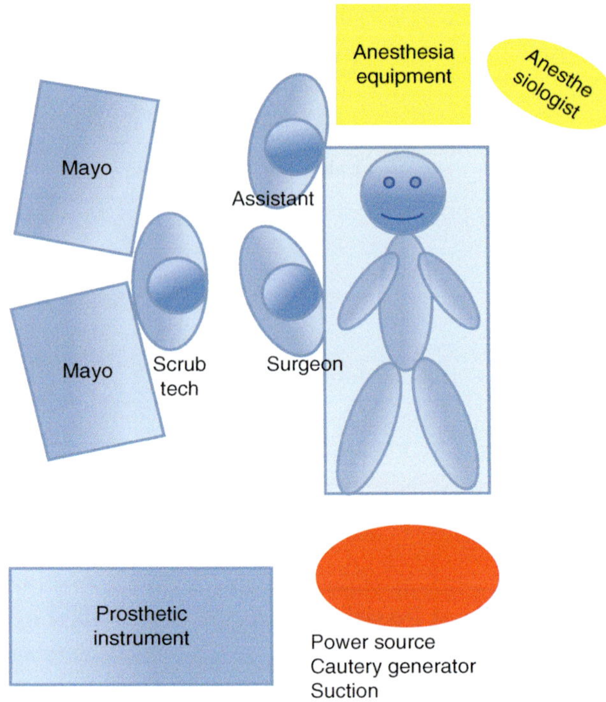

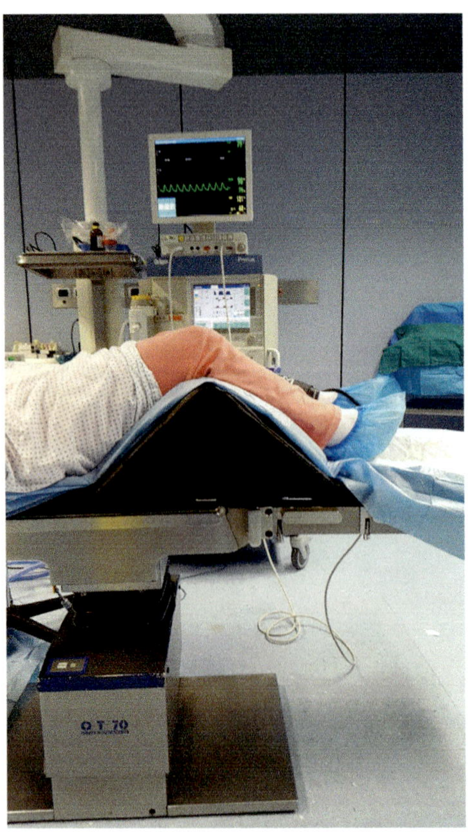

Fig. 17.2 Patient in the beach chair position

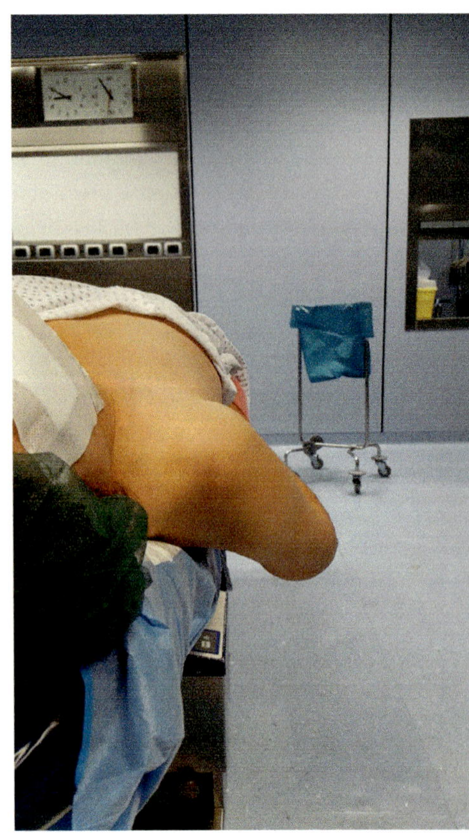

Fig. 17.3 Patient is positioned laterally with the arm out of the operating table

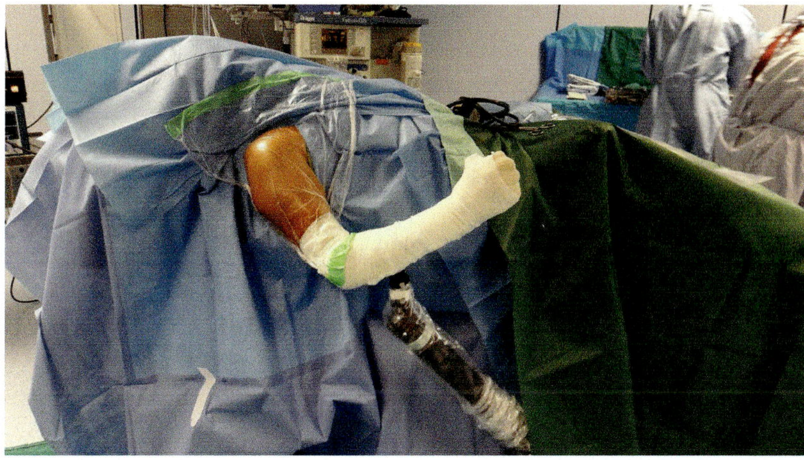

Fig. 17.4 Arm assistant helping during surgery

placed inferiorly and superiorly; finally, a Betadine-impregnated adhesive drape is placed to cover completely the skin.

17.3 Staff Position

The anesthesiologist is located at the head of the operating table, the surgeon stands facing the patient's axilla, the assistant stands behind the shoulder, and the surgical technician stands on the operative side of the patient, between the surgeon and assistant (Fig. 17.1).

17.4 Surgical Instrumentation

Generally used two Mayo tables there are the most commonly instrument to performed a shoulder prosthesis (List 1)

List 1: Knife, Mayo needle holder, forceps, scissors, retractors, clamps, saw and drill, osteotome, rongeur, syringe, and mallet (Fig. 17.5a, b)

On the second Mayo table, there are specific prosthetic equipment (List 2).

List 2: Humeral lateralization set (Fig. 17.6a) and glenoid set (Fig. 17.6b) Equinoxe

Humeral without lateralization set (Fig. 17.7a, b) and glenoid set (Fig. 17.7c) (Johnson & Johnson)

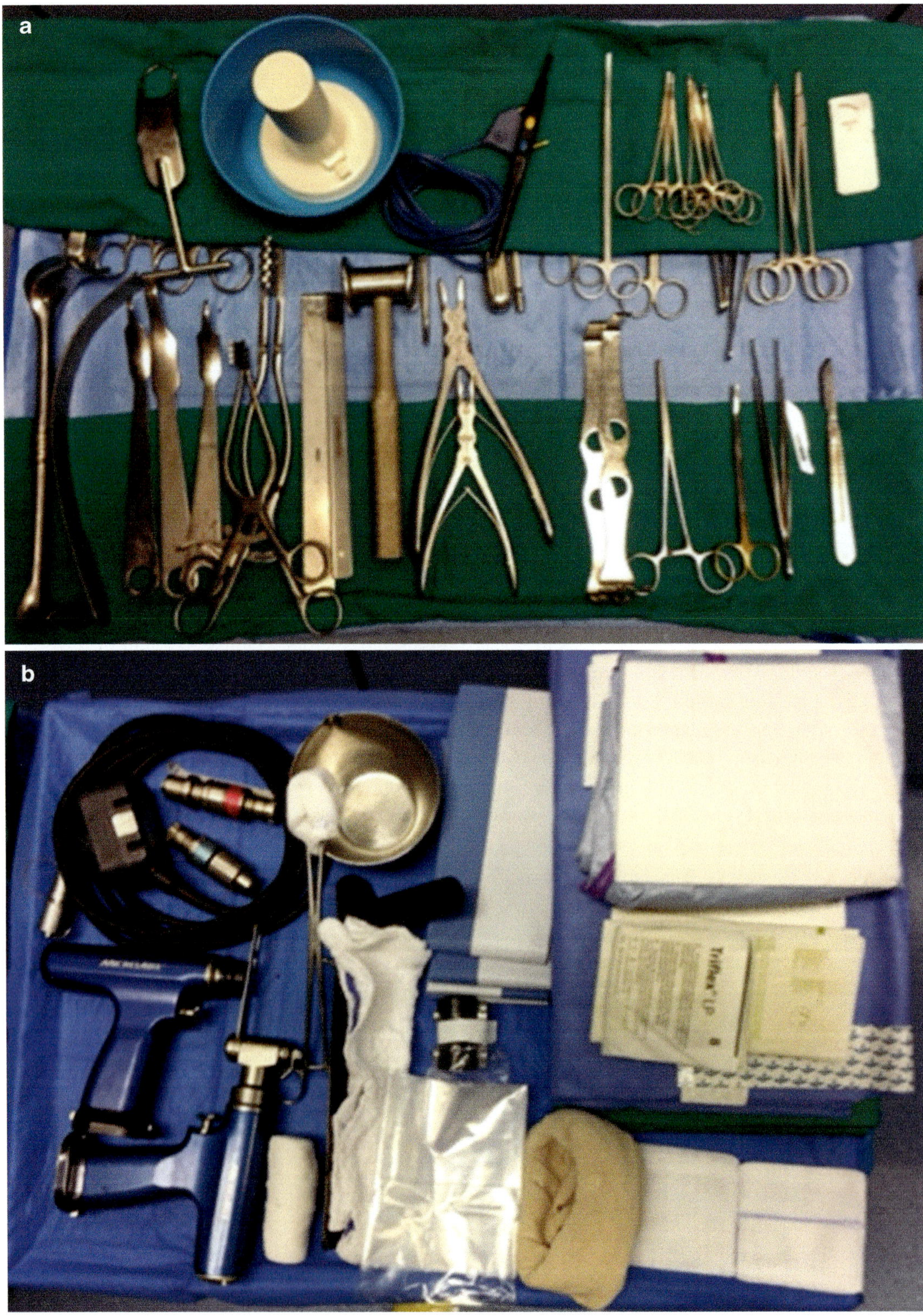

Fig. 17.5 Arrangement of instruments on the Mayo table

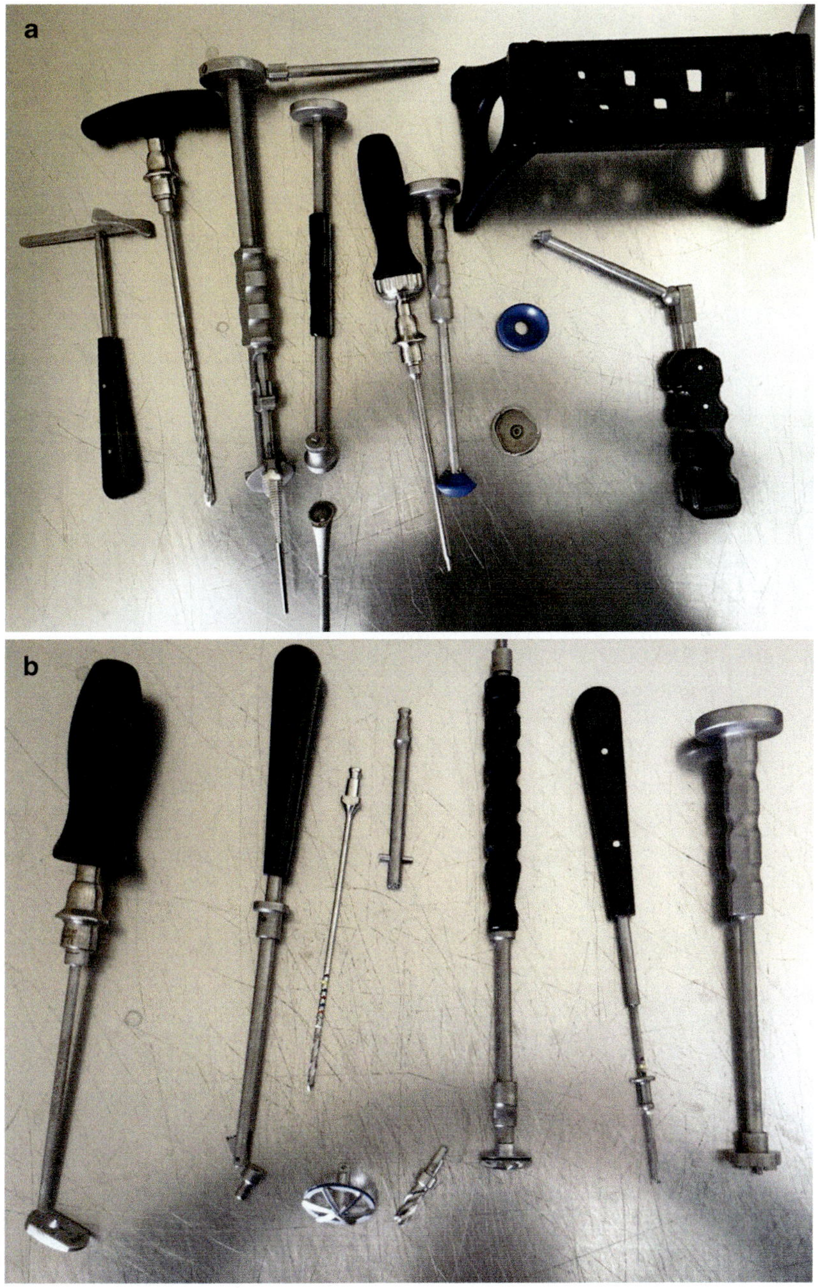

Fig. 17.6 Arrangement of lateralization prosthetic equipment

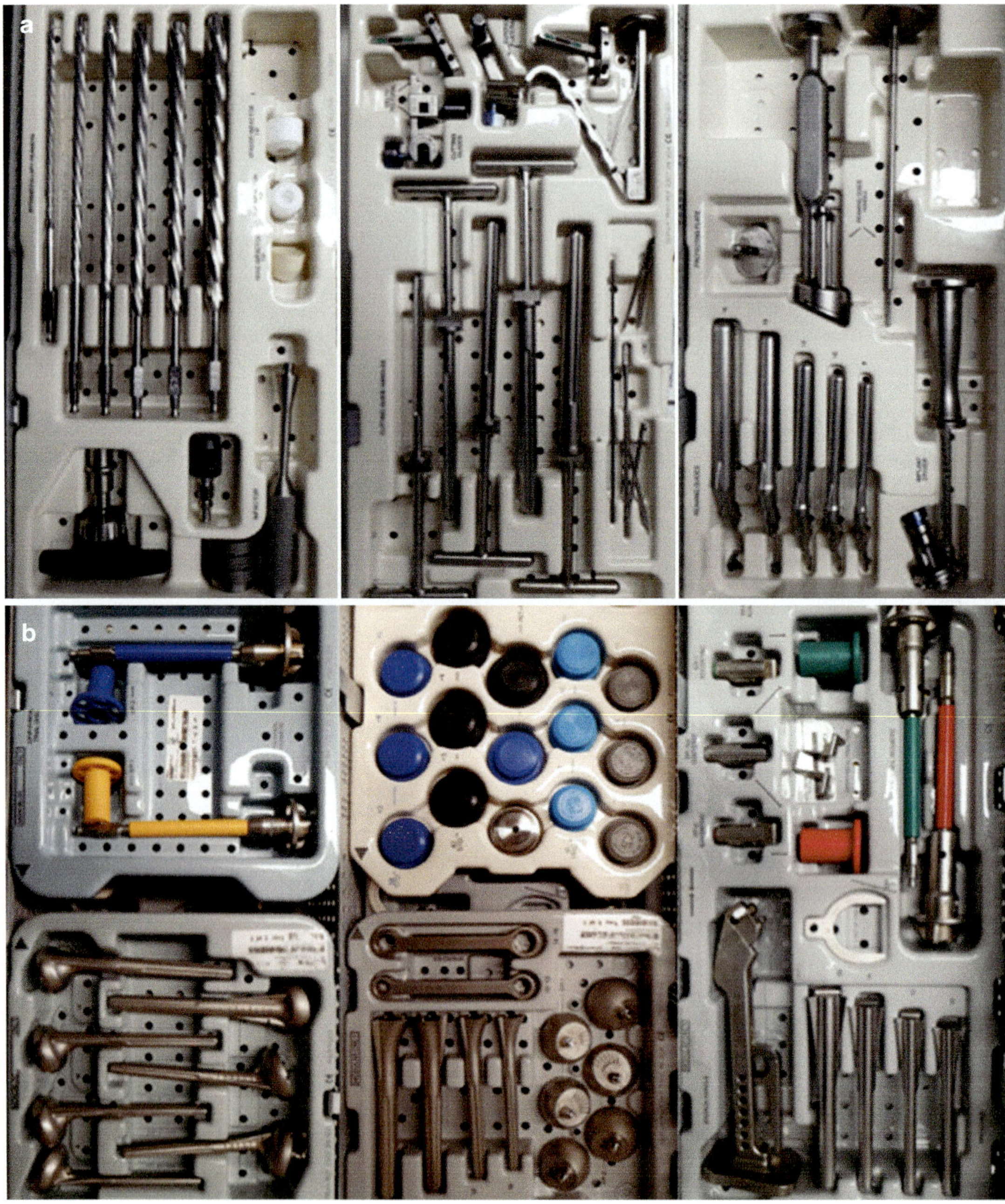

Fig. 17.7 Arrangement of non lateralization prosthetic equipment

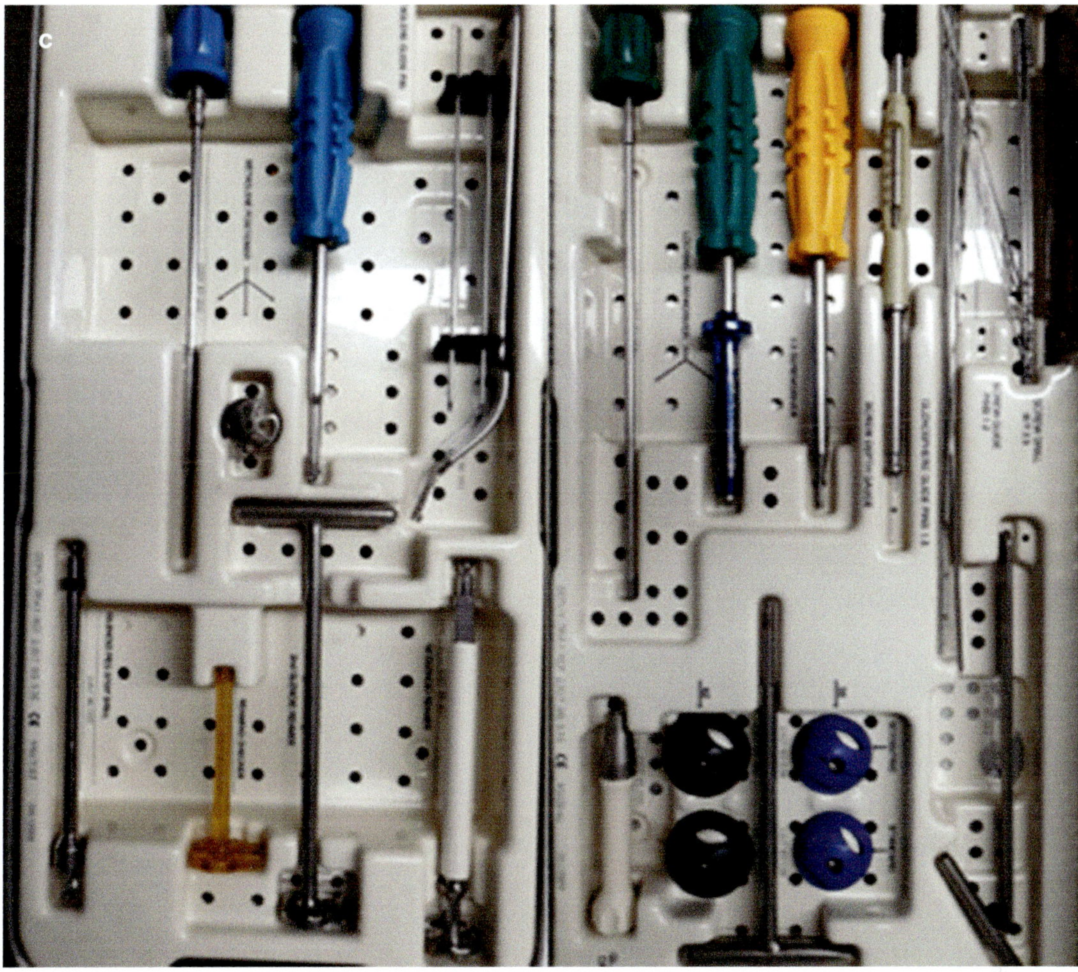

Fig. 17.7 (continued)

18 Anesthesiological Techniques

Fabrizio Fattorini and Alessandro Rocco

The association of general "light" anesthesia and the peripheral brachial plexus block seems to be the most suitable anesthesiological technique during shoulder prosthesis, both for patients' needs and surgeon requirements. Even if locoregional anesthesia potentially allows the surgical intervention by itself, its application is likely to be limited by several factors. The intraoperative position assumed by the patient—beach chair or lateral—associated with a prolonged surgical procedure often causes a discomfort that can sometimes require the switch to general anesthesia during intervention. Being general anesthesia for shoulder surgical interventions not different from that adopted in other types of surgery, only locoregional anesthesiological procedures will be described in this chapter.

18.1 Locoregional Anesthesia

In the last decades, locoregional anesthesia underwent a progressive development, especially in orthopedic surgery: a better safety and analgesia are improved, especially during surgical interventions performed in day surgery setting. Several clinical studies demonstrate the efficacy of peripheral blocks not only for their effective control of intra- and postoperative acute pain but also for their use during the rehabilitation and functional recovery [1, 2]. It is in fact possible to prolong the analgesic effect of peripheral block during postoperative period (continuous nervous blocks) by continuous perineural infusion of local anesthetics. Furthermore, the introduction of ultrasonography to identify nerves makes the peripheral blocks more selective and safer.

Locoregional anesthesia is based on the pharmacological action of specific drugs (local anesthetics) able to temporarily block the conduction of nervous impulse. This effect can be obtained in each region of the body in which nerves can be reached by percutaneous injection. In orthopedic surgery locoregional anesthesia is widely used, as it guarantees both intraoperative anesthesia and postoperative analgesia. Before performing any locoregional technique, the patient must be evaluated with the same accuracy that is used for general anesthesia. Any absolute contraindication (documented allergy to topical anesthetics, infection in the treated region) must be excluded, and any relative contraindication (hemorrhagic diathesis, systemic clinically stable neurological diseases, and local nervous damage) must be carefully considered in terms of risk/benefit ratio. Lastly, an informed consent concerning the planned anesthesiological technique must be signed by the patient [3, 4].

F. Fattorini (✉) · A. Rocco
Anesthesia and Intensive Care Medicine, Policlinico Umberto I Hospital, Sapienza University of Rome, Rome, Italy
e-mail: Fabrizio.fattorini@uniroma1.it

S. Gumina et al. (eds.), *Reverse Shoulder Arthroplasty*, https://doi.org/10.1007/978-3-319-97743-0_18

The electroneurostimulator (ENS) is a direct current generator that permits to localize a nerve by releasing tunable current, applied to an exploratory needle. ENS determines the depolarization of the motor component of afferent muscles (myoclonic) when the needle is near to the nervous fiber. Maximal muscle contraction obtained with minimal current intensity indicates the maximal proximity between the nerve and needle.

ENS allows:

(a) Low risk of nervous lesions
(b) Reduced amount of required local anesthetic
(c) Performing selective blocks
(d) Performing blocks on non-collaborative patients

The introduction of ENS made the peripheral block techniques easy to perform and safe and usable. However, it should be considered that searching nerves with ENS is a blind technique that is error-prone and may cause neurological damages. Indeed, the electroneurostimulation sometimes results in false negatives: the needle is correctly located in the perineural space without eliciting muscle contraction. This results in a useless needle redirection, with an increased risk of nerve lesions and discomfort for patient.

Moreover, locoregional anesthesia of the superior arm has been profoundly influenced by the use of ultrasounds. Beyond showing nerves, echography shows also vessels, muscles, pleura, and all the structures that have to be identified to perform blocks. As well, echography shows anatomical individual variations—not assessed by ENS alone—that could make difficult performing blocks [5].

Echography (or ultrasonography) is an extremely user-friendly procedure since it does not use ionizing radiations, is not invasive, is repeatable, and allows a real-time imaging of anatomical structures closely following the diagnostic and therapeutic procedures. Linear high-frequency probes can be used for imaging superficial structures, such as in the interscalenic, supraclavear, and axillary approaches to brachial plexus. The propagation of sound waves shows different echogenicity in relation to density of tissue that it encounters. Therefore, the higher is the intensity of reflection, the higher is the brightness (hyperechogenicity). On the other hand, the higher the absorbance by tissues, the lower the brightness of echo on the screen (hypoechogenicity). A structure totally lacking of echoes is defined as anechogenic. At roots (e.g., brachial plexus), nerves are hypoechogenic. When nerves progressively approach periphery, they become hyperechogenic ("aspect of honeycomb") due to a higher level of myelination. The anatomy of involved structures (nerves, blood vessels) can be studied by two levels of scanning: longitudinal (long axis) and transversal (short axis). The relationship between visualized anatomic structures and the exploratory needle is the function of the reciprocal position of the probe and the needle. This latter is entirely visible if it is parallel to the long axis of the probe (IN-PLANE technique); on the other hand, only the tip is visible if the needle is introduced perpendicularly to the probe (OUT-OF-PLANE technique) [6].

Echography brought a revolution in locoregional anesthetic procedures, since it permits to:

- Directly visualize various nerves, also those exclusively sensitive.
- Follow the needle movement, thus reducing the risk of nervous lesions.
- Observe the spread of the anesthetic around the nerve, thus minimizing the risk of intravascular and/or pneumothorax injection.
- Guide the positioning of perineural catheter.
- Have a quicker onset time and a longer duration of action.
- Perform the block without pain due to muscle contraction (particularly discomforting when fractures are present).
- Reduce the dose and volume of local anesthetics (30–40% less than those with ENS technique), thus reducing the risk of adverse reactions [7].
- Reduce the incidence of complications and increase the number of success.
- Perform the block also in the presence of serious anatomic abnormalities.

However, we think that echography does not substitute neurostimulation, but rather integrates it and helps to increase both success rate and safety.

18.2 Blocks for Shoulder Surgery

18.2.1 Interscalene Block (Fig. 18.1)

The interscalene brachial plexus block represents the gold standard of shoulder anesthesia, since it involves the lateral two-thirds of the clavicle, proximal humerus, and glenohumeral joint. With this procedure, the brachial plexus is reached in correspondence of its roots, thus delivering the local anesthetic to C5–C6 or the superior trunk. Depending on the amount of anesthetic used, also the roots of C7 and C8 can be involved, while ulnar roots are mainly saved (C8 and T1) [8, 9]. The block can be performed by a single injection (single shot) or continuous block, both assisted by ENS and echograph.

The patient is positioned supine with the head rotated controlaterally to the side of the block and the arm in neutral position along the body. An echographic probe at high frequency regulated at 12–18 MHz and stimulating 50 mm needles (22 G) are used. The brachial plexus can be easily visualized by ultrasounds in correspondence of the posterior interscalene space. The search for the brachial plexus starts laterally to the larynx, passing through the thyroid, carotid artery, and internal jugular vein. Then, moving the probe more externally and downward along the lateral edge of the sternocleidomastoid muscle, the nervous structures become visible in transversal vision as oval or circular hypoechogenic areas are delimited by the anterior and medium scalene muscles. The roots of brachial plexus (C5, C6, and C7) are located immediately behind the anterior scalene muscle and appear as round hypoechogenic structures, sometimes "traffic light-shaped" [10]. By ultrasonography, both the needle movement through the interscalene space and the diffusion of the local anesthetic can be monitored. Most complications associated with the block of brachial plexus, continuous or not, are transient and do not have any consequence; however, extreme caution should be given during the procedure due to the proximity between the exploratory needle and neurovascular structures. Common complications of the interscalene brachial plexus block include the block of homolateral phrenic nervous (consensual hemi-diaphragmatic paralysis), Horner's syndrome due to the block of stellate ganglion (enophthalmos, palpebral ptosis), recurrent block of laryngeal nerve (dysphonia), and vascular cut (hematomas). Rare complications, but potentially severe, are carotid and intervertebral cuts, pneumothorax, subarachnoidal or intraforaminal cut (cause of spinal anesthesia and cervical epidural, respectively), and direct nervous lesion. In continuous blocks, perineural catheters can infect, kneel, tie, or become imprisoned [11, 12].

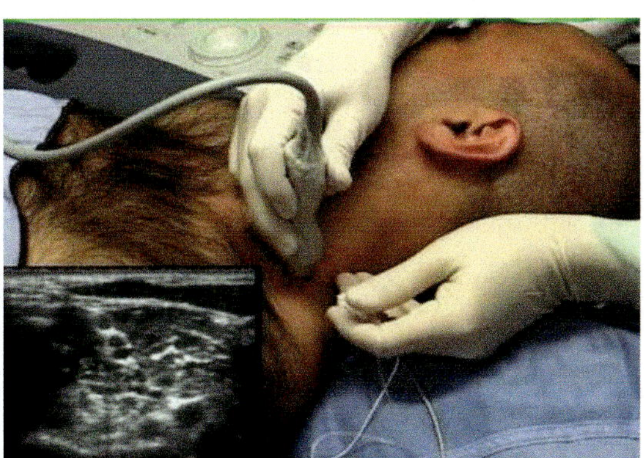

Fig. 18.1 Interscalene block: clinical approach and echographic aspect of brachial plexus ("traffic light-shaped")

18.2.2 Supraclavear Block

The use of ultrasounds allows to easily perform anesthetic procedures which were associated with a high risk up to date. This is the case of supraclavear block that was progressively neglected in clinical practice due to the high incidence of pneumothorax dependent on close relationship between neurovascular structures and the lung. The introduction of echography has drastically reduced those risks, making this block feasible also in pediatric patients [13]. In patients who are not eligible to general anesthesia—even if light—the association of supraclavear and interscalene blocks allows the intervention on shoulder in totally conscious patient. The patient is positioned supine with the head rotated controlaterally to the side of the block and the arm in neutral position along the body. An echographic probe at high frequency set between 12 and 18 MHz is positioned into the supraclavear groove, in parallel to the third medium of clavicle and with the ultrasound beam in caudal direction. Then, the probe is laterally and medially slid to search for the subclavian artery that will appear, over the short axis, as a hypoechogenic and pulsatile structure; color Doppler can be used to confirm the vascular nature (especially when the anatomy is abnormal). The subclavian vein is more superficial and medially located with respect to the artery. Behind the artery, the surface of the first rib will appear as a hyperechogenic line with an underlying hypoanechogenic shadow, since the bone surface totally reflects ultrasounds. The first rib and its posterior shadow interrupt the continuity of an underlying hyperechogenic line which represents the parietal pleura that—unlike the rib—is passed by ultrasounds, thus generating reflection artifacts. These artifacts, defined as "comet tail," are typical of the tissue-air interface that represents pulmonary parenchyma. The patient may be asked to take a deep breath in order to show the sliding of layers of parietal and visceral pleura. In most patients, the skin-pleura distance at supraclavear level is far less than 3 cm. The plexus is identified laterally, behind, and in cephalic position with respect to the artery. When it is visualized over the short axis, it appears as a complex of hypoechogenic, round, and oval structures in a number ranging 2–12 (according to patients' characteristics and the level of analysis). The most superficial nerves usually innervate the proximal extremity of the superior limb (shoulder and proximal part of the arm), while the deepest nerves, near to the first rib, innervate the distal part (elbow, forearm, hand). A lateral-medial approach is usually preferred over medial-lateral approaches, since with this approach it is possible to avoid the subclavian vein that alternatively could collapse because of probe pressure and lead to a missing identification of the intravascular injection. In our opinion, for a supraclavear block, the in-plane approach is more suitable, thanks to its safety (the needle should be always followed to reduce the risk of pneumothorax). After skin disinfection, the probe is positioned to the image of the artery in the center of the screen. Then, the needle is inserted using the in-plane approach and slowly moves to contact the sheath that envelops nerves. After this, the band is pierced by slightly pressing the needle. In this way, it is possible to enter into the virtual space that hosts nervous structures. When the desired location is reached, the needle can be connected to the ENS in order to have a further confirmation of its exact position. After aspiration, a local anesthetic solution is injected, and its diffusion around nervous structures is observed. When the diffusion of the anesthetic cannot be observed, the procedure should be suspended and the needle repositioned. The correct position is confirmed by the anesthetic spread around the nerve (sign of "ring-shaped cake") (Fig. 18.2).

18.2.3 Continuous Interscalene Block

The advantages of interscalene block are likely to be prolonged onward natural duration of single-shot anesthetics by positioning a catheter nearby plexus roots. Shoulder surgery is associated with moderate to severe pain, and good analgesia is very important for functional recovery of the patients and for early discharge [14, 15]. Prospective randomized study comparing continuous interscalene and continuous subacromial infusion for arthroscopic rotator cuff repair

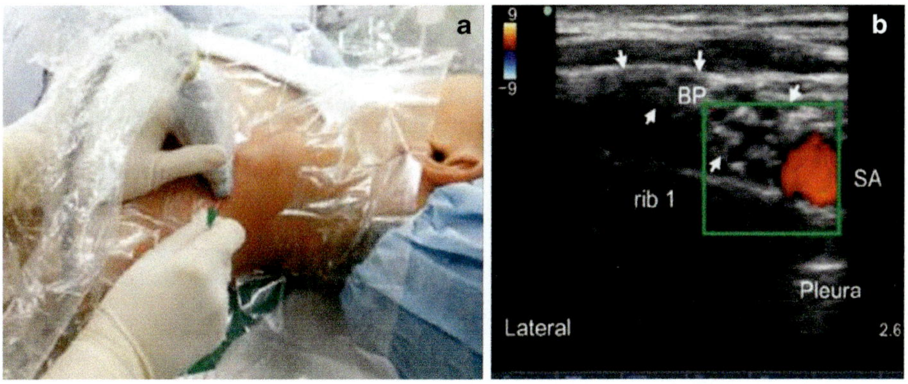

Fig. 18.2 Supraclavear block: clinical approach and echogenic aspect (*BP* brachial plexus, *SA* subclavian artery)

showed better analgesia in the interscalene group. There are various approaches for interscalene catheters (anterior, anterolateral, and posterior). The use of ultrasound has been shown to be associated with improved success rate and less number of needle passes. For shoulder surgery it is really important the catheter is placed near C5/6 root (superior trunk) and use of ultrasound facilitates this. In a randomized controlled study, comparing catheter placement with ultrasound and neurostimulation showed the former is associated with improved success [16]. The patient is supine or semi-sitting with the head facing away from the side to be blocked. It is often easier to perform the procedure standing behind the patient at the head end. It is important all equipment is prepared in advance as any small movement will easily dislodge the needle. The Tuohy needle insertion may be in-plane or out-of-plane. In the in-plane technique, it is important to visualize the whole length of the needle when advancing. The out-of-plane technique is preferred for the placement of nerve catheter. The needle is advanced by hydrodissection with 0.5–1 mL of local anesthetic to open the fascial plane. The local anesthetic should spread anteriorly and posteriorly to the nerve structures and surround them as doughnut-shaped hypoechoic areas. Injection up to 10 mL of local anesthetic distends the interscalene groove in order to facilitate the advancement of catheter. The catheter is advanced at least 3–5 cm beyond the tip of the needle, and the needle is carefully withdrawn as the catheter can easily dislodge being superficial [17, 18].

18.3 Comparison Between Echographic and ENS Approaches

Echography provides an anatomical visualization, reduces complications, increases the success rate of blocks, and limits anesthetic doses. However, interscalene block performed by ENS is an established technique, with high success rate, low complication rate, more rapid, and less expensive than echography. In a prospective randomized study on 230 patients, Liu demonstrated that ENS reduces the duration of the anesthetic procedure and the onset of the block. Moreover, no difference was shown between the two techniques with respect to the incidence of block failure, patient satisfaction, or severity of postoperative neurological symptoms [19]. In a similar trial on 160 patients, Kapral reported a surgical anesthetic rate of 99%, in an echo-guided group in comparison to the 91% reported in the ENS group ($p < 0.01$). Sensitive and motor extension appears higher in the first group [20]. According to available evidence and our experience, the gold standard approach to perineural blocks is represented by echographic imaging

Table 18.1 Local anesthetics: dosages and concentrations

Anesthetic (for interscalene or supraclavear block)	Single-shot block concentration (0.3–0.4 mL/kg)	Continuous block concentration (5–7 mL/h)
Lidocaine	1.5–2%	
Mepivacaine	1.5–2%	
Ropivacaine	0.5–0.75%	0.2%
Levobupivacaine	0.5%	0.125%

with the exploratory needle connected to ENS and a parallel evocation of muscle twitch.

18.4 Local Anesthetics

Several local anesthetics are currently available; each drug presents advantages and disadvantages due to its specific pharmacokinetic and pharmacodynamic characteristics. Some of these (lidocaine, mepivacaine) have a short onset of action (and a shorter duration of action, as well) and others longer onset, but with prolonged duration of action (bupivacaine, levobupivacaine, ropivacaine). Bupivacaine is poorly used in blocks for its high cardiotoxicity. For a continuous block, only local anesthetics with long-term action are used (ropivacaine and levobupivacaine) (Table 18.1).

References

1. Kehlet H. Multimodal approach to control postoperative pathophysiology and rehabilitation. Br J Anaesth. 1997;78:606–17.
2. Kehlet H, Dahl J. Anaesthesia, surgery, and challenges in postoperative recovery. Lancet. 2003;362:1921–8.
3. Bowens C, Sripada R. Regional blockade of the shoulder approaches and outcomes. Anesthesiol Res Pract. 2012;2012:971963.
4. Beecroft C, Coventry DM. Anaesthesia for shoulder surgery. Contin Educ Anaesth Crit Care Pain. 2008;8(6):193–8.
5. Marhofer P, Greher M, Kapral S. Ultrasound guidance in regional anaesthesia. Br J Anaesth. 2005;94(1):7–17.
6. Marhofer P. Ultrasound guidance for nerve blocks. Principles and practical implementation. Oxford: Oxford University Press; 2008.
7. McNaught A, Shastri U, Carmichael N, et al. Ultrasound reduces the minimum effective local anaesthetic volume compared with peripheral nerve stimulation for interscalene block. Br J Anaesth. 2011;106:124–30.
8. Borgeat A, Ekatodramis G. Anaesthesia for shoulder surgery. Best Pract Res. 2002;16(2):211–25.
9. Winnie AP. Interscalene brachial plexus block. Anesth Analg. 1970;49(3):455–66.
10. Chan VW. Applying ultrasound imaging to interscalene brachial plexus block. Reg Anesth Pain Med. 2003;28(4):340–3.
11. Borgeat A, Ekatodramis G, Kalberer F, Benz C. Acute and nonacute complications associated with interscalene block and shoulder surgery. Anesthesiology. 2001;95(4):875–80.
12. Benumof JL. Permanent loss of cervical spinal cord function associated with interscalene block performed under general anesthesia. Anesthesiology. 2000;93(6):1541–4.
13. Kapral S, Krafft P, Eibenberger K, Fitzgerald R, Gosch M, Weinstabl C. Ultrasound-guided supraclavicular approach for regional anesthesia of the brachial plexus. Anesth Analg. 1994;78:507–13.
14. Meier G, Bauereis C, Heinrich C. The interscalene brachial plexus catheter for anaesthesia and postoperative pain management. Experience with a modified technique. Anaesthesist. 1997;46(8):715–9.
15. Fanelli G, Casati A, Chelly JE, Bertini L. Blocchi periferici continui. Milano: Mosby Italia srl; 2001.
16. Fredrickson MJ, Ball CM, Dalgleish AJ. A prospective randomized comparison of ultrasound guidance versus neurostimulation for interscalene catheter placement. Reg Anesth Pain Med. 2009;34:590–4.
17. Chelly JE, Ghisi D, Fanelli A. Continuous peripheral nerve blocks in acute pain management. Br J Anaesth. 2010;105(Suppl 1):i86–96.
18. Tognù A, Bonarelli S, Borghi B, Gullotta S. Tecniche di Anestesia Locoregionale Ecoguidate. Milano: Elsevier; 2010.
19. Liu SS, Zayas VM, Gordon MA, et al. A prospective, randomized, controlled trial comparing ultrasound versus nerve stimulator guidance for interscalene block for ambulatory shoulder surgery for postoperative neurological symptoms. Anesth Analg. 2009;109(1):265–71.
20. Kapral S, Greher M, Huber G, et al. Ultrasonographic guidance improves the success rate of interscalene brachial plexus blockade. Reg Anesth Pain Med. 2008;33(3):253–8.

19 What Do the Companies Propose?

Celeste Bertone and Dario Petriccioli

19.1 Introduction

The history of shoulder arthroplasty was revolutionized by Paul Grammont in 1985 with his new semiconstrained "ball and socket" implant [1]. While this modern widely accepted reverse shoulder arthroplasty (RSA) is relatively recent, the concept of RSA is not new as several RSA devices were originally developed in the early 1970s. These devices did not gain widespread acceptance, and only limited case studies or book chapters are reported in the literature [2–6]. To this day none of these devices are on the market with the exception of the Bayley-Walker prosthesis, a modified version of the original Kessel design [6, 7].

The two major innovations introduced in the RSA by Paul Grammont were a large glenoid hemisphere with no neck and a small almost horizontally inclined (155°) humeral component covering less than half of the hemisphere [8, 9].

Fundamental biomechanical advantages of this reverse prosthesis are as follows: (1) the large ball offers greater arc motion and more stability than a small ball, (2) the small lateral offset (absence of neck) places the center of rotation directly in contact with the glenoid surface and reduces the torque at the point of fixation of the glenoid component, (3) medializing the center of rotation recruits more deltoid fibers for elevation or abduction, and (4) lowering the humerus increases tension on the deltoid. These biomechanical properties may lead to better functioning of the deltoid by an increase of its lever arm and action moment, compensating for rotator cuff deficiency [1, 8, 9].

Since Grammont's first RSA prototype composed of a ceramic cemented two-thirds of a sphere for the glenosphere and an inverted polyethylene cemented humeral stem (Fig. 19.1), numerous parameter design modifications have been executed in order to optimize the clinical results and minimize complications [1, 10–14]. While RSA has been utilized primarily in elderly patients with cuff tear arthropathy (Fig. 19.2), there is an expansion in indications including acute proximal humeral fractures in the older patients with poor bone or cuff quality, fracture sequelae with tuberosity nonunion or irreparable rotator cuff tear, tumors, and revision shoulder arthroplasty. Due to widespread use, in 2017 not less than 30 model designs are currently available on the market [15, 16].

The aim of this chapter is to compare different prosthetic designs in order to analyze those parameters that can influence biomechanic and kinematic of the RSAs. To evaluate the numerous

C. Bertone (✉) · D. Petriccioli
Gruppo Ospedaliero San Donato, Istituti Ospedalieri Bresciani, Milano, Italy

Istituto Clinico Sant'Anna, Brescia, Italy

UO Ortopedia, Chirurgia della Spalla e del Gomito, Brescia, Italy

S. Gumina et al. (eds.), *Reverse Shoulder Arthroplasty*, https://doi.org/10.1007/978-3-319-97743-0_19

design parameters defining the RSA geometry, we identify four separate prosthetic elements: baseplate, glenosphere, polyethylene, and humeral component.

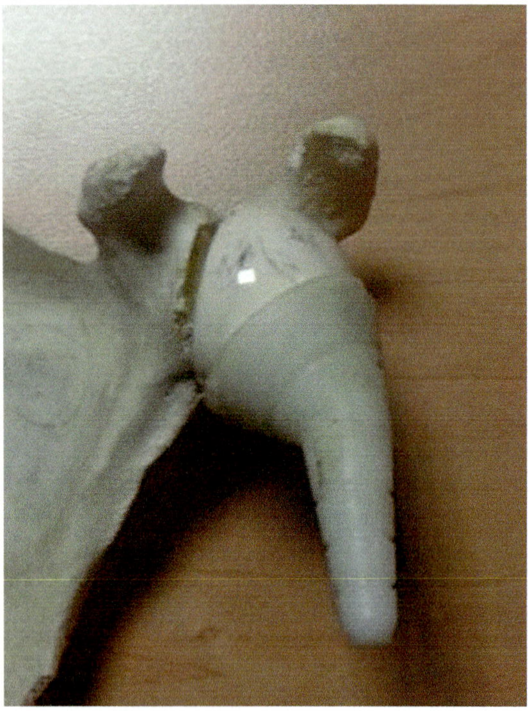

Fig. 19.1 The reverse shoulder prosthesis "Trompette" designed by Paul Grammont in 1985 (Dijon, France)

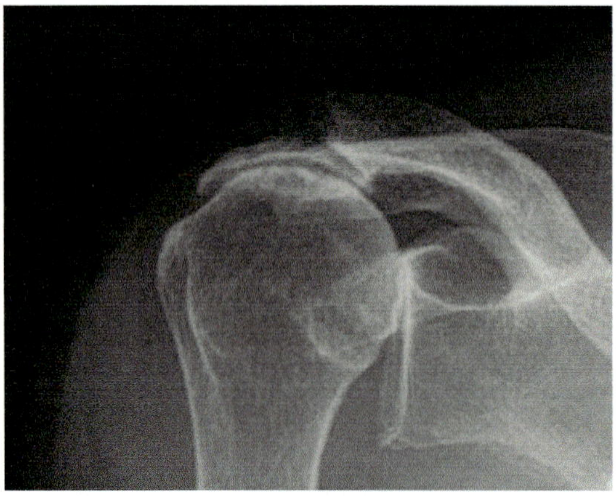

Fig. 19.2 Glenohumeral eccentric osteoarthritis with acromial acetabularization (Hamada and Fukuda stage 4b) (Hamada K., Fukuda H., Mikasa M., Kobayashi Y. Roentgenographic findings in massive rotator cuff tears. A long-term observation. Clin Orthop Relat Res 1990;254:92–6)

19.2 Baseplate

Multiple manufacturers have developed different RSA glenoid designs over the past decade. Although many share similar characteristics, the baseplates available on the market can be differentiated according to:

- Shape: oval or circular
- Backside geometry: flat or convex
- Type of fixation: pegged or screwed baseplate
- Surface finish to improve bone ingrowth (secondary stability)
- Thickness: standard or augmented

Since Grammont's introduction, the commonly used baseplate had a circular shape with a 29-mm diameter [9] (Fig. 19.3). During the RSA procedure, because of glenoid wear or small glenoid size, glenoid surface area could be insufficient to fix the commonly used 29-mm-diameter baseplate. In small glenoids, the standard glenoid implant (29 mm) is larger than

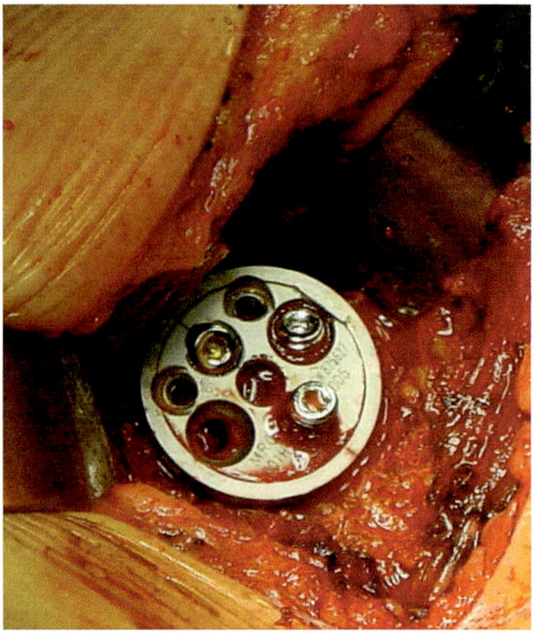

Fig. 19.3 Based on Grammont's original design, a 29-mm-diameter circular glenoid baseplate with a central peg and three circumferential adjustable screws

glenoid bone stock, which results in insufficient screw fixation in anterior or posterior aspect of glenoid itself [17]. Facing this uncertainty, some manufacturers have developed baseplates with a smaller diameter (25 mm), and their use is increasing especially among small females and Asian patients [18, 19]. Chae et al. stated that the use of a smaller baseplate (25 mm) is beneficial in improving initial stability of glenoid component fixation and thereby increasing impingement-free range of motion in small glenoids, compared with the commonly used baseplate (29 mm) [18].

Other companies have developed oval baseplates (Fig. 19.4). Roche et al. tested, in vitro, the fixation strength of four generic baseplates, attached to a low-density bone-substitute polyurethane substrate model. They suggested that oval baseplates (25 × 34 mm) show better fixation characteristics than circular ones (25 mm) [20]. A round baseplate, on the other hand, has the advantage of simplifying the surgical technique because a reamer with a smaller diameter can be used and the longitudinal axis of the glenoid does not have to be defined.

Middernacht et al. also suggested the use of a circular baseplate with a smaller radius than currently used to avoid scapular notching, considering the varied size of the infraglenoid tubercle. They recommended using a smaller baseplate in order to move the center of rotation even lower on the glenoid face [21, 22] (Fig. 19.5).

Despite several authors suggesting the use of a smaller baseplate to reduce scapular notching or to manage a small glenoid, oval baseplates are currently available with an inferior extension to protect the inferior part of the scapula as a shield [23] (Fig. 19.6).

An ideal glenoid baseplate implant must match the size, shape, and congruity of the glenoid surface. A perfect fit between the congruity of implant and glenoid improves load transfer and reduces deformation and displacement of the implant. The backside of a baseplate can be flat or convex. Curved back components have a biomechanical advantage

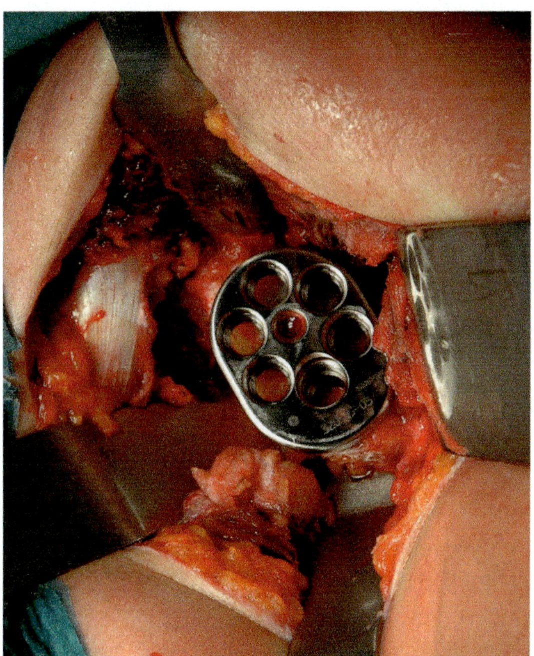

Fig. 19.4 Equinoxe® oval glenoid baseplate (Exactech; Gainesville, FL, USA). An oval design increases the surface contact area and the number of screw option positions from four to six to provide surgeons with additional intraoperative flexibility

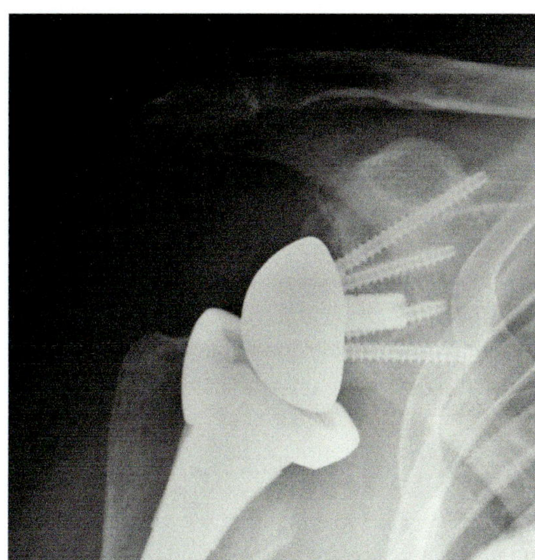

Fig. 19.5 DELTA XTEND® implant design (Depuy Synthes; Warsaw, IN, USA) offers a smaller circular baseplate diameter (27 mm) allowing the surgeon to position the metaglene axis as lower as possible to prevent scapular notching

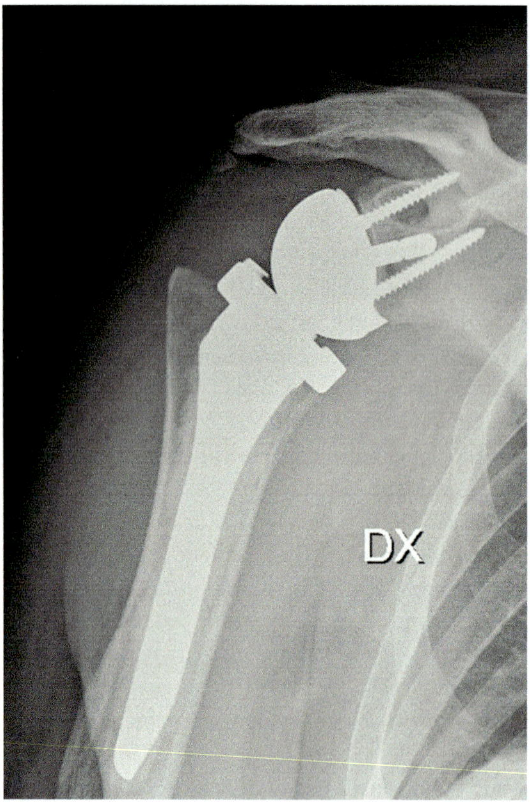

Fig. 19.6 The Duocentric® prosthesis glenoid baseplate (Aston Medical, Saint-Étienne, France) presents a spherical inferior integrated overhang that places a protective resurfacing shield over the scapular pillar

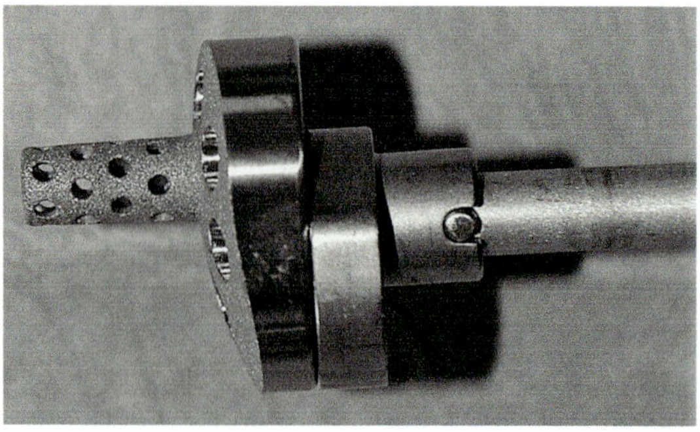

Fig. 19.7 Equinoxe® glenoid baseplate (Exactech; Gainesville, FL, USA) has curved back surface preserving the glenoid bone stock and increasing cortical bone contact to maximize baseplate support. It is designed with an eccentric single cage peg that fills the central bone defect left by an explanted glenoid implant in case of revision

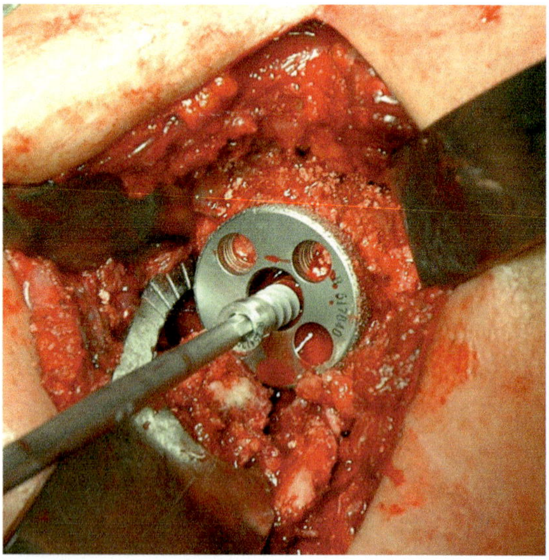

Fig. 19.8 The Biomet Comprehensive® RSA baseplate (Zimmer Biomet; Warsaw, IN, USA) has a large central hole to accommodate a modular 6.5-mm screw for rigid compression into the glenoid vault

over flat glenoids with a larger contact area and a better spreading of pressure [24, 25] (Fig. 19.7).

As a consequence flat and convex reamers can be used to prepare the glenoid. Flat reaming will remove more bone than convex reaming in uniconcave glenoids (type A2 according to Walch classification). In contrast, flat reaming removes less bone in biconcave glenoids (type B2 according to Walch classification). However, this difference is minimal [26–28]. Careful reaming of the glenoid surface is critical; Sutton et al. reported that 5 mm of reaming decreases glenoid surface area by 28% and the amount of the glenoid in contact with the baseplate by 27% [29].

Other differences can be found in terms of glenoid preparing. There are systems with pin-guided reamers, as well as systems using a nipple-guided technique. A recent study showed that both techniques are equally accurate [26]. Furthermore, a reduced reamer diameter could facilitate the reaming process, although scientific evidence is not yet available for this.

Regarding the type of fixation, there are screwed (Fig. 19.8) single or double pegged baseplates. Most implants use peg fixation, usually central; in other implants the peg is above center (Fig. 19.7); some have two pegs or a blade. The choice of an eccentric glenoid peg was therefore made to provide better positioning of the glenoid baseplate while still enabling the distal translation of the glenoid sphere. There is yet no scientific evidence for a difference in stability or fixation between these different types of baseplates. According to the literature, baseplate fixation is multifactorial, with screw fixation playing the most important role; to obtain a stable fixation, the peg should be anchored as deeply as possible into the native scapula bone stock [30–32]. Frankle et al. suggest that baseplates with a central screw have better primary stability than pegged ones do to the compressive forces between the bone and the baseplate; this primary stability represents an ideal environment for osseous integration (secondary stability) [33].

All current baseplates offer the possibility of positioning extra screws for fixation. These screws can be locking or non-locking screws. There are no studies promoting the use of variable angle locking screws, although this does seem to be useful for baseplate fixation. James et al. investigated the number of screws needed for initial stability [31] and suggested that only two locking screws provide sufficient stability and extra screws have no added value. These extra screws become more important when the depth of the central peg anchorage is reduced. If possible, four metaglene screws should be used in those cases of uncontained bone loss to guarantee the highest stability [32].

The backside coating is crucial for baseplate osseous ingrowth for secondary stabilization. Most of the available components have a roughened hydroxyapatite-coated surface. A difference can be made between regrowth of bone on prosthesis surface or ingrowth of bone into the prosthesis. This latter form can be expected to be more stable but may complicate potential revision surgery in the future (Fig. 19.9).

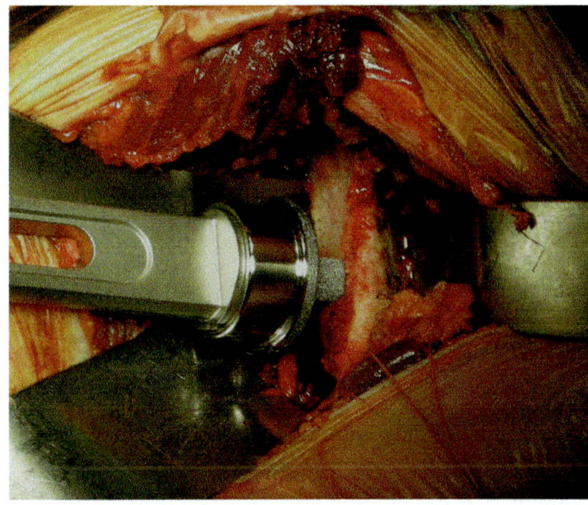

Fig. 19.9 The Zimmer Trabecular Metal® RSA baseplate (Zimmer Biomet; Warsaw, IN, USA) has a highly porous tantalum structure to support bony ingrowth

The mediolateral length of the glenoid components (baseplate + glenosphere) represents a crucial point in RSA design. This parameter, with the neck-shaft angle of the humeral component, determines the center of rotation and ultimately influences the final position of the humerus [34]. In adduction, a more medial rotation center may allow the medial aspect of the polyethylene socket to impinge on the inferior portion of the scapular neck (scapular notching). Some implants are designed with a thicker baseplate in order to lateralize the center of rotation and reduce the risk of notching by creating a longer scapular neck but potentially increase shear stresses at the bone-prosthesis interface and thus the risk of loosening [35–37].

Finally, there are also augmented baseplates, specially developed for bony defects of the glenoid. These should make it possible to place the baseplate in a correct position, ideally perpendicular to the scapular plane, even in difficult cases: i.e., glenoid with superior erosion, type E2 or E3, according to Levigne and Favard classification [38, 39] (Fig. 19.10).

For these difficult cases, baseplates with a long peg are available; the central peg must be long enough for native glenoid bone anchorage. If necessary these options can all be combined with bone grafting to overcome bony defects (Fig. 19.11a–c).

19.3 Glenosphere

The glenosphere morphology may be characterized by several different parameters. The glenosphere can be designed as:

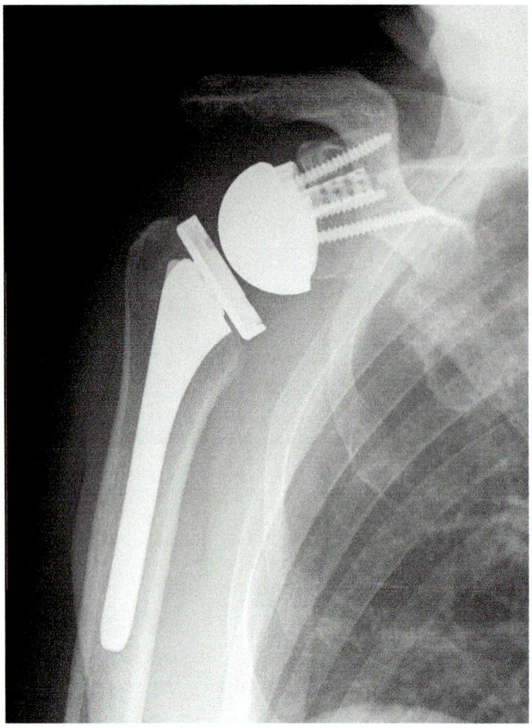

Fig. 19.10 X-ray showing a case of superior augmented baseplate using the Equinoxe® RSA (Exactech; Gainesville, FL, USA)

- Hemisphere, but it can also be more or less than half sphere
- Concentric or eccentric

A glenosphere of more than half sphere will allow a lateralization of the rotation center. This morphology (lateral offset) would restore the deltoid contour and tension the remaining rotator cuff muscles [40–42]. Using a virtual computer simulation, Werner et al. have shown that lower humeral neck-shaft angle and glenoid lateralization are effective for improvement in range of motion after onlay design RSA. The use of the 135° model with 5 mm of glenoid lateralization provided the best results in impingement-free range of motion, except for abduction [43]. In adduction, the lateral offset would reduce impingement on the inferior scapular neck, thereby reducing scapular notching. Based on a systematic literature review, Lawrence et al. demonstrated that scapular notching rates were higher in the traditional Grammont-style implant group compared to the lateralized group. In their conclusions, the authors stated that these differences could be the result of different morphologies of the polyethylene component, different humeral stem neck-shaft angles, and differences in glenosphere offset as well patient factors such as body mass index. It is important also to underline that Grammont systems evaluated in this systematic review were designed with a 155° neck-shaft angle, whereas the lateralized prosthesis had a 135° neck-shaft angle, which could also explain the higher rates of notching in the traditional group [44].

Further, there are also eccentric glenospheres that are placed in a lowered, off-centered position, in order to reduce the incidence of scapular notching [45]. An increased lateral offset and an inferior glenosphere overhang of >3.5 mm prevented notching, but there will be a greater stress on the baseplate in this position with a higher probability of loosening [45–47] (Fig. 19.12). The maximum stress that occurs at the base of the inferior screw elucidates the direct contact failure mode in the middle of the inferior screw. The use of an eccentric glenosphere or a low position of the glenosphere in the vertical plane allows satisfactory deltoid re-tensioning.

The prevalence of peripheral nerve lesions following primary RSA is thus common, but most lesions are subclinical, and most clinically apparent lesions are temporary [48]. A cadaveric study examined the relationship of the axillary nerve in RSA. The axillary nerve is not in close proximity to the glenosphere, with a distance between the nerve and the glenosphere that was systematically greater than 15 mm. Inferior glenosphere overhanging did not appear to decrease the distance to the axillary nerve. Rather, it seems that lengthening of the arm after a RSA leads to a lowering and lateralization of the nerve and protects it from impingement with the glenosphere component. Therefore, the position of the glenosphere in the vertical plane is probably not related to the development of a neurological lesion due to direct contact, but it is rather related to the proximity of the axillary nerve to the posterior metaphysis or humeral implant [49].

As far as the importance of the size of the glenosphere, it has been shown that a larger

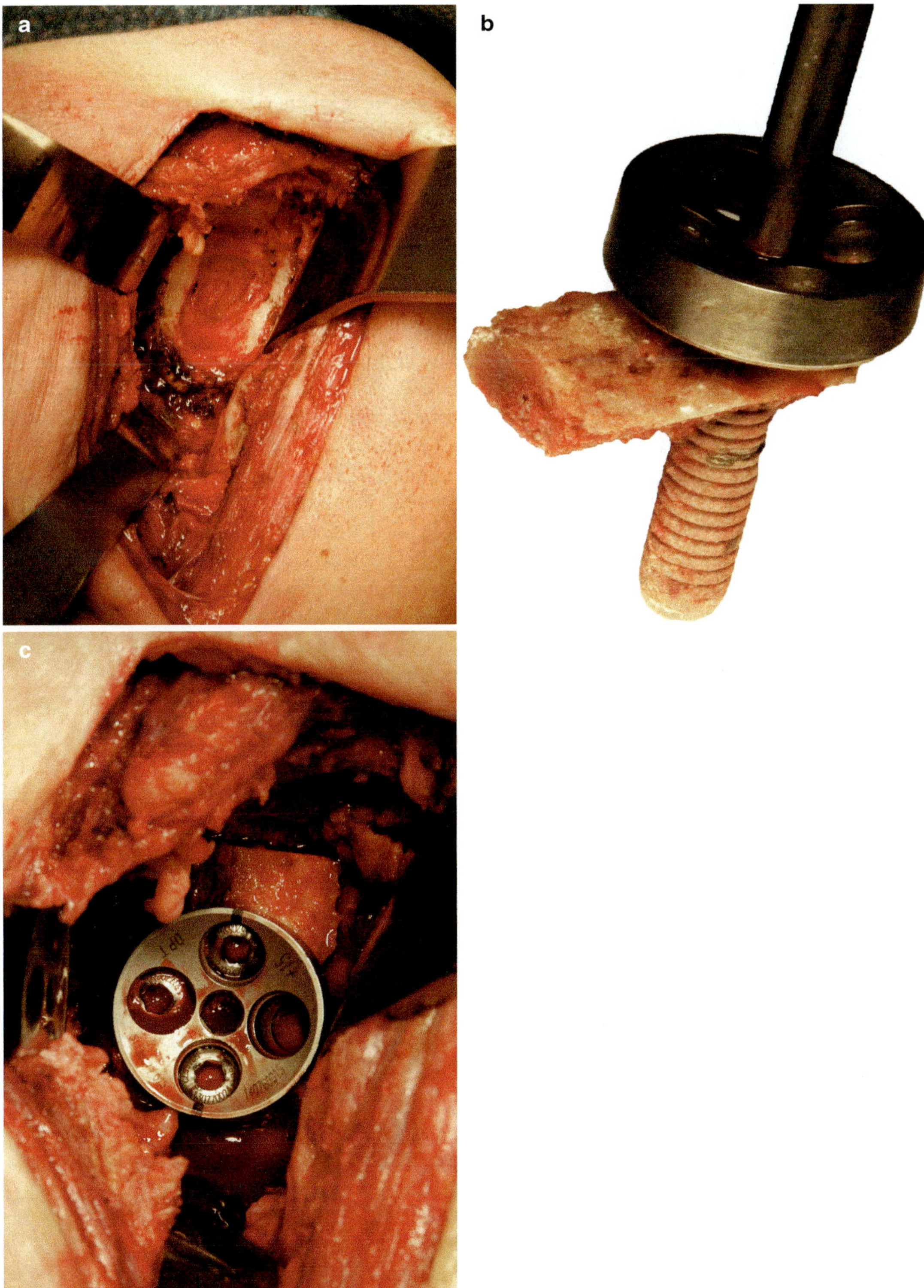

Fig. 19.11 (**a**) Severe central glenoid bone defect according to Antuna classification (Antuna SA, Sperling JW, Cofield RH, Rowland CM Glenoid revision surgery after total shoulder arthroplasty. J Shoulder Elbow Surg. 2001 May–Jun;10(3):217–24). (**b**) Tricortical iliac crest bone graft implanted on a longer central peg baseplate. (**c**) In RSA with glenoid bone grafting, it's crucial to ensure that the baseplate fixation extends into the native glenoid

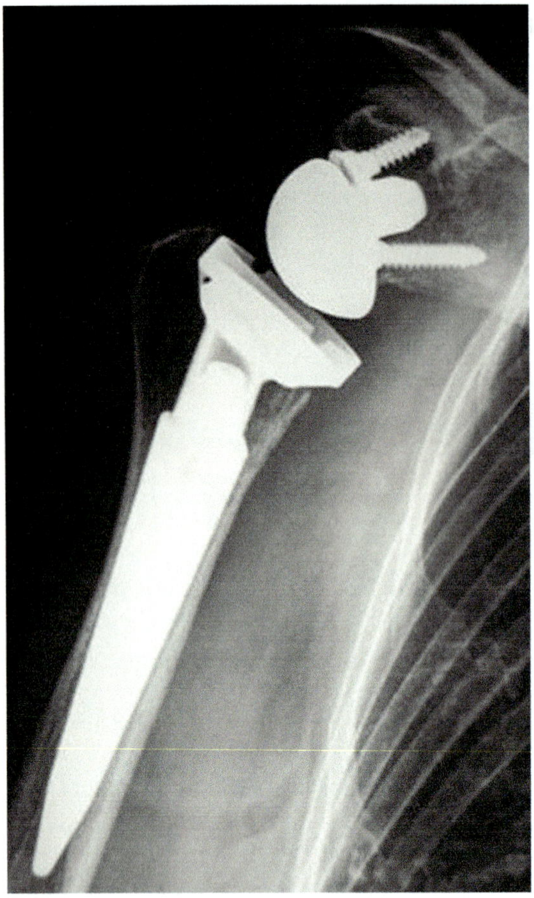

Fig. 19.12 X-ray showing a case of an eccentric glenosphere using the Promos® RSA (Smith and Nephew, Andover, MA, USA). An eccentric glenosphere places the inferior aspect of the sphere below the lateral pillar of the scapula and glenoid neck, reducing the chance of scapular notching

glenosphere increases the range of motion and prevents inferior scapular notching [50–52]. A disadvantage of a larger glenosphere is that it complicates the surgery because it is technically more difficult to put in place. Gerber et al. [53] showed in laboratory environment that reverse shoulder prostheses with small glenospheres would be more stable. In vivo, however, stability of the prosthesis is a multifactorial concept. Deltoid function, localization of the rotation center, soft tissue stiffness, and glenosphere size are influencing factors for stability of the prosthetic joint [53]. Although several biomechanical studies show that increasing the glenosphere diameter significantly increases the joint load and deltoid force, the clinical impact of these changes is presently unclear.

Inferior tilting of the glenosphere is also known to help preventing scapular notching [54–56]. Simovitch et al. validated the importance of glenosphere inferior position in clinical practice, providing the rational for glenosphere designs with a small amount of inferior tilt or offset [57]. Following this principle, Duocentric prosthesis (Aston Medical, Saint-Étienne, France), which was developed by the engineers of the Delta III prosthesis and the successors of Grammont, has a glenosphere with a built-in inferior inclination of 10°. This configuration should lead less impingement, though this has not yet been proven. This varus tilt also ensures that less subchondral bone will be removed at the glenoid when a slight varus position is the goal. If a built-in varus tilt is implanted, the surgeon needs to realize that this lateralizes the center of rotation and thus increases the loads on the glenoid component [10].

Finally, glenospheres with an inferior extension are available. This extension could prevent inferior impingement. However, a lateralized and lowered center of rotation resulting in off-axis shear forces across the bone-prosthesis interface may compromise the fixation of the glenoid baseplate [46].

The type of glenosphere (size and eccentricity) allows adjustment of arm length by only several millimeters, about 1% of arm length defined as the length from the acromion to the epicondylar axis (humeral length plus acromiohumeral distance). Consequently, the key factors for arm length are the height of the stem, type of stem, polyethylene thickness, and the use of an augment or spacer. Collectively, these factors allow arm lengthening by up to several centimeters (about 10% of arm length) [48, 49].

There are a few ways to fix the glenosphere on to the baseplate. Due to the failures with threaded glenospheres (Fig. 19.13), fixation of the glenosphere on the metaglene is generally obtained with a Morse taper [9]. Very often

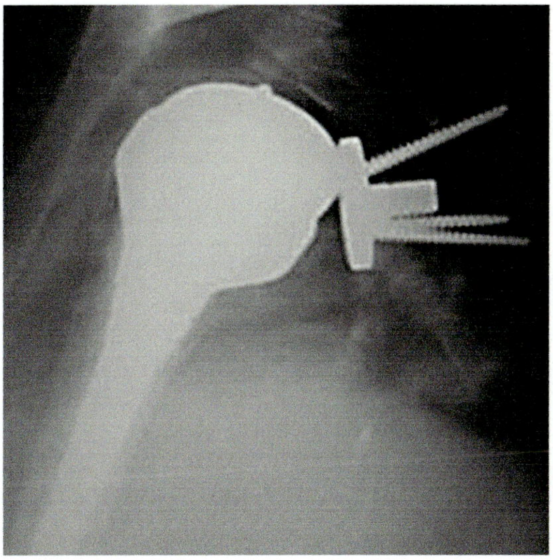

Fig. 19.13 X-ray showing a glenosphere disengagement in a non-Morse taper RSA design

loosening was seen after time with this type of fixation. Today most companies obtain the fixation with a Morse taper, after prior axial screwing, or with direct impaction. As this connection is made in vivo, it is important to avoid soft tissue interposition. Glenosphere disengagement, using a correct technique, fortunately is rare (1.7–5%) [22–58]. The use of a central screw should ease the placement of the glenosphere in the optimal position and can be used without damaging the humeral polyethylene [58].

Regarding the material of the glenosphere, different options are available: polished Cr-Co-Ni alloy, all-polyethylene, or titanium (nickel-free solution for allergic patients). Some companies reversed the materials and manufactured a polyethylene glenosphere and a metallic cup (Affinis reversed, Mathys Ltd., Bettlach, Switzerland; SMR Lima, Villanova di San Daniele del Friuli, Italy) (Fig. 19.14). This modification did not solve the mechanical conflict, but a polyethylene glenosphere combined with a metal or ceramic humeral liner has the advantage that it creates less polyethylene debris when scapular notching would occur. Theoretically, this will induce less active osteolysis [59–62]. However, this remains to be proven in long-term clinical studies.

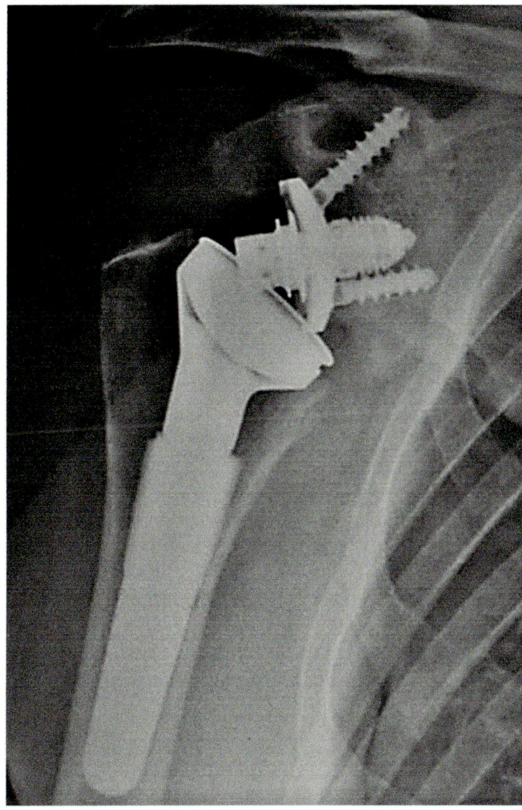

Fig. 19.14 The SMR® Reverse Shoulder System (Lima Ltd., Villanova di San Daniele del Friuli, Italy) provides a new design solution to avoid the impingement of the polyliner and the consequent debris generating osteolysis: the inversion of the materials. The solution consists in the creation of a polyethylene glenosphere articulating with a metal liner

19.4 Polyethylene Insert

Regarding the polyethylene insert of the humeral component, several variations can be found. It is important to underline that the stability of the prosthesis depends on the amount of surface of the glenosphere that is in contact with the polyethylene inlay [15, 52, 53, 63].

Some companies make a distinction between an inlay with minimal contact surface (high-mobility) and intermediate and maximal contact (constraint or retentive). High-mobility polyethylene insert offers reduced polyethylene cup depth in order to improve the range of motion in any direction (adduction, abduction, and internal and

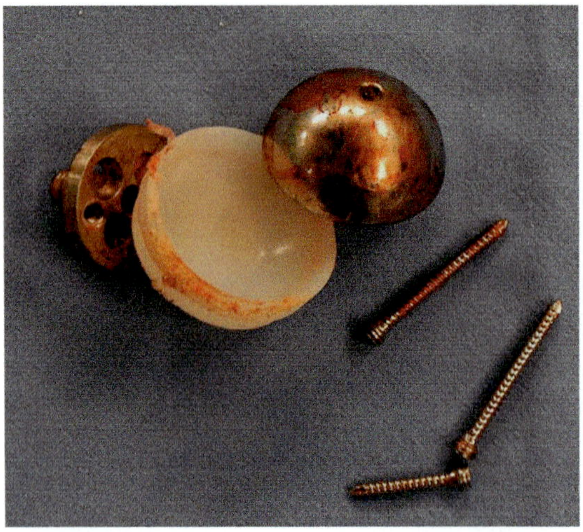

Fig. 19.15 Photograph of a retrieved RSA (implantation time: 7 years); retentive polyethylene humeral insert rim damage due to bony scapular impingement or screw contact

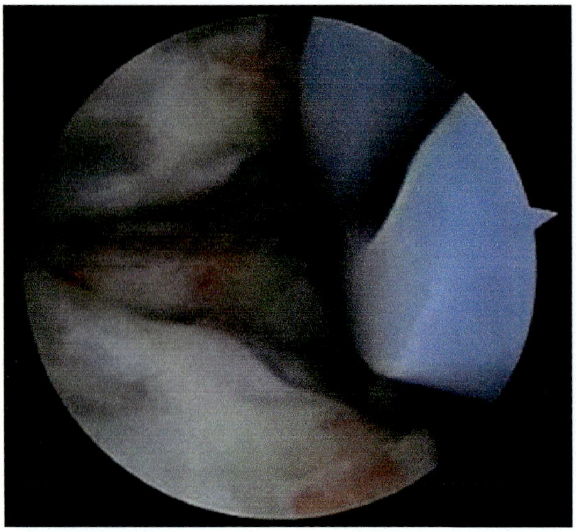

Fig. 19.16 Arthroscopic view from posterior portal showing (on the right) a blunt polyethylene humeral insert

external rotation). It has been shown that a reduction of 3 mm in the depth of the polyethylene inlay results in a gain of range of motion of 12° [64]. This design option slightly reduces the stability and should only be used if the correct joint stability is achieved during intraoperative trials.

The use of different thickness polyethylene insert could help to achieve optimal stability and lateralization, but the surgeon should take care not to overstuff the joint creating negative effects on deltoid force and joint loading [41]. There is interadaptibility available so that most sizes of humeral components can be combined with most sizes of glenospheres.

If implant instability occurs during intraoperative trials, a constrained insert could also be used. The advantage of the deeper socket is improved stability by increasing the translational force necessary to dislocate the glenosphere from the socket. However, it results in medialization of the humeral component and less lateral offset, thereby increasing the potential for subsequent polyethylene wear-induced aseptic loosening [63, 65] (Fig. 19.15). In a computer-simulated model, Gutiérrez et al. established a hierarchy of surgical- and implant-related factors for impingement-free abduction and adduction following RSA [65, 66]. The hierarchy of factors associated with increased impingement-free abduction were lateral offset, glenosphere inferior placement and tilt, humeral neck-shaft angle, and prosthetic size. With respect to impingement-free adduction, the factors were neck-shaft angle, glenosphere inferior placement and size, and lateral offset [65, 66].

Knowing that inferior rim damage is the predominant cause of polyethylene wear and that this wear can induce mechanical loosening of the glenoid component [67], a polyethylene insert with a notch between 3 and 9 o'clock may lead to decreased contact between the humeral cup and the scapula neck or the inferior glenoid screw, although this has not yet been clinically proven [68] (Fig. 19.16).

19.5 Humeral Component

RSA requires placement of a polyethylene socket on a well-fixed humeral stem. A variety of proximal implant geometries has been developed to achieve this goal. The original Grammont-style humeral implants typically have a more valgus (155°; horizontal) metaphyseal inclination (neck-shaft angle) than the native humerus, thereby optimizing stability [9]. However, this larger neck-shaft angle is associated with greater humeral medialization that leads to impingement between the humeral liner and scapula neck. In order to reduce adduction impingement, scapular notching, and polyethylene wear, many recent systems have a more varus (vertical) metaphyseal inclination [63, 66, 68, 69].

A reduction of the inclination to 135° in an onlay configuration also lateralizes the humerus, optimizing the muscle tension and range of motion [70, 71]. These advantages have to be weighed out to the loss of stability in the initial abduction, as confirmed in laboratory conditions by Oh et al. [72]. For designs with an inclination of 155°, this study describes an increased incidence of scapulohumeral conflict but a higher stability in internal rotation (the most critical position for anterior stability) [72].

However, the recent introduction of the platform systems allowing a conversion from an anatomical to a reverse prosthesis opens up the discussion concerning the optimal neck-shaft angle inclination. Revision from hemiarthroplasty or total shoulder arthroplasty to RSA is occasionally necessary. The humeral stem is frequently well-fixed in these patients, and its removal is the most common source of intraoperative complications [73]. To avoid these complications, humeral stems without removal of their fixed portion have been developed [74–77].

The ideal humeral metaphyseal stem inclination for RSA is still under discussion. Therefore, platform stems must include modularity that optimizes the implant position for both arthroplasty designs, anatomic and reverse. Recently Tornier, Inc., has developed a modular system that reduces scapular notching by utilizing a fixed 145° angle by summation of the stem and polyethylene liner angles. This angle has been shown to minimize scapular impingement while optimizing elevation and internal and external rotation through virtual implantation studies [78] (Fig. 19.17).

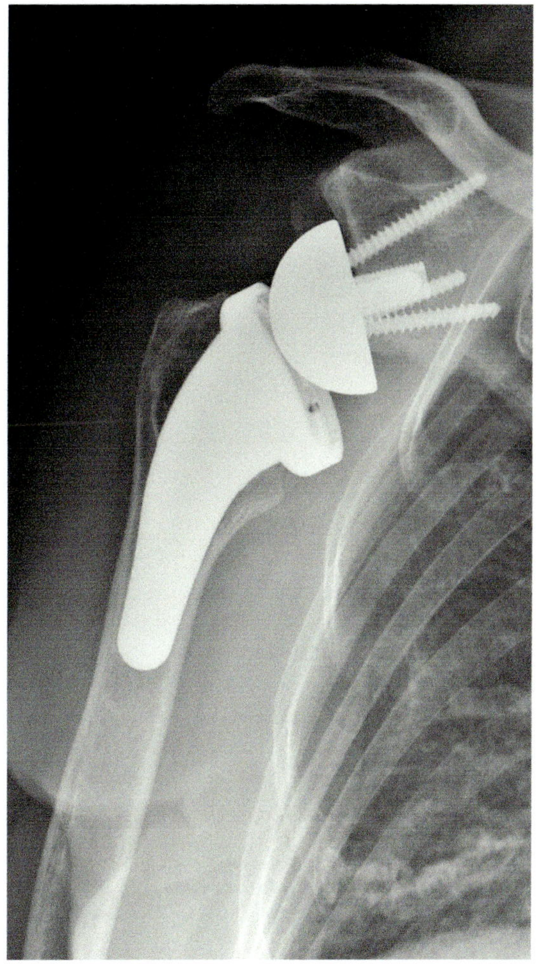

Fig. 19.17 X-ray showing the Aequalis Ascend Flex RSA (Wright Tornier Inc., Memphis, TN, USA) onset design with 145° neck-shaft angle

The humeral component can be stemmed, short stemmed, or stemless [69]. The series with stemless prostheses present equal results as the stemmed ones [79–85]. Advantages of short stemmed or stemless implants include a potential reduction in the risk of periprosthetic fracture, preservation of proximal humeral bone, and the uncoupling of implant location and diaphyseal endosteal canal location. The latter issue may be particularly relevant in patients with proximal humeral deformity (Fig. 19.18), existing hardware, and extreme anatomic variants.

Stemless implants render the concept of neck-shaft angle essentially a surgical technical problem. Because these implants are placed without reference to the diaphyseal canal, it is possible for a less experienced surgeon to place the implant in a position that is widely divergent from the required position [79, 83]. Implant manufacturers have developed short-stemmed implants as a compromise between stemless and standard

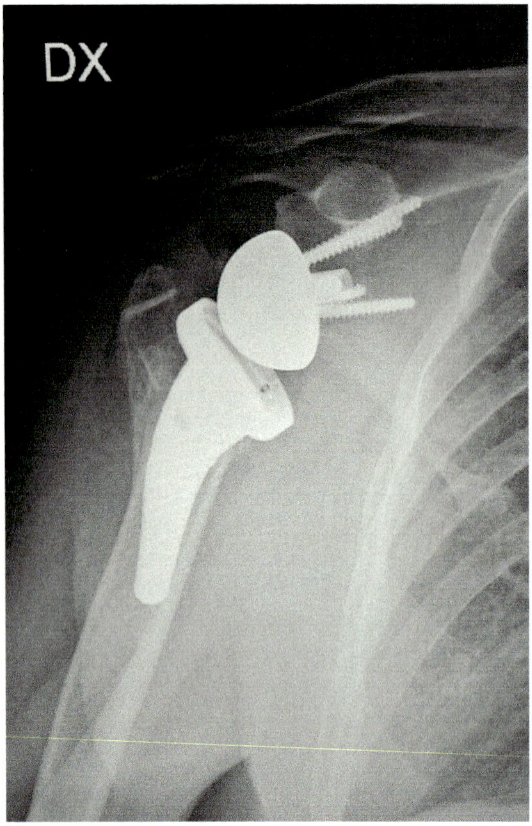

Fig. 19.18 A short humeral stem allows freedom of implant position aside from intramedullary restrictions as in fracture sequelae

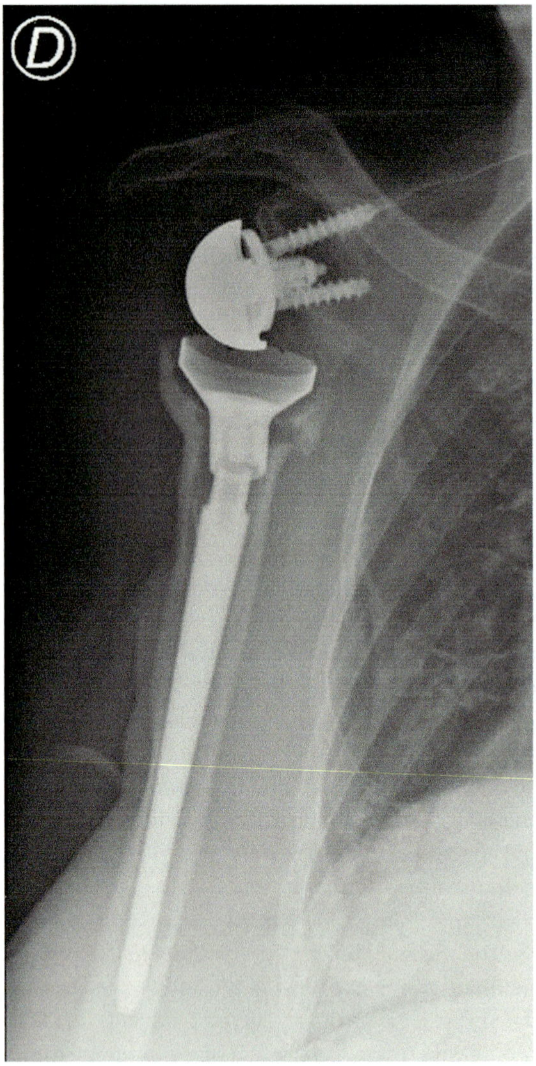

Fig. 19.19 X-ray showing humeral stem disassembly in a shoulder modular prosthesis

stemmed implants, but limited evidence is available regarding these devices [80–82, 84, 85].

Stemmed implants continue to be specifically indicated instead of stemless or short stemmed in patients with proximal humeral bone loss as in fracture cases. In these scenarios, a windowed dedicated trauma stem could be an option and seems to enhance the ingrowth of the tuberosities [86–90].

With stemmed prostheses, the surgeon can choose between monoblock and modular humeral devices. Monoblocks should prevent dissociation of the prosthetic components (Fig. 19.19) in patients where no reconstruction of a viable bony proximal humerus can be expected [70]. In this situation additional modularity could be a potential site of fretting, metallosis, and implant breakage (Figs. 19.20 and 19.21).

Stemmed prostheses can be press-fit or cemented. Both provide similar radiographic and functional outcomes [91]. The most recent press-fit humeral component has a proximal metaphyseal fixation; advantages include better vascularity potentially allowing more rapid ingrowth, easier stem removal during revision, reduced stress shielding rate and incidence of periprosthetic fractures, and lower rates of radiographic loosening [74–92].

In patients where the bone stock cannot provide adequate stability (e.g., fractures, elderly), a

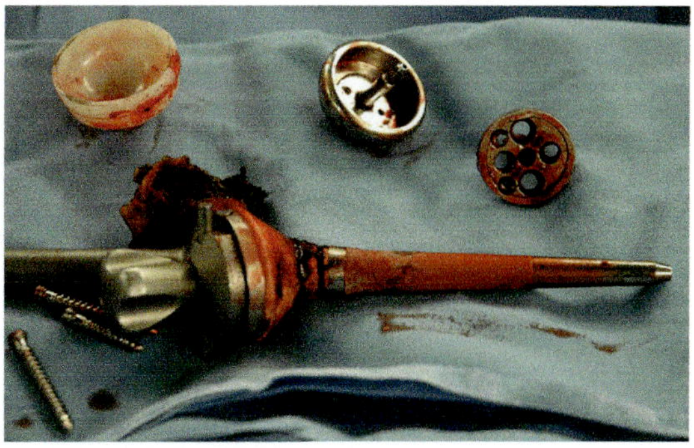

Fig. 19.20 Retrieved RSA implanted in a 73-year-old female with rotator cuff insufficiency, revised after 4 years for humeral stem loosening. Damage of the modular humeral junction consisted of mild to moderate fretting of the stem

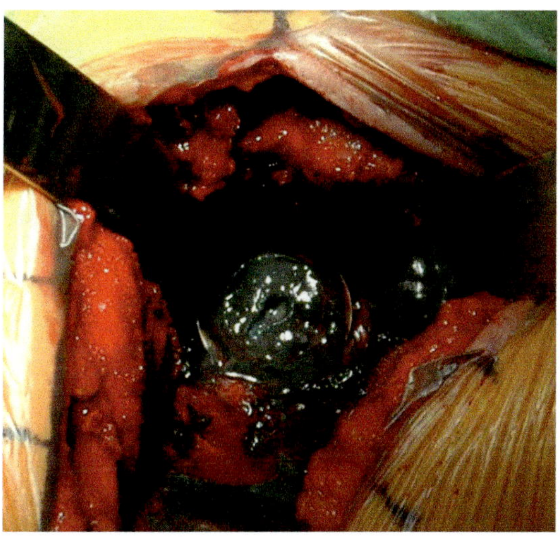

Fig. 19.21 Intraoperative image of the case in Fig. 19.20. Extensive metallosis was found with blackening of intra-articular tissues

cemented prosthesis may be necessary. In case of revision, if the humeral component removal is required, a cemented stem will create more bone loss than can be expected for a press-fit humeral component [93] (Fig. 19.22a, b).

At the level of the epiphysis, it is possible to place an epiphyseal component with or without offset. An eccentric component allows to center the reverse epiphysis in the middle of the humeral head osteotomy, preserving the anterior cortical bone of the humerus. Positioning the humeral tray with posterior offset offers a biomechanical advantage by increasing the internal rotational moment arm of the subscapularis, without creating inferior impingement [94, 95]. However, Onstot et al. observed that a posterior offset reverse shoulder was to have more impingement than the non-offset design. The authors suggested that a posterior-superior offset RSA design may provide better teres minor function and rotational strength and may decrease the incidence of acromial stress fractures relative to the non-offset design [96].

19.6 Conclusions

RSA design has changed considerably as a result of increased understanding of the biomechanics of the prosthesis. Implants have evolved in order to limit the rate of all complications reported in early designs.

The original monoblock Grammont design has changed in new modular implants, with numerous variable components and the possibility to convert an anatomic implant in a reverse one.

Surgeons experience plays a significant role in decreasing perioperative and postoperative problems, along with careful selection of the ideal implant for all the evolving applications. In this scenario, computerized planning software and patient-specific instruments could help the surgeons in the next future. Investigations into computer planning for RSA are in the early stages. Stubing et al. reported in a cadaveric study that glenoid baseplate positioning in the axial plane was improved by the use of three-dimensional navigation, with a mean deviation of 1.6° in the navigated procedure and 11.5° using conventional methods. However, they did not find a significant difference in the coronal plane [97]. Similarly in a cadaveric study, Venne et al. showed that computer planning and navigation allowed improved accuracy and precision of screw and baseplate placement [98].

One of the main challenges currently with three-dimensional planning or templating for RSA is understanding how conventional two-dimensional

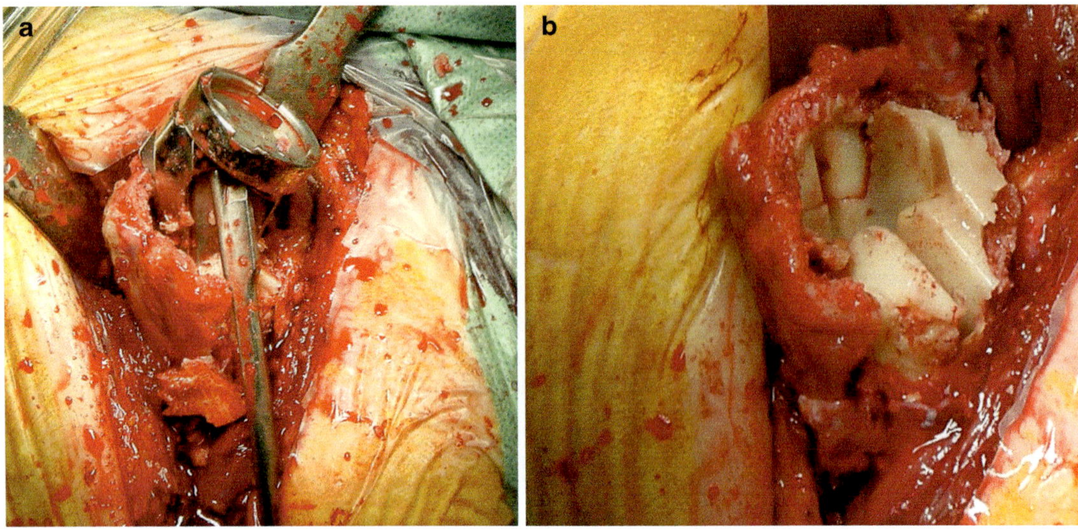

Fig. 19.22 Revision arthroplasty. (**a**) Removal of a well-fixed cemented humeral stem. (**b**) Loose cement has to be removed, and the canal has to be opened with a significant metaphyseal bone loss

measurements correlate with three-dimensional measurements. The development of three-dimensional imaging techniques and computerized planning for shoulder arthroplasty helps surgeons with planning for surgery; however, the development of patient-specific instrumentation has been introduced to optimize surgical procedure.

In RSA, the evidence for patient-specific instrumentation is limited to cadaveric anatomic studies. Levy et al. used patient-specific guides in 15 cadaveric shoulders for glenoid baseplate placement and found them to be very accurate at reproducing a three-dimensional preoperative plan. However, they did not compare this to standard instrumentation [99]. Throckmorton et al. randomized cadaver shoulders to standard versus patient-specific guides and found no significant difference in guide pin position between the groups [100].

Currently, there are several companies that provide tools for preoperatively planning and then create patient-specific instrumentation to direct implantation. Most systems require a CT scan of certain specifications to be performed, and then three-dimensional reconstruction can be rendered for planning.

Despite the theoretical benefits of improved accuracy of implant placement, clinical data supporting improved patient-reported outcomes and implant survivorship over the long term are lacking. Further study is needed to confirm cost-benefit analysis and to determine whether this technology should be widely adopted or whether it should be reserved for selected patients with major severe deformity.

In conclusion, in both the planning and execution phase of the process, the role of the surgeon remains crucial and cannot be replaced by technology. Preoperative planning using computer software requires surgical experience that cannot be outsourced. The intraoperative execution using patient-specific instruments cannot completely control the variability, and the surgeon's intuition remains cardinal in the preparation and final component implantation.

References

1. Grammont P, Trouilloud P, Laffay JP, Deries X. Etude et realisation d'une nouvelle prothese d'epaule. Rhumatologie. 1987;39(10):407–18.
2. Buechel FF, Pappas MJ, DePalma AF. "Floating-socket" total shoulder replacement: anatomical, biomechanical, and surgical rationale. J Biomed Mater Res. 1978;12(1):89–114.
3. Fenlin JM Jr. Total glenohumeral joint replacement. Orthop Clin North Am. 1975;6(2):565–83.

4. Reeves B, Jobbins B, Flowers F, Dowson D, Wright V. Some problems in the development of a total shoulder endo-prosthesis. Ann Rheum Dis. 1972;31(5):425–6.
5. Laurence M. Replacement arthroplasty of the rotator cuff deficient shoulder. J Bone Joint Surg Br. 1991;73(6):916–9.
6. Kessel L, Bayley I. Prosthetic replacement of shoulder joint: preliminary communication. J R Soc Med. 1979;72(10):748–52.
7. Ahir SP, Walker PS, Squire-Taylor CJ, Blunn GW, Bayley JI. Analysis of glenoid fixation for a reversed anatomy fixed-fulcrum shoulder replacement. J Biomech. 2004;37(11):1699–708.
8. Grammont PM, Baulot E. The classic: Delta shoulder prosthesis for rotator cuff rupture. 1993. Clin Orthop Relat Res. 2011;469(9):2424. https://doi.org/10.1007/s11999-011-1960-5.
9. Boileau P, Watkinson DJ, Hatzidakis AM, Balg F. Grammont reverse prosthesis: design, rationale, and biomechanics. J Shoulder Elb Surg. 2005;14(1 Suppl S):147S–61S.
10. Roche C, Flurin PH, Wright T, Crosby LA, Mauldin M, Zuckerman JD. An evaluation of the relationships between reverse shoulder design parameters and range of motion, impingement, and stability. J Shoulder Elb Surg. 2009;18(5):734–41. https://doi.org/10.1016/j.jse.2008.12.008.
11. Boileau P, Watkinson D, Hatzidakis AM, Hovorka I. Neer award 2005: the Grammont reverse shoulder prosthesis: results in cuff tear arthritis, fracture sequelae, and revision arthroplasty. J Shoulder Elb Surg. 2005;15(5):527–40.
12. Sirveaux F, Favard L, Oudet D, Huquet D, Walch G, Molé D. Grammont inverted total shoulder arthroplasty in the treatment of glenohumeral osteoarthritis with massive rupture of the cuff. Results of a multicentre study of 80 shoulders. J Bone Joint Surg Br. 2004;86(3):388–95.
13. Guery J, Favard L, Sirveaux F, Oudet D, Molé D, Walch G. Reverse total shoulder arthroplasty. Survivorship analysis of eighty replacements followed for five to ten years. J Bone Joint Surg Am. 2006;88(8):1742–7.
14. Zumstein MA, Pinedo M, Old J, Boileau P. Problems, complications, reoperations, and revisions in reverse total shoulder arthroplasty: a systematic review. J Shoulder Elb Surg. 2011;20(1):146–57. https://doi.org/10.1016/j.jse.2010.08.001.
15. Middernacht B, Van Tongel A, De Wilde L. A critical review on prosthetic features available for reversed total shoulder arthroplasty. Biomed Res Int. 2016;2016:3256931. https://doi.org/10.1155/2016/3256931.
16. Sachinis NP, Athanasiadou P. Current designs and trends in reverse shoulder arthroplasty. OA Orthopaedics. 2013;1(3):24–31.
17. Frankle MA, Teramoto A, Luo ZP, Levy JC, Pupello D. Glenoid morphology in reverse shoulder arthroplasty: classification and surgical implications. J Shoulder Elb Surg. 2009;18(6):874–85. https://doi.org/10.1016/j.jse.2009.02.013.
18. Chae SW, Kim SY, Lee H, Yon JR, Lee J, Han SH. Effect of baseplate size on primary glenoid stability and impingement-free range of motion in reverse shoulder arthroplasty. BMC Musculoskelet Disord. 2014;15:417. https://doi.org/10.1186/1471-2474-15-417.
19. Athwal S, Faber KJ. Outcomes of reverse shoulder arthroplasty using a mini 25-mm glenoid baseplate. Int Orthop. 2016;40(1):109–13. https://doi.org/10.1007/s00264-015-2945-x.
20. Roche CP, Stroud NJ, Flurin PH, Wright TW, Zuckerman JD, DiPaola MJ. Reverse shoulder glenoid baseplate fixation: a comparison of flat-back versus curved-back designs and oval versus circular designs with 2 different offset glenospheres. J Shoulder Elb Surg. 2014;23(9):1388–94. https://doi.org/10.1016/j.jse.2014.01.050.
21. Middernacht B, De Roo PJ, Van Maele G, De Wilde LF. Consequences of scapular anatomy for reversed total shoulder arthroplasty. Clin Orthop Relat Res. 2008;466(6):1410–8. https://doi.org/10.1007/s11999-008-0187-6.
22. Middernacht B, De Wilde L, Molé L, Favard L, Debeer P. Glenosphere disengagement: a potentially serious default in reverse shoulder surgery. Clin Orthop Relat Res. 2008;466(4):892–8. https://doi.org/10.1007/s11999-007-0090-6.
23. Trouilloud P, Gonzalvez M, Martz P, Charles H, Handelberg F, Nyffeler RW, Baulot E, Duocentric® Group. Duocentric reversed shoulder prosthesis and personal fit templates: innovative strategies to optimize prosthesis positioning and prevent scapular notching. Eur J Orthop Surg Traumatol. 2014;24(4):483–95. https://doi.org/10.1007/s00590-013-1213-2.
24. Checroun AJ, Hawkins C, Kummer FJ, Zuckerman JD. Fit of current glenoid component designs: an anatomic cadaver study. J Shoulder Elb Surg. 2002;11(6):614–7. https://doi.org/10.1067/mse.2002.126099.
25. Szabo I, Buscayret F, Edwards TB, Nemoz C, Boileau P, Walch G. Radiographic comparison of flat-back and convex-back glenoid components in total shoulder arthroplasty. J Shoulder Elb Surg. 2005;14(6):636–42. https://doi.org/10.1016/j.jse.2005.05.004.
26. Karelse A, Leuridan S, Van Tongel A, Piepers IM, Debeer P, De Wilde LF. A glenoid reaming study: how accurate are current reaming techniques? J Shoulder Elb Surg. 2014;23(8):1120–7. https://doi.org/10.1016/j.jse.2013.11.023.
27. Walch G, Badet R, Boulahia A, Khoury A. Morphologic study of the glenoid in primary glenohumeral osteoarthritis. J Arthroplast. 1999;14(6):756–60.
28. Bercik MJ, Kruse K 2nd, Yalizis M, Gauci MO, Chaoui J, Walch G. A modification to the Walch classification of the glenoid in primary glenohumeral

osteoarthritis using three-dimensional imaging. J Shoulder Elb Surg. 2016;25(10):1601–6. https://doi.org/10.1016/j.jse.2016.03.010.
29. Sutton LG, Werner FW, Jones AK, Close CA, Nanavati VN. Optimization of glenoid fixation in reverse shoulder arthroplasty using 3-dimensional modeling. J Shoulder Elb Surg. 2010;19(5):664–9. https://doi.org/10.1016/j.jse.2009.12.003.
30. Parsons BO, Gruson KI, Accousti KJ, Klug RA, Flatow EL. Optimal rotation and screw positioning for initial glenosphere baseplate fixation in reverse shoulder arthroplasty. J Shoulder Elb Surg. 2009;18(6):886–91. https://doi.org/10.1016/j.jse.2008.11.002.
31. James J, Allison MA, Werner FW, McBride DE, Basu NN, Sutton LG, Nanavati VN. Reverse shoulder arthroplasty glenoid fixation: is there a benefit in using four instead of two screws? J Shoulder Elb Surg. 2013;22(8):1030–6. https://doi.org/10.1016/j.jse.2012.11.006.
32. Königshausen M, Jettkant B, Sverdlova N, Ehlert C, Gessmann J, Schildhauer TA, Seybold D. Influence of different peg length in glenoid bone loss: a biomechanical analysis regarding primary stability of the glenoid baseplate in reverse shoulder arthroplasty. Technol Health Care. 2015;23(6):855–69. https://doi.org/10.3233/THC-151031.
33. Frankle M, Siegal S, Pupello D, Saleem A, Mighell M, Vasey M. The reverse shoulder prosthesis for glenohumeral arthritis associated with severe rotator cuff deficiency: a minimum two-year follow-up study of sixty patients. J Bone Joint Surg Am. 2005;87(8):1697–705.
34. Streit JJ, Shishani Y, Gobezie R. Medialized versus lateralized center of rotation in reverse shoulder arthroplasty. Orthopedics. 2015;38(12):e1098–103. https://doi.org/10.3928/01477447-20151120-06.
35. Valenti P, Sauzières P, Katz D, Kalouche I, Kilinc AS. Do less medialized reverse shoulder prostheses increase motion and reduce notching? Clin Orthop Relat Res. 2011;469(9):2550–7. https://doi.org/10.1007/s11999-011-1844-8.
36. Gutiérrez S, Walker M, Willis M, Pupello DR, Frankle MA. Effects of tilt and glenosphere eccentricity on baseplate/bone interface forces in a computational model, validated by a mechanical model, of reverse shoulder arthroplasty. J Shoulder Elb Surg. 2011;20(5):732–9. https://doi.org/10.1016/j.jse.2010.10.035.
37. Nerot C, Ohl X. Primary shoulder reverse arthroplasty: surgical technique. Orthop Traumatol Surg Res. 2014;100(1 Suppl):S181–90. https://doi.org/10.1016/j.otsr.2013.06.011.
38. Gilot GJ. Addressing glenoid erosion in reverse total shoulder arthroplasty. Bull Hosp Jt Dis (2013). 2013;71(Suppl 2):S51–3. Review.
39. Lévigne C, Boileau P, Favard L, Garaud P, Molé D, Sirveaux F, Walch G. Scapular notching in reverse shoulder arthroplasty. J Shoulder Elb Surg. 2008;17(6):925–35. https://doi.org/10.1016/j.jse.2008.02.010.
40. Greiner S, Schmidt C, König C, Perka C, Herrmann S. Lateralized reverse shoulder arthroplasty maintains rotational function of the remaining rotator cuff. Clin Orthop Relat Res. 2013;471(3):940–6. https://doi.org/10.1007/s11999-012-2692-x.
41. Giles JW, Langohr GD, Johnson JA, Athwal GS. Implant design variations in reverse total shoulder arthroplasty influence the required deltoid force and resultant joint load. Clin Orthop Relat Res. 2015;473(11):3615–26. https://doi.org/10.1007/s11999-015-4526-0.
42. Hoenecke HR Jr, Flores-Hernandez C, D'Lima DD. Reverse total shoulder arthroplasty component center of rotation affects muscle function. J Shoulder Elb Surg. 2014;23(8):1128–35. https://doi.org/10.1016/j.jse.2013.11.025.
43. Werner BS, Chaoui J, Walch G. The influence of humeral neck shaft angle and glenoid lateralization on range of motion in reverse shoulder arthroplasty. J Shoulder Elb Surg. 2017;26(10):1726–31. https://doi.org/10.1016/j.jse.2017.03.032.
44. Lawrence C, Williams GR, Namdari S. Influence of glenosphere design on outcomes and complications of reverse arthroplasty: a systematic review. Clin Orthop Surg. 2016;8(3):288–97. https://doi.org/10.4055/cios.2016.8.3.288.
45. Poon PC, Chou J, Young SW, Astley T. A comparison of concentric and eccentric glenospheres in reverse shoulder arthroplasty: a randomized controlled trial. J Bone Joint Surg Am. 2014;96(16):e138. https://doi.org/10.2106/JBJS.M.00941.
46. Chou J, Malak SF, Anderson IA, Astley T, Poon PC. Biomechanical evaluation of different designs of glenospheres in the SMR reverse total shoulder prosthesis: range of motion and risk of scapular notching. J Shoulder Elb Surg. 2009;18(3):354–9. https://doi.org/10.1016/j.jse.2009.01.015.
47. Yang CC, Lu CL, Wu CH, Wu JJ, Huang TL, Chen R, Yeh MK. Stress analysis of glenoid component in design of reverse shoulder prosthesis using finite element method. J Shoulder Elb Surg. 2013;22(7):932–9. https://doi.org/10.1016/j.jse.2012.09.001.
48. Lädermann A, Lubbeke A, Melis B, Stern R, Christofilopoulos P, Bacle G, Walch G. Prevalence of neurologic lesions after total shoulder arthroplasty. J Bone Joint Surg Am. 2011;93(14):1288–93. https://doi.org/10.2106/JBJS.J.00369.
49. Lädermann A, Stimec BV, Denard PJ, Cunningham G, Collin P, Fasel JH. Injury to the axillary nerve after reverse shoulder arthroplasty: an anatomical study. Orthop Traumatol Surg Res. 2014;100(1):105–8. https://doi.org/10.1016/j.otsr.2013.09.006.
50. Berhouet J, Garaud P, Favard L. Evaluation of the role of glenosphere design and humeral component retroversion in avoiding scapular notching during reverse shoulder arthroplasty. J Shoulder Elb Surg. 2014;23(2):151–8. https://doi.org/10.1016/j.jse.2013.05.009.
51. Langohr GD, Giles JW, Athwal GS, Johnson JA. The effect of glenosphere diameter in reverse shoulder

arthroplasty on muscle force, joint load, and range of motion. J Shoulder Elb Surg. 2015;24(6):972–9. https://doi.org/10.1016/j.jse.2014.10.018.
52. Müller AM, Born M, Jung C, Flury M, Kolling C, Schwyzer HK, Audigé L. Glenosphere size in reverse shoulder arthroplasty: is larger better for external rotation and abduction strength? J Shoulder Elb Surg. 2018;27:44–52. https://doi.org/10.1016/j.jse.2017.06.002. [Epub ahead of print].
53. Gerber C, Pennington SD, Nyffeler RW. Reverse total shoulder arthroplasty. J Am Acad Orthop Surg. 2009;17(5):284–95.
54. Lévigne C, Garret J, Boileau P, Alami G, Favard L, Walch G. Scapular notching in reverse shoulder arthroplasty: is it important to avoid it and how? Clin Orthop Relat Res. 2011;469(9):2512–20. https://doi.org/10.1007/s11999-010-1695-8.
55. Nyffeler RW, Werner CM, Gerber C. Biomechanical relevance of glenoid component positioning in the reverse Delta III total shoulder prosthesis. J Shoulder Elb Surg. 2005;14(5):524–8.
56. Gutiérrez S, Levy JC, Frankle MA, Cuff D, Keller TS, Pupello DR, Lee WE 3rd. Evaluation of abduction range of motion and avoidance of inferior scapular impingement in a reverse shoulder model. J Shoulder Elb Surg. 2008;17(4):608–15. https://doi.org/10.1016/j.jse.2007.11.010.
57. Simovitch RW, Zumstein MA, Lohri E, Helmy N, Gerber C. Predictors of scapular notching in patients managed with the Delta III reverse total shoulder replacement. J Bone Joint Surg Am. 2007;89(3):588–600.
58. Fuller CB, Gregorius SF, Lim EK. Glenosphere disengagement in a reverse total shoulder arthroplasty with a non-Morse taper design. Int Orthop. 2015;39(2):305–8. https://doi.org/10.1007/s00264-014-2653-y.
59. Vaupel ZM, Baker KC, Kurdziel MD, Wiater JM. Wear simulation of reverse total shoulder arthroplasty systems: effect of glenosphere design. J Shoulder Elb Surg. 2012;21(10):1422–9. https://doi.org/10.1016/j.jse.2011.10.024.
60. Kohut G, Dallmann F, Irlenbusch U. Wear-induced loss of mass in reversed total shoulder arthroplasty with conventional and inverted bearing materials. J Biomech. 2012;45(3):469–73. https://doi.org/10.1016/j.jbiomech.2011.11.055.
61. Irlenbusch U, Kääb MJ, Kohut G, Proust J, Reuther F, Joudet T. Reversed shoulder arthroplasty with inversed bearing materials: 2-year clinical and radiographic results in 101 patients. Arch Orthop Trauma Surg. 2015;135(2):161–9. https://doi.org/10.1007/s00402-014-2135-0.
62. Ackland DC, Patel M, Knox D. Prosthesis design and placement in reverse total shoulder arthroplasty. J Orthop Surg Res. 2015;10:101. https://doi.org/10.1186/s13018-015-0244-2.
63. Gutiérrez S, Luo ZP, Levy J, Frankle MA. Arc of motion and socket depth in reverse shoulder implants. Clin Biomech (Bristol, Avon). 2009;24(6):473–9. https://doi.org/10.1016/j.clinbiomech.2009.02.008.
64. De Wilde LF, Poncet D, Middernacht B, Ekelund A. Prosthetic overhang is the most effective way to prevent scapular conflict in a reverse total shoulder prosthesis. Acta Orthop. 2010;81(6):719–26. https://doi.org/10.3109/17453674.2010.538354.
65. Gutiérrez S, Keller TS, Levy JC, Lee WE 3rd, Luo ZP. Hierarchy of stability factors in reverse shoulder arthroplasty. Clin Orthop Relat Res. 2008;466(3):670–6. https://doi.org/10.1007/s11999-007-0096-0.
66. Gutiérrez S, Comiskey CA 4th, Luo ZP, Pupello DR, Frankle MA. Range of impingement-free abduction and adduction deficit after reverse shoulder arthroplasty. Hierarchy of surgical and implant-design-related factors. J Bone Joint Surg Am. 2008;90(12):2606–15. https://doi.org/10.2106/JBJS.H.00012.
67. Day JS, MacDonald DW, Olsen M, Getz C, Williams GR, Kurtz SM. Polyethylene wear in retrieved reverse total shoulder components. J Shoulder Elb Surg. 2012;21(5):667–74. https://doi.org/10.1016/j.jse.2011.03.012.
68. Lädermann A, Gueorguiev B, Charbonnier C, Stimec BV, Fasel JH, Zderic I, Hagen J, Walch G. Scapular notching on kinematic simulated range of motion after reverse shoulder arthroplasty is not the result of impingement in adduction. Medicine (Baltimore). 2015;94(38):e1615. https://doi.org/10.1097/MD.0000000000001615.
69. Keener JD, Chalmers PN, Yamaguchi K. The humeral implant in shoulder arthroplasty. J Am Acad Orthop Surg. 2017;25(6):427–38. https://doi.org/10.5435/JAAOS-D-15-00682.
70. Jeon BK, Panchal KA, Ji JH, Xin YZ, Park SR, Kim JH, Yang SJ. Combined effect of change in humeral neck-shaft angle and retroversion on shoulder range of motion in reverse total shoulder arthroplasty—a simulation study. Clin Biomech (Bristol, Avon). 2016;31:12–9. https://doi.org/10.1016/j.clinbiomech.2015.06.022.
71. Lädermann A, Denard PJ, Boileau P, Farron A, Deransart P, Terrier A, Ston J, Walch G. Effect of humeral stem design on humeral position and range of motion in reverse shoulder arthroplasty. Int Orthop. 2015;39(11):2205–13. https://doi.org/10.1007/s00264-015-2984-3.
72. Oh JH, Shin SJ, McGarry MH, Scott JH, Heckmann N, Lee TQ. Biomechanical effects of humeral neck-shaft angle and subscapularis integrity in reverse total shoulder arthroplasty. J Shoulder Elb Surg. 2014;23(8):1091–8. https://doi.org/10.1016/j.jse.2013.11.003.
73. Wright TW. Revision of humeral components in shoulder arthroplasty. Bull Hosp Jt Dis (2013). 2013;71(Suppl 2):77–81.
74. Wieser K, Borbas P, Ek ET, Meyer DC, Gerber C. Conversion of stemmed hemi- or total to reverse total shoulder arthroplasty: advantages of a modular stem design. Clin Orthop Relat Res. 2015;473(2):651–60. https://doi.org/10.1007/s11999-014-3985-z.

75. Werner BC, Dines JS, Dines DM. Platform systems in shoulder arthroplasty. Curr Rev Musculoskelet Med. 2016;9(1):49–53. https://doi.org/10.1007/s12178-016-9317-z.
76. Crosby LA, Wright TW, Yu S, Zuckerman JD. Conversion to reverse total shoulder arthroplasty with and without humeral stem retention: the role of a convertible-platform stem. J Bone Joint Surg Am. 2017;99(9):736–42. https://doi.org/10.2106/JBJS.16.00683.
77. Kirsch JM, Khan M, Thornley P, Gichuru M, Freehill MT, Neviaser A, Moravek J, Miller BS, Bedi A. Platform shoulder arthroplasty: a systematic review. J Shoulder Elb Surg. 2018;27:756–63. https://doi.org/10.1016/j.jse.2017.08.020. [Epub ahead of print].
78. Edwards TB, Morris BJ, Hodorek B. Tornier Aequalis Ascend™ Flex Convertible Shoulder System. In: Frankle M, et al., editors. Reverse shoulder arthroplasty. Cham: Springer International Publishing; 2016. p. 441–8. https://doi.org/10.1007/978-3-319-20840-4_44.
79. Kadum B, Mafi N, Norberg S, Sayed-Noor AS. Results of the total evolutive shoulder system (TESS): a single-centre study of 56 consecutive patients. Arch Orthop Trauma Surg. 2011;131(12):1623–9. https://doi.org/10.1007/s00402-011-1368-4.
80. Giuseffi SA, Streubel P, Sperling J, Sanchez-Sotelo J. Short-stem uncemented primary reverse shoulder arthroplasty: clinical and radiological outcomes. Bone Joint J. 2014;96-B(4):526–9. https://doi.org/10.1302/0301-620X.96B3.32702.
81. Atoun E, Van Tongel A, Hous N, Narvani A, Relwani J, Abraham R, Levy O. Reverse shoulder arthroplasty with a short metaphyseal humeral stem. Int Orthop. 2014;38(6):1213–8. https://doi.org/10.1007/s00264-014-2328-8.
82. Levy O, Narvani A, Hous N, Abraham R, Relwani J, Pradhan R, Bruguera J, Sforza G, Atoun E. Reverse shoulder arthroplasty with a cementless short metaphyseal humeral implant without a stem: clinical and radiologic outcomes in prospective 2- to 7-year follow-up study. J Shoulder Elb Surg. 2016;25(8):1362–70. https://doi.org/10.1016/j.jse.2015.12.017.
83. Moroder P, Ernstbrunner L, Zweiger C, Schatz M, Seitlinger G, Skursky R, Becker J, Resch H, Krifter RM. Short to mid-term results of stemless reverse shoulder arthroplasty in a selected patient population compared to a matched control group with stem. Int Orthop. 2016;40(10):2115–20.
84. Schnetzke M, Preis A, Coda S, Raiss P, Loew M. Anatomical and reverse shoulder replacement with a convertible, uncemented short-stem shoulder prosthesis: first clinical and radiological results. Arch Orthop Trauma Surg. 2017;137(5):679–84. https://doi.org/10.1007/s00402-017-2673-3.
85. Wagner ER, Statz JM, Houdek MT, Cofield RH, Sánchez-Sotelo J, Sperling JW. Use of a shorter humeral stem in revision reverse shoulder arthroplasty. J Shoulder Elb Surg. 2017;26(8):1454–61. https://doi.org/10.1016/j.jse.2017.01.016.
86. Reuther F, Kohut G, Nijs S. Newly developed modular reverse fracture endoprosthesis in non-reconstructable humeral head fracture in old people. Oper Orthop Traumatol. 2014;26(4):369–82.; ; quiz 382–4. https://doi.org/10.1007/s00064-013-0250-7.
87. Garofalo R, Flanagin B, Castagna A, Lo EY, Krishnan SG. Reverse shoulder arthroplasty for proximal humerus fracture using a dedicated stem: radiological outcomes at a minimum 2 years of follow-up-case series. J Orthop Surg Res. 2015;10:129. https://doi.org/10.1186/s13018-015-0261-1.
88. Szerlip BW, Morris BJ, Edwards TB. Reverse shoulder arthroplasty for trauma: when, where, and how. Instr Course Lect. 2016;65:171–9.
89. Grubhofer F, Wieser K, Meyer DC, Catanzaro S, Beeler S, Riede U, Gerber C. Reverse total shoulder arthroplasty for acute head-splitting, 3- and 4-part fractures of the proximal humerus in the elderly. J Shoulder Elb Surg. 2016;25(10):1690–8. https://doi.org/10.1016/j.jse.2016.02.024.
90. Gigis I, Nenopoulos A, Giannekas D, Heikenfeld R, Beslikas T, Hatzokos I. Reverse shoulder arthroplasty for the treatment of 3 and 4-part fractures of the humeral head in the elderly. Open Orthop J. 2017;11:108–18. https://doi.org/10.2174/1874325001711010108.
91. King JJ, Farmer KW, Struk AM, Wright TW. Uncemented versus cemented humeral stem fixation in reverse shoulder arthroplasty. Int Orthop. 2015;39(2):291–8. https://doi.org/10.1007/s00264-014-2593-6.
92. Raiss P, Edwards TB, Deutsch A, Shah A, Bruckner T, Loew M, Boileau P, Walch G. Radiographic changes around humeral components in shoulder arthroplasty. J Bone Joint Surg Am. 2014;96(7):e54. https://doi.org/10.2106/JBJS.M.00378.
93. Zavala JA, Clark JC, Kissenberth MJ, Tolan SJ, Hawkins RJ. Management of deep infection after reverse total shoulder arthroplasty: a case series. J Shoulder Elb Surg. 2012;21(10):1310–5. https://doi.org/10.1016/j.jse.2011.08.047.
94. Berhouet J, Kontaxis A, Gulotta LV, Craig E, Warren R, Dines J, Dines D. Effects of the humeral tray component positioning for onlay reverse shoulder arthroplasty design: a biomechanical analysis. J Shoulder Elb Surg. 2015;24(4):569–77. https://doi.org/10.1016/j.jse.2014.09.022.
95. Roche CP, Hamilton MA, Diep P, Flurin PH, Routman HD. Design rationale for a posterior/superior offset reverse shoulder prosthesis. Bull Hosp Jt Dis (2013). 2013;71(Suppl 2):S18–2.
96. Onstot BR, Jacofsky MC, Hansen ML. Muscle force and excursion requirements and moment arm analysis of a posterior-superior offset reverse total shoulder prosthesis. Bull Hosp Jt Dis (2013). 2013;71(Suppl 2):S25–30.
97. Stübig T, Petri M, Zeckey C, Hawi N, Krettek C, Citak M, Meller R. 3D navigated implantation of

the glenoid component in reversed shoulder arthroplasty. Feasibility and results in an anatomic study. Int J Med Robot. 2013;9(4):480–5. https://doi.org/10.1002/rcs.1519.
98. Venne G, Rasquinha BJ, Pichora D, Ellis RE, Bicknell R. Comparing conventional and computer-assisted surgery baseplate and screw placement in reverse shoulder arthroplasty. J Shoulder Elb Surg. 2015;24(7):1112–9. https://doi.org/10.1016/j.jse.2014.10.012.
99. Levy JC, Everding NG, Frankle MA, Keppler LJ. Accuracy of patient-specific guided glenoid baseplate positioning for reverse shoulder arthroplasty. J Shoulder Elb Surg. 2014;23(10):1563–7. https://doi.org/10.1016/j.jse.2014.01.051.
100. Throckmorton TW, Gulotta LV, Bonnarens FO, Wright SA, Hartzell JL, Rozzi WB, Hurst JM, Frostick SP, Sperling JW. Patient-specific targeting guides compared with traditional instrumentation for glenoid component placement in shoulder arthroplasty: a multi-surgeon study in 70 arthritic cadaver specimens. J Shoulder Elb Surg. 2015;24(6):965–71. https://doi.org/10.1016/j.jse.2014.10.013.

Part V

Surgical Technique

Surgical Technique for Cuff Tear Arthropathy

20

Stefano Gumina, Kamal I. Bohsali, and Michael A. Wirth

Prior to surgical intervention, a thorough history and physical exam should be performed. Particular attention must be paid to previous or remote history of infection, prior shoulder surgery, and medical comorbidities which may contribute to a suboptimal outcome for the patient. The physical exam should focus on evaluation of the soft tissue envelope, integrity of the deltoid and teres minor, and coexisting cervical spine issues which may affect the ability to achieve pain relief and improved function after reverse shoulder arthroplasty. Appropriate imaging with plain radiographs and CT scan will allow for preoperative templating (Fig. 20.1a, b). Unless otherwise contraindicated, all anticoagulant and antiplatelet therapy should be discontinued at least 5–7 days prior to intervention. Glycemic control should be optimized to reduce the risk of postoperative infection. Perioperative IV antibiotics such as a first-generation cephalosporin or vancomycin (for patients allergic to penicillin) are administered within an hour of intervention.

The patient after induction is placed in the Semi-Fowler position on the operative table utilizing a commercially available beach chair positioner that permits unencumbered access to the shoulder (Fig. 20.2). The operative extremity is prepped and draped free for the intervention (Fig. 20.3).

A majority of surgeons utilize the delto-pectoral approach, though the European experience has demonstrated viability with the superior-lateral technique. Each approach has its proponents, opponents, advantages, and disadvantages. With regard to the superior-lateral approach, the subscapularis remains intact as the deltoid is split to gain access to the glenohumeral joint through a probable massive rotator cuff tear. Some reports have indicated reduced risk of anterior instability with this approach due to the intact subscapularis. Opponents cite difficulty with glenoid visualization, decreased postoperative external rotation, and an inability to address revision scenarios that require component extraction, tendon transfers, and bone grafting [1]. Our preference is the delto-pectoral approach, as this exposure may be extended for revision cases and allows for improved visualization of the glenoid and identification and safeguarding of the axillary nerve.

The skin incision begins from the inferior border of the clavicle and transverses over the cora-

S. Gumina (✉)
Department of Orthopaedics and Traumatology, Sapienza University of Rome, Rome, Italy
e-mail: stefano.gumina@uniroma1.it

K. I. Bohsali
BOSM, Jacksonville, FL, USA

M. A. Wirth
Orthopaedic Surgery, University of Texas HSC-San Antonio, San Antonio, TX, USA

S. Gumina et al. (eds.), *Reverse Shoulder Arthroplasty*,
https://doi.org/10.1007/978-3-319-97743-0_20

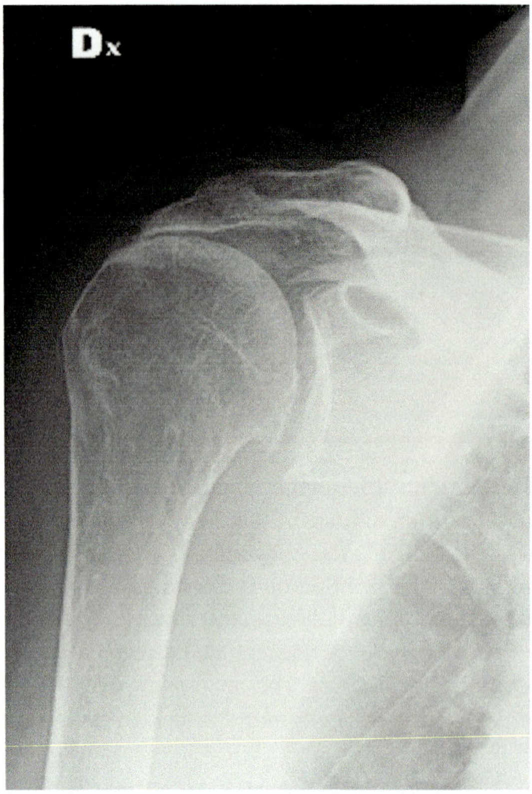

Fig. 20.1 (**a**, **b**) AP radiograph demonstrating stereotypical changes of rotator cuff arthropathy with proximal humeral head migration, femoralization of the humeral head, acetabularization of the acromion

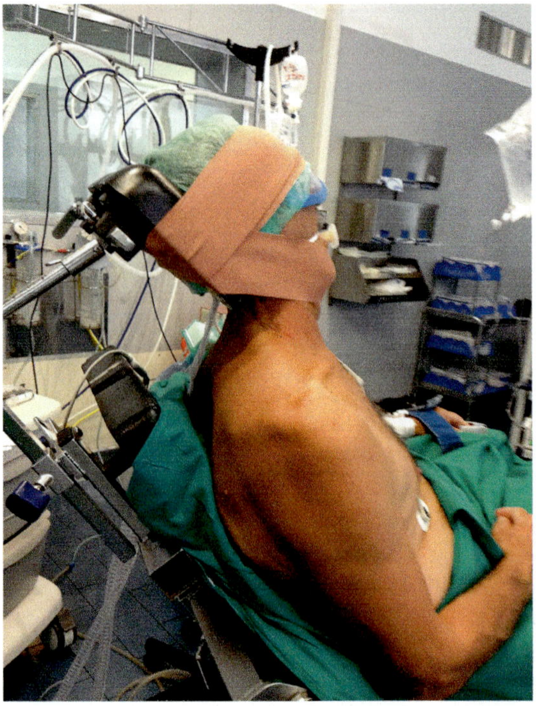

Fig. 20.2 A commercially available beach chair positioner allows for safe positioning of the neck and head, as well as facile access to the shoulder during shoulder arthroplasty

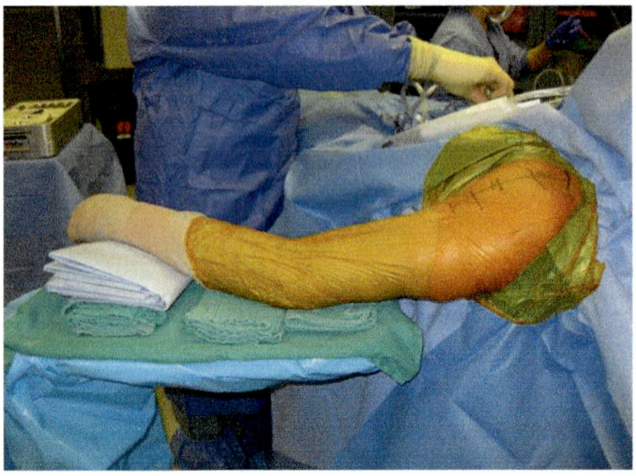

Fig. 20.3 The operative shoulder is draped free for the procedure. Surgical preference dictates whether a padded Mayo stand or commercially available arm positioner is utilized during the intervention

coid process and toward the deltoid insertion (Fig. 20.4). The subcutaneous tissue planes are elevated to identify the cephalic vein which is mobilized laterally in a majority of cases. Incise the clavipectoral fascia from the coracoacromial ligament to the superior border of the pectoralis major insertion (Fig. 20.5a, b). Humeroscapular interface will need to be released with careful blunt and sharp dissection. Adhesions posterior to the conjoint tendon should also be carefully released and the musculocutaneous nerve identified. Palpate the axillary nerve at the anterior-inferior border of the subscapularis. Intermittent reassessment of the nerve should be performed to confirm its integrity. The anterior humeral circumflex vessels should be ligated with electrocautery (Fig. 20.6).

The subscapularis is either tenotomized or "peeled" from the lesser tuberosity and later reapproximated or allowed to medialize without reattachment. Advocates of repair cite improved internal rotation and reduced incidence of anterior instability [2]. However, Mole and Favard in their multicenter study of 484 patients who had undergone reverse total shoulder arthroplasty did not demonstrate statistically different outcomes when comparing subscapularis repair versus tenotomy without repair [3]. Additionally, Clark and coauthors performed a retrospective cohort study of 120 patients, of which 55 underwent repair of the subscapularis during reverse total shoulder arthroplasty. They concluded that reattachment of the subscapularis did not have any positive effect on complication rate, dislocation rate, pain relief, and range of motion gains [4]. Despite these reports, we currently advocate primary repair of the subscapularis when technically feasible to reduce the potential risk of anterior instability and improve the potential for internal rotation.

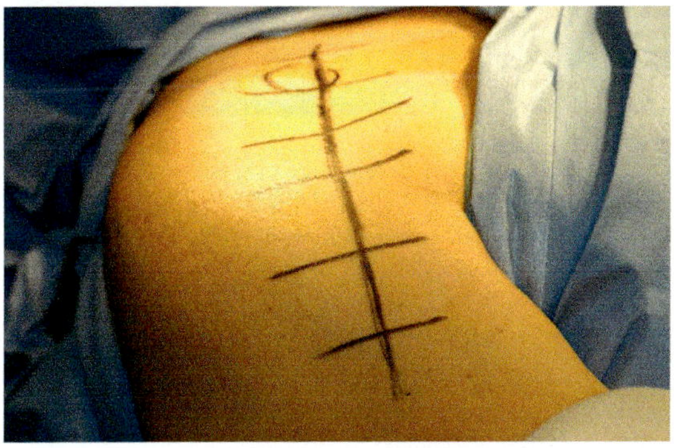

Fig. 20.4 Delto-pectoral approach: the skin incision begins from the inferior border of the clavicle and transverses over the coracoid process and toward the deltoid insertion

A Darrach retractor is placed inferiorly at the humeral insertion of the capsule. A fishtail elevator and knife are used to release the capsule to the 6 o'clock position. The humeral head should be easily dislocated with gentle extension and adduction of the arm (Fig. 20.7). With the shoulder dislocated, position the starting reamer at the most superior-lateral location, and create a pilot hole to gain intramedullary access to the humerus (Fig. 20.8).

The tendon of the long head of the biceps tendon is tenodesed adjacent to the pectoralis major tendon insertion.

The humeral head is generally osteotomized in neutral to slight retroversion to preserve internal rotation. More recent studies have suggested resecting the humeral head in native version for the patient to maximize active external rotation [5]. The humeral head resection is performed with

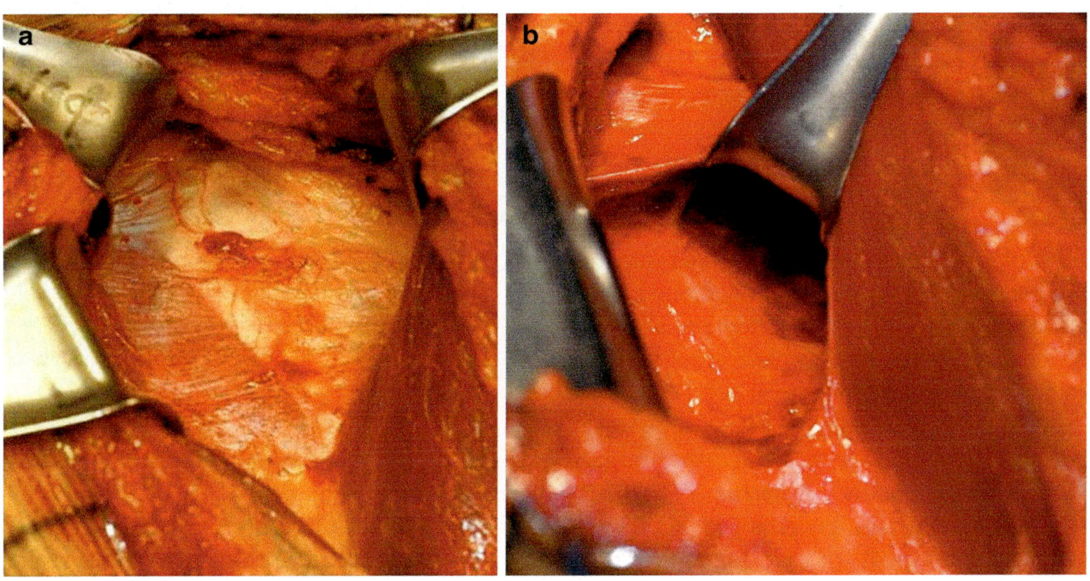

Fig. 20.5 (**a**, **b**) After identification of the cephalic vein, the deltoid muscle is mobilized laterally, allowing for visualization of the pectoralis major tendon insertion. At this point, the clavipectoral fascia is incised and the biceps tendon transected or tenodesed adjacent to the pectoralis major tendon insertion (**a**). The pectoralis major insertion may require partial release for exposure purposes screws (**b**)

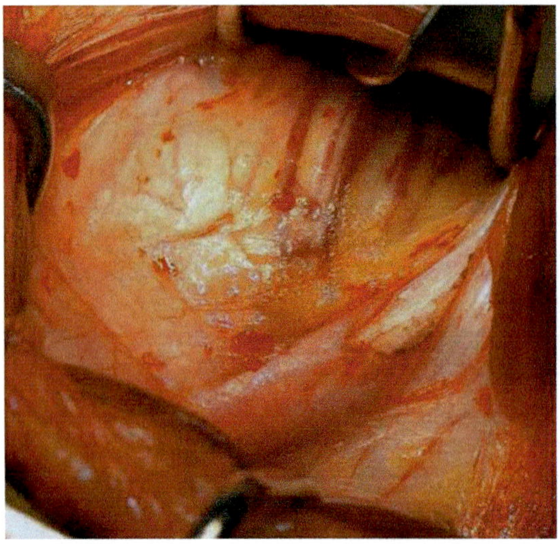

Fig. 20.6 Gentle digital or blunt dissection should occur posterior to the conjoint tendon taking care to identify and protect the musculocutaneous nerve. The anterior circumflex vessels are encountered and will need to be ligated or cauterized prior to release of the subscapularis. The axillary nerve should be routinely visualized and palpated prior to release of the subscapularis

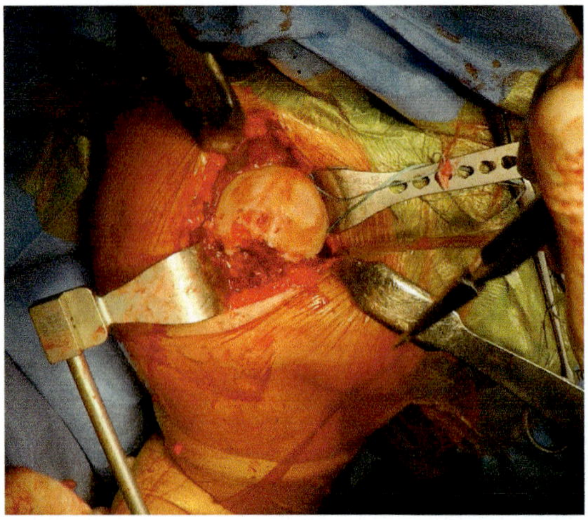

Fig. 20.7 Following release of the subscapularis and capsule, the humeral head should be readily dislocated with gentle extension and adduction of the arm screws

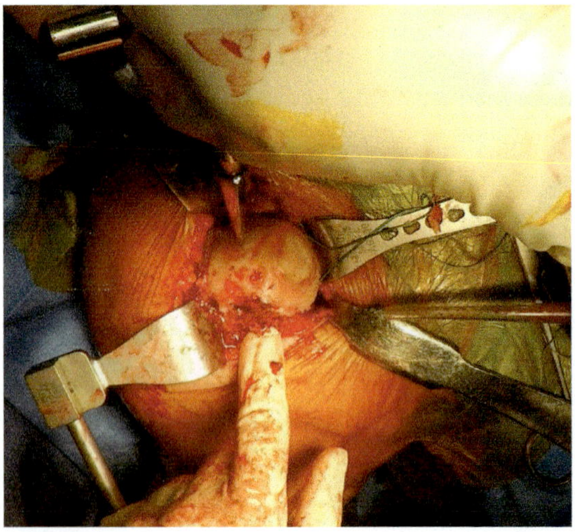

Fig. 20.8 With the shoulder dislocated, position the starting reamer at the most superior-lateral location, and create a pilot hole to gain intramedullary access to the humerus. Do not use power to ream the humeral canal to avoid iatrogenic injury

a sagittal saw (Fig. 20.9a–c). Neck-shaft inclination varies depending upon the implant system with Grammont-based implants reliant upon the 155° angle [6]. A metallic cover plate is then placed to protect the osteotomy site (Fig. 20.10).

Glenoid exposure is of paramount importance for proper positioning of the glenosphere. The remaining labrum and biceps tendon origin are excised sharply (Fig. 20.11). A 360° release of the subscapularis, if intact, is performed. The posterior, inferior, and superior capsule are released with careful attention paid to the location of the axillary nerve at all times. To adequately visualize the lateral pillar of the glenoid, the origin of the long head of the triceps tendon may be partially released. A forked retractor or modified Sonnabend is then utilized to displace the proximal humerus (Fig. 20.12). All osteophytes may be removed with small osteotomes or small rongeur. Metaglene position should be chosen to obtain adequate glenoid fixation while minimizing the risk of mechanical impingement. Careful attention must be paid to the native version of the glenoid and the amount of glenoid vault available for baseplate fixation. Some systems require placement of a central guidewire from which glenoid reaming is based. It is critical to avoid

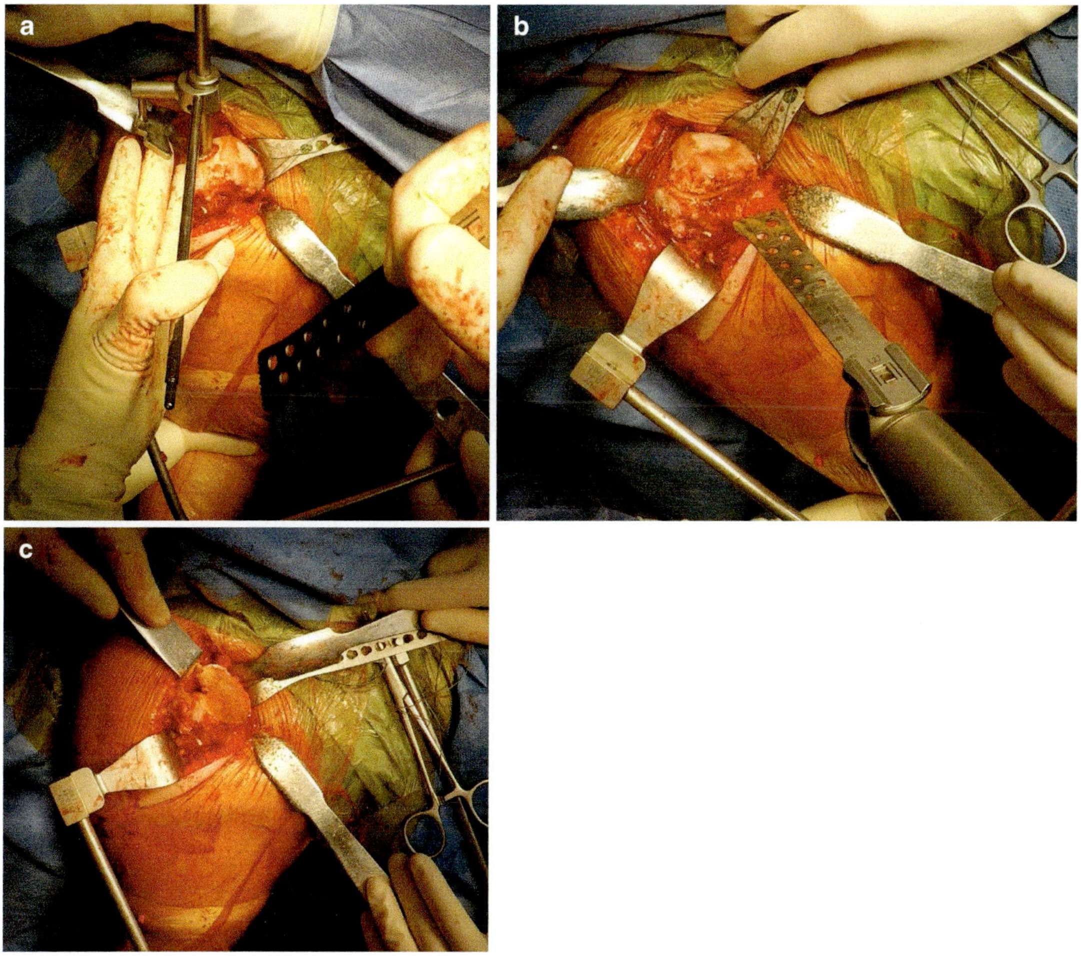

Fig. 20.9 The humeral head is osteotomized using an intramedullary guide in native version (**a**). The osteotomy is completed without the guide (**b**, **c**). We generally place the humeral component in neutral version to preserve internal rotation

excessive medialization, superior tilt, and version (anterior or posterior) of the glenoid during the reaming step. Some authors have advocated inferior tilt with baseplate positioning to reduce the incidence of scapular notching, whereas others have indicated minimal benefit with this technique and similar patient outcomes with or without inferior tilt of the glenoid component [7–10]. Most surgeons agree that the baseplate must be placed as inferior as possible on the glenoid face, but not beyond the glenoid rim, to minimize notching and to allow for improved adduction of the arm.

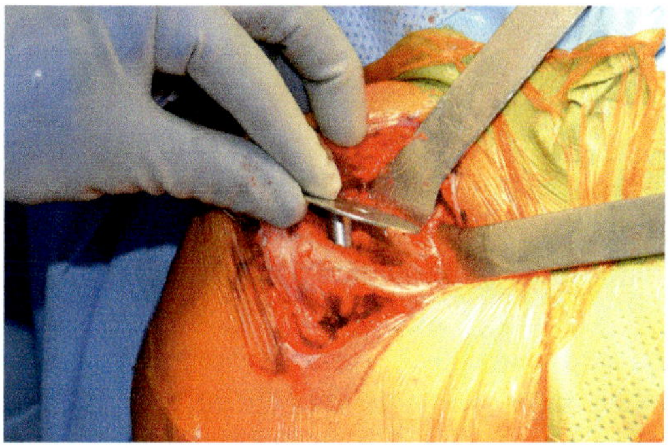

Fig. 20.10 A metallic cover plate is then placed to protect the osteotomy site

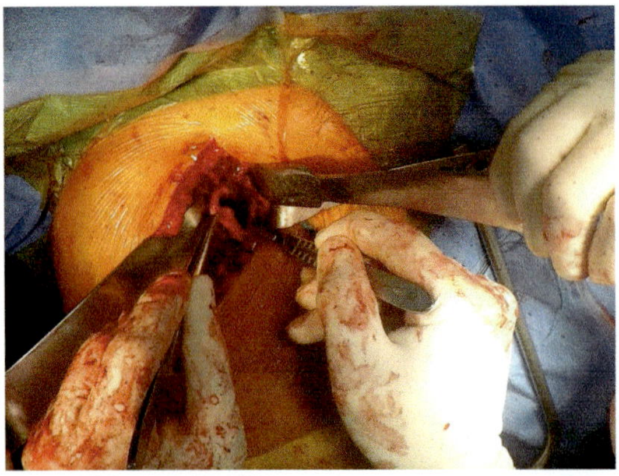

Fig. 20.11 The remaining labrum and biceps tendon origin are excised in order to achieve an adequate glenoid exposure

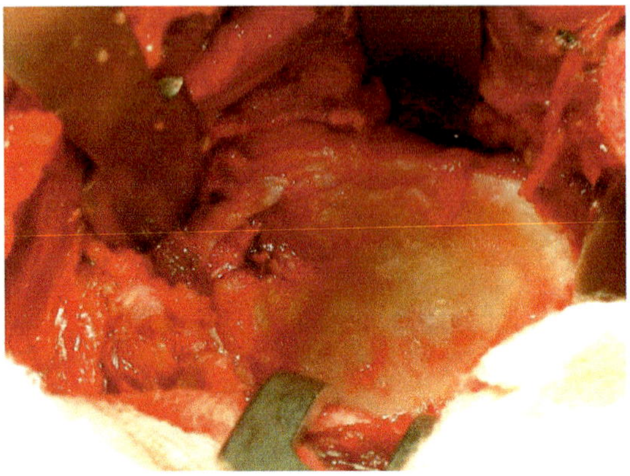

Fig. 20.12 Sequential capsular releases should afford an appropriate view of the glenoid face for metaglene and glenosphere placement. Common retractors include a forked retractor or modified Sonnabend, Hohmann, and anterior glenoid retractor

The metaglene central peg ought to be positioned posterior and inferior to the intersection of the glenoid axis. Particular attention should be given to pain to glenoid morphology on preoperative imaging studies, as metaglene position will need to be adjusted based upon adequacy and screw and postfixation. The metaglene positioner is placed flush with the inferior glenoid rim, and a guide pin is advanced perpendicular to the glenoid face. Avoid superior tilt of the pin placement which may result in suboptimal positioning of the metaglene and glenosphere (Fig. 20.13a, b). A two-step reaming process allows for appropriate preparation of the glenoid followed by a central cannulated drill bit to prepare for the metaglene post (Fig. 20.14a, b). Implant the final metaglene into position using autograft to address minor deficiencies in the glenoid surface. The metaglene rotation should be positioned to allow for inferior screw placement within the scapular neck and superior screw placement within the coracoid base [11] (Fig. 20.15a, b). We will generally place the final glenosphere which comes from 36–38 mm to 40–42 mm diameters and standard/eccentric sphericities (Fig. 20.16a, b). The 40 mm glenosphere provides improved range of motion and stability, but may not be feasible to use in patients with smaller glenoids.

Correct positioning of the glenoid component, however, can be challenging because of variable scapular anatomy and glenoid bone loss. Three-dimensional preoperative planning and patient-specific instrumentation have been introduced for shoulder arthroplasty to better deal with glenoid deformity and bone loss. Before surgery, patients undergo a preoperative thin-cut CT scan of the shoulder. The two-dimensional images in the digital imaging and communications in medicine format are loaded in a 3D image processing software system and are reformatted into accurate 3D models of the scapulae. The scapular plane is defined by three points: the glenoid center point, the scapula trigonum, and the inferior angle of the scapula. This patient-specific 3D model of the scapula is then uploaded into an interactive surgical planning software program, enabling the surgeon to virtually preoperatively plan the ideal position of the glenoid component. From this surgical plan, patient-specific polyamide guides were manufactured to intraoperatively control the position and orientation of the central glenoid guide pin. In addition to this glenoid guide, a patient-specific glenoid replica was also created to allow the surgeon to visualize the optimal guide position during the surgery.

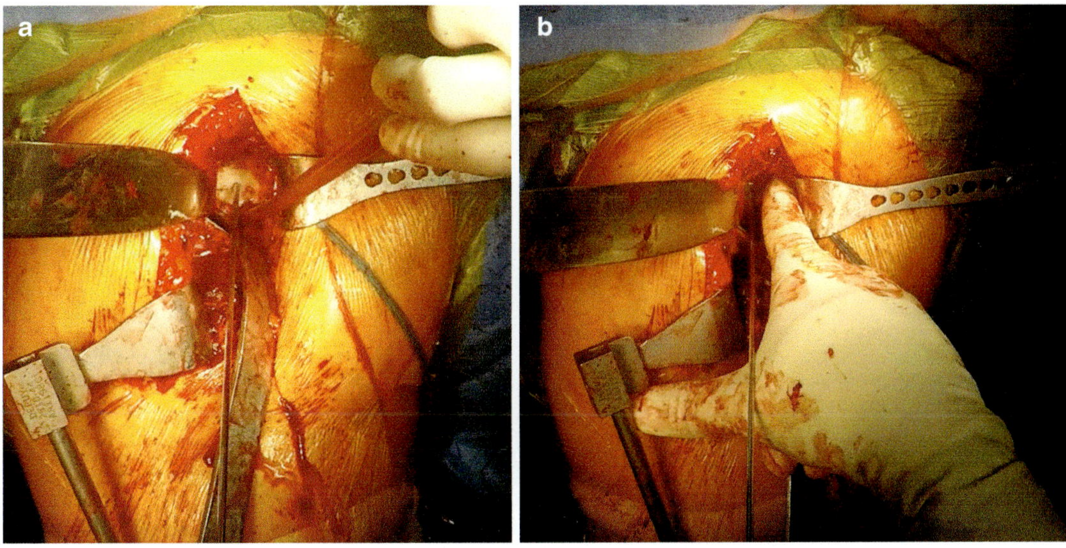

Fig. 20.13 (**a**, **b**) The metaglene guide pin should be placed slightly inferior and posterior to the intersection of the glenoid axes (**a**). The correct version is confirmed intraoperatively by palpating the anterior surface of the scapula neck (**b**)

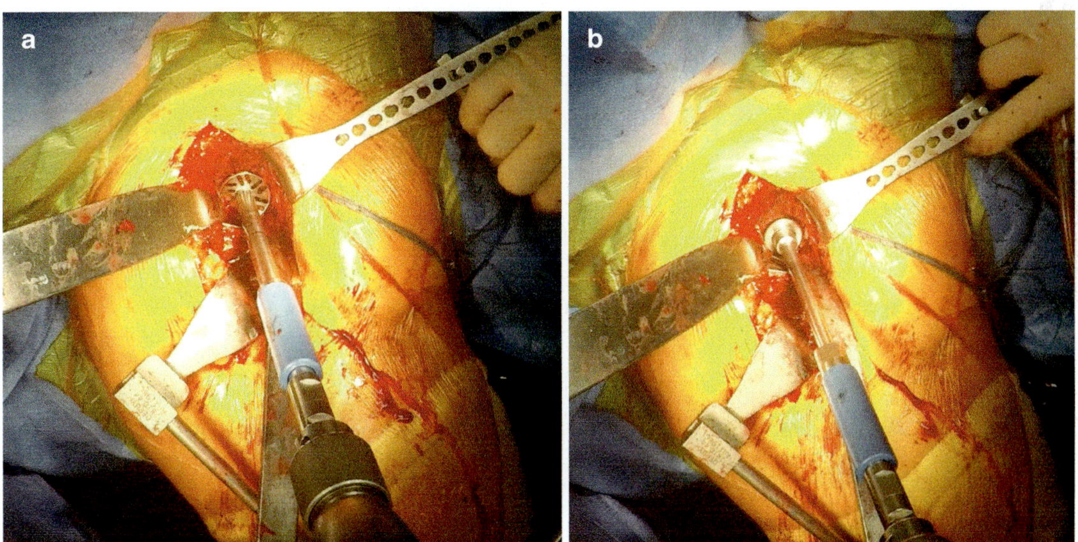

Fig. 20.14 (**a**, **b**) A two-step reaming process (**a**) allows for appropriate preparation of the glenoid followed by a central cannulated drill bit to prepare for the metaglene post (**b**)

After final glenosphere implantation, the shoulder is re-dislocated for proximal humerus preparation. The humeral side is reamed, broached, and prepared for humeral component implantation (Fig. 20.17a–d). Modern reverse shoulder arthroplasty designs demonstrate modularity that allows for press-fit reconstruction. Controversy remains regarding the amount of version necessary to maximize range of motion and functional outcome. Mole and Favard's study

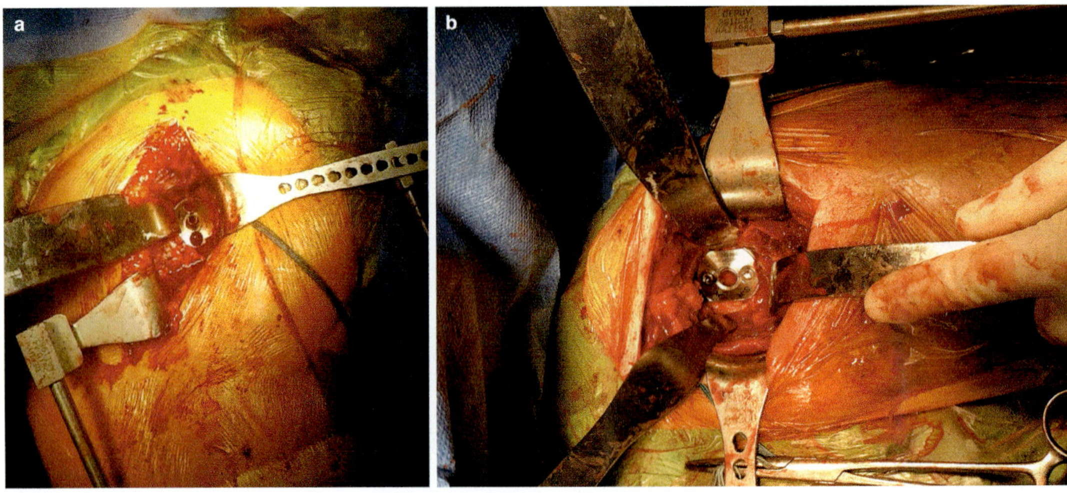

Fig. 20.15 The metaglene rotation should be positioned to allow for inferior screw placement within the scapular neck and superior screw placement within the coracoid base (**a**, **b**)

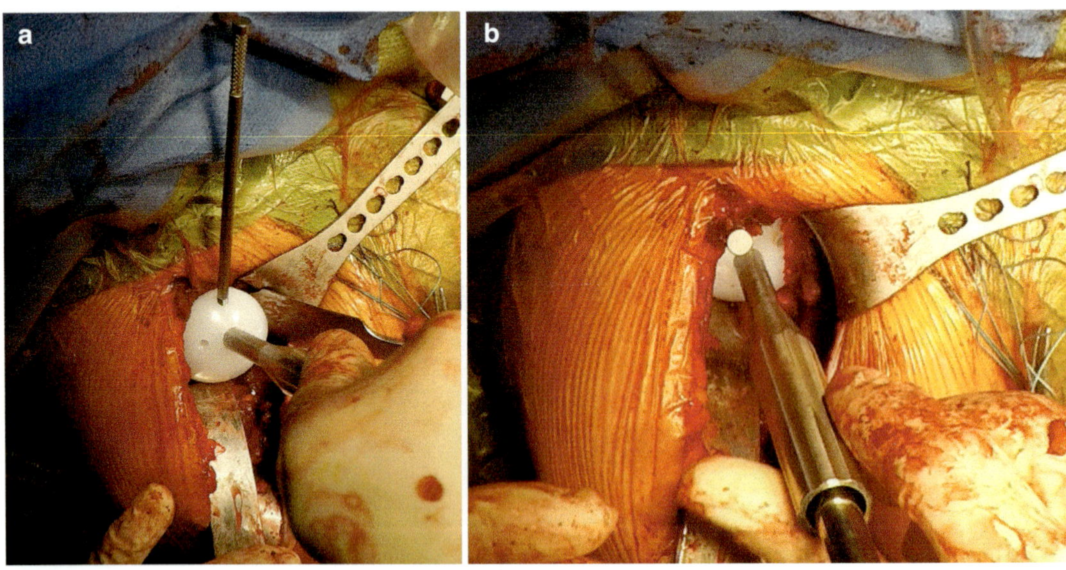

Fig. 20.16 (**a**, **b**) The glenosphere is initially advanced over a central guide wire (**a**). Clockwise rotation with intermittent impaction will result in locking of the Morse taper. The scapula should begin to rotate when the glenosphere has seated completely (**b**)

in 2007 recommended neutral version based upon better outcomes involving activities of daily living, strength, Constant scores, and implant failure rate [3]. More recently, Favard et al. noted diminished inferior impingement and scapular notching rates with near anatomic version of the humerus. The authors cautioned regarding the adoption of this technique as the effects on external rotation, internal rotation, and anterior-posterior impingement have not been clearly defined [5]. Humeral cup liner depths vary based upon implant systems, but most allow for multiple thicknesses, degrees

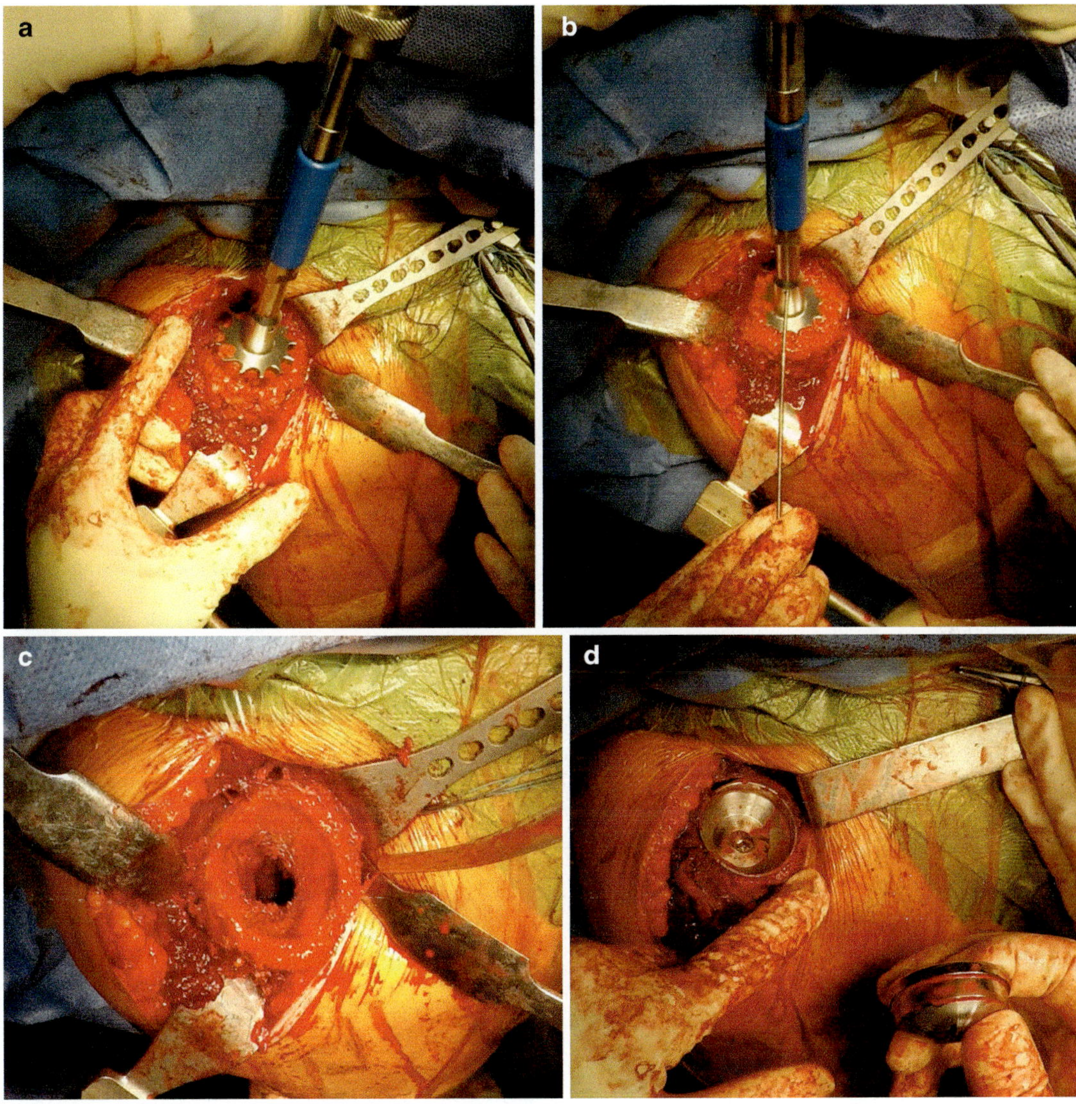

Fig. 20.17 (**a**–**d**) Preparation of the humeral component implant

of constraint, and metallic spacers for revision situations. Intraoperative reduction is generally accomplished by gentle longitudinal traction and downward push on the humerus. Stability and assessment of soft tissue tensioning remain a qualitative analysis. We will generally perform the following assessments to assure appropriate stability of the construct: the conjoint tendon should demonstrate increased but not excessive tension (i.e., bowstring); dislocation with abduction and internal rotation of the arm should not occur; minimal gapping should occur with adduction of the arm; and humeral cup glenosphere dissociation should not occur with longitudinal traction of the arm. If subluxation or frank instability occurs with any of these steps, stability may be improved by increasing humeral cup liner depth, removing soft tissue or osseous structures that cause impingement, changing to a 42–44 mm glenosphere or use of the humeral spacer.

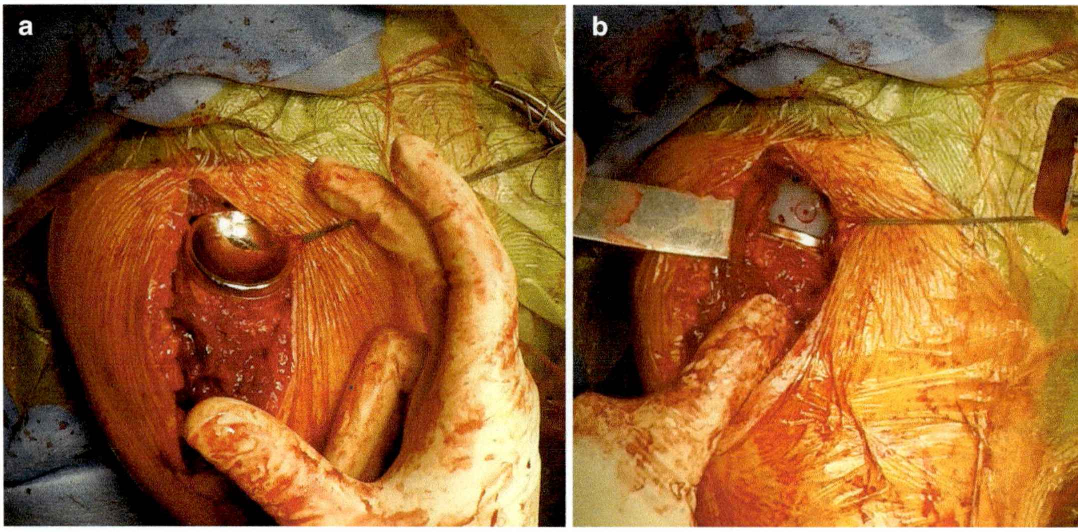

Fig. 20.18 (**a**, **b**) Humeral cap liner has been tested (**a**) so that shoulder could be reduced by gentle longitudinal traction and downward push on the humerus (**b**) and the assessment to assure appropriate stability starts

Once satisfied with the stability of the construct, the final humeral cup liner is inserted followed by glenohumeral reduction (Fig. 20.18a, b). In the event that the subscapularis can be repaired, we will place three to four drill holes through the proximal humerus approximately 1 cm below the osteotomy level for suture management purposes (Fig. 20.19). The subscapularis is reapproximated to the remaining portion of the lesser tuberosity with the previously placed #2 nonabsorbable sutures. The axillary nerve's integrity is reconfirmed. The soft tissues are closed in layers over a suction drain to reduce the risk of hematoma formation.

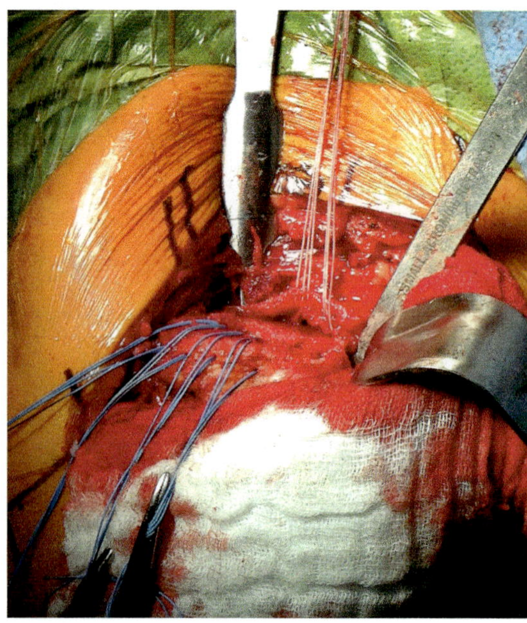

Fig. 20.19 The subscapularis is repaired with the use of drill holes and nonabsorbable passing sutures through the proximal humerus approximately 1 cm distal to the osteotomy site

The patient's operative extremity is immobilized in a sling or similar device. Active elbow, wrist, and digital exercises are allowed postoperative day 1. Pendulum, passive forward flexion, and passive abduction exercises are permitted at 2 weeks postoperatively. Active range of motion exercises, including isometrics, are allowed at 6 weeks. The patient should be cautioned to avoid internal rotation and "push-off" activities for the first 6 weeks to reduce the risk of an instability event. The patient should additionally understand that shoulder function is highly dependent on compliance with therapy protocols and to expect incremental functional improvement for up to 1 year after surgery.

20.1 Indications for Concomitant Latissimus and Teres Major Tendon Transfers

Several authors have advocated latissimus and teres major tendon transfers in the setting of reverse shoulder arthroplasty for rotator cuff arthropathy associated with loss of external rotation [12–14]. The loss of external rotation may be due to structural or functional deficiency of the infraspinatus and teres minor. Simovitch and coauthors demonstrated lower Constant scores and negative external rotation arcs in patients who underwent reverse shoulder arthroplasty with preoperative evidence of teres minor fatty atrophy [15]. Boileau et al. demonstrated improved forward flexion and external rotation in a series of 17 patients through a single delto-pectoral approach [14]. More recently, Gerber and others demonstrated durability of the combined transfer at a mean follow-up of 53 months in the setting of reverse shoulder arthroplasty. One of us has utilized the single delto-pectoral approach as described by Boileau in patients undergoing reverse shoulder arthroplasty with a preoperative external lag sign or hornblower's sign. The delto-pectoral approach affords direct access to the combined insertion of the latissimus and teres major, once the proximal portion of the pectoralis major tendon is released. Careful dissection should allow adequate visualization and protection of the radial and axillary nerves. Subperiosteal detachment of the combined insertion is followed by gentle release of adhesions in a lateral to medial direction, not to exceed 6 cm. Boileau and coauthors have estimated 3–5 cm of tendon excursion with this technique [14]. The tendon ends are tagged with #5 nonabsorbable suture (Fig. 20.20a–d). The final glenosphere has already been implanted. The trial humeral stem is dislocated, and the tendons are transferred to the remaining greater tuberosity or humeral shaft through a soft tissue window posterior to the humeral diaphysis. Drill holes are placed in the humeral diaphysis at the same level of the native latissimus and teres major tendon insertions. The drill holes are directed from the bicipital groove toward the posterolateral humeral cortex. One suture limb is delivered from posterior to anterior and hand tied to the corresponding suture partner (Fig. 20.21a–c). As an alternative, commercially available suture anchors may be utilized rather than bone tunnels for reapproximation of the transferred tendon complex. The final humeral implant and liner are impacted into appropriate position. The pectoralis major tendon is repaired, and the subscapularis is reapproximated in a manner previously described. Layered wound closure is performed over a drain.

Postoperatively, the patient is placed into an abduction-external rotation brace. For the first 6 weeks, only elbow, wrist, and digital exercises are permitted. The patient then begins physician-directed therapy with a focus on passive forward flexion, abduction, and external rotation. Internal rotation is restricted to neutral rotation for 6–9 weeks and to the greater trochanter from weeks 9 to 12. At 3 months, the strengthening may be allowed. Maintenance exercises should be performed for 6–12 months after surgery.

20.1.1 Posterior Glenoid Bone Loss

Rotator cuff tears can alter glenohumeral mechanics and predispose the glenoid to abnormal wear patterns [16]. The technical aspect of joint replacement increases in complexity with increasing bone loss and posterior glenohumeral subluxation [17–19], especially in cases of type B glenoid morphology according to Walch's classification (Fig. 20.22) [20].

Assessing the preoperative glenoid morphology and correcting it are fundamental for the surgical procedure since posterior glenoid erosion is not only a risk factor for glenoid loosening, but also it results in worse function outcomes and pain [21–23]. In this situation, the theoretical goal of shoulder surgeons performing an arthroplasty is to restore native joint biomechanics by improving glenoid version and maintaining or restoring the glenohumeral joint line.

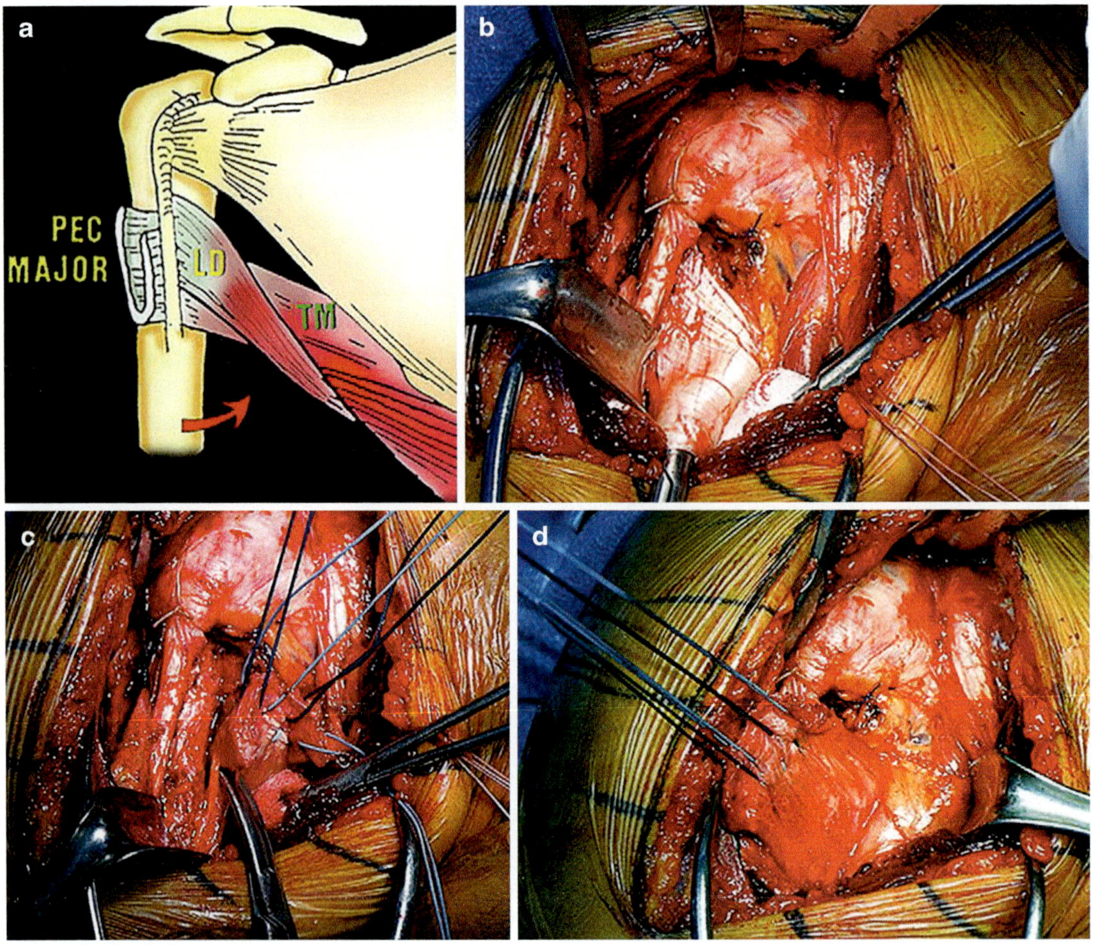

Fig. 20.20 (**a–d**) A portion of the pectoralis major insertion must be released to visualize the latissimus dorsi and teres major tendons (**a**); identification of the axillary and radial nerves is required prior to release of the latissimus and teres major tendon complex (**b**); adhesions are released bluntly under direct vision to gain excursion of the released tendons (**c**); the tendon complex is then captured with a modified Mason-Allen or equivalent suture configuration using large caliber nonabsorbable suture (**d**) (Reproduced, with permission from Elsevier, from: Boileau P, Rumian AP, Zumstein MA. Reversed shoulder arthroplasty with modified L'Episcopo for combined loss of active elevation and external rotation. J Shoulder Elbow Surg 2010;19: 20–30)

20.1.1.1 Biomechanics of Glenoid Retroversion and Posterior Bone Loss

Shoulder biomechanics is inevitably altered by glenoid bone loss, resulting in humeral head displacement and eccentric stresses placed on the glenoid component leading to polyethylene wear, component loosening, or instability. Posterior glenoid bone loss results in altered net humeral joint reaction forces which pass outside the effective glenoid arc, creating joint instability (Fig. 20.23). Bryce et al. [24] studying the relationship between glenoid wear and humeral head subluxation in their cadaveric biomechanical model demonstrated that subluxation is steadily present already with 2.5° of glenoid retroversion. The degree of bone loss and glenoid retroversion directly influence both glenohu-

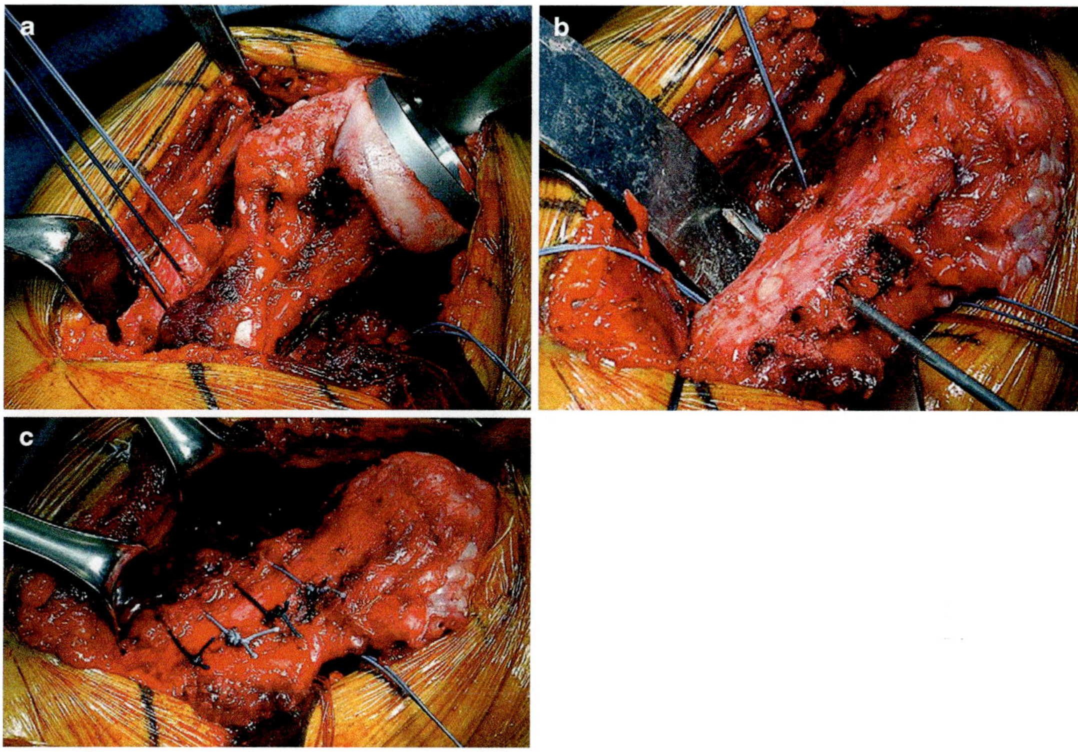

Fig. 20.21 (**a–c**) The tendon complex is passed posterior to the dislocated proximal humerus at the meta-diaphyseal region (**a**); drill holes are placed just lateral to the bicipital groove with the arm internally rotated to allow for exit at the desired location for the tendon transfer (**b**); one suture limb from each pair is brought through the drill hole, whereas the corresponding limb travels posterior to the proximal humerus. Sutures are tied with the arm in slight internal rotation (**c**) (Reproduced, with permission from Elsevier, from Boileau P, Rumian AP, Zumstein MA. Reversed shoulder arthroplasty with modified L'Episcopo for combined loss of active elevation and external rotation. J Shoulder Elbow Surg 2010;19: 20–30)

meral forces and humeral head displacement; every 4° increase in retroversion resulted in a 2° shift of joint reactive forces away from the glenoid midline [23]. This condition causes approximately 0.5 mm of posterior humeral head displacement for every corresponding degree of glenoid retroversion. Altered joint forces cause humeral head subluxation which can lead to eccentric loading of the glenoid component, mechanism described as "rocking horse," and be associated with high tensile forces across the glenoid component-bone interface [24, 25].

Farron et al. [26] using three-dimensional finite element analysis stated that retroversion of 20° created a posterior contact point on the glenoid, increasing stresses within the cement mantle and glenoid bone by 326% and 162%, respectively. Retroversion of just 10° resulted in an increase in micromotion at the bone-cement interface of >700%, and they concluded that retroversion beyond this point should be corrected. Placing the glenoid implant in 15° of retroversion (in cadaveric shoulders), Shapiro et al. [27] evaluated the effects of a glenoid component version on joint biomechanics. This procedure significantly decreased the glenohumeral contact area, increased contact pressures, and decreased inferior and posterior glenohumeral forces.

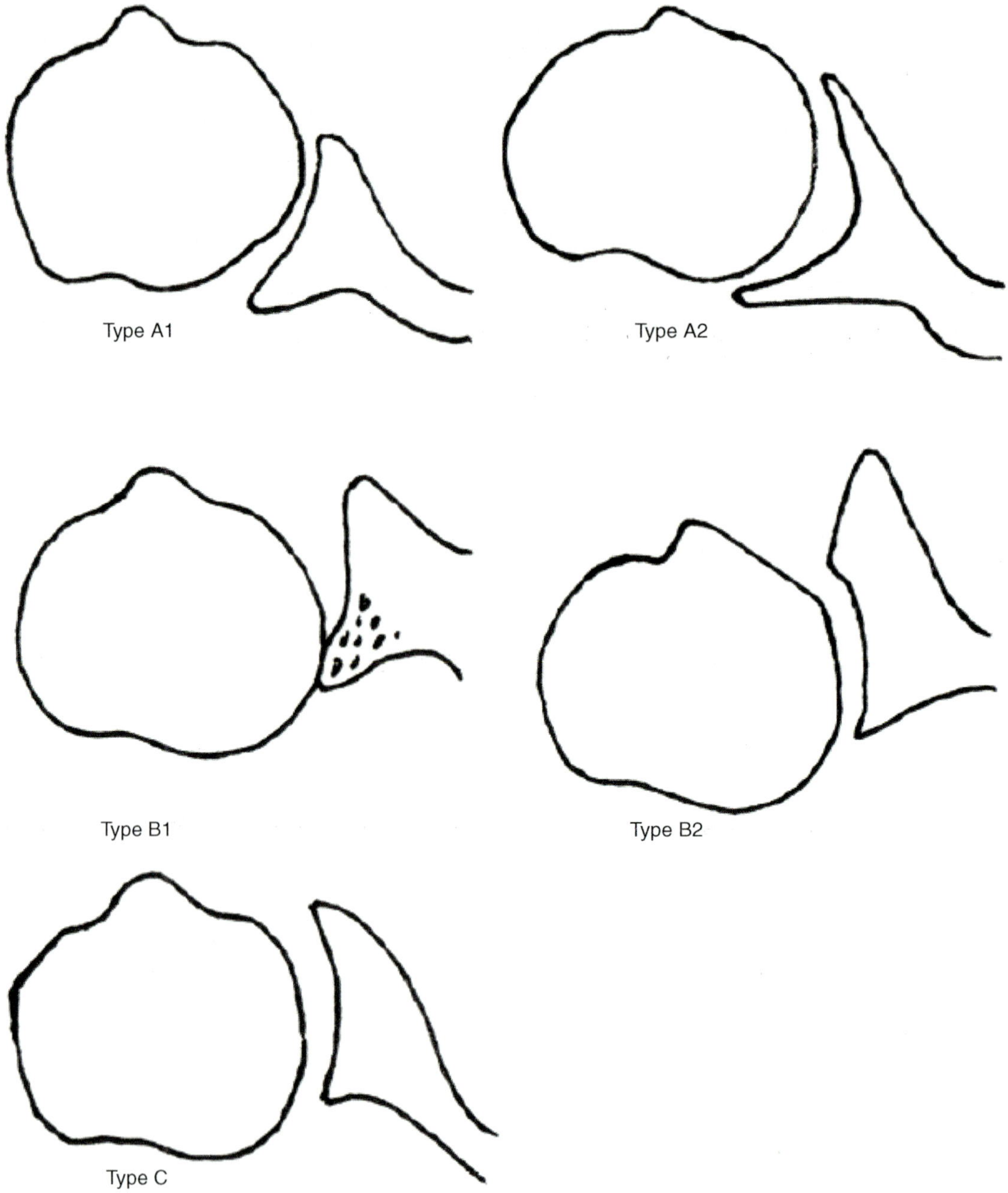

Fig. 20.22 Glenoid morphology according to Walch's classification [20]

20.2 Treatment Options

20.2.1 Eccentric Reaming

Eccentric reaming is a common procedure performed prior to component insertion with the aim to improve excessive glenoid retroversion. An excessive reaming can reduce the subchondral bone available for implant support, medialize the joint line, and allow cortical perforation of the polyethylene implant.

Walch et al. [28] found that motorized reaming was significantly associated with glenoid loosening for both subsidence and posterior tilt

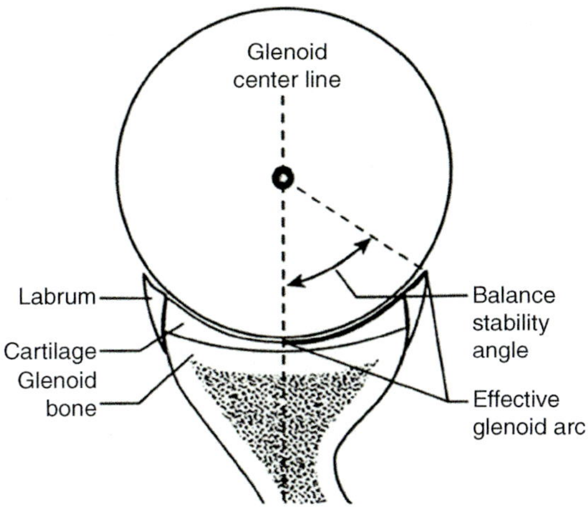

Fig. 20.23 Principles of biomechanics in the absence of posterior glenoid bone loss. From Rockwood CA, et al.: The shoulder, ed. 4, Philadelphia, 2010, Saunders

and so suggested that subchondral bone be preserved to provide sufficient osseous support to withstand the stresses experienced by the glenoid implant.

Many studies have been performed with the aim to define the limits of eccentric reaming in order to minimize the removal of subchondral bone while maximizing version correction. Attempting to correct 15° of retroversion, Gillespie et al. [29] found implant peg penetration or inadequate bone support in four of eight cadaveric specimens studied. Correcting even 10° of version, a significant decrease in anteroposterior glenoid diameter was found. Clavert et al. [30] reamed to neutral version five cadaveric scapulae in which they have previously created posterior glenoid defects and placed a pegged glenoid component. The result was one peg perforation in all five specimens and one fracture of the anterior glenoid rim leading the authors to conclude that if version exceeds 15°, the surgeon should consider alternatives to reaming the anterior aspect of the glenoid, such as posterior deficiency bone grafting.

Computer software has allowed investigators to simulate the effect that reaming has on glenoid component implantation.

Iannotti et al. [31], using a three-dimensional surgical simulator, compared ideal versus actual retroversion correction and joined the conclusion that retroversion of >19° would have been associated to peg perforation if ideal component placement had been performed.

Nowak et al. [32] considered a version <12° as optimal to implant a standard glenoid component, while version of >18° resulted in peg penetration. However, it is important to note that glenoid perforation after a short-term follow-up period is not correlated to adverse clinical effects or radiographic findings, lacking the literature of long-term follow-up studies.

In summary, an eccentric reaming is restricted by the available bone stock and should be limited to mild defects with no more than 10–15° of glenoid retroversion; an excessive reaming should be avoided to reduce the risk of loss of subchondral bone support, cortical perforation, and consequent implant loosening.

20.2.2 Glenoid Bone Grafts

When posterior glenoid bone loss is too excessive, bone grafting is a valid method to improve version, reestablish the joint line, and restore glenoid bone deficiency with the potential for biologic incorporation.

Bone grafting is a valid method when there is insufficient bone stock for component fixation or an inability to correct component position with glenoid reaming as it would result in an incorrect glenoid implant in cases of retroversion >15° [33–35]. The aim of bone grafting is that of improving version, reestablishing the joint line, and restoring glenoid bone deficiency with the potential for biologic incorporation. Problems connected to this procedure are nonunion, resorption, or subsidence, in addition to the technical demand of graft placement and fixation [34, 36, 37].

Few studies evaluated the clinical and radiological outcomes of reverse shoulder arthroplasty using bone grafting for excessive glenoid retroversion.

Mizuno et al. [38] studied 27 reverse shoulder replacements performed for the treatment of primary glenohumeral osteoarthritis with a biconcave glenoid; retroversion (mean, 32°) and humeral head subluxation (mean, 87%) were not such as to be corrected by asymmetric reaming. Ten patients required a bone graft if version could not be corrected to within 10° of neutral or when the baseplate surface contact was <80%. Constant score increased from 31 to 76 points ($p < 0.0001$). In 4 (15%) of 27 patients, a complication occurred, with 3 patients having neurologic issues and 1 patient having early glenoid loosening. At the latest follow-up evaluation (mean FU, 44 months), 25 patients (93%) were either very satisfied or satisfied with their results. No radiolucent lines were observed around the central peg or screws; no recurrence of posterior instability was found. The authors concluded that reverse shoulder arthroplasty offers a viable solution for the treatment of severe static posterior glenohumeral instability and severe glenoid erosion. Wall et al. reviewed the results of reverse total shoulder arthroplasty in 240 patients (mean age, 72 years) according to different surgical indication [39]. Of those patients, 33 underwent reverse total shoulder arthroplasty because of severe posterior glenoid bone loss and posterior humeral head subluxation. The mean Constant score after a mean FU of 38 months passed from 24.7 to 65.1 points and mean shoulder flexion from 77° to 115°. A rapid loosening of both the graft and implant was found, and this patient needed surgery for conversion to a cuff tear arthroplasty.

20.2.3 Our Experience

In our practice, each patient submitted to reverse shoulder prosthesis undergoes preoperative evaluation with standard Rx examination (true AP and axillary view) and CT scan (with 3D reconstructions) in order to obtain a detailed surgical planning. In case of glenoid retroversion <15°, we perform an eccentric reaming in order to restore a correct joint congruity and the right glenoid version. If retroversion is >15°, we utilize a bone grafting using the humeral head bone (Fig. 20.24a–d).

20.2.4 Augmented Glenoid Components

As an alternative to eccentric reaming and bone grafting, augmented glenoid components were designed.

Clinical and radiological outcomes regarding this technique are controversial. Rice et al. [40] reviewing 14 shoulders treated with an asymmetric wedge-shaped posteriorly augmented glenoid component (mean FU, 60 months) found only 2 clinical unsatisfactory results. However, more than half of the glenoid components demonstrated radiolucent lines, and one-third demonstrated moderate or severe posterior glenohumeral subluxation, although no revision surgery was performed.

Rice et al. concluded that the contribution of the modified glenoid component to overall correction of glenoid bone wear and humeral subluxation seemed marginal, and the use of this implant was discontinued.

In the last years, we have seen the development of a stepped, posteriorly augmented glenoid design that places the component perpendicular to the vector of joint forces and allows for improved biomechanical properties [41–43]. Iannotti et al. [43] compared the resistance to anterior glenoid lift-off of four different all-polyethylene augmentation designs, under both compressive and eccentric loads. The stepped glenoid resulted in having lower initial and final lift-off values compared with the augmentation designs, although not all reached significance.

Glenoid implant augmentation can improve glenoid version while preventing implant perforation, joint line medialization, and subchondral bone loss. However, more clinical studies are needed. Furthermore, augmented glenoid implantation is technically a demanding procedure; a precise creation of a glenoid bone bed to seat the augmented component is essential. High rate of micromotion and the risk of loosening are reported [44].

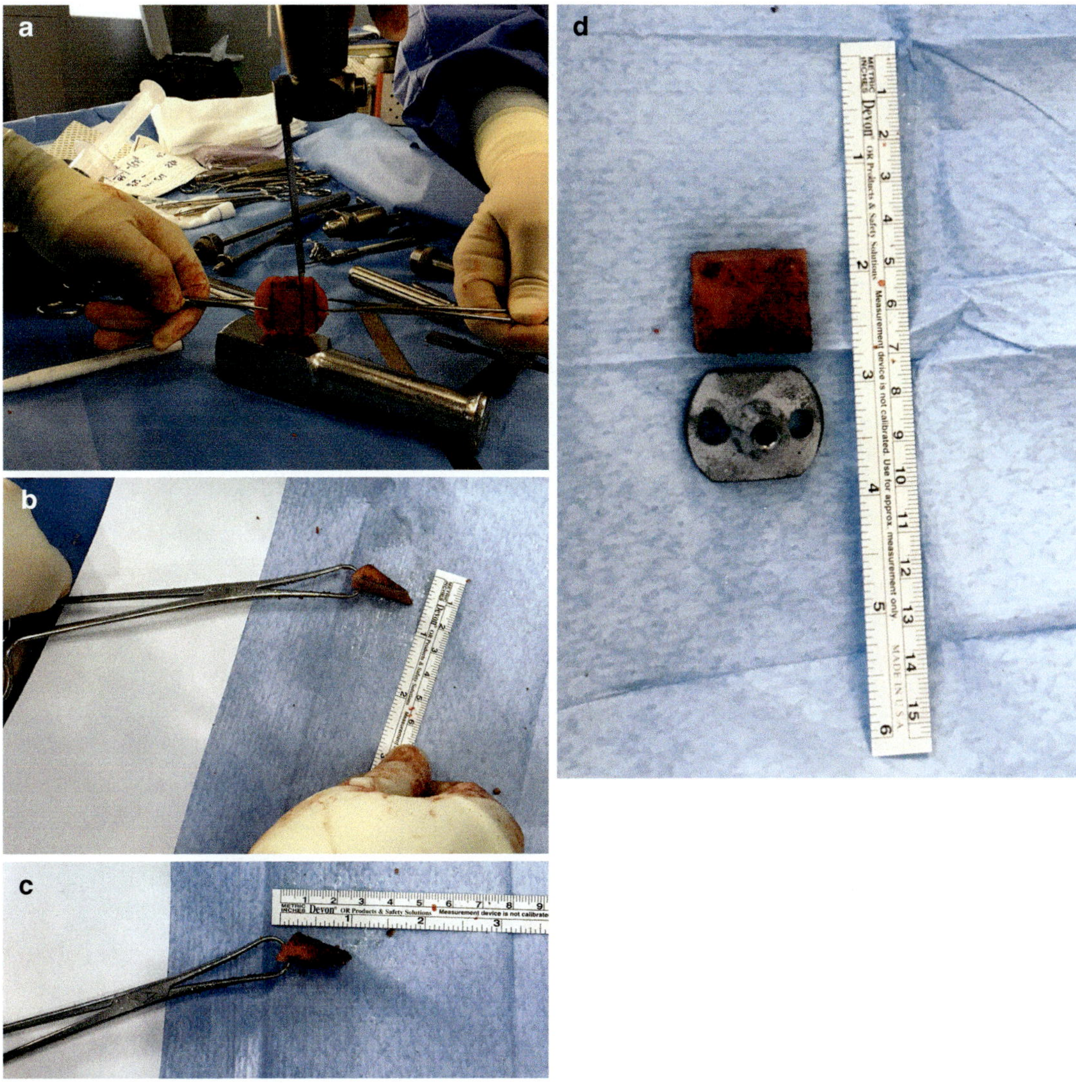

Fig. 20.24 (**a**–**d**) Bone grafting using the humeral head bone. Intraoperative phases (**a**–**d**)

20.2.5 Lateralization of the Center of Rotation in Reverse Shoulder Prosthesis

The Grammont-style reverse shoulder prosthesis had two biomechanical principles: medialization of the glenohumeral center of rotation and the lowering of the humerus [45]. These principles reduce torque on the glenoid component and increase the deltoid lever arm, overcoming the weakness or the absence of rotator cuff tendons [5, 46].

Many studies reported problems and complications attributed to this design [2, 47–51]. The scapular notching is the most frequent, ranging from 50% to 96% in post-op radiograms [25–28] (Fig. 20.25). It consists of the inferomedial impingement of the humeral component against the scapular neck during arm adduction and rotation responsible for bone erosion and polyethylene wear. Prosthetic instability is a further complication consequent to humeral medialization because of glenohumeral impingement and the poor soft tissue tension; it has been observed in 3–6% of cases [2, 5, 52]. Finally, patients submitted to reverse shoulder prosthesis complain of cosmetic concerns, related to the loss of their normal shoulder contour [5, 45] (Fig. 20.26).

With the attempt to overcome these problems, many authors have proposed different surgical techniques to obtain an increased-offset RSA. Metallic lateralization, increasing the offset of the glenosphere and/or baseplate, is an option. Historically, experience with lateralized offset prostheses led to unsatisfactory outcomes, because of high rate of glenoid loosening and screw breakage due to the increasing torque or shear force applied to the glenoid component [53, 54]. More recently, Frankle et al. [55] have demonstrated the beneficial results of metallic lateralization in reducing the scapular notching. However, in their study, they reported 12% rate of glenoid loosening after a mean follow-up of 21 months, all requiring revision. Biomechanical studies demonstrated the greater risk of baseplate-related complications after increased-offset reversed prostheses [56]. Harman et al. [56] observed that, during eccentric loading, the motion of a +7-mm increased-offset baseplate was four times greater than that observed with the Grammont-medialized prosthesis. The results of both clinical and biomechanical studies led Frankle et al. to modify their initial lateral offset design, using 5-mm locking screws to increase baseplate stability and enhance glenoid component fixation. Cuff et al. [57] reported encouraging early clinical results using such design.

Boileau et al. obtained the lateralization using bony increased-offset reverse shoulder arthroplasty (BIO-RSA) [58]. According to this technique, the lateralization is obtained by placing an autogenous bone graft harvested from the humeral head on a specifically designed baseplate with a long central peg.

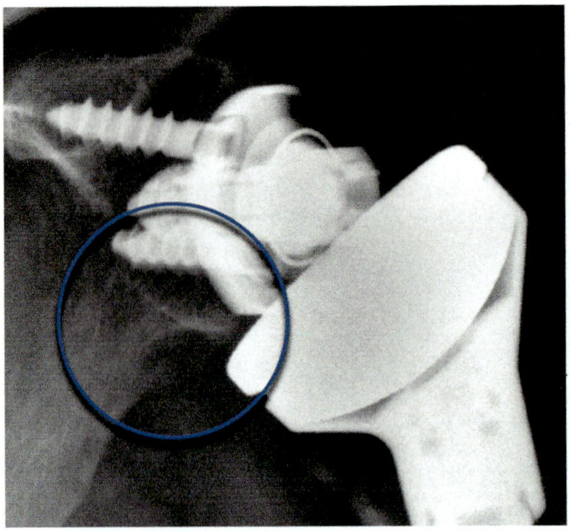

Fig. 20.25 Reverse shoulder arthroplasty: scapular notching

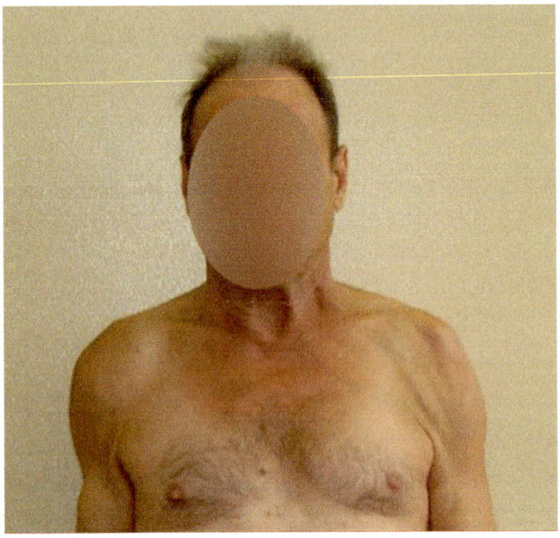

Fig. 20.26 Loss of the normal shoulder contour in a male patient submitted to a left reverse shoulder arthroplasty

Once the bone graft has healed to the native scapula, the articular center of rotation is maintained at the bone-prosthesis interface. In 2011, Boileau et al. [58] published the clinical and

Fig. 20.27 Outcomes comparison between Grammont and BIO-RSA according to Boileau et al. [58]

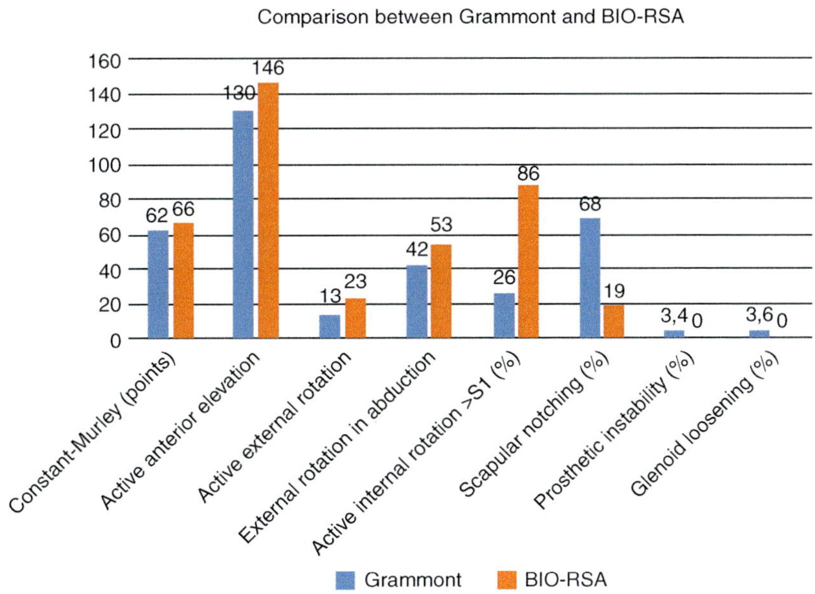

radiological outcomes of a series of 42 patients submitted to BIO-RSA. Outcomes were equivalent to or even better than those reported with the standard medialized Grammont RSA for cuff tear arthropathy (Fig. 20.27) [2, 39, 59, 60].

The effect of lateralization on shoulder motion is still a motive for discussion. In their biomechanical study, Costantini et al. [61] stated that lateralization of the center of rotation leads to an increase in the overall joint contact forces across the glenosphere. Most of this increased loading occurred through compression, although increases in anterior-posterior and superior-inferior shear were also observed. Moment arms of the deltoid consistently decreased, and bending moments at the implant interface increased with lateralization. Progressive lateralization resulted in improved stability. Greiner et al. [62] stated that in patients with lateralized RSA, the subscapularis and teres minor maintained their length and rotational moment arms; their flexion forces were increased and abduction capability decreased explaining why in their series they found improved rotation in lateralized RSA compared with standard implant.

Scapular notching remains the most frequent complication associated to RSA. For this reason, 19% rate of Boileau's series [58] is not entirely satisfactory. Recently, De Wilde et al. [63] have evaluated which is the optimal way to overcome the scapular notching during an RSA implantation choosing among six different solutions (change of the angle of humeral neck-shaft inclination, change in the depth of the polyethylene cup, lateralization of the center of rotation, downward glenoid inclination, increase in glenosphere radius, creation of an inferior prosthetic overhang to the glenoid bone). The authors concluded that a prosthetic overhang of about 2.5 mm created the biggest gain in notch angle.

In our surgical practice, the optimal configuration to reduce the rate of scapular notching and to produce favorable compressive forces on the glenoid bone graft is the lateralization of the implant (Fig. 20.28a–h) together with the positioning of the glenosphere flush to the inferior glenoid margin associated to an inferior tilt, sometimes through the help of an asymmetrical reaming and/or the use of asymmetrical bone graft.

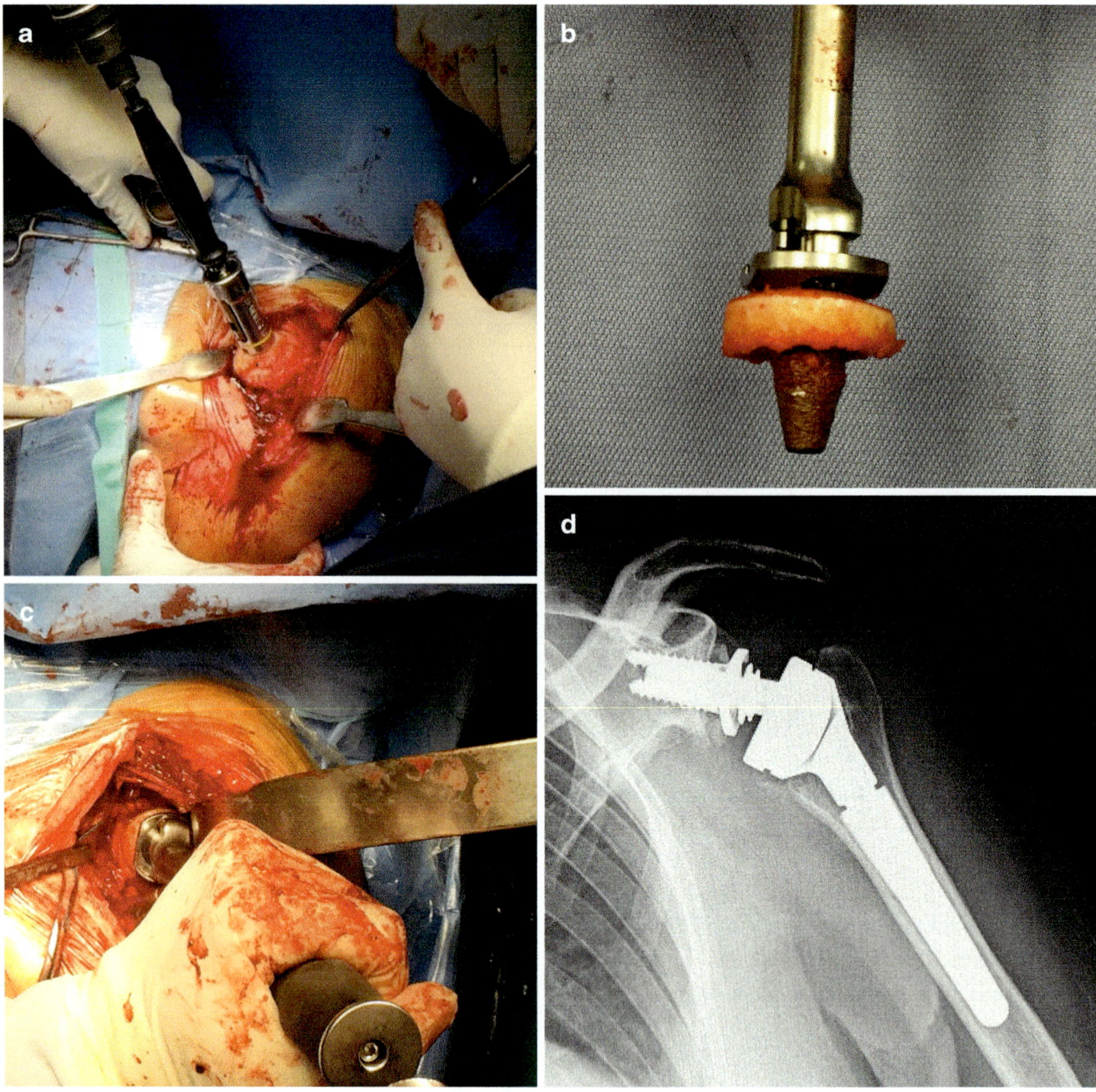

Fig. 20.28 (**a**–**h**) Right BIO-RSA in a 71-year-old female. Intraoperative phases (**a**–**c**); radiological (**d**) and clinical (**e**–**h**) outcomes

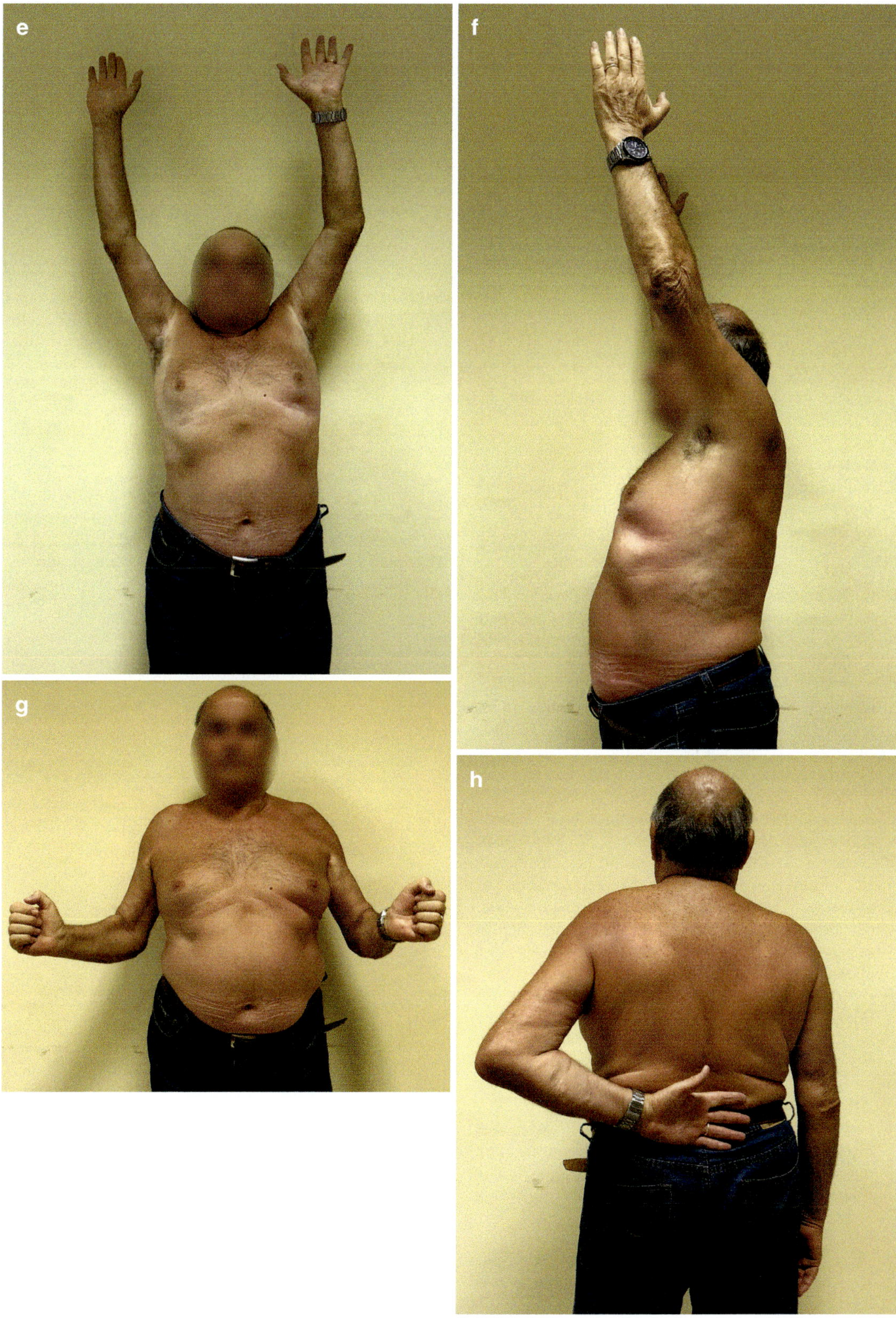

Fig. 20.28 (continued)

References

1. Walch G, Wall B, Mottier F. Complications and revision of the reverse prosthesis, a multicenter study of 457 cases. In: Walch G, Boileau P, Mole D, Favard L, Levigne C, Sirveaux F, editors. Reverse shoulder arthroplasty: clinical results, complications, revision. Montpellier: Sauramps Medical; 2006. p. 335–52.
2. Gerber C, Pennington SD, Nyffeler RW. Reverse Total Shoulder Arthroplasty. J Am Acad Orthop Surg. 2009;17:284–95.
3. Mole D, Favard L. Excentered scapulohumeral osteoarthritis [French]. Rev Chir Orthop Reparatrice Appar Mot. 2007;93(6 suppl):37–94.
4. Clark JC, Ritchie J, Song FA, Kissenberth MJ, Tolan SF, Hart ND, Hawkins RJ. Complication rates, dislocation, pain, and postoperative range of motion after reverse shoulder arthroplasty in patients with and without repair of the subscapularis. J Shoulder Elb Surg. 2012;21:36–41.
5. Berhouet J, Garaud P, Favard L. Evaluation of the role of glenosphere design and humeral component retroversion in avoiding scapular notching during reverse shoulder arthroplasty. J Shoulder Elb Surg. 2014;23:151–8. https://doi.org/10.1016/j.jse.2013.05.009.
6. Boileau P, Watkinson DJ, Hatzidakis AM, Baig F. Grammont reverse prosthesis: design, rationale, and biomechanics. J Shoulder Elb Surg. 2005;14(1 Suppl S):147S–61S.
7. Nyffeler RW, Werner CW, Gerber C. Biomechanical relevance of glenoid component positioning in the reverse Delta III total shoulder prosthesis. J Shoulder Elb Surg. 2005;14:524–8.
8. Simovitch RW, Zumstein MA, Lohri E, Helmy N, Gerber C. Predictors of scapular notching in patients managed with the Delta III reverse total shoulder replacement. J Bone Joint Surg Am. 2007;89:588–600.
9. Gutierrez S, Comiskey CA 4th, Luo ZP, Pupello DR, Frankle MA. Range of impingement-free abduction and adduction deficit after reverse shoulder arthroplasty. Hierarchy of surgical and implant design-related factors. J Bone Joint Surg Am. 2008;90:2606–15.
10. Edwards TB, Trappey GJ, Riley C, O'Connor DP, Elkousy HA, Gartsman GM. Inferior tilt of the glenoid component does not decrease scapular notching in reverse shoulder arthroplasty: results of a prospective randomized study. J Shoulder Elb Surg. 2012;21:641–6.
11. Parsons BO, Gruson KI, Accousti KJ, Klug RA, Flatow EL. Optimal rotation and screw positioning for initial glenosphere baseplate fixation in reverse shoulder arthroplasty. J Shoulder Elb Surg. 2009;18:886–91.
12. Gabor PJ, Catanzaro S, Gerber C. Clinical outcome of reverse total shoulder arthroplasty combined with latissimus dorsi transfer for the treatment of chronic combined pseudoparesis of elevation and external rotation of the shoulder. J Shoulder Elb Surg. 2014;23:49–57.
13. Favre P, Loeb MD, Helmy N, Gerber C. Latissimus dorsi transfer to restore external rotation with reverse shoulder arthroplasty: a biomechanical study. J Shoulder Elb Surg. 2008;17:650–8.
14. Boileau P, Rumian AP, Zumstein M. Reversed shoulder arthroplasty with modified L'Episcopo for combined loss of active elevation and external rotation. J Shoulder Elb Surg. 2010;19:20–30.
15. Simovitch RW, Helmy N, Zumstein MA, Gerber C. Impact of fatty infiltration of the teres minor muscle on the outcome of reverse total shoulder arthroplasty. J Bone Joint Surg Am. 2007;89:934–9.
16. Frankle MA, Teramoto A, Luo ZP, Levy JC, Pupello D. Glenoid morphology in reverse shoulder arthroplasty: classification and surgical implications. J Shoulder Elb Surg. 2009;18(6):874–85. Epub 2009 May 30.
17. Neer CS 2nd, Watson KC, Stanton FJ. Recent experience in total shoulder replacement. J Bone Joint Surg Am. 1982;64(3):319–37.
18. Norris TR, Iannotti JP. Functional outcome after shoulder arthroplasty for primary osteoarthritis: a multicenter study. J Shoulder Elb Surg. 2002;11(2):130–5.
19. Singh JA, Sperling JW, Cofield RH. Revision surgery following total shoulder arthroplasty: analysis of 2588 shoulders over three decades (1976 to 2008). J Bone Joint Surg Br. 2011;93(11):1513–7.
20. Walch G, Badet R, Boulahia A, Khoury A. Morphologic study of the glenoid in primary glenohumeral osteoarthritis. J Arthroplasty 1999;14(6):756–760.
21. Iannotti JP, Norris TR. Influence of preoperative factors on outcome of shoulder arthroplasty for glenohumeral osteoarthritis. J Bone Joint Surg Am. 2003;85(2):251–8.
22. Walch G, Moraga C, Young A, Castellanos-Rosas J. Results of anatomic nonconstrained prosthesis in primary osteoarthritis with biconcave glenoid. J Shoulder Elb Surg. 2012;21(11):1526–33. Epub 2012 Mar 23.
23. Nyffeler RW, Sheikh R, Atkinson TS, Jacob HAC, Favre P, Gerber C. Effects of glenoid component version on humeral head displacement and joint reaction forces: an experimental study. J Shoulder Elb Surg. 2006;15(5):625–9.
24. Bryce CD, Davison AC, Okita N, Lewis GS, Sharkey NA, Armstrong AD. A biomechanical study of posterior glenoid bone loss and humeral head translation. J Shoulder Elb Surg. 2010;19(7):994–1002. Epub 2010 Jul 24.
25. Matsen FA 3rd, Clinton J, Lynch J, Bertelsen A, Richardson ML. Glenoid component failure in total shoulder arthroplasty. J Bone Joint Surg Am. 2008;90(4):885–96.
26. Farron A, Terrier A, Büchler P. Risks of loosening of a prosthetic glenoid implanted in retroversion. J Shoulder Elb Surg. 2006;15(4):521–6.
27. Shapiro TA, McGarry MH, Gupta R, Lee YS, Lee TQ. Biomechanical effects of glenoid retroversion

in total shoulder arthroplasty. J Shoulder Elb Surg. 2007;16(3 Suppl):S90–5. Epub 2006 Dec 12.
28. Walch G, Young AA, Boileau P, Loew M, Gazielly D, Mol'e D. Patterns of loosening of polyethylene keeled glenoid components after shoulder arthroplasty for primary osteoarthritis: results of a multicenter study with more than five years of follow-up. J Bone Joint Surg Am. 2012;94(2):145–50.
29. Gillespie R, Lyons R, Lazarus M. Eccentric reaming in total shoulder arthroplasty: a cadaveric study. Orthopedics. 2009;32(1):21.
30. Clavert P, Millett PJ, Warner JJ. Glenoid resurfacing: what are the limits to asymmetric reaming for posterior erosion? J Shoulder Elb Surg. 2007;16(6): 843–8.
31. Iannotti JP, Greeson C, Downing D, Sabesan V, Bryan JA. Effect of glenoid deformity on glenoid component placement in primary shoulder arthroplasty. J Shoulder Elb Surg. 2012;21(1):48–55. Epub 2011 May 20.
32. Nowak DD, Bahu MJ, Gardner TR, Dyrszka MD, Levine WN, Bigliani LU, Ahmad CS. Simulation of surgical glenoid resurfacing using three-dimensional computed tomography of the arthritic glenohumeral joint: the amount of glenoid retroversion that can be corrected. J Shoulder Elb Surg. 2009;18(5):680–8. Epub 2009 May 31.
33. Friedman RJ, Hawthorne KB, Genez BM. The use of computerized tomography in the measurement of glenoid version. J Bone Joint Surg Am. 1992;74(7):1032–7.
34. Hill JM, Norris TR. Long-term results of total shoulder arthroplasty following bone-grafting of the glenoid. J Bone Joint Surg Am. 2001;83(6):877–83.
35. Sabesan V, Callanan M, Ho J, Iannotti JP. Clinical and radiographic outcomes of total shoulder arthroplasty with bone graft for osteoarthritis with severe glenoid bone loss. J Bone Joint Surg Am. 2013;95(14):1290–6.
36. Friedman RJ, Hawthorne KB, Genez BM. Glenoid augmentation for total shoulder arthroplasty. Orthop Trans. 1992;16:66.
37. Cheung EV, Sperling JW, Cofield RH. Reimplantation of a glenoid component following component removal and allogenic bone-grafting. J Bone Joint Surg Am. 2007;89(8):1777–83.
38. Mizuno N, Denard PJ, Raiss P, Walch G. Reverse total shoulder arthroplasty for primary glenohumeral osteoarthritis in patients with a biconcave glenoid. J Bone Joint Surg Am. 2013;95(14):1297–304.
39. Wall B, Nové-Josserand L, O'Connor DP, Edwards TB, Walch G. Reverse total shoulder arthroplasty: a review of results according to etiology. J Bone Joint Surg Am. 2007;89(7):1476–85.
40. Rice RS, Sperling JW, Miletti J, Schleck C, Cofield RH. Augmented glenoid component for bone deficiency in shoulder arthroplasty. Clin Orthop Relat Res. 2008;466(3):579–83. Epub 2008 Jan 8.
41. Sabesan V, Callanan M, Sharma V, Iannotti JP. Correction of acquired glenoid bone loss in osteoarthritis with a standard versus an augmented glenoid component. J Shoulder Elb Surg. 2014;23(7):964–73. Epub 2014 Jan 7.
42. Kirane YM, Lewis GS, Sharkey NA, Armstrong AD. Mechanical characteristics of a novel posterior-step prosthesis for biconcave glenoid defects. J Shoulder Elb Surg. 2012;21(1):105–15. Epub 2011 Mar 21.
43. Iannotti JP, Lappin KE, Klotz CL, Reber EW, Swope SW. Liftoff resistance of augmented glenoid components during cyclic fatigue loading in the posterior-superior direction. J Shoulder Elb Surg. 2013;22(11):1530–6. Epub 2013 Mar 22.
44. Allen B, Schoch B, Sperling JW, Cofield RH. Shoulder arthroplasty for osteoarthritis secondary to glenoid dysplasia: an update. J Shoulder Elb Surg. 2014;23(2):214–20. Epub 2013 Aug 9.
45. Boileau P, Watkinson D, Hatzidakis AM, Hovorka I. Neer Award 2005: the Grammont reverse shoulder prosthesis: results in cuff tear arthritis, fracture sequelae, and revision arthroplasty. J Shoulder Elb Surg. 2006;15:527–40.
46. Terrier A, Reist A, Merlini F, Farron A. Simulated joint and muscle forces in reversed and anatomic shoulder prostheses. J Bone Joint Surg Br. 2008;90:751–6.
47. Guery J, Favard L, Sirveaux F, Oudet D, Mole D, Walch G. Reverse total shoulder arthroplasty: survivorship analysis of eighty replacements followed for five to ten years. J Bone Joint Surg Am. 2006;88:1742–7.
48. Levigne C, Boileau P, Favard L, Garaud P, Molé D, Sirveaux F, Walch G. Scapular notching in reverse shoulder arthroplasty. In: Walch G, Boileau P, Molé D, Favard L, Lévigne C, Sirveaux F, editors. Reverse shoulder arthroplasty. Montpellier: Sauramps Medical; 2006. p. 353–72.
49. Matsen FA 3rd, Boileau P, Walch G, Gerber C, Bicknell RT. The reverse total shoulder arthroplasty. Instr Course Lect. 2008;57:167–74.
50. Vanhove B, Beugnies A. Grammont's reverse shoulder prosthesis for rotator cuff arthropathy: a retrospective study of 32 cases. Acta Orthop Belg. 2004;70:219–25.
51. Werner CM, Steinmann PA, Gilbart M, Gerber C. Treatment of painful pseudoparesis due to irreparable rotator cuff dysfunction with the Delta III reverse-ball-and-socket total shoulder prosthesis. J Bone Joint Surg Am. 2005;87:1476–86.
52. Nové-Josserand L, Walch G. Instability after reverse shoulder arthroplasty. In: Walch G, Boileau P, Molé D, Favard L, Lévigne C, Sirveaux F, editors. Reverse shoulder arthroplasty. Montpellier: Sauramps Medical; 2006. p. 81–101.
53. Gilbart MK, Gerber C. Comparison of the subjective shoulder value and the Constant score. J Shoulder Elb Surg. 2007;16:717–21.
54. Valenti P, Sauzieres P, Cogswell L, O'Toole G, Katz D. The reverse shoulder prosthesis: surgical technique. Tech Hand Up Extrem Surg. 2008;12: 46–55.
55. Frankle M, Levy JC, Pupello D, Siegal S, Saleem A, Mighell M, Vasey M. The reverse shoulder prosthesis

for glenohumeral arthritis associated with severe rotator cuff deficiency: a minimum two-year follow-up study of sixty patients: surgical technique. J Bone Joint Surg Am. 2006;88(Suppl 1):178–90.
56. Harman M, Frankle M, Vasey M, Banks S. Initial glenoid component fixation in 'reverse' total shoulder arthroplasty: a biomechanical evaluation. J Shoulder Elb Surg. 2005;14(1 Suppl S):162S–7S.
57. Cuff D, Pupello D, Virani N, Levy J, Frankle M. Reverse shoulder arthroplasty for the treatment of rotator cuff deficiency. J Bone Joint Surg Am. 2008;90:1244–51.
58. Boileau P, Moineau G, Roussanne Y, O'Shea K. Bony increased-offset reversed shoulder arthroplasty minimizing scapular impingement while maximizing glenoid fixation. Clin Orthop Relat Res. 2011;469:2558–67.
59. Sirveaux F, Favard L, Oudet D, Huguet D, Lautman S. Grammont inverted total shoulder arthroplasty in the treatment of glenohumeral osteoarthritis with massive and non repairable cuff rupture. In: Walch G, Boileau P, Mole D, editors. 2000 Shoulder prostheses: two to ten year follow-up. Montpellier: Sauramps Medical; 2001. p. 247–52.
60. Boulahia A, Edwards TB, Walch G, Baratta RV. Early results of a reverse design prosthesis in the treatment of arthritis of the shoulder in elderly patients with a large rotator cuff tear. Orthopedics. 2002;25:129–33.
61. Costantini O, Choi DS, Kontaxis A, Gulotta LV. The effects of progressive lateralization of the joint center of rotation of reverse total shoulder implants. J Shoulder Elb Surg. 2015;24(7):1120–8. https://doi.org/10.1016/j.jse.2014.11.040.
62. Greiner S, Schmidt C, König C, Perka C, Herrmann S. Lateralized reverse shoulder arthroplasty maintains rotational function of the remaining rotator cuff. Clin Orthop Relat Res. 2013;471(3):940–6. https://doi.org/10.1007/s11999-012-2692-x.
63. de Wilde LF, Poncet D, Middernacht B, Ekelund A. Prosthetic overhang is the most effective way to prevent scapular conflict in a reverse total shoulder prosthesis. Acta Orthop. 2010;81(6):719–26. https://doi.org/10.3109/17453674.2010.538354.

RSA for Proximal Humeral Fractures

21

Federico A. Grassi

During the last decade, reverse shoulder arthroplasty (RSA) has gained popularity for the surgical treatment of proximal humeral fractures, and its use is projected to increase steadily in the next years.

Fractures of the proximal humerus are common injuries, especially among the elderly population with osteopenia. Most of these injuries are successfully treated with conservative methods, but a remarkable number of fractures require surgery in order to prevent shoulder pain and loss of function.

Several treatment options are available, and the choice should be tailored according to fracture pattern as well as to patients' conditions and needs.

Shoulder replacement for proximal humeral fractures was popularized by Neer in the 1950s [1]. He reported satisfactory clinical outcomes with anatomic hemiarthroplasty (HA), and his experience was decisive for the acceptance of this technique as an alternative to conservative treatment or fixation for complex fractures. However, subsequent clinical experiences could not unanimously reproduce Neer's results [2].

In the majority of elderly patients, the loss of shoulder function after HA is common, because of the coexistence of negative prognostic factors, such as tuberosity comminution, rotator cuff degeneration and tears, low compliance and/or lack of logistic support for performing adequate rehabilitation.

RSA was proposed as an alternative option to overcome the limits of HA [3, 4]. The main advantages provided by RSA for fracture include the fixed fulcrum mechanics of the glenohumeral joint, in case of tuberosity or cuff failure, and the less demanding rehabilitation program after surgery.

Several clinical studies and literature reviews have been carried out to compare RSA and HA for the treatment of proximal humeral fractures, and most of the collected data are now in favor of RSA [5]. Biomechanical research, surgical experience, and improvement in implant designs were critical factors for the worldwide success of RSA for fracture.

Data indicating the superiority of RSA on HA need to be interpreted with caution in order to avoid over-indications of RSA in patients that can be successfully treated with alternative methods. Table 21.1 summarizes the author's indications for RSA in patients with fractures of the proximal humerus requiring shoulder replacement.

Loss of tuberosities invariably leads to poor functional outcomes with HA [6], while results with RSA are less dependent on tuberosity position and healing. Nonetheless, it has been reported that improved function with RSA, especially with regard to external rotation, is observed when consolidation of the tuberosities occurs [7].

F. A. Grassi (✉)
Department of Orthopaedics and Traumatology, Hospital "Maggiore della Carità", University of East Piedmont, Novara, Italy
e-mail: federico.grassi@med.uniupo.it

S. Gumina et al. (eds.), *Reverse Shoulder Arthroplasty*,
https://doi.org/10.1007/978-3-319-97743-0_21

Table 21.1 Author's indications for RSA in patients with proximal humerus fractures requiring shoulder replacement

Elderly patients	♀ > 65–70 (osteopenia) ♂ > 70–75
Patients ≥ 60	– Large rotator cuff tear
	– Comminuted tuberosities and/or poor blood supply (diabetes, smoking)
	– Need to replace the glenoid (Fx-dislocations, osteoarthritis)
	– Limited functional demands
	– Low compliance for rehabilitation

While reconstruction of the greater tuberosity/posterior cuff should always be performed for preserving external rotation, there is no consensus about the necessity of repairing the lesser tuberosity with the subscapularis tendon [8].

Even though subscapularis repair might play a stabilizing role for the prosthesis, it might also have biomechanical drawbacks on RSA, especially for the potential loss of external rotation [9]. Owing to humeral lowering in RSA, the anterior tension resulting from reconstruction of the lesser tuberosity/subscapularis can jeopardize recovery of external rotation in elderly patients, who already exhibit muscular weakness if not extensive rotator cuff tears. The role of subscapularis repair in RSA for fracture should be brought into focus by randomized controlled trials.

Complications of RSA for fracture do not differ from those observed in RSA implanted for other conditions. The rate of complications varies considerably among studies published in literature, with instability being the most common major complication, followed by infection. Correct positioning of RSA is crucial for avoiding specific complications of this implant, such as scapular notching (whose long-term consequences are still not clear) and acromial or scapular spine fractures (mainly related to excessive tensioning of RSA).

21.1 Surgical Technique

The surgical technique of RSA for fracture is variable from surgeon to surgeon. The main differences are related to the surgical approach (anterior deltopectoral vs. anterosuperior transdeltoid), the management of the subscapularis tendon, the version of the humeral component, and soft tissue tension after reduction.

For the majority of orthopedic surgeons, the deltopectoral is the standard approach to the shoulder. It provides excellent exposure of proximal humerus and glenoid and can be easily extended distally in case of need. Some difficulties with this approach may arise from exposure and reduction of the greater tuberosity.

The anterosuperior approach requires detachment of the deltoid from the acromion as well as particular care to avoid axillary nerve injuries with distal split of the muscle. Potential advantages include the easier access to the greater tuberosity and more favorable working conditions for periprosthetic reconstruction of the tuberosities.

Even though the choice of the exposure influences some steps of the surgical procedure, the technique of implantation does not differ substantially between the two surgical approaches. In the author's experience, the preferred technique uses a deltopectoral approach and is described hereafter.

The printed figures refer to a 78-year-old lady, who suffered a four-part valgus impacted fracture of the right humerus following an accidental fall (Figs. 21.1 and 21.2). Noteworthy features of this injury included significant osteopenia with comminution of the greater tuberosity and a concomitant tear of the supraspinatus tendon.

The patient is placed in the beach chair position with the head firmly secured. The superior limb is included in the operative field and overhangs the edge of the table to allow extension and adduction of the shoulder. The arm

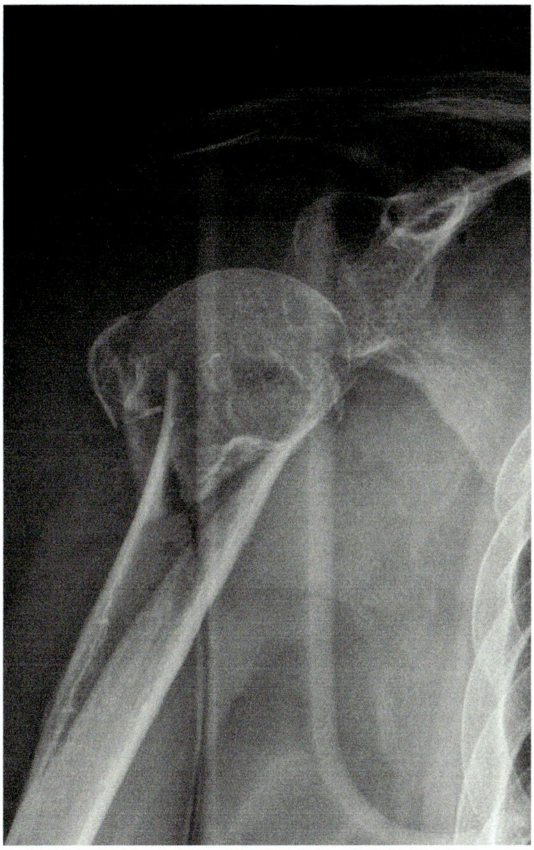

Fig. 21.1 Anteroposterior radiograph of the right shoulder: four-part valgus impacted fracture of the proximal humerus

must be easily mobilized by an assistant or a mechanical positioner throughout the procedure. The shoulder is covered by an adhesive surgical drape with iodine. The skin incision starts at the coracoid tip and runs distally and laterally for about 10 cm in the direction of deltoid insertion (Fig. 21.3).

A standard deltopectoral approach is used for exposing the fracture site. The cephalic vein is retracted laterally along with the deltoid muscle, which is separated from the pectoralis major (Fig. 21.4). The deep layer of the deltoid is released from the underlying subacromial bursa and rotator cuff tendons with a Cobb elevator.

The deep aspect of the conjoined muscle tendon unit is palpated in order to prepare a site for retraction as well as to identify the position of the musculocutaneous nerve. A self-retaining retractor can be placed between the deltoid and the conjoined tendon. The coracoacromial ligament can be sectioned to improve surgical exposure of the subacromial space (Fig. 21.4).

The tendon of the long head of the biceps (LHB) is identified and can be tenodesed at the level of the pectoralis major tendon.

The LHB is an excellent landmark and can be followed proximally to identity the rotator interval and separate the subscapularis from the supraspinatus tendon (Fig. 21.5). This incision gives access to the articular space. The portion of LHB proximal to the tenodesis is resected. The anterior circumflex vessels are ligated or cauterized in order to avoid bleeding.

Stay sutures are passed through the subscapularis tendon (Fig. 21.5). If the subscapularis is not repaired at the end of the procedure, as routinely done by the author, it can be resected with the lesser tuberosity and anterior capsule. Once the anterior tissues are removed, the glenohumeral joint and the remaining fracture fragments of the proximal humerus are easily exposed.

The humeral head is disengaged and removed through the created gap (Fig. 21.6). It is important to check the complete removal of the articular surface: any residual portion of the articular surface still attached to either tuberosity must be removed.

The supraspinatus tendon is resected to avoid superior pull on the tuberosity fragment. Strong nonabsorbable sutures are passed at the tendon-bone posteriorly (greater tuberosity/infraspinatus) (Fig. 21.6). If tuberosity comminution is present, the sutures are firmly secured to the tendons.

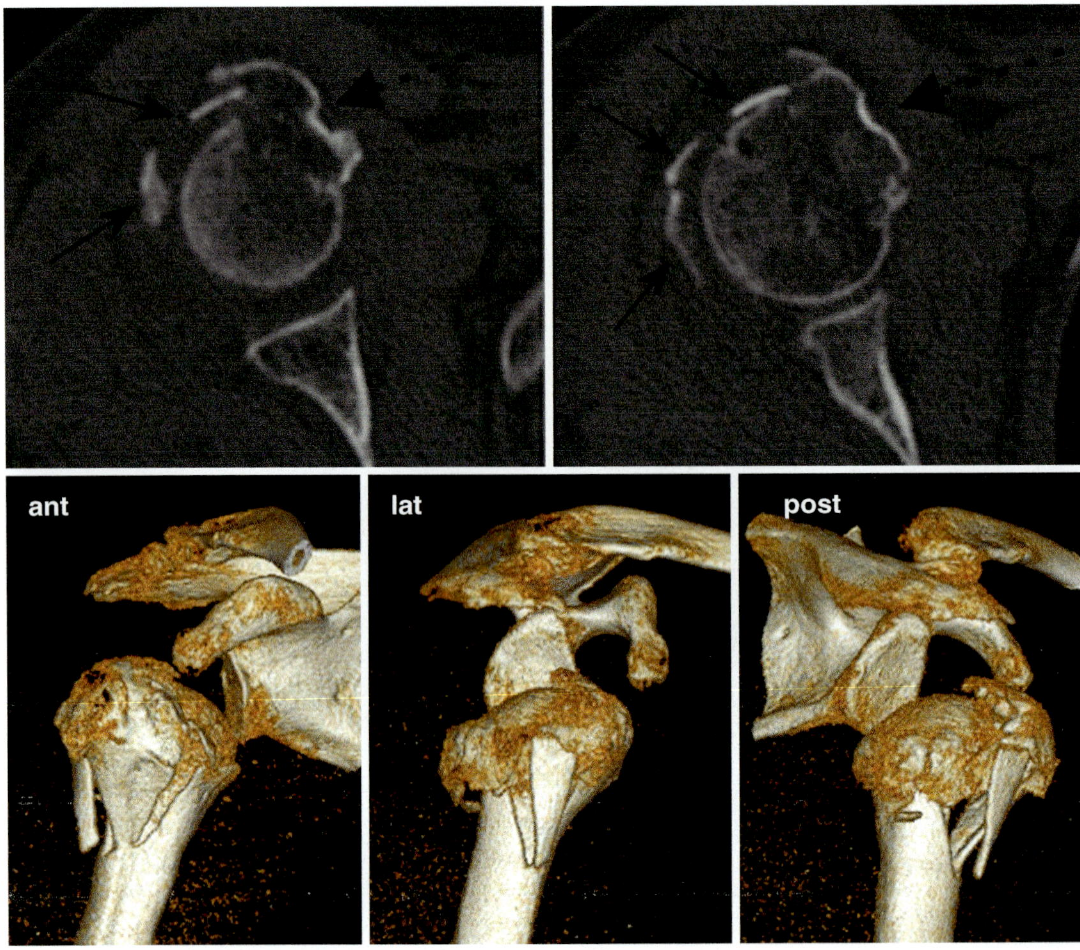

Fig. 21.2 CT imaging of the fracture. Axial scans show posterior comminution of the greater tuberosity (arrows) and separation of the lesser tuberosity with bicipital groove and anterior part of the greater tuberosity (dotted arrow). Three-dimensional reconstructions better define fracture pattern in different viewpoints

The glenoid components of the reverse prosthesis are implanted according to the standard technique. The labrum is removed from the glenoid rim by sharp dissection, and the inferior capsule is released to palpate the long head of the triceps and the lateral pillar of the scapula. Retractors (Hohmann or Rowe's "dinner fork") are placed on the anterior, posterior, and inferior aspect of the scapular neck in order to achieve perfect visualization of the glenoid (Fig. 21.7).

After having determined the correct position of the baseplate, a centering pin is inserted in the glenoid as a guide for reaming (Fig. 21.7). As well known, superior placement and superior tilt of the baseplate must be imperatively avoided. Since the glenoid is well preserved in most proximal humeral fractures, this step is not particularly challenging.

The glenoid is reamed, and the baseplate is implanted and fixed with at least two screws according to the system used (Figs. 21.8, 21.9, and 21.10). The glenosphere is assembled securely on the baseplate (Fig. 21.11). The author's preference is to use a glenosphere size that matches patient's dimensions (most commonly a 38-mm diameter).

Keeping the arm adducted and extended, the humeral canal is reamed manually until a delicate bite is felt on the inner wall of the humeral shaft (Fig. 21.12). This allows to provide an adequate

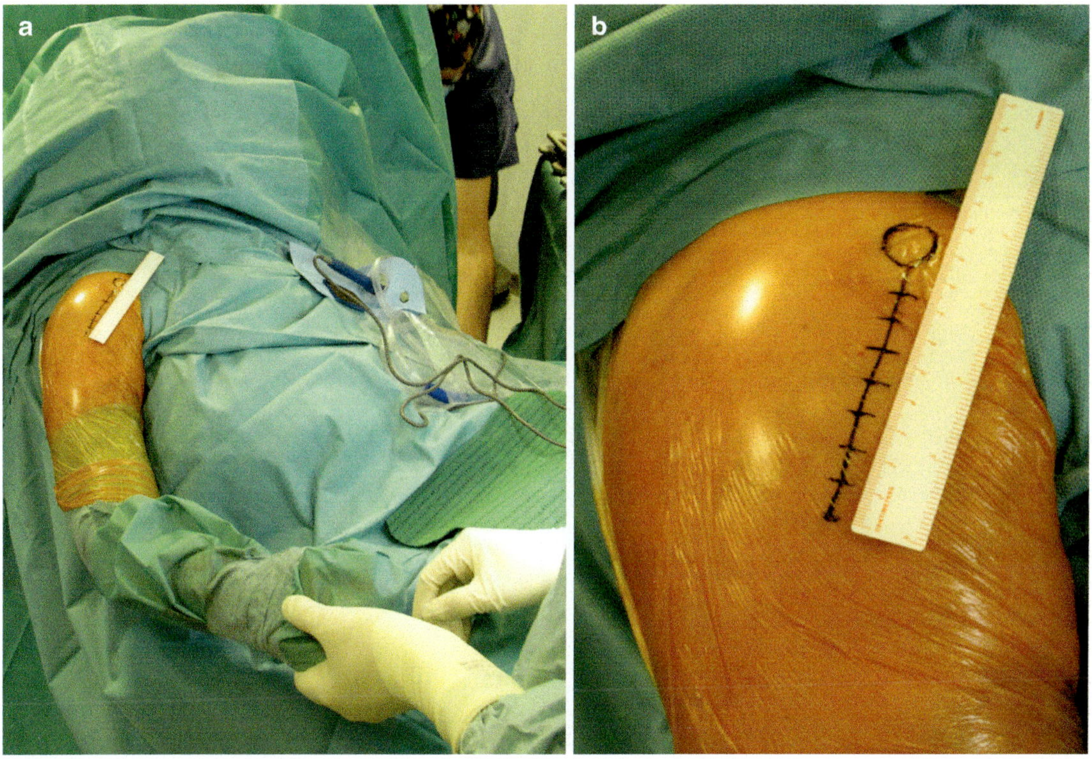

Fig. 21.3 (**a**) Patient covered by surgical drapes in the beach chair position. The upper limb overhangs the table edge so that the shoulder can be easily extended. (**b**) Close-up of skin incision running from the coracoid to the middle portion of the deltoid

cement mantle if a cemented stem is used; alternative reaming technique can be adopted if a cementless stem is used. In the author's opinion, the use of a cemented stem is advisable because cementation helps in achieving a correct implant position minimizing the risk of intraoperative fractures of the humeral shaft in osteopenic patients. Some authors suggest the use of antibiotic loaded cement for humeral component fixation in RSA, but there are no definitive data in support of this choice.

Two 2-mm holes are drilled in the humeral shaft laterally to the bicipital groove (Fig. 21.12): strong nonabsorbable sutures are passed through these holes for vertical fixation of the greater tuberosity at the time of reconstruction. If also the lesser tuberosity is repaired, additional two holes are drilled medially to the bicipital groove.

There is no consensus about the degree of retroversion of the humeral component. Some surgeons prefer to implant the humeral component in neutral version, as described originally by Grammont, while others reproduce the anatomical retroversion. Using the deltopectoral approach, the author suggests to place the implant in 20° of retroversion, using the forearm axis as landmark for orientation (Fig. 21.13). Most RSA implants have ancillary instruments that hold alignment rods to provide a reference with the forearm.

Restoration of proper humeral length is a critical factor for preventing RSA dislocation. This step can be challenging in fractures with severe shaft comminution.

The criteria described in literature for establishing the correct height of the humeral component in HA rely on pectoralis major tendon insertion (approximately 5.6 cm caudal to the top of the humeral head) [10] or on anatomical matching of the tuberosity fragments on the

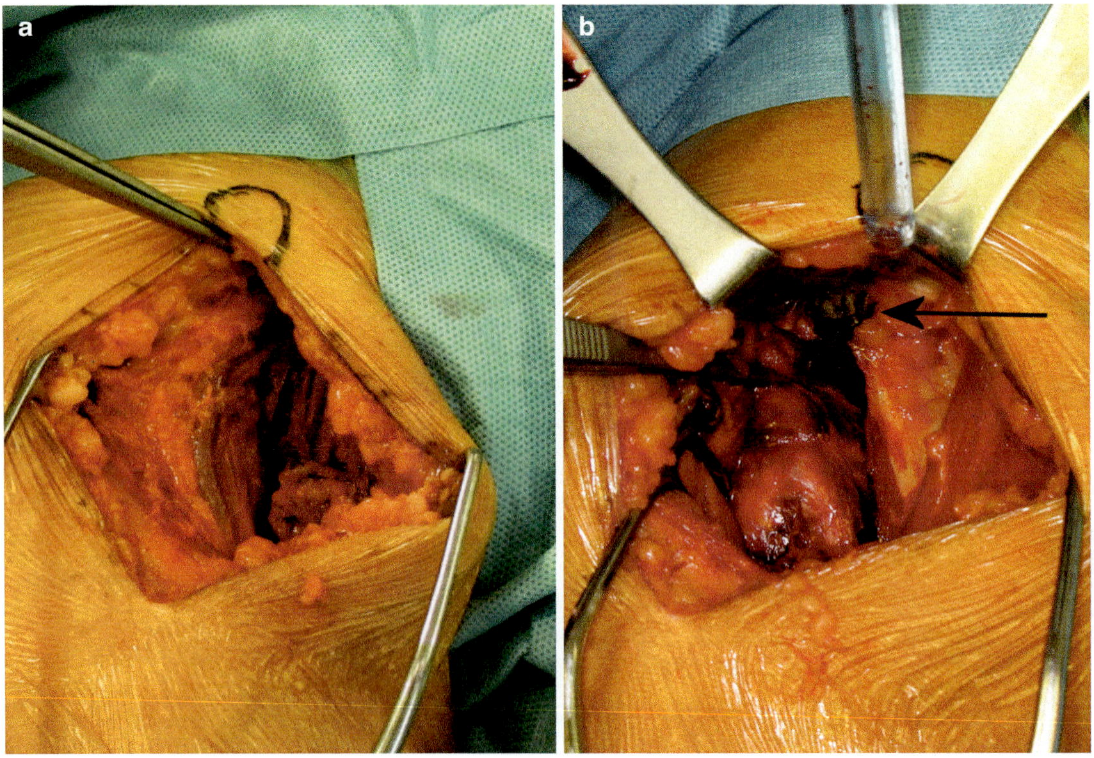

Fig. 21.4 (**a**) Deltopectoral approach with the cephalic vein retracted laterally. (**b**) The coracoacromial ligament is sectioned with electrocautery at the coracoid insertion (arrow) for improving visualization of the subacromial space

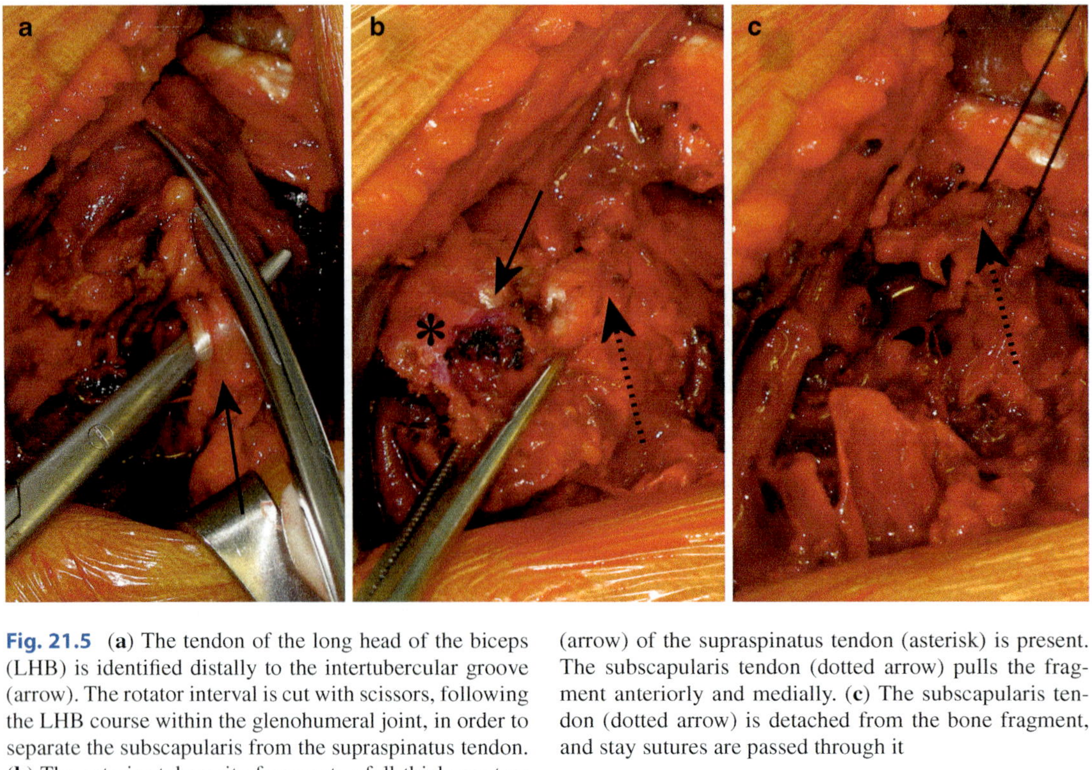

Fig. 21.5 (**a**) The tendon of the long head of the biceps (LHB) is identified distally to the intertubercular groove (arrow). The rotator interval is cut with scissors, following the LHB course within the glenohumeral joint, in order to separate the subscapularis from the supraspinatus tendon. (**b**) The anterior tuberosity fragment: a full-thickness tear (arrow) of the supraspinatus tendon (asterisk) is present. The subscapularis tendon (dotted arrow) pulls the fragment anteriorly and medially. (**c**) The subscapularis tendon (dotted arrow) is detached from the bone fragment, and stay sutures are passed through it

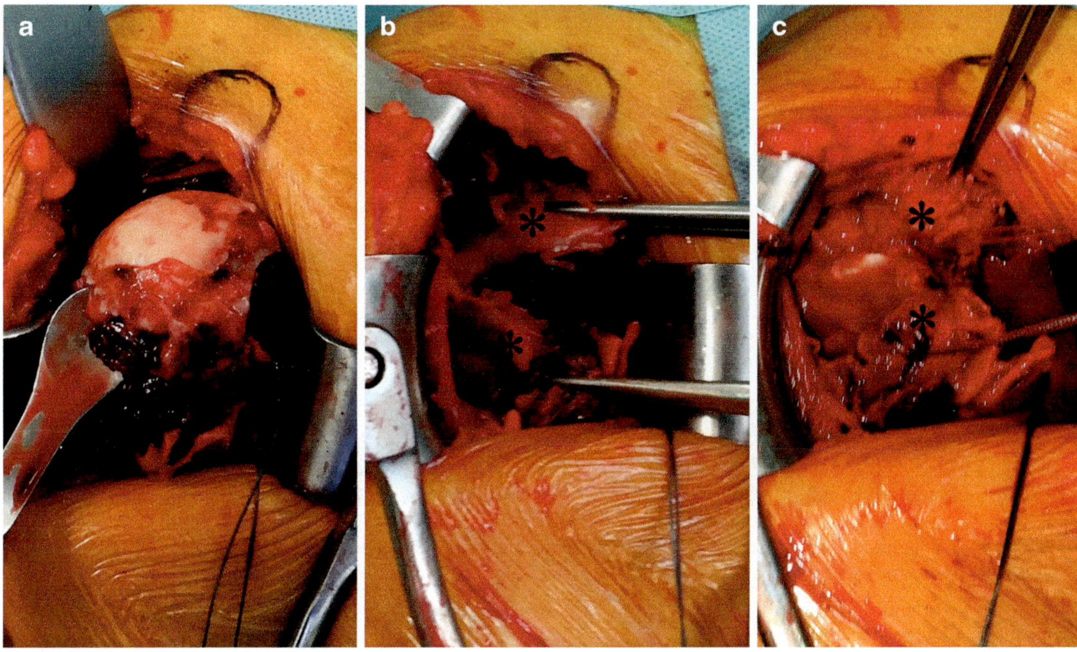

Fig. 21.6 (**a**) The humeral head fragment is disengaged and removed. (**b**) Posterior fragments of the greater tuberosity (asterisk) are identified. (**c**) Strong nonabsorbable sutures are passed at the bone-tendon junction of the posterior cuff for subsequent periprosthetic reconstruction

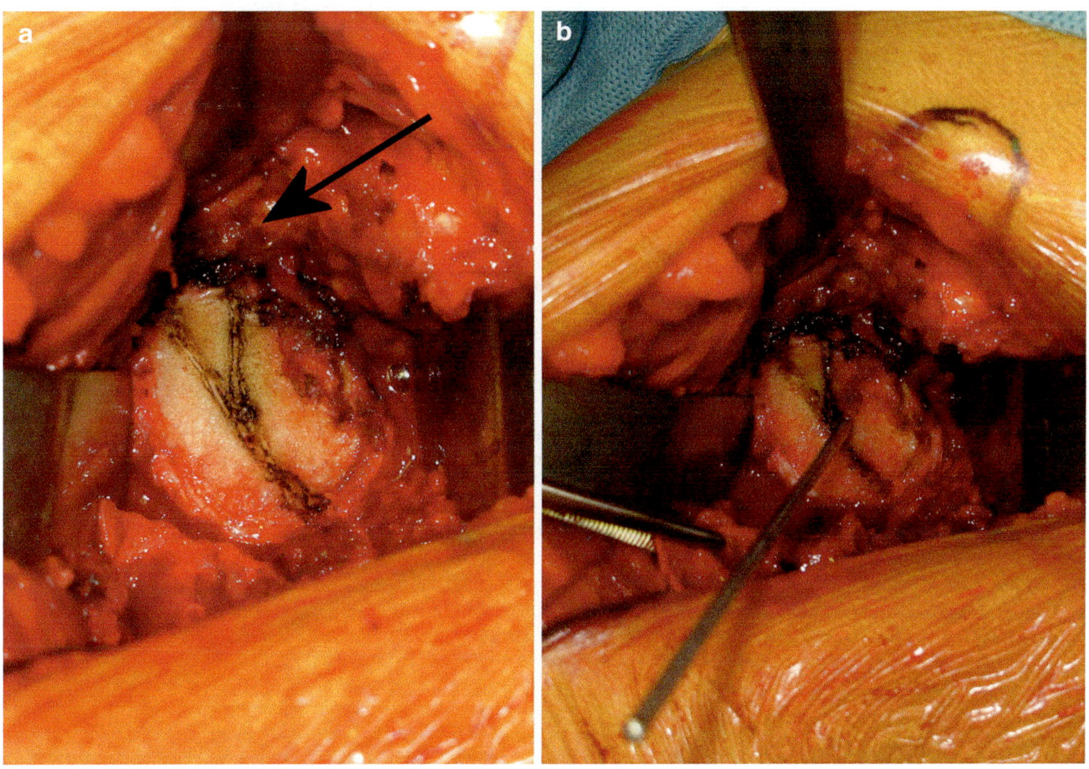

Fig. 21.7 (**a**) Exposure of the glenoid with electrocautery markings showing supero-inferior diameter and base of the coracoid at "1 o'clock" (arrow). In left shoulders, the base of the coracoid is at "11 o'clock." (**b**) Centering pin for guided preparation of the glenoid

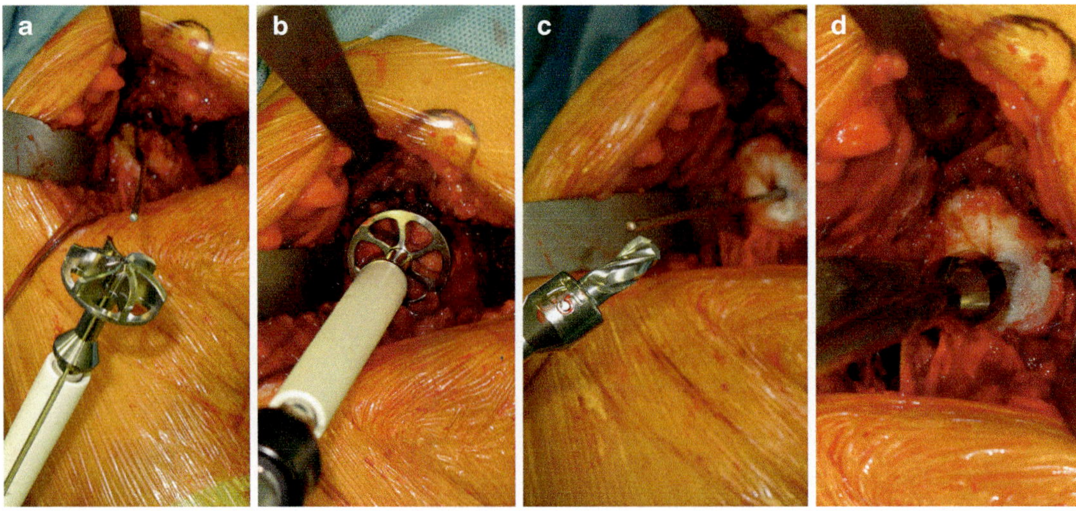

Fig. 21.8 (**a**) Cannulated reamer for the glenoid. (**b**) Glenoid reaming. (**c**) Cannulated 7.5-mm drill for the glenoid. (**d**) Hole drilling for the central peg of the glenoid component

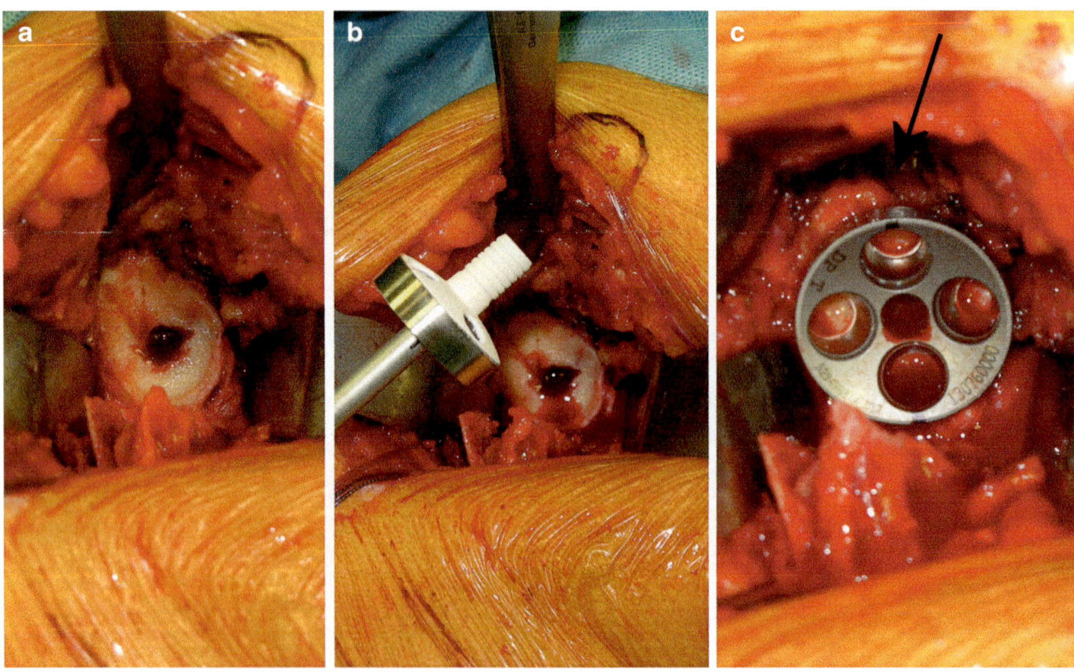

Fig. 21.9 (**a**) Glenoid appearance before baseplate implantation. (**b**) Baseplate (metaglene) mounted to the holder driver for insertion. (**c**) Positioning of the baseplate: the superior hole is directed toward the base of the coracoid (arrow) for optimal bone purchase of the superior screw

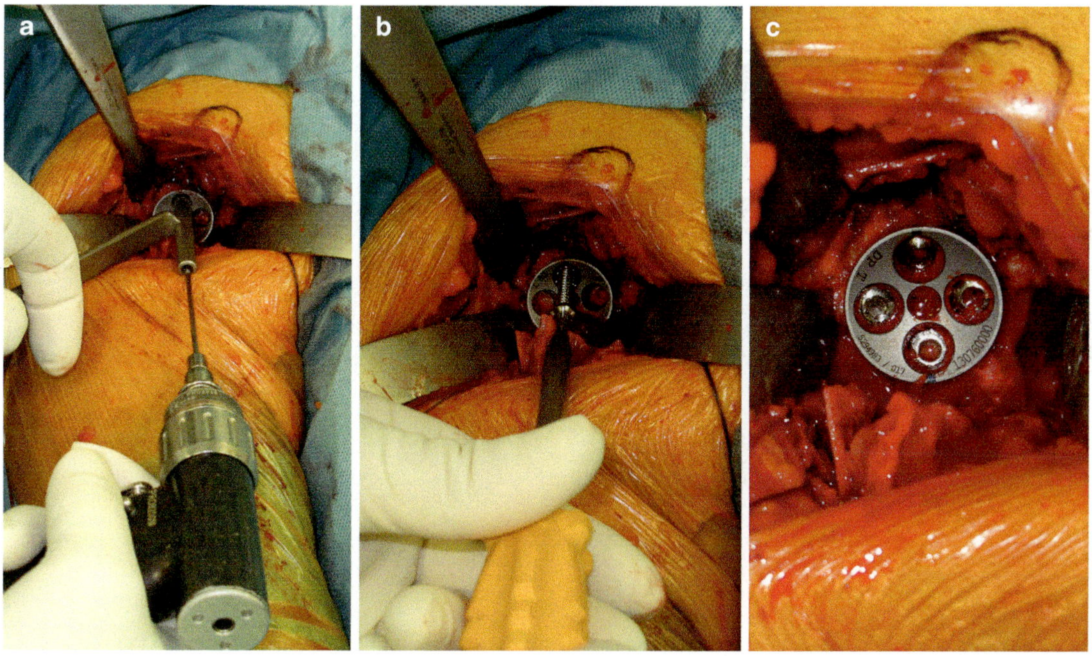

Fig. 21.10 (**a**) Drilling of the superior screw hole into the base of the coracoid. (**b**) Insertion of the superior screw. (**c**) Final fixation of the baseplate with four screws

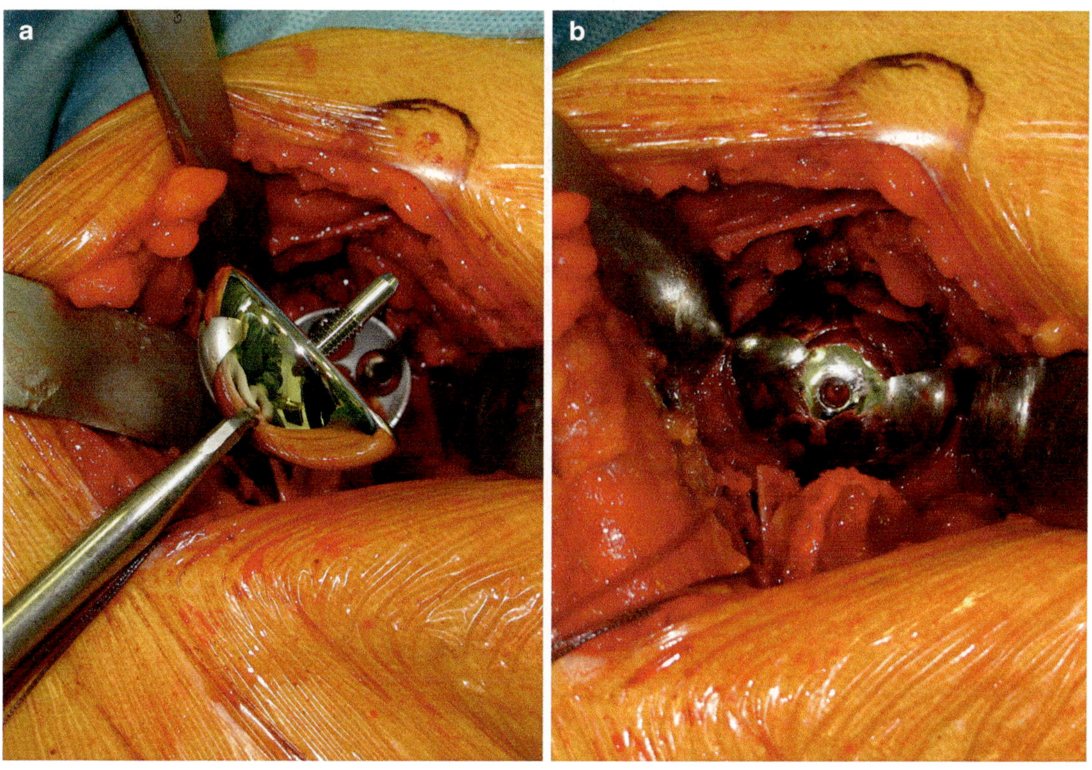

Fig. 21.11 (**a**) Glenosphere mounted to the screwdriver for insertion. (**b**) Final appearance of the glenoid component of the reverse prosthesis

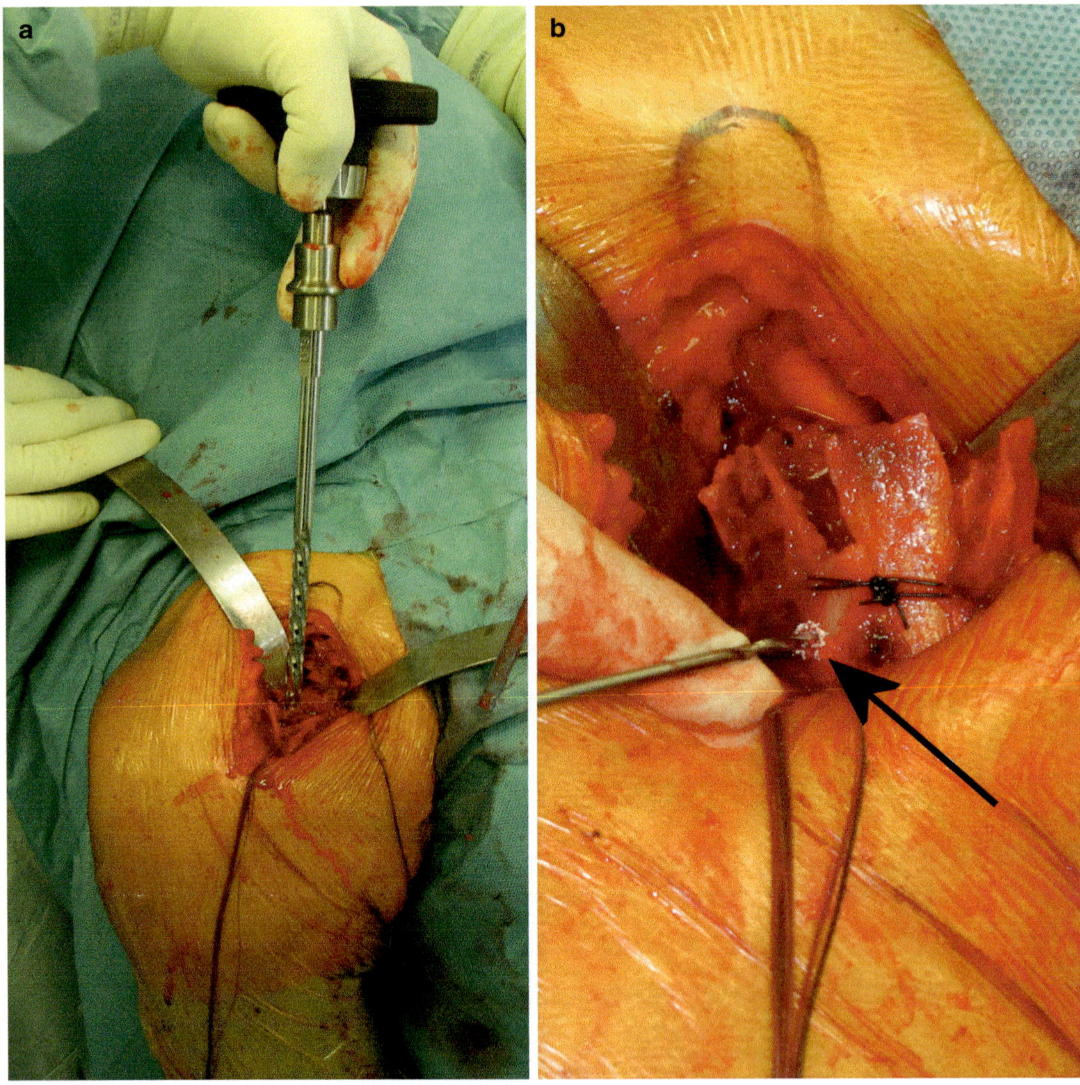

Fig. 21.12 (**a**) Manual reaming of the humeral canal. Gentle bite of the canal indicates the correct size of the stem: it is useless to risk potential iatrogenic fractures with aggressive reaming, considering that this stem will be cemented. (**b**) Drilling of 2-mm holes at the proximal end of the diaphyseal fragment for subsequent fixation of the tuberosity with vertical sutures

diaphysis. These criteria can be helpful in RSA, too.

Radiograms of the opposite humerus with radiographic markers can also assist the surgeon in determining height. However, many surgeons rely on the subjective assessment of the reduced trial for establishing the final position: tension of the conjoined tendon and deltoid muscle can be evaluated as well as joint stability and mobility.

RSA must be stable before tuberosity reconstruction, but overlengthening (>2.5 cm) should be avoided in order to decrease the risk of postoperative complications (acromial or spine fractures, neurological injuries).

In the technique adopted by the author, the position of the humeral component is assessed empirically during the surgical procedure by means of an extramedullary jig that firmly

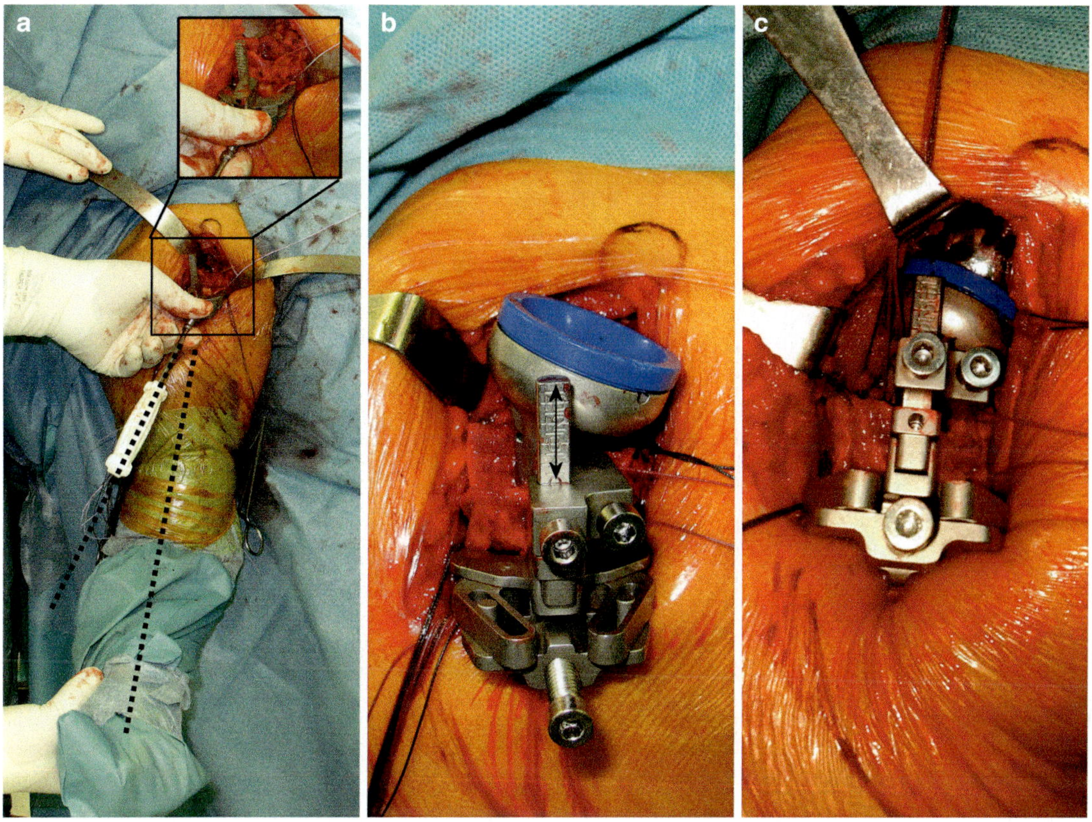

Fig. 21.13 (**a**) Application of a positioning jig that assists the surgeon in implanting the humeral component. The alignment of the screwdriver with the forearm axis determines the degree of retroversion (in this case retroversion is set at 20°). (**b**) The trial component is inserted in the canal and fixed to the jig. A sliding mechanism (double arrow) allows to modify the height of the humeral component. (**c**) Once retroversion and height are decided, the trial prosthesis is reduced with the jig in place. Mobility and stability can be assessed before implanting the definitive component

stabilizes the trial implant to the diaphysis (Fig. 21.13) [11]. Without performing any additional dissection, it is possible to reduce the trial prosthesis and evaluate shoulder stability, mobility, and soft tissue tension before implanting the definitive stem. After removal of the trial humeral component, the jig is left in place in order to allow a precise reproduction of the predefined position with the final implant (Fig. 21.14). If a cemented stem is used, the jig is useful for preventing accidental displacement of the humeral component while cement is polymerizing. It also allows to remove excess cement at the proximal end of the diaphyseal fragment (Fig. 21.14).

After humeral insert assembly and joint reduction (Fig. 21.15), secure tuberosity and cuff reconstruction around the humeral stem must be achieved. Autologous graft retrieved from the humeral head is placed at the interface between the tuberosities and the shaft to enhance bone healing (Fig. 21.16).

The reconstruction technique reproduces the pattern of horizontal and vertical sutures normally adopted for HA [12]. The transverse sutures passed at the tendon-bone junction of the tuberosities are tied around the implant and to each other (horizontal sutures). The sutures passed in the holes drilled in the humeral shaft are passed through the respective tuberosities/

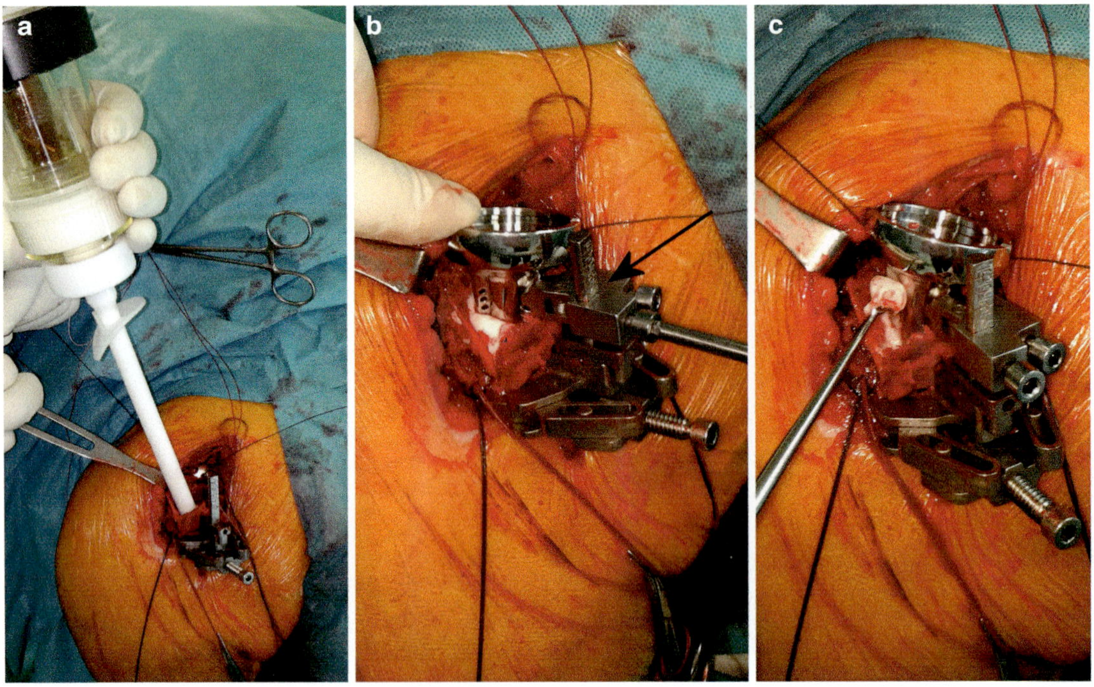

Fig. 21.14 (**a**) Cement is inserted in the humeral canal. (**b**) The humeral component is inserted in the humeral canal: the jig allows to reproduce the exact position (arrow) of the previously tested trial. (**c**) Excess cement is removed at the proximal end of the diaphysis

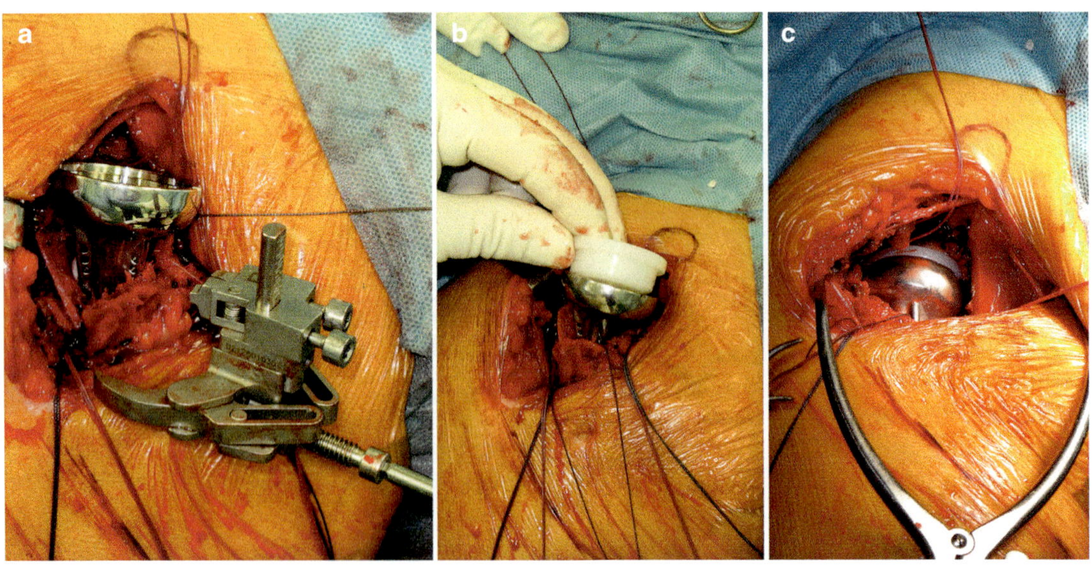

Fig. 21.15 (**a**) The jig is removed after cement polymerization. (**b**) The polyethylene humeral cup is assembled into the stem. (**c**) Final reduction of the prosthesis

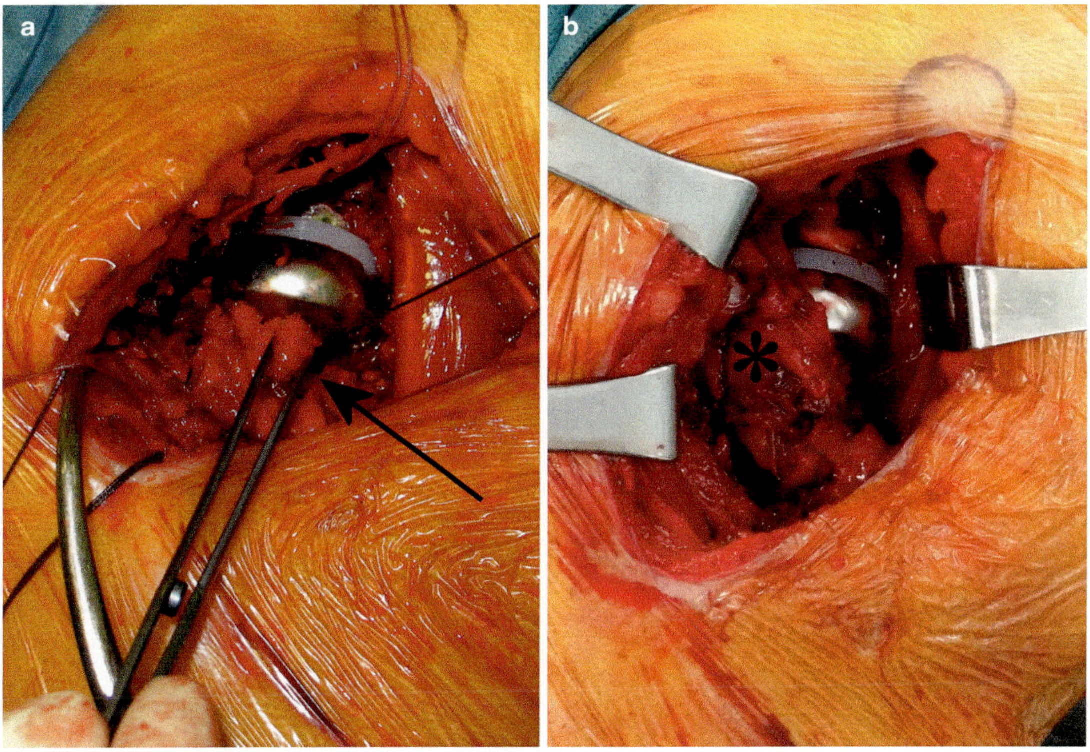

Fig. 21.16 (**a**) Autologous bone chips (arrow) retrieved from the humeral head are placed at the proximal end of the diaphysis to enhance tuberosity healing. (**b**) Periprosthetic repair of greater tuberosity fragments and posterior cuff (asterisk) is carried out by means of horizontal and vertical sutures. Since the lesser tuberosity and subscapularis tendon are not repaired, there is not any coverage of the anterior aspect of the prosthesis

tendons and then tied (vertical sutures). Some variants of this general scheme can be adopted according to individual conditions and implant designs.

If the subscapularis is not repaired, as in the author's technique, horizontal and vertical sutures are placed for exclusive fixation of the greater tuberosity and posterior cuff (Fig. 21.16).

Once reconstruction is completed, the shoulder is mobilized in forward elevation and external rotation for verifying strut strength and joint mobility.

A suction drain is placed deeply under the deltoid before wound closure and is removed 24–48 h after surgery (Fig. 21.17). Postoperative radiograms are taken to verify the position of prosthetic components and tuberosity fragments (Fig. 21.18).

In the postoperative period, the arm is kept in a sling (or in a brace in 30° of abduction and neutral rotation) for 1 month in order to protect healing of the tuberosities. Assisted passive mobilization of the shoulder (elevation on the scapular plane and external rotation) is usually started 2 weeks after surgery. Active shoulder motion for light daily activities (eating, personal care) below shoulder level is allowed after 3 weeks. At 1 month, X-rays are taken, and the patient is encouraged to use the arm as tolerated. Rehabilitation is focused on recovery of active shoulder motion with a normal scapulohumeral rhythm (i.e., correction of scapular dyskinesia).

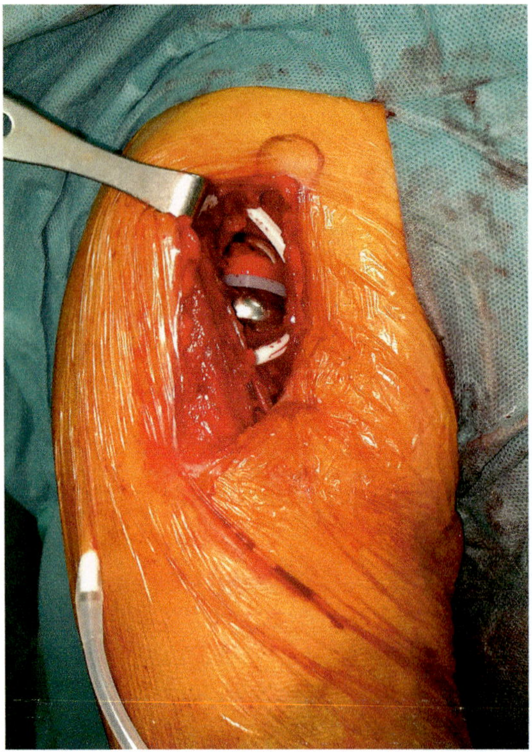

Fig. 21.17 A suction drain is placed below the conjoined tendon

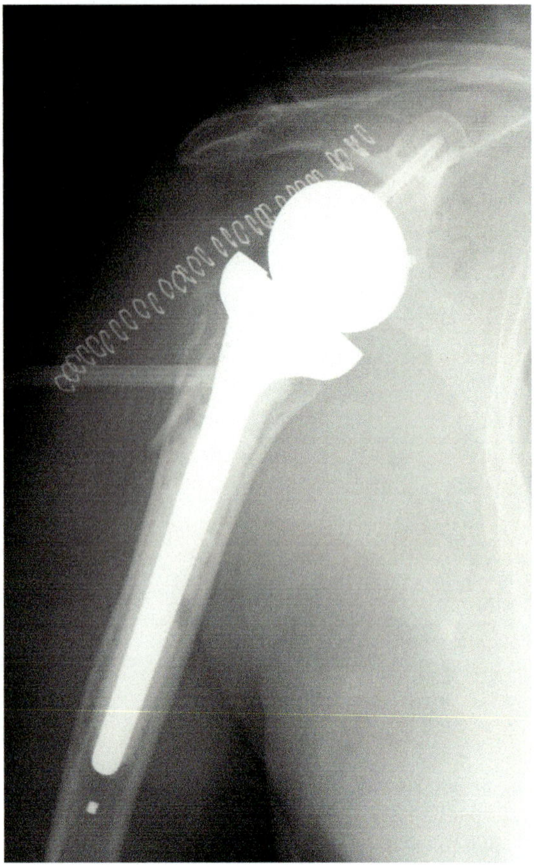

Fig. 21.18 Postoperative radiograph showing periprosthetic reconstruction of the comminuted greater tuberosity. It is also evident the position of the superior screw of the baseplate inside the coracoid base

References

1. Neer CS. Indications for replacement of the proximal humeral articulation. Am J Surg. 1955;89:901–7. https://doi.org/10.1016/0002-9610(55)90160-4.
2. Kontakis G, Koutras C, Tosounidis T, Giannoudis P. Early management of proximal humeral fractures with hemiarthroplasty: a systematic review. J Bone Joint Surg Br. 2008;90:1407–13. https://doi.org/10.1302/0301-620X.90B11.21070.
3. Cazeneuve JF, Cristofari DJ. Grammont reversed prosthesis for acute complex fracture of the proximal humerus in an elderly population with 5 to 12 years follow-up. Rev Chir Orthop Reparatrice Appar Mot. 2006;92:543–8. (in French)
4. Bufquin T, Hersan A, Hubert L, Massin P. Reversed shoulder arthroplasty for the treatment of three- and four-part fractures of the proximal humerus in the elderly. A prospective review of 43 cases with a short-term follow-up. J Bone Joint Surg Br. 2007;89:516–20. https://doi.org/10.1302/0301-620X.89B4.18435.
5. Wang J, Zhu Y, Zhang F, Chen W, Tian Y, Zhang Y. Meta-analysis suggests that reverse shoulder arthroplasty in proximal humerus fractures is a better option than hemiarthroplasty in the elderly. Int Orthop. 2016;40:531–9. https://doi.org/10.1007/s00264-015-2811-x.
6. Boileau P, Krishnan SG, Tinsi L, Walch G, Coste JS, Mole D. Tuberosity malposition and migration: reasons for poor outcomes after hemiarthroplasty for displaced fractures of the proximal humerus. J Shoulder Elb Surg. 2002;11:401–12. https://doi.org/10.1067/mse.2002.124527.
7. Gallinet D, Adam A, Gasse N, Rochet S, Obert L. Improvement in shoulder rotation in complex shoulder fractures treated by reverse shoulder arthroplasty. J Shoulder Elb Surg. 2013;22:38–44. https://doi.org/10.1016/j.jse.2012.03.011.

8. Vourazeris JD, Wright TW, Struk AM, King JJ, Farmer KW. Primary reverse total shoulder arthroplasty outcomes in patients with subscapularis repair versus tenotomy. J Shoulder Elb Surg. 2017;26:450–7. https://doi.org/10.1016/j.jse.2016.09.017.
9. Routman HD. The role of subscapularis repair in reverse total shoulder arthroplasty. Bull Hosp Jt Dis. 2013;71(Suppl 2):S108–12.
10. Murachovsky J, Ikemoto RY, Nascimento GP, Fujiki EN, Milani C, Warner JP. Pectoralis major tendon reference (PMT): a new method for accurate restoration of humeral length with hemiarthroplasty for fracture. J Shoulder Elb Surg. 2006;15:675–8. https://doi.org/10.1016/j.jse.2005.12.011.
11. Grassi FA, Zorzolo I. Reverse shoulder arthroplasty without subscapularis repair for the treatment of proximal humeral fractures in the elderly. Musculoskelet Surg. 2014;98(Suppl 1):S5–13. https://doi.org/10.1007/s12306-014-0321-4.
12. Boileau P, Walch G, Krishnan S. Tuberosity osteosynthesis and hemiarthroplasty for four-part fractures of the proximal humerus. Tech Shoulder Elbow Surg. 2000;1:96–109.

Scapular Notching in Reverse Shoulder Arthroplasty

22

Giulia Nicolaci, Andrea Pautasso, Michel Calò, and Filippo Castoldi

22.1 Introduction

Initially described by Grammont in 1987, reverse total shoulder arthroplasty was proposed in patients with cuff tear arthropathy, failed total shoulder arthroplasty, and sequelae of trauma in order to improve function and pain relief. The satisfactory clinical results and advances in technology have led to an expansion of the indications such as in proximal humerus fractures in the elderly and in reconstruction after tumor resection.

Since its introduction, many modifications of the original reverse shoulder prosthetic design have been proposed, focusing mainly on the positioning of the glenoid baseplate, on both vertical and horizontal plane, its tilt, and the humeral socket inclination. These variations modified the stability of the glenoid implant and the range of movement of the shoulder. However, there are a number of concerns regarding the design, and the ideal implantation technique still remains controversial.

Furthermore, the complication rate associated with reverse shoulder arthroplasty has been decreasing since its introduction but still remains significant and includes scapular notching. Scapular notching is actually considered one of the most frequent complications after reverse total shoulder arthroplasty, occurring in 44–96% of patients, particularly within the first few months [1, 2]. In a recent systematic analysis of complications in reverse shoulder arthroplasty, scapular notching accounted for 52% of all complications [3].

22.2 Definition

Firstly described by Sirveaux in 1997, it has been defined as the glenoid neck erosion resulting from the repeated contact of the humeral stem with the inferior scapular neck during the adduction of the arm. This is the so-called abutment-type impingement [1].

The same author proposed a classification system based on the radiographic evidence of bone loss (Table 22.1 and Fig. 22.1).

Furthermore, the following studies presented scapular notching also as the effect of a rotational friction during internal and external rotation: this mechanism has been called "frictional impingement" [4]. Nyffeler, in 2004, demonstrated how this recurrent contact between the humeral stem and the scapular neck might cause polyethylene wear and scapular notching as a consequence: the

G. Nicolaci (✉) · A. Pautasso · M. Calò · F. Castoldi
Orthopaedics and Traumatology Unit,
San Luigi Gonzaga Hospital, Orbassano, Torino, Italy
e-mail: giulia.nicolaci@edu.unito.it; andrea009@alice.it; filippo.castoldi@unito.it

S. Gumina et al. (eds.), *Reverse Shoulder Arthroplasty*,
https://doi.org/10.1007/978-3-319-97743-0_22

Table 22.1 Sirveaux's scapular notching classification

Grade 1	Bone defect within the inferior pillar of the scapular neck
Grade 2	Bone defect under the level of the glenosphere baseplate inferior screw
Grade 3	Bone loss over the inferior fixation screw
Grade 4	Bone defect at the level of the central peg

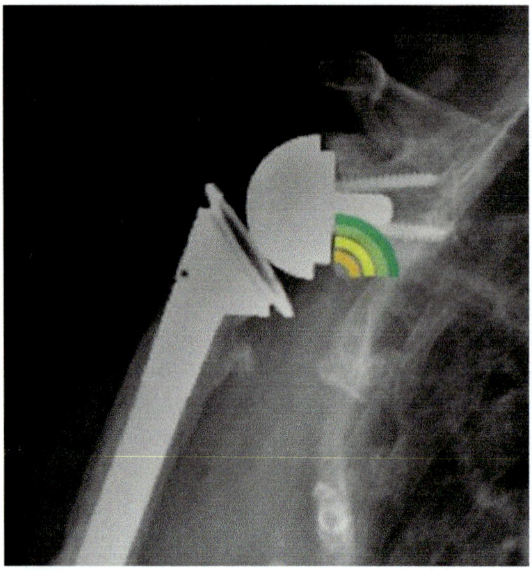

Fig. 22.1 Sirveaux's classification on a shoulder AP radiograph

released fragments induce inflammation of the joint capsule with granulomatous cells and osteolysis [5].

The clinical consequences of scapular notching still appear controversial: for some authors [3, 6], the radiographic image does not have any significant clinical effect; for other physicians [7–9] on the contrary, it is related to reduced strength, reduced range of motion, implant loosening, and possible joint instability. Boileau, in a retrospective study about revision arthroplasty after failed rotator cuff surgery, observed notching in 74% of cases, but neither the presence nor the size of the notching influenced the clinical scores after 4 years of follow-up [10]. Sirveaux analyzed the clinical results obtained after 80 TSA followed for a mean period of 44 months: in 63% of patients, scapular notching was diagnosed, and it significantly affected the Constant score when it was grade 4 or extensive, according to the classification proposed by the same author [1].

Levigne et al. [11] did not find any correlation between scapular notching and pain; nevertheless, a significant reduction in strength and in passive and active anterior elevation was observed.

Despite the small numbers of patients included in Delloye's case report, a correlation was observed between notching and glenoid baseplate loosening at 6 years of follow-up [12].

Similarly, there is no consensus on the progression of the erosion: in some studies [6, 7], the radiographic evolution of notching seemed to reach a plateau (Werner followed his patients for 1 year after the operation; at that time, 79% of patients did not show any progression); other authors [11, 13, 14] found that bone erosion after TSA could worsen with the length of follow-up.

22.3 Risk Factors

Among the factors associated with the development of notching, there are prosthetic design, surgical approach, positioning of the glenosphere, preoperative diagnosis, and the possible pattern of the glenoid wear occurring during the degenerative process [15].

22.3.1 Preoperative Phase

Regarding preoperative factors, it seems that E2 glenoid morphology (Favard's classification) and a shorter scapular neck have a higher risk of notching [11]. Similarly, a higher grade of infraspinatus muscle atrophy, according to the Goutallier classification, has been associated to Sirveaux grade 3 and 4 scapular neck erosion [16]. Furthermore, the diagnosis affects significantly the incidence of notching: an eccentric osteoarthritis with cuff tear arthropathy has been related to a higher risk of scapular notching.

22.3.2 Intraoperative Phase

The anterolateral approach has been demonstrated to lead to a higher risk of notching (86% of notching compared to 56% with the deltopectoral approach). The anterolateral approach implies the deltoid splitting and offers a poorer exposure of the glenoid surface, the posterior structures, and the humerus, leading potentially to an incorrect baseplate position and an excessive humeral resection.

22.4 How to Avoid Scapular Notching

22.4.1 Glenoid Reaming and Baseplate Positioning

One of the main factors that have been demonstrated to influence the risk of scapular notching, as well the stability of the implant, is the glenoid baseplate positioning and inclination.

In 2005, Nyffler et al. [17] demonstrated a significant improvement in the adduction and abduction range of motion and a reduction of notching when the metaglene was positioned flushed with the inferior rim: in this case, the glenosphere extended almost 4 mm beyond the scapular neck. Moreover, these authors underlined the inferior position of the glenoid as the most important factor preventing notching.

After Nyffler, several studies obtained similar results. In 2008, Kelly et al. [18] proposed a precise CT-guided measurement for the correct metaglene position during surgery: the central peg, in their opinion, was to be placed 12 mm above the inferior rim of the unreamed glenoid. As underlined in their study, this measure can be considered effective only with a specifically designed baseplate, and another possible limitation is the need of CT-templating softwares.

In our experience, the easiest method to place the metaglene flushed with the inferior rim consists initially in the release of the long head of the triceps, in order to obtain a full exposure of the inferior pole of the glenoid. Afterward, the glenoid bone is reamed until the surface of cancellous bone becomes flat. The center of the reamed surface is then marked with electrocautery, and the central peg is placed slightly inferior to it, in the middle of the inferior radius of curvature. The glenoid version is chosen according to the scapular neck anatomy that needs to be previously checked.

If preoperative glenoid inclination is directed inferiorly, because of inferior erosion or constitutional inferior tilt, the baseplate is placed without attempting to change the orientation. Otherwise, if preoperative glenoid inclination is directed superiorly, preferential reaming is performed inferiorly to restore a more vertical glenoid inclination. The inferior "smile sign" after reaming confirms the correct tilt (Fig. 22.2).

In order to gain a better stability of the metaglene, screw fixation is recommended. Some authors believe in the "three-column theory" proposed by Humphrey and colleagues [19]: an optimal fixation can be achieved if screws are oriented in the three areas of thicker bone. These areas are represented by the coracoid process (first column), the scapular spine (second column), and, inferiorly, the scapular pillar (third column). The area between these columns, in fact, is thinner, and this theory can be easily applicable with variable-angle locking screws.

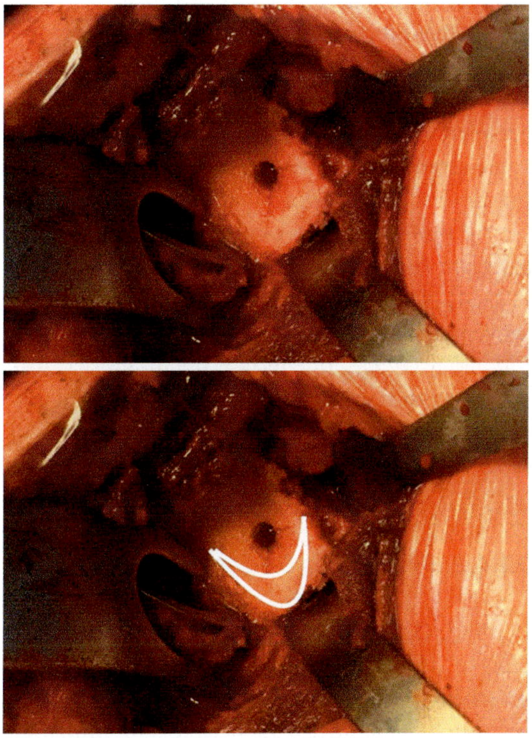

Fig. 22.2 The inferior "smile sign" after reaming confirms the correct tilt

Concerning the neutral or inferior tilting of the baseplate, results appear to be controversial: several studies [11, 20] seem to support inferior tilted implants, with a demonstrated significant reduction in scapular notching rates compared to neutral or superiorly tilted baseplates. In their retrospective study, Huri et al. [21] found how, for each degree of increase in the angle of glenoid inclination, there was a 7% reduction in the risk of developing notching. Furthermore, for each millimeter of increase between the PEG and the inferior margin of the rimmed glenoid, the risk of scapular notching rose by 34%.

In addition, it has been demonstrated that with a slight inclination, compressive forces under the baseplate are higher; therefore, the amount of micro-movements is inferior. Gutièrrez et al. [20] underlined how the inferior tilt offers the most even distribution of forces directed on the baseplate and a greater impingement-free arc of motion, if the glenoid implant has a concentric-PEG design; with an eccentric-PEG design, on the contrary, the inferior inclination might be counterproductive in terms of stability.

On the other hand, however, there are few authors [7, 22, 23] who did not find significant differences in scapular notching frequency between neutral and inferior tilting. Moreover, in some studies on prosthesis biomechanics, it seems that the inferior placement of the glenosphere was even more effective than the inferior tilting in reducing the risk of scapular notching [17, 24]. Finally, Chae et al. analyzed the micromovement rates of the baseplate between a neutral and a 10° inferior tilting, obtaining opposite results to the ones of Gutièrrez et al., assuming therefore that tilting could affect the longevity of the prosthesis [25].

22.4.2 Prosthesis Design

In 1985, Grammont altered the widely endorsed idea of shoulder arthroplasty proposing a new prosthetic model whose functioning was based on the deltoid muscle action, overcoming the rotator cuff deficiency.

In a normal shoulder, the rotator cuff stabilizes the joint by compressing the humeral head against the glenoid: the torque created by internal and external rotators acts as a resistance to the upward shear force generated by the deltoid.

Consequently, in a rotator cuff-deficient shoulder, the deltoid action led the humeral head to migrate superiorly.

The distance between the center of rotation and the bone-implant interface is equal to a lever arm through which destabilizing forces act on the glenosphere to create a torque. In Grammont's model, the absence of a neck in the glenoid component, its hemisphere shape, and the humeral cut ensured a medialization of the center of rotation, as well as its lowering (Fig. 22.3).

This modifies both the length of the deltoid arm and the recruitment of its anterior and posterior fibers, improving, as a result, the shoulder elevation and abduction and reducing the muscular effort for movement such as lifting and pushing [26].

Despite the remarkable innovation of this design and the reduction in glenoid loosening due to mechanical stress, in the following years, the medialized reverse arthroplasty was linked to complications such as acromial and scapular fractures, reduction in internal and external rotation, and shoulder instability, as well as scapular notching.

Regarding scapular notching, with the aim of reducing its incidence, several authors have proposed new prosthetic models.

Frankle et al. proposed a lateralized glenosphere design with a metal-bone interface at the scapular neck: moving the joint center of rotation laterally creates a greater impingement-free adduction movement; on the other side, higher rates of glenoid loosening have been observed, due to increased shear forces at bone-implant interface [27–29] (Fig. 22.3).

Boileau et al. [30] studied prosthetic models with biologic tissue at the glenoid baseplate in order to reduce both notching and implant loosening: in the BIO-RSA (bony increased offset), the humeral head removed during surgery is used again to create an autologous graft plate in which a longer baseplate peg is inserted.

There are still disagreements about the comparison of clinical results between medialized

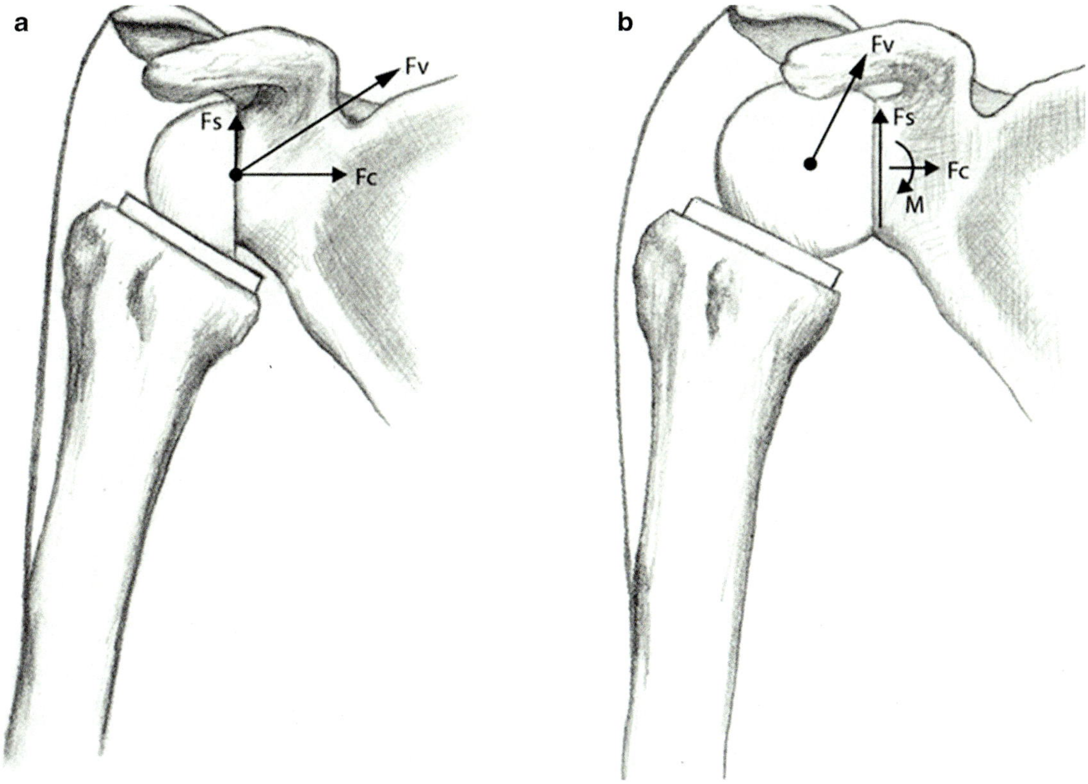

Fig. 22.3 (**a**) The resultant force vector (Fv) is obtained with both compressive (Fc) and shear (Fs) forces, all of them acting on the center of rotation located at the bone-implant interface on the surface of the glenoid [24]. (**b**) The lateralization of the center of rotation results in a reduction in compressive forces, a longer lever arm for destabilizing shear forces, and a new moment (M) at the bone-implant interface. Lateralization also provides for a larger impingement-free range of motion (Illustrations by Julianne Ho)

prosthesis and lateralized models: authors in favor of a medialized center of rotation glenosphere design point out the decreased forces on the glenoid baseplate and therefore the concomitant decreased rates of glenosphere loosening. They dismiss the scapular notching as largely avoidable with a lower baseplate placement, as well as questioning the actual clinical relevance of notching. On the other hand, authors preferring a lateralized design have underlined the greater impingement-free range of motion and the lower baseplate loosening rates obtained with locking screw fixation. Finally, advocates for the BIO-RSA have pointed out the high rate of graft incorporation and favorable bone-implant forces but must concede that this approach is more recent and has less supporting data in literature.

Nevertheless, the scientific community agrees in underlining the reduction of notching with the lateralized models.

In a recent systematic review by Lawrence et al., published in 2016, scapular notching was revealed in 44.9% of patients where a traditional 155° head-shaft angle was used, compared to 5.4% of patients where a more lateralized 135° head-shaft angle was used. However, the same authors claimed that the rate of clinically significant glenoid loosening was 1.8% in the traditional group and 8.8% with the lateralized implant. Finally, active external rotation was significantly increased in the lateralized group compared to the traditional group [29].

A possible alternative to the lateralization of the center of rotation, in order to avoid the risk of shear stress on the glenoid implant, consists in the humeral lateralization. Humeral lateralization has been defined as the difference between the humeral pivot point and the diaphyseal axis.

As Walch et al. [31] underlined, the humeral lateralization depends on elements like the shape of the humeral stem, the neck-shaft angle, and the onlay or inlay of the polyethylene spacer. The aim of the introduction of these new implants was the reduction of the notching, as well as the reduction of tuberosity and metaphyseal bone resorption.

Firstly, the humeral offset with a curved stem is increased compared to a straight stem, and this leads to an increase in the adduction range of movement.

Moreover, it has been well demonstrated that valgus implant designs, with a 155° neck-shaft angle, were related with a higher incidence of scapular notching compared to more varus neck-shaft angles, ranging from 135° to 143° [22, 32–34]; this effect may be increased by using thicker polyethylene insert. Finally, Walch obtained a higher lateralization construct with an outlay polyethylene, located outside the humerus (above the humerus cut): because of the height of the liner and the collar of the tray, in fact, a minimum 6 mm of lateralization is achieved.

In all these conditions, the center of rotation is shifted inferiorly, increasing, as a result, the adduction range of movement.

The glenosphere diameter may also contribute to humeral lateralization, to adduction improvement, and therefore to a reduction of the incidence of scapular notching. Although Gutièrrez et al. [35] demonstrated its minor role compared to the offset of the center of rotation and the glenoid position, the same authors established how larger glenospheres allow better range of motion without worsening the risk of dislocation. In fact, the jumping distance and the dislocation force do not increase as the diameter grows, as demonstrated through mechanical measurements. Therefore, the use of larger glenosphere can represent a valuable option to obtain better joint stability and reduce scapular notching.

Although we also use this option in our current practice, the major disadvantage of the humeral lateralization lies on the loss of the abduction range of motion due to acromial impingement.

22.5 Conclusion

The scientific community generally agrees on how the rate of complication after reverse shoulder arthroplasty relies on a correct surgical indication at first and afterward on the surgical technique.

Medialized and lateralized implants have demonstrated both advantages and disadvantages; the choice of implant therefore must depend on the patient clinical status, his everyday activities, and his expectations.

Biomechanical analysis [33, 36] has demonstrated that both humeral neck-shaft angle and glenosphere placement play the most important role in the reduction of scapular notching incidence and the increase of the range of motion in adduction (Fig. 22.4).

Procedures		Possible risks
Lateralization of the center of rotation		Increased glenoid loosening
Lateralization of the humerus	Stem design	
	Reducing humeral neck-shaft angles	
Baseplate inferior positioning		
Glenosphere inferior tilting		Reduce the longevity of the prosthesis
Increased Glenosphere diameter		

Fig. 22.4 Possible procedures to adopt in order to decrease the risk of scapular notching. Biomechanical analysis has demonstrated that both humeral neck-shaft angle and glenosphere placement play the most important role

There is still no consensus in literature on the correlation between scapular notching and poorer clinical results, as demonstrated by a systematic review published in 2015 [37, 38]. Nevertheless, the lack of studies with long-term follow-up makes further researches essential.

References

1. Sirveaux F, Favard L, Oudet D, et al. Grammont inverted total shoulder arthroplasty in the treatment of glenohumeral osteoarthritis with massive rupture of the cuff—results of a multicentre study of 80 shoulders. J Bone Joint Surg. 2004;86-B:388–95.
2. Nicholson GP, Strauss EJ, Sherman SL. Scapular notching recognition and strategies to minimize clinical impact. Clin Orthop Relat Res. 2011;469:2521–30.
3. Li X, Dines J, Warren R, et al. Inferior glenosphere placement reduces scapular notching in Reverse Total Shoulder Arthroplasty. Orthopedics. 2015;38(2):e88–93.
4. Ladermann A, Gueorguiev B, Charbonnier C, et al. Scapular notching on kinematic simulated range of motion after Reverse Shoulder Arthroplasty is not the result of impingement in adduction. Medicine. 2015;94(38):e1615.
5. Nyffeler RW, Werner CML, Simmen BR, et al. Analysis of a retrieved Delta III total shoulder prosthesis. J Bone Joint Surg. 2004;86-B:1187–91.
6. Werner CM, Steinmann PA, Gilbart M, Gerber C. Treatment of painful pseudoparesis due to irreparable rotator cuff dysfunction with the Delta III reverse-ball-and-socket total shoulder prosthesis. J Bone Joint Surg Am. 2005;87:1476–86.
7. Simovitch RW, Zumstein MA, Lohri E, et al. Predictors of scapular notching in patients managed with the Delta III reverse total shoulder replacement. J Bone Joint Surg Am. 2007;89:588–600.
8. Mollon B, Mahure SA, Roche CP, Zuckermann JD. Impact of scapular notching on clinical outcomes after reverse total shoulder arthroplasty: an analysis of 476 shoulders. J Shoulder Elb Surg. 2007;26:1253–61.
9. Boulahia A, Edwards TB, Walch G, Baratta RV. Early results of a reverse design prosthesis in the treatment of arthritis of the shoulder in elderly patients with a large rotator cuff tear. Orthopedics. 2002;25(2):129–33.
10. Boileau P, Gonzalez JF, Chuinard C, et al. Reverse total shoulder arthroplasty after failed rotator cuff surgery. J Shoulder Elb Surg. 2009;18(4):600–6.
11. Levigne C, Garret J, Boileau P, et al. Scapular notching in reverse shoulder arthroplasty:is it important to avoid it and how? Clin Orthop Relat Res. 2011;469:2512–20.
12. Delloye C, Joris D, Colette A, et al. Mechanical complications of total shoulder inverted prosthesis. Rev Chir Orthop Reparatrice Appar Mot. 2002;88(4):410–4.
13. Levigne C, Boileau P, Favard L, et al. Scapular notching in reverse shoulder arthroplasty. J Shoulder Elbow Surg. 2008;17:925–35.
14. Grassi FA, Murena L, Valli F, Alberio R. Six-year experience with the Delta III reverse shoulder prosthesis. J Orthop Surg. 2009;17(2):151–6.
15. Taliaferro JP, Crosby LA. Scapular notching in reverse total shoulder arthroplasty: now what? Semin Arthroplast. 2014;25:44–7.
16. Paisley KC, Kraeutler MJ, Lazarus MD, et al. Relationship of scapular neck length to scapular notching after reverse total shoulder arthroplasty by use of plain radiographs. J Shoulder Elb Surg. 2014;23:882–7.
17. Nyffeler RW, Werner CML, Gerber C. Biomechanical relevance of glenoid component positioning in the reverse Delta III total shoulder prosthesis. J Shoulder Elb Surg. 2005;14:524–8.
18. Kelly JD, Humphrey CS, Norris TR. Optimizing glenosphere position and fixation in reverse shoulder arthroplasty, Part One: The twelve-mm rule. J Shoulder Elb Surg. 2008;17:589–94.
19. Humphrey CS, Kelly JD, Norris TR. Optimizing glenosphere position and fixation in reverse shoulder arthroplasty, Part Two: The three-column concept. J Shoulder Elb Surg. 2008;17(4):595–601.
20. Gutierrez S, Walker M, Willis M, et al. Effects of tilt and glenosphere eccentricity on baseplate/bone interface forces in a computational model, validated by a mechanical model, of reverse shoulder arthroplasty. J Shoulder Elb Surg. 2011;20:732–9.
21. Huri G, Familiari F, Salari N, et al. Prosthetic design of reverse shoulder arthroplasty contributes to scapular notching and instability. World J Orthop. 2016;7(11):738–45.
22. Kempton LB, Balasubramaniam M, Ankerson E, Wiater JM. A radiographic analysis of the effects of glenosphere position on scapular notching following reverse total shoulder arthroplasty. J Shoulder Elb Surg. 2011;20:968–74.
23. Edwards TB, Trappey GJ, Riley C, et al. Inferior tilt of the glenoid component does not decrease scapular notching in reverse shoulder arthroplasty: results of a prospective randomized study. J Shoulder Elb Surg. 2012;21:641–6.
24. Berliner JL, Regalado-Magdos A, Ma CB, Feeley BT. Biomechanics of reverse total shoulder arthroplasty. J Shoulder Elb Surg. 2015;24:150–60.
25. Chae SW, Leeb J, Hanc SH, Kimd SY. Inferior tilt fixation of the glenoid component in reverse total shoulder arthroplasty: a biomechanical study. Orthop Traumatol Surg Res. 2015;101:421–5.
26. Ackland DC, Patel M, Knox D. Prosthesis design and placement in reversetotal shoulder arthroplasty. J Orthop Surg Res. 2015;10:101.
27. Frankle M, Siegal S, Pupello D, et al. The reverse shoulder prosthesis for glenohumeral arthritis associated with severe rotator cuff deficiency. A minimum two-year follow-up study of sixty patients. J Bone Joint Surg Am. 2005;87(8):1697–705.

28. Cuff D, Pupello D, Virani N, et al. Reverse shoulder arthroplasty for the treatment of rotator cuff deficiency. J Bone Joint Surg Am. 2008;90(6):1244–51.
29. Lawrence C, Williams GR, Namdari S. Influence of glenosphere design on outcomes and complications of reverse arthroplasty: a systematic review. Clin Orthop Surg. 2016;8:288–97.
30. Boileau P, Moineau G, Roussanne Y, O'Shea K. Bony increased-offset reversed shoulder arthroplasty minimizing scapular impingement while maximizing glenoid fixation. Clin Orthop Relat Res. 2011;469:2558–67.
31. Ladermann A, Denard PJ, Boileau P, et al. Effect of humeral stem design on humeral position and range of motion in reverse shoulder arthroplasty. Int Orthop. 2015;39:2205–13.
32. Kowalsky MS, Galatz LM, Shia DS, et al. The relationship between scapular notching and reverse shoulder arthroplasty prosthesis design. J Shoulder Elb Surg. 2012;21:1430–41.
33. Gutierrez S, Comiskey CA, Luo Z, et al. Range of impingement-free abduction and adduction deficit after Reverse Shoulder Arthroplasty : hierarchy of surgical and implant-design-related factors. J Bone Joint Surg Am. 2008;90:2606–15.
34. Erickson BJ, Frank RM, Harris JD, et al. The influence of humeral head inclination in reverse total shoulder arthroplasty: a systematic review. J Shoulder Elb Surg. 2015;24(6):988–93.
35. Gutierrez S, Keller TS, Levy JC, et al. Hierarchy of stability factors in reverse shoulder arthroplasty. Clin Orthop Relat Res. 2008;466:670–6.
36. Virani NA, Cabezas A, Gutierrez S, et al. Reverse shoulder arthroplasty components and surgical techniques that restore glenohumeral motion. J Shoulder Elb Surg. 2013;22:179–87.
37. Samitier G, Alentorn-Geli E, Torrens C, Wright TW. Reverse shoulder arthroplasty. Part 1: Systematic review of clinical and functional outcomes. Int J Shoulder Surg. 2015;9(1):24–31.
38. Samitier G, Alentorn-Geli E, Torrens C, Wright TW. Reverse shoulder arthroplasty. Part 2: Systematic review of reoperations, revisions, problems, and complications. Int J Shoulder Surg. 2015;9(2):60–7.

Fractures Sequelae

23

Chiara Fossati, Alessandra Menon,
Nicolò Cosmelli, and Pietro Randelli

23.1 Fractures Sequelae

Glenohumeral fractures, depending on the patient's general and local clinical situation, may hesitate in numerous complications.

They have different incidence and different clinical impact and consequently may involve different types of treatment.

23.1.1 Stiffness

Stiffness is the most frequent complication after a glenohumeral fracture mainly due to several combined factors, such as capsular contracture, mal-union, mechanical impingement or rotator cuff tears [1].

In capsular contracture pattern, the clinical situation might resemble a "frozen shoulder", and rotation and abduction are usually the most limited movements [1].

C. Fossati · A. Menon (✉) · N. Cosmelli · P. Randelli
Laboratory of Applied Biomechanics, U.O.C.
1st Department, Azienda Socio Sanitaria Territoriale
Centro Specialistico Ortopedico Traumatologico
Gaetano Pini-CTO, Milan, Italy

Department of Biomedical Sciences for Health,
University of Milan, Milan, Italy
e-mail: pietro.randelli@unimi.it

S. Gumina et al. (eds.), *Reverse Shoulder Arthroplasty*,
https://doi.org/10.1007/978-3-319-97743-0_23

23.1.2 Avascular Necrosis (AVN)

Osteonecrosis, also called avascular necrosis (AVN), is an infarction of bone marrow and bone tissue. It may be idiopathic or secondary. Secondary AVN is divided in traumatic and atraumatic, according to the aetiology. Post-traumatic AVN, which usually occurs in the humeral head, is a rare condition closely associated to multifragmentary fractures of the proximal humerus, and its presence may affect the functional recovery after such injuries [2]. In any case, AVN is caused by an impairment of the physiological blood supply.

The blood supply to the proximal humerus is guaranteed by the circumflexed anterior and posterior arteries. Most of the humeral head is vascularized by the arcuate artery, continuation of the falling branch of the anterior circumflex artery.

Post-traumatic AVN may also occur in the tuberosities which can "disappear" on an X-ray. The vascularization of the fractured tuberosities is guaranteed by the periosteal flow and by the rotator cuff attachments.

Immunocompromission, use of corticosteroids, heavy tobacco use and alcohol abuse are the principle predisposing factors for this disease.

Hertel et al. have shown that different fracture patterns are related to the possibility of developing AVN. In particular, they identify two anatomical criteria of fracture that have a high prognostic significance on necrosis: the length of the metaphysial calcar attached to the fractured head (bad if less than 8 mm) and the integrity of the medial hinge. The possibility of necrosis in complex fractures can reach 60%; therefore consider carefully whether reconstructing a complex fracture or proceeding with a primary prosthetic replacement [3].

In undisplaced fractures in valgus, where the medial hinge is, at least, partially preserved, osteosynthesis procedures are better tolerated with less chance of AVN [4].

Operative fixation of proximal humerus fractures (PHFs), compared to conservative treatment, has a significantly higher risk of development of AVN than conservative treatment [5]. The clinical features of AVN usually are functional impairment, pain and stiffness after a "latent period". The diagnosis is confirmed radiologically: collapse and resorption of the humeral head are usually shown with standard X-rays, but, in most of the cases, further investigations with magnetic resonance imaging (MRI) and computed tomography (CT) scans are needed.

It is possible to diagnose AVN when it is still asymptomatic and with initial radiological findings.

23.1.3 Positioning/Mobilization of Implants

In patients with poor bone quality, implant loosening is quite frequent. Modern systems with angular stability surely have advantages, but the correct position and length of implanted components (in particular screws in the humeral head) should always be very carefully checked intraoperatively using image intensifier (Fig. 23.1).

Factors that predispose the mobilization of the implant are osteoporosis and Parkinson's disease [1].

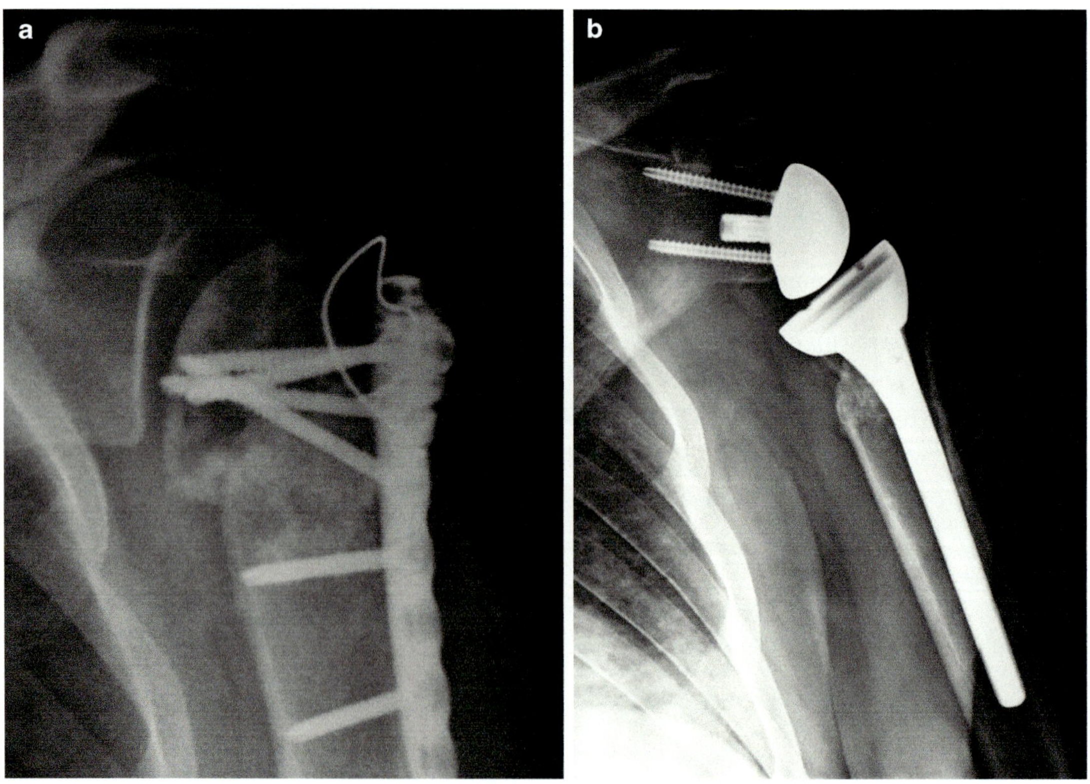

Fig. 23.1 Mobilization of the screws of the humeral head due to head collapse: preoperative (**a**) and postoperative (**b**) X-rays

An effective and rapid system for assessing bone quality was proposed by Tingart et al. They observed how the sum of medial and lateral humerus cortical thicknesses is significantly correlated to the degree of osteoporosis. A total thickness of less than 4 mm is a highly predictive of a low bone density value [6].

23.1.4 Nonunion

Nonunion is defined as a mobile fracture site 4–6 months post-injury. This complication is a rare occurrence at the proximal humerus level, but the presence of predisposing factors including immunocompromission, rheumatoid arthritis (RA), tumour malignancies, therapy with corticosteroids, heavy tobacco use and alcohol abuse can increase the risk of developing this sequelae [7].

Clinically, the shoulder is "pseudoparalytic", the range of motion (ROM) is painful, and, radiologically, there is an area of resorption at the level of the fracture line.

23.1.5 Mal-union

Mal-union after multifragmentary PHF results from both nonoperative and operative treatments. It is important to underline that a certain degree of displacement is a common finding after conservative treatment [7].

Two types of scenarios are the most common mal-union complications:

1. Mal-union of the head on the shaft: the epiphysis might heal impacted, angulated or translated. This pattern is usually well tolerated, and it is seldom a cause of secondary surgical intervention.
2. Mal-union of the tuberosities: the forces generated by the rotator cuff muscles are the cause of displaced healing of PHFs involving the tuberosities. Old patients usually well tolerate such extra-articular mal-unions unlike young subjects. Stronger muscles lead to malposition of the tuberosities during the healing process, hesitating in pain and functional impairments.

23.1.6 Nerve Lesions

The circumflexed (or axillary) nerve is the most frequently damaged nervous structure at this anatomical level, both for traumatic anterior dislocations and for intraoperative manoeuvring.

It innervates the deltoid muscles, the skin covering it and the teres minor. Its path is anterior and inferior to the margin of the glenoid. For this reason, it can often be involved during glenohumeral fracture-luxation. According to Visser et al., the incidence rises from 59% in composite fractures to 82% in displaced fractures. Fortunately, only few fractures result in permanent nerve damage, while in most of the other cases, nerve recovery is usually expected [8].

23.1.7 Infections

Peri-implant infections at the shoulder level are rare because vascularization of this area is good and the implants are deep, under generous soft tissues. An infection is even rarer in a patient who has been treated conservatively.

Diabetes, rheumatoid arthritis, corticosteroids, immunosuppression and metastatic tumours are the main predisposing factors [1, 7].

23.2 Treatment Options for Fractures Sequelae

As we saw above, fractures sequelae include many clinical scenarios and, consequently, many therapeutic options.

Treatment options for stiffness are multiple, from stretching to implant removal and from mobilization in narcosis to arthroscopic release. Manipulations under anaesthesia should be performed in a very gentle way in order to avoid humerus fractures, brachial plexus palsies and rotator cuff tears.

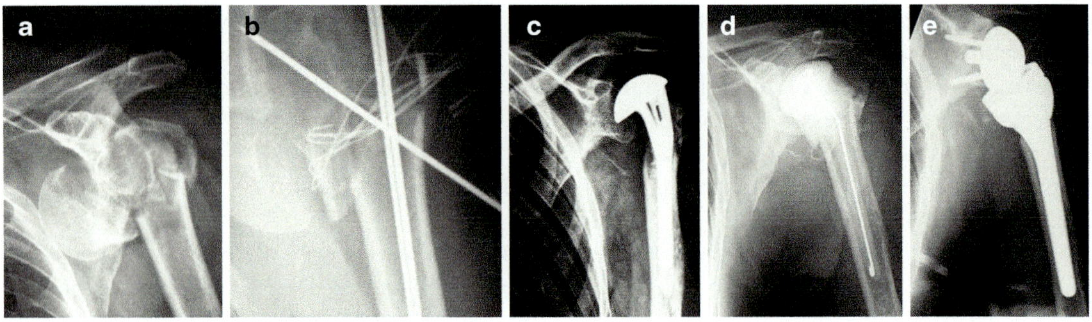

Fig. 23.2 Infection of the implant: X-rays of the (**a**) complex fracture of the proximal humerus with the head fragment dislocation, (**b**) failure of the fixation with k-wires, (**c**) infection of hemiarthroplasty, (**d**) two-stage treatment of the infection with spacer added with antibiotics and (**e**) final revision with RSA. RSA: reverse shoulder arthroplasty

Table 23.1 Classification of complications of PHFs and their recommended treatment [9]

Grade	Description	Recommended treatment
I	Osteonecrosis of the humeral head	Conventional arthroplasty
II	Neglected (locked) fracture dislocation	Conventional arthroplasty
III	Nonunion of the head-neck segment	Plate/bone graft if possible or RSA
IV	Head-tuberosity nonunion/mal-union	RSA

PHF proximal humerus fractures, *RSA* reverse shoulder arthroplasty

In case of peri-prosthetic infections, characterized by pathogens organized in biofilm, therapy should be aggressive. Removal of the implanted components, accurate debridement, intraoperative culture swabs, empirical antibiotic therapy and subsequent targeted antibiotic therapy are the basic steps in the treatment of peri-implant infections. Eventually, infection on the prosthetic implant can be treated in either one-stage or two-stage surgeries depending on the clinical case (Fig. 23.2).

Boileau et al. analysed the major complications and associated them to the most correct surgical option (Table 23.1) [9].

In the event of AVN of the humeral head isolated without loss of bone stock in the glenoid and with a functioning rotator cuff, if the conservative approach (the use of bisphosphonates, anticoagulants and vasodilators, hyperbaric therapy, core decompression, etc.) fails, the first surgical choice is an anatomical total shoulder prosthesis.

The spectrum of treatment in mal-unions is wide, and, for older patients, a conservative treatment with physiotherapy and pain management is often preferred.

When the surgical treatment is necessary, nonunions are usually treated with open reduction and internal fixation (ORIF) and eventually bone grafts if:

- An infection is excluded.
- There is adequate humeral head bone stock.
- There is no severe tuberosity mal-union.
- There are no signs of degenerative changes/collapse of the humeral articular surface.

In patients with insufficient bone stock and signs of osteoarthritis, a reverse shoulder arthroplasty (RSA) needs to be studied with appropriate preoperative planning [10].

When evaluating replacement, careful evaluation of the fracture and sequelae pattern is essential to predict the proper functioning of the rotator cuff [11].

Its correct behaviour is strictly necessary in a well-functioning anatomical total shoulder arthroplasty. Therefore, when there is the nonunion/mal-union of the head tuberosity, it is necessary to use a RSA in order to bypass the rotator cuff which is usually damaged at its insertion on the tuberosities (Figs. 23.3 and 23.4) [12–15].

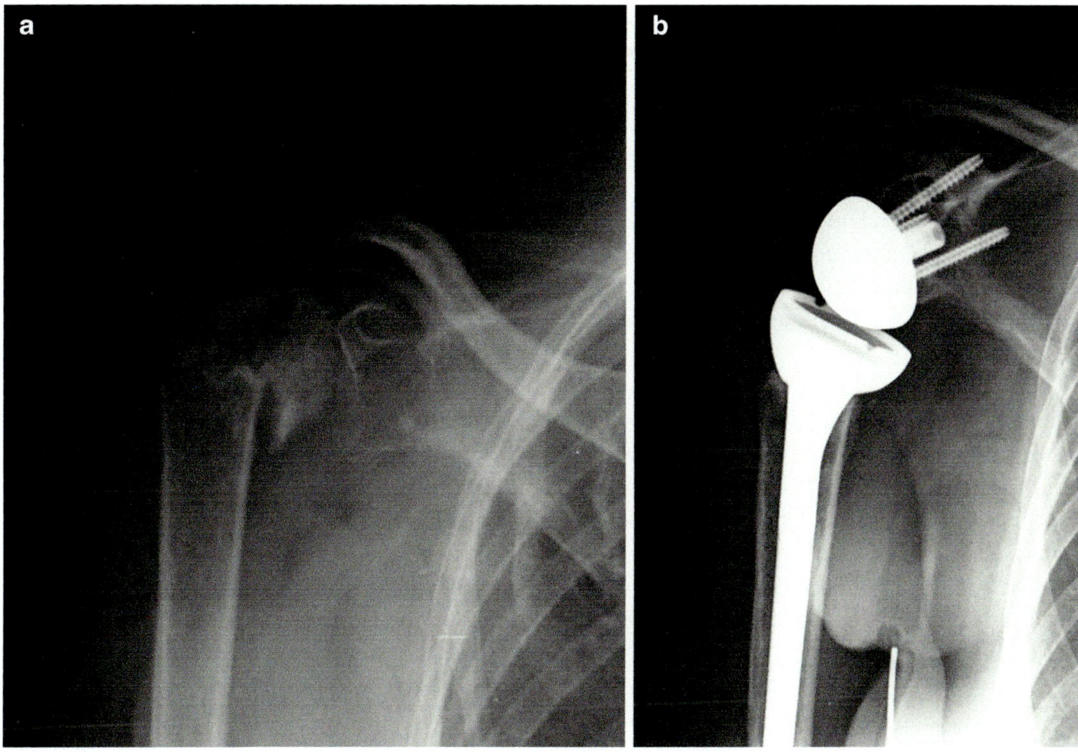

Fig. 23.3 Nonunion and avascular necrosis of the humeral head and tuberosities: preoperative (**a**) and postoperative (**b**) X-rays

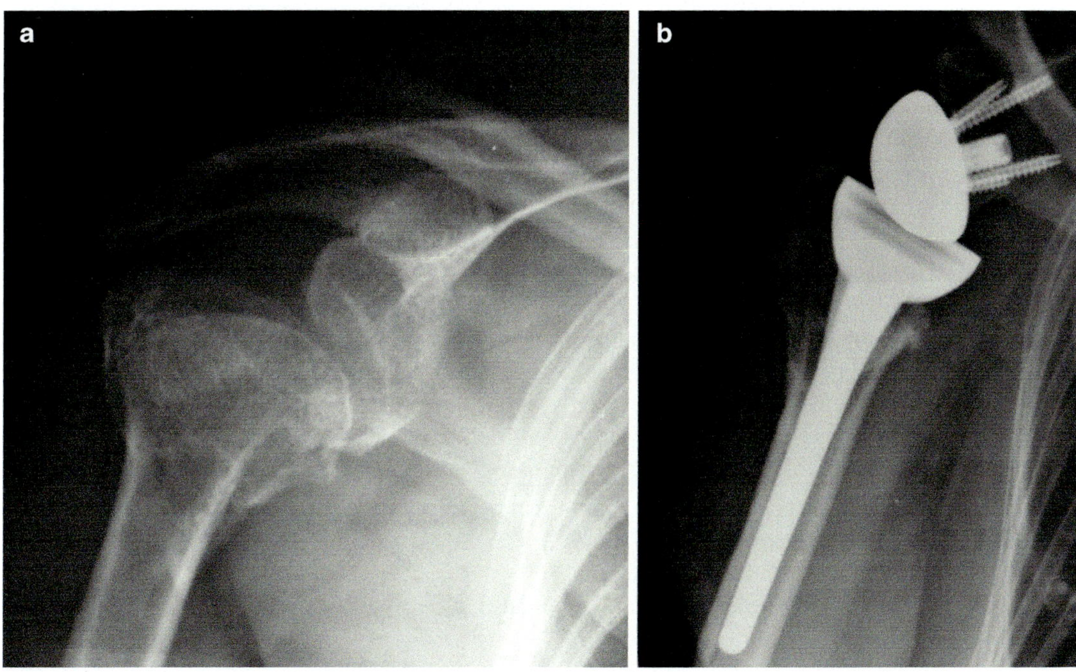

Fig. 23.4 Mal-union of the head and tuberosities: preoperative (**a**) and postoperative (**b**) X-rays

23.3 Reverse Shoulder Arthroplasty in Glenohumeral Fractures Sequelae

23.3.1 Imaging and Planning

For a correct approach to RSA in the treatment of sequelae, an accurate customized preoperative planning is extremely important.

Therefore, the radiological investigations must include:

- Standard X-rays: calculation of angles of deformity and the evaluation of the glenohumeral arthritis. It is suggested to obtain a scaled X-ray of both shoulders in order to analyse shortenings or medialization of bone fragments.
- MRI: a careful evaluation of the rotator cuff.
- CT: assessment of possible bone loss with 3D reconstructions.

An appropriate bone stock is not always guaranteed, and failing to address glenoid bone loss may complicate the execution of surgery, resulting in later dislocation or scapular notching [16].

Some authors described humeral bone defects as a predictor of revision RSA outcome. Patients with great metaphyseal bone loss (>3 cm) had a significant lower Constant score. These findings were correlated to degenerative conditions of the teres minor muscle [17].

In order to prevent malalignment and loosening of the prosthetic components, bone grafts can be used [18]. In the vast majority of cases, RSA and bone grafting are performed as a single one-stage procedure.

The surgeon may choose between several options:

1. Autograft
    - Humeral head: the addition of this bone graft to the implant is named the "bio-RSA". It is used in the majority of cases with good results [16]. The obvious advantages are no additional incisions or sources of pain and short surgical time loss. It is not advisable to harvest the humeral head in an AVN setting for obvious reasons [16, 18].
    - Tricortical iliac crest: The technique of harvesting this autograft has been described by Norris et al. It is advised to implant the baseplate directly on the crest obtaining an immediate solid fixation of the implant on the graft. The graft is harvested, and, subsequently, both implant and graft are fixated to the scapula [19]. Local iliac pain after the osteotomy is the main disadvantage to this procedure.
2. Allograft

    If the surgeon faces large bone defects and humeral head quality is poor or when it is advisable to avoid iliac crest autograft morbidity, allografts can be used. The femoral neck is one of the preferred options due to its anatomical similarity to native glenoid [20].

23.3.2 Surgical Approach

There are mainly two surgical approaches for RSA surgery: the antero-superior and the delto-pectoral approach.

There is no unanimous consensus on the effect that the approach can have on the prosthetic implant in terms of baseline positioning or scapular notching [21].

In the authors' experience, the delto-pectoral approach guarantees a better control on the glenoid version while preserving the deltoid muscle, the main actor in the RSA functioning.

23.3.3 Positioning

The patient is placed in beach-chair decubitus, with the trunk raised at 30° and hips and knees flexed at 45°. The head is slightly inclined towards the opposite side and the upper limb is free [21].

23.3.4 Anaesthesia

Surgery is usually performed under a general anaesthetic with an interscalene block.

23.3.5 Surgical Technique

The incision is vertical, starting from the apex of the coracoid process and reaching to the anterior axillary angle. In the case of a previous surgical scar, we suggest to use the same surgical route.

Cicatricial adhesions may alter the physiological surgical findings described below. It is important to perform a wide lysis of scar tissue, proceeding with caution in order to avoid damage of axillary nerve.

After haemostasis, the deltoid-pectoral sulcus is identified. It is easier to identify in the upper part of the incision due to the different path of muscle fibres.

Cephalic vein can be either moved or bound, preferring to do so at the proximal level, before its anastomosis with axillary vein (authors prefer to move it laterally).

The incision of the clavi-pectoral fascia is performed along the lateral edge of the conjoint tendon which is retracted medially.

The subscapularis tendon is highlighted, and by placing the limb in external rotation, the upper and lower margins are identified.

Along the lower margin, you should pay attention to the anterior circumflex arteries along the lower edge, which must be tied and cauterized in order to avoid acute and delayed bleeding.

The subscapular tendon is cut at about 1 cm from its insertion on the small tuberosity, with vertical incision. A vertical anterior capsulotomy is performed, paying attention to the axillary nerve.

With a gentle external rotation and extension, the front humeral head can be displaced.

For the cutting guide positioning, the bicipital groove or the transepicondylar axis can be used as a reference point.

Perform a retroversion calculation according to the preoperative planning on CT imaging and surgeon's preferences.

Diaphysis is prepared with progressive cutters.

One challenging aspect of the humeral preparation in sequelae secondary surgeries is the tuberosities condition. As previously described, there might be a selective AVN of the tuberosities or a consistent mal-union, and the normal anatomical references can be altered.

In order to perform the correct humeral cuts, it is advisable to take accurate measures on the X-ray of the contralateral side.

The glenoid is accurately exposed with debridement of osteophytes and is prepared with special cutters.

We proceed with the metaglene and glenosphere implant, and then it's back to the humeral side where a proof stem is implanted.

The stability of the implant is challenging due to a lack of anatomical references and is often link to the sensibility and experience of the surgeon. We suggest to choose the final stem and tray with an evaluating of the conjoint tendon tension, with an "index test" (the capacity of implant dislocation with the surgeon index finger) and with the shoulder ROM.

The ROM is tested mimicking the movements of patient daily activity, as combing (abduction and extra-rotation) and performing intimate hygiene (adduction, extension and intra-rotation).

The sutures, which are to be used to reattach the tuberosities, are inserted at the supraspinatus tendo-osseous junction or through the greater tuberosity fragment before the insertion of the humeral implant.

Excessive tightening when fixing the tuberosities must be avoided in order to prevent limitation of external or internal rotation which might result from over-reduction of, respectively, lesser or greater tuberosities.

After the implant of definitive stem and tray, new stability and movement tests are performed. Authors suggest to carefully suture the tendon of subscapularis with non-absorbable sutures. At the end of the procedure, a drain is placed and usually removed the day after surgery.

23.3.6 Postoperative Management

We performed a standard postoperative protocol with a shoulder immobilization for 28 days in 30° abduction with early mobilization of the elbow, wrist, hand and scapula-thoracic plane. Antithrombotic and antibiotic prophylaxis is administered postoperatively.

Gentle passive physiotherapy starts after 28 days, while active exercises of the shoulder start after 2 months. Clinical examination and imaging examination are taken at 2 and 6 months of follow-up.

23.4 Conclusions

The management of glenohumeral fractures (GHFs) is complicated, and the clinical outcomes might be not satisfying for both patient and physician.

The sequelae are different and must be faced with an accurate customized surgical plan which must include extensive imaging examinations.

RSA is certainly a valid option in the treatment of GHF complications. It allows to solve the most difficult cases in different clinical situations, such as post-traumatic arthritis in rotator cuff failure, AVN and nonunions/mal-unions [22].

Current literature is focusing on the timing of RSA for GHFs, comparing acute/primary arthroplasty for fracture management and late/secondary arthroplasty for sequelae.

Even if both "acute" and "late" RSA can obtain a postoperative pain relief and significant functional improvement compared with their preoperative condition, late RSA shows lower functional scores and higher complication rates [23, 24]. In particular, secondary RSA results in higher rates of scapular notching and in worse active external rotation motion [25]. These different results can be explained by the fact that an easier and more accurate great tuberosity reconstruction is obtainable in acute RSA [26].

Conflict of Interest Prof. Pietro Randelli is consultant for DePuy and Arthrex. The other authors declare no commercial associations (e.g. consultancies, stock ownership, equity interest, patent/licensing arrangements, etc.) that might pose a conflict of interest in connection with the submitted manuscript.

References

1. Ruedi T, Buckley R, Moran CG. AO principles of fracture management. New York: George Thieme Verlag; 2007.
2. Patel S, Colaco HB, Elvey ME, Lee MH. Post-traumatic osteonecrosis of the proximal humerus. Injury. 2017;46:1878–84.
3. Hertel R, Hempfing A, Stiehler M, Leunig M. Predictors of humeral head ischemia after intracapsular fracture of the proximal humerus. J Shoulder Elb Surg. 2004;13:427–33.
4. Jakob R, Miniaci A. Four-part valgus impacted fractures of the proximal humerus. J Bone Joint Surg Br. 1991;73:295–8.
5. Xu J, Zhang C, Wang T. Avascular necrosis in proximal humeral fractures in patients treated with operative fixation: a meta-analysis. J Orthop Surg Res. 2014;9:31.
6. Tingart MJ, Apreleva M, von Stechow D, Zurakowski D, Warner JJ. The cortical thickness of the proximal humeral diaphysis predicts bone mineral density of the proximal humerus. J Bone Joint Surg Br. 2003;85(4):611–7.
7. Buchholz, R.W., Court-Brown, C.M, Heckman, JD, Tornetta, P, E. Rockwood and green's fractures in adults. 7th ed. Lippincott Williams Wilkins Philadelphia 2010.
8. Visser CPJ, Coene LNJEM, Brand R, Tavy DLJ. Nerve lesions in proximal humeral fractures. J Shoulder Elb Surg. 2001;10:421–7.
9. Boileau P, Chuinard C, Le Huec JC, Walch G, Trojani C. Proximal humerus fracture sequelae: impact of a new radiographic classification on arthroplasty. Clin Orthop Relat Res. 2006;442:121–30.
10. Grubhofer F, et al. Reverse total shoulder arthroplasty for failed open reduction and internal fixation of fractures of the proximal humerus. J Shoulder Elb Surg. 2017;26:92–100.
11. Hattrup SJ, Waldrop R, Sanchez-Sotelo J. Reverse total shoulder arthroplasty for posttraumatic sequelae. J Orthop Trauma. 2016;30:e41–7.
12. Gigis I, Nenopoulos A, Giannekas D, Heikenfeld R, Beslikas T, Hatzokos I. Reverse shoulder arthroplasty for the treatment of 3 and 4- part fractures of the humeral head in the elderly. Open Orthop J. 2017;11:108–18.
13. Holton J, Yousri T, Arealis G, Levy O. The role of reverse shoulder arthroplasty in management of proximal humerus fractures with fracture sequelae: a systematic review of the literature. Orthop Rev (Pavia). 2017;9:27–31.
14. Raiss P, Edwards TB, da Silva MR, Bruckner T, Loew M, Walch G. Reverse shoulder arthroplasty for the treatment of nonunions of the surgical neck of the proximal part of the humerus (type-3 fracture sequelae). J Bone Joint Surg Am. 2014;96:2070–6.
15. Schliemann B, Theisen C, Kösters C, Raschke MJ, Weimann A. Reverse total shoulder arthroplasty for type I fracture sequelae after internal fixation of proximal humerus fractures. Arch Orthop Trauma Surg. 2017;137(12):1677–83.
16. Seidl AJ, Williams GR, Boileau P. Challenges in reverse shoulder arthroplasty: addressing glenoid bone loss. Orthopedics. 2016;39:14–23.

17. Greiner S, et al. The metaphyseal bone defect predicts outcome in reverse shoulder arthroplasty for proximal humerus fracture sequelae. Arch Orthop Trauma Surg. 2014;134:755–64.
18. Garofalo R, Brody F, Castagna A, Ceccarelli E, Krishnan SG. Reverse shoulder arthroplasty with glenoid bone grafting for anterior glenoid rim fracture associated with glenohumeral dislocation and proximal humerus fracture. Orthop Traumatol Surg Res. 2016;102:989–94.
19. Norris TR, Kelly JD, Humphrey CS. Management of glenoid bone defects in revision shoulder arthroplasty: a new application of the reverse total shoulder prosthesis. Tech Shoulder Elb Surg. 2007;8:37–46.
20. Bateman E, Donald SM. Reconstruction of massive uncontained glenoid defects using a combined autograft-allograft construct with reverse shoulder arthroplasty: preliminary results. J Shoulder Elb Surg. 2012;21:925–34.
21. Bentley G. European surgical orthopaedics and traumatology. In: The EFORT textbook. Heidelberg: Springer; 2014.
22. Alentorn-Geli E, Guirro P, Santana F, Torrens C. Treatment of fracture sequelae of the proximal humerus: comparison of hemiarthroplasty and reverse total shoulder arthroplasty. Arch Orthop Trauma Surg. 2014;134:1545–50.
23. Nikola C, Hrvoje K, Nenad M. Reverse shoulder arthroplasty in acute fractures provides better results than in revision procedures for fracture sequelae. Int Orthop. 2014;39:343–8.
24. Sebastia-Forcada E, et al. Outcomes of reverse total shoulder arthroplasty for proximal humeral fractures: primary arthroplasty versus secondary arthroplasty after failed proximal humeral locking plate fixation. J Orthop Trauma. 2017;31(8):e236–40.
25. Lévigne C, et al. Scapular notching in reverse shoulder arthroplasty. J Shoulder Elb Surg. 2008;17:925–35.
26. Seidl A, et al. Early versus late reverse shoulder arthroplasty for proximal humerus fractures: does it matter? Arch Bone Joint Surg. 2017;5(4):213–20.

Proximal Humerus Neoplasia

24

Raimondo Piana, Nicola Ratto, Andrea Ferro, and Michele Boffano

24.1 Introduction

The reconstruction of the proximal humerus following a tumor resection remains a big challenge for the orthopedic surgeon. The glenohumeral joint functionality depends on a complex stabilization system both static and dynamic including the periarticular soft tissues that are often sacrificed during the resection because it is invaded by the tumor. As a result, the joint function is impaired by a limitation of the articular range of motion and an increased instability of the shoulder. The purpose is obviously different depending on tumor malignancy: in primary bone sarcomas, the oncological outcome prevails over the function, and an amputation rate of about 5% has already been a great achievement in recent years [1].

On the other side, when soft tissue tumors invade the bone in the upper extremity as anywhere else in the body, they require a bone resection to obtain clear margins, according to Enneking's principles [2]; therefore, in a simplified way from a surgical point of view, they could be considered as bone sarcomas with soft tissue invasion.

The proximal humerus is also a very common site of metastasis for carcinomas. Following US and Canadian surveys, metastatic bone disease involves 50% of all patients with a primitive cancer and 30% of patients with a new diagnosis of carcinoma along their life [3, 4]. Most metastatic patients require nonsurgical or minimally invasive surgical treatments. Nevertheless, an early cancer diagnosis and new chemotherapy protocols determine an improvement in overall long-term survival, sometimes obtaining a chronicization of the oncologic disease with a subsequent need for surgical interventions to guarantee an acceptable quality of life. Extensive bone resections comparable to those for primitive bone tumors are increasingly performed in patients with solitary metastatic lesions to reduce the tumor burden and improve survival [5]. As a general rule for metastatic surgery, "the reconstruction should survive the patient" because it is always very difficult to revise an implant after several years, in an older patient, with a probable progression of disease.

The age and comorbidities of the patient are other factors influencing the choice of the treatment.

Many different options have been described to reconstruct the shoulder after a proximal humerus resection, and these should respect the following goals:

- Stability of the glenohumeral joint, allowing the functionality of the elbow and the hand
- Pain control
- Restoration of passive and active mobility

R. Piana (✉) · N. Ratto · A. Ferro · M. Boffano
Orthopedic Oncologic Surgery, CTO Hospital, AOU Città della Salute e della Scienza, Torino, Italy
e-mail: rpiana@cittadellasalute.to.it

S. Gumina et al. (eds.), *Reverse Shoulder Arthroplasty*, https://doi.org/10.1007/978-3-319-97743-0_24

In some cases, an allograft or an autograft arthrodesis is preferred, because even though it cannot grant a wide arch of mobility, it restores a stable shoulder, allowing a satisfactory elbow and hand function for the common daily activities.

The restoration of a mobile joint can be obtained with endoprosthetic replacements (EPR – tumor prosthesis), osteoarticular allografts, and allograft-prosthetic composites. Although all of these reconstructive methods are in use and there are some situations where only one approach might be appropriate for a particular patient, there are many scenarios in which all of them are potential options.

While there is still no consensus about the best technique of the proximal humerus reconstruction, the use of a reverse shoulder arthroplasty (RSA) associated or not to an allograft seems to provide the best functional results [6, 7]. However, sometimes the residual anatomy after the tumor resection can help in the decision process for the reconstruction.

24.2 Anatomical Considerations

The main problem for the surgeon facing a proximal humerus tumor is the complex anatomy of the shoulder. To obtain an adequate resection with wide margins, the resection of the rotator cuff and/or deltoid muscles and the axillary nerve is often necessary. A detailed physical preoperative examination and an accurate imaging study assist the surgeon to establish the best planning for both resection and reconstruction phases. The physical examination may suggest a neurovascular involvement or compression by abnormal neurovascular findings or by a decreased pulse and an involvement of the glenohumeral joint by the presence of pain or by a reduced range of motion.

A complete imaging study includes standard radiographs, a computed tomography (CT), and a magnetic resonance imaging (MRI). While MRI is useful to determine the soft tissue involvement and the tumor extension into the joint, CT scan is preferred to evaluate cortical bone changes, invasion, or destruction. Tc99 bone scan or FDG PET/CT may help to evaluate the intraosseous tumor extension and to detect other bone or visceral metastases. Although vessels can be well visualized using MRI, an arteriography or even better a CT angiography is essential to study the relationship between the tumor and the main vessels and whether or not they are included in the neoplasm. For example, the extension of a bone sarcoma in the axillary fossa and the involvement of the major vascular-nerve axes impose a shoulder disarticulation or a forequarter amputation in order to obtain adequate margins.

On the other hand, a tumor that spreads from the lower part of the capsule and from the humeral neck may frequently invade or involve the posterior circumflex branch and the axillary nerve, and consequently the resection would cause a loss of function of the deltoid muscle.

An accurate study of the bone and the articular surfaces of the glenohumeral joint is mandatory during preoperative planning and allows to classify the lesion according to the surgical system described by Malawer [8]. According to his classification, the humeral head is always resected in bone tumors of the shoulder joint. However, it is important to know if the tumor invades the joint. In these cases, an en bloc resection of the proximal humerus, the joint capsule, and the glenoid, called extra-compartmental resection (type V resection according to Malawer's classification), is necessary. When there is no joint extension of the tumor and the scapular glenoid can be spared, an intra-compartmental resection can be performed (type I resection). Obviously, in an extra-compartmental resection, the remaining scapula prevents the implantation of a glenoid component and the possibility of a functional reconstruction.

Finally, it is necessary to evaluate the extension of the neoplasm in the soft tissues. The articular capsule and the rotator cuff muscle tendons, which ensure joint stability and allow active shoulder mobility, are often sacrificed. The excision of most of the deltoid muscle affects the glenohumeral joint function and questions the indication to RSA.

24.3 Principles of Reconstruction

The reconstruction of the shoulder after tumor resection takes into account the bone, the joint, and the periarticular soft tissues.

The bone can be replaced with a modular or one-block custom-made prosthesis or with a massive humeral allograft from the local musculoskeletal bone bank. A recycled autograft (autoclave, nitrogen cryotherapy, external irradiation) is nowadays seldom used in the Western countries.

Different options are described for the reconstruction of the glenohumeral joint. The key factors, which influence the choice, are the preservation of the rotator cuff tendons and/or the axillary nerve, as shown in Fig. 24.1.

A completely biological reconstruction is performed with an osteoarticular allograft including the articular cartilage, allowing the direct suture of the capsule and the donor tendons to the soft tissue around the shoulder. However, the observed early cartilage degeneration over time dealt to a gradual dismissal of this exclusive technique [9].

The current trend is to use the allograft associated with a resurfacing prosthesis or a conventional long-stemmed endoprosthesis to fix the allograft to the residual bone. This solution called allograft-prosthetic composite (APC) combines a more durable reconstruction of the articular surfaces with a prosthesis and allows to reattach the patient's tendons.

As well as in patients with irreparable rotator cuff degenerative tears, in patients with excision of the rotator cuff for oncologic margins, the preferred functional solution is a RSA.

This mechanical concept in contrast to the normal anatomy provides a degree of stability even in the absence of soft tissue reconstruction and an active motility by means of the deltoid muscle even in the absence of rotator cuff. To guarantee a functional RSA reconstruction, the resection should be intra-compartmental and preserve the circumflex nerve and a relevant amount of the deltoid muscle.

A RSA can be implanted as a proximal humerus endoprosthetic replacement or in association with an allograft forming an APC.

The lack of function of deltoid muscle is not an absolute contraindication. The partial resection of the anterior part of the axillary nerve leads to the loss of the only anterior muscle fibers resulting in loss of active forward flexion, but maintaining good function on the other planes.

Streitbuerger obtained a better function in patients with RSA and partial deltoid function than in patients with a conventional anatomical prosthesis and intact deltoid function [10].

In selected cases the complete absence of the deltoid muscle may be supplied with a latissimus dorsi muscle transfer either pedicled or as a free flap.

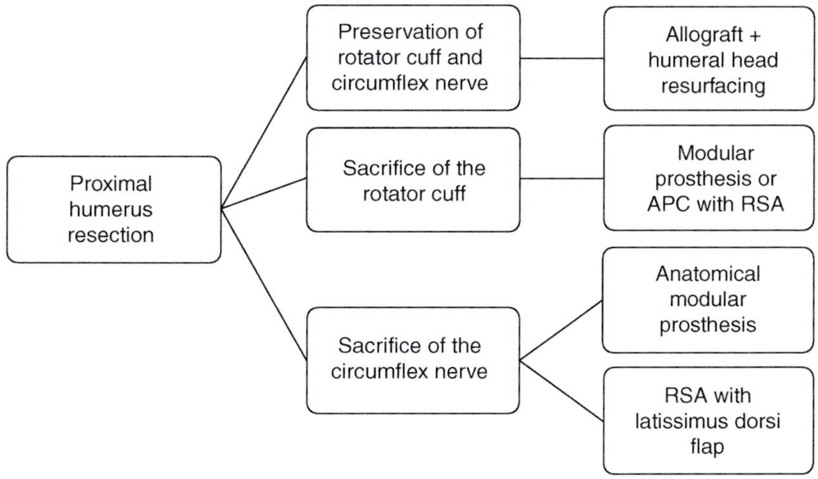

Fig. 24.1 Schematic diagram representing the possible reconstructive solutions based on the type of resection and surrounding soft tissue involvement

When a RSA is not indicated, an anatomical prosthesis can be implanted as an endoprosthetic replacement or as an APC with a conventional long-stemmed prosthesis. In the first case, the shoulder function is similar to a spacer and limited because the reinsertion of rotator cuff tendons at the prosthesis does not represent an efficient and durable reconstruction [11].

The tendons and the capsule can be sutured in an anatomical APC, but usually the abduction is limited to a maximum of 70° [12].

24.4 Surgical Technique for Reverse Prostheses

The first surgical step in orthopedic oncology is the biopsy. Although often underestimated, the biopsy is crucial, because its tract must be carefully excised with the tumor at the time of the definitive surgery. Following the general biopsy principles, the deltopectoral interval should not be used for the risk to contaminate two different anatomical compartments. An approach through the anterior fibers of the deltoid muscle is usually used. To prevent the removal of a large portion of the deltoid and therefore allow a good residual functionality, the biopsy should be through the deltoid muscle but as near as possible to the deltopectoral interval.

As already mentioned, a preoperative complete imaging study is mandatory to evaluate the extension of the tumor. A coronal image of the entire humerus is necessary to determinate the correct length of the bone and soft tissue resection.

Proximally the incision generally begins from the acromioclavicular joint area continuing distally to include the biopsy tract. The skin incision should be extended till the area of the distal bone resection. The dissection continues through the deltoid muscle, which is always split, leaving the contaminated tissue with the resected tumor and preserving the cephalic vein.

Each tumor has its own localization and expansion, which makes each intervention different from the other.

The major vascular-nerve bundle should always be under surgeon's control to guarantee an accurate dissection (adventitia and perineurium are generally excellent barriers to tumor extension) and to avoid an excessive stretching during tumor removal or prosthesis implantation.

In an intra-compartmental resection, the articular surface is reached after the dissection of the subscapularis muscle, the pectoralis muscles, and the anterior capsule, leaving a safe margin from the humerus and the tumor. Similarly a conservative capsulotomy should be completed; the rotator cuff and the posterior portion of the latissimus dorsi and teres major muscles should be dissected, leaving a safe margin but preserving the maximum possible length. The tendons and the capsule portions are singularly armored with nonabsorbable stitches before their sectioning. If it is planned to use a RSA, the axillary nerve should be identified and protected along the inferior edge of the subscapularis muscle. After separating the humerus from the glenoid, the dissection proceeds distally to isolate the humerus and the tumor by ensuring wide margins. The goal is to preserve as much as possible muscular tissue and all the vascular and nerve structures. If the humerus resection is distal to the insertion of the deltoid muscles, its tendinous insertion should be spared for later repair. Then, the humerus is resected distally as planned with preoperative imaging, carefully protecting the radial nerve and the vascular structures. A frozen histological examination of the distal bone marrow could be performed to confirm the absence of pathological tissue and consequently the right extension of resection. At this point, the tumor is excised en bloc and sent for pathology and the reconstructive phase may start.

Differently if an extra-compartmental articular resection is needed, the capsule should be excised entirely, and the glenohumeral joint should not be opened. The proximal surgical access is prolonged medially to identify the neck of the scapula and the coracoid process. One or two Hohmann retractors are placed on the neck of the scapula, and the scapular resection is performed. A particular attention should be paid to the major neurovascular structures at the base of the coracoid: the axillary nerve, the axillary artery, and the lateral cord of the brachial plexus.

The reconstruction can start either distally on the residual humeral shaft or proximally on the scapula.

The most used modular prostheses can switch from a reverse to an anatomical proximal component any time during surgery according to the intrinsic stability and the spared muscular structures. If the surgeon is in doubt on which reconstruction to perform, it would be better to start with the distal humerus preparation. The humeral shaft is reamed with progressively growing manual or motorized rasps according to the available instrumentation till the desired diameter to implant the right size of a cemented or an uncemented stem. The usual length of the stem of a proximal humerus tumor prosthesis ranges from 8 to 10 cm. Some modular prostheses used to have an external flange plate to increase the fixation with one or two screws going from the plate to the other cortex passing through the stem.

If an APC reconstruction is performed, the distal humerus is prepared or not according to the preferred fixation whether with the distal portion of a long-stemmed prosthesis or a plate. On a separate table, the humeral allograft is prepared by cutting the humeral head in a standard way and resecting the humeral shaft at least 1 cm longer than the measured resection. The humeral lengthening allows a better pretension of the deltoid muscle, but if necessary a distal recut is still possible. The allograft and the host bone osteotomies have to match accurately. This junction can be either represented by two transverse plain surfaces or a proper dovetail connection. A dovetail technique is recently preferred because of its intrinsic increased stability.

An osteosynthesis with plate and a humeral short-stemmed implant is more prone to end with a mechanical failure due to the torsional forces as described in the clinical case in Fig. 24.2.

The use of a long stem that goes beyond the host bone-allograft junction ensures greater stability. In this case, the humeral allograft and the distal native canal are sequentially reamed and then broached, before testing with the trial components. The allograft is usually over-reamed compared with the native humerus to allow a better fit at the host bone-allograft junction. Once the stability and the soft tissue tension appear to be appropriate, the definitive reconstruction of the proximal humerus is carried out by maintaining the correct retroversion. The prosthesis stem is usually cemented both in the allograft and in the host bone shafts, as shown in the clinical case presented in Fig. 24.3. Some authors add a unicortical plate while the cement is hardening in order to neutralize the rotational forces and enhance compression at the host bone-allograft junction [13].

The glenoid implant is similar to any conventional RSA facilitated by a wider exposure due to the absence of the resected proximal humerus. Every prosthesis has its instrumentation to guide the implantation of the glenoid component usually fixed into the bone with a peg and one or two screws. The use of a lateralized glenosphere is more advisable in case of partial deltoid muscle loss or any concern for deltoid dysfunction. The lateralization of the glenosphere will change the natural humeral center of rotation, but creating a more compressive force from the deltoid.

When a modular EPR is implanted, the choice between a cemented and an uncemented stem depends on the age and the bone quality of the patient but often on the surgeon's beliefs and habits. A modular implant allows to change the stem whether cemented or uncemented and the reconstruction length according not only to the resection but also to the right tension of the soft tissues. If the EPR is custom-made, the choice of the stem and the length must be decided 3–4 weeks preoperatively, and no intraoperative changes are possible.

After the implantation of the definitive prosthesis, all the muscular tendons, which have been spared, should be singularly reattached. The rotator cuff and the deltoid tendons may be sutured to the corresponding allograft tendon insertions using nonabsorbable suture wires. In orthopedic oncology, the posterior components of the rotator cuff are easier to reattach than in standard RSA,

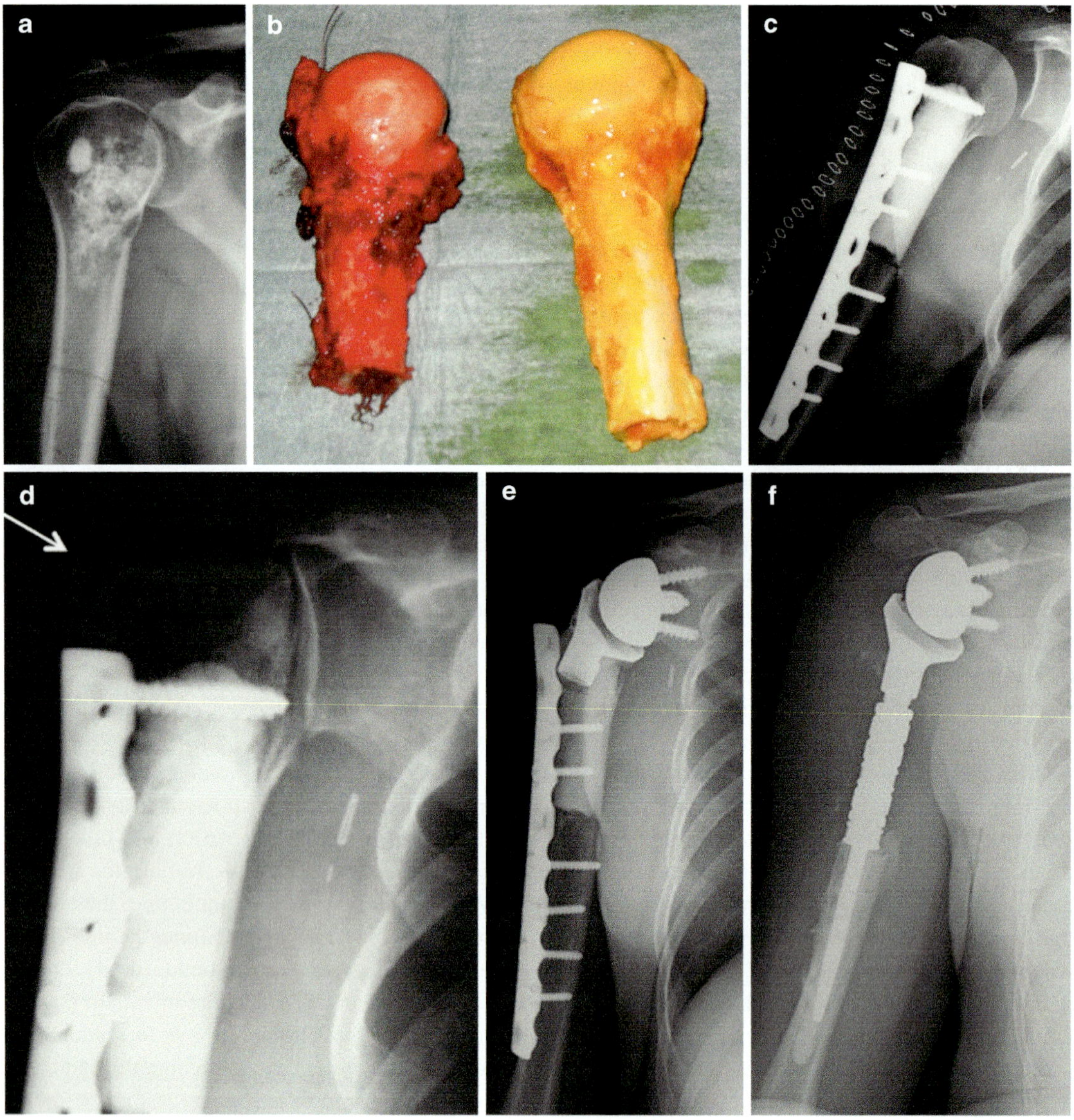

Fig. 24.2 A 41-year-old woman treated several years before for a central chondrosarcoma of the proximal humerus. (**a**) X-ray of the lesion. (**b**) On the left the specimen of the tumor resection, on the right the proximal humerus allograft. (**c**, **d**) The osteochondral reconstruction failed due to the bone reabsorption. The deformity of the humeral head caused a progressive arm dysfunction requiring a conversion to a RSA after about 3 years from the first implant. (**e**) The use of a short stem led to a new failure after only 1 year. (**f**) The last picture shows X-ray control at 8 years from revision prosthetic reconstruction resulting in a fair function of the upper limb during daily life activities over the years

thanks to the wide exposure for tumor excision. If the tendons should be attached to the prostheses, it can be performed directly to the prosthesis or through an attachment tube. Several prostheses are provided with holes to pass the suture wires to anchor the tendons or with special porous surfaces (e.g., Trabecular Metal™) and an overlying fixation plate. Synthetic attachment tubes, usually made by polyethylene terephthalate, are available off the shelves to be fixed on the prosthetic shaft to allow the tendon fixation and to increase the implant stability by a capsular suture.

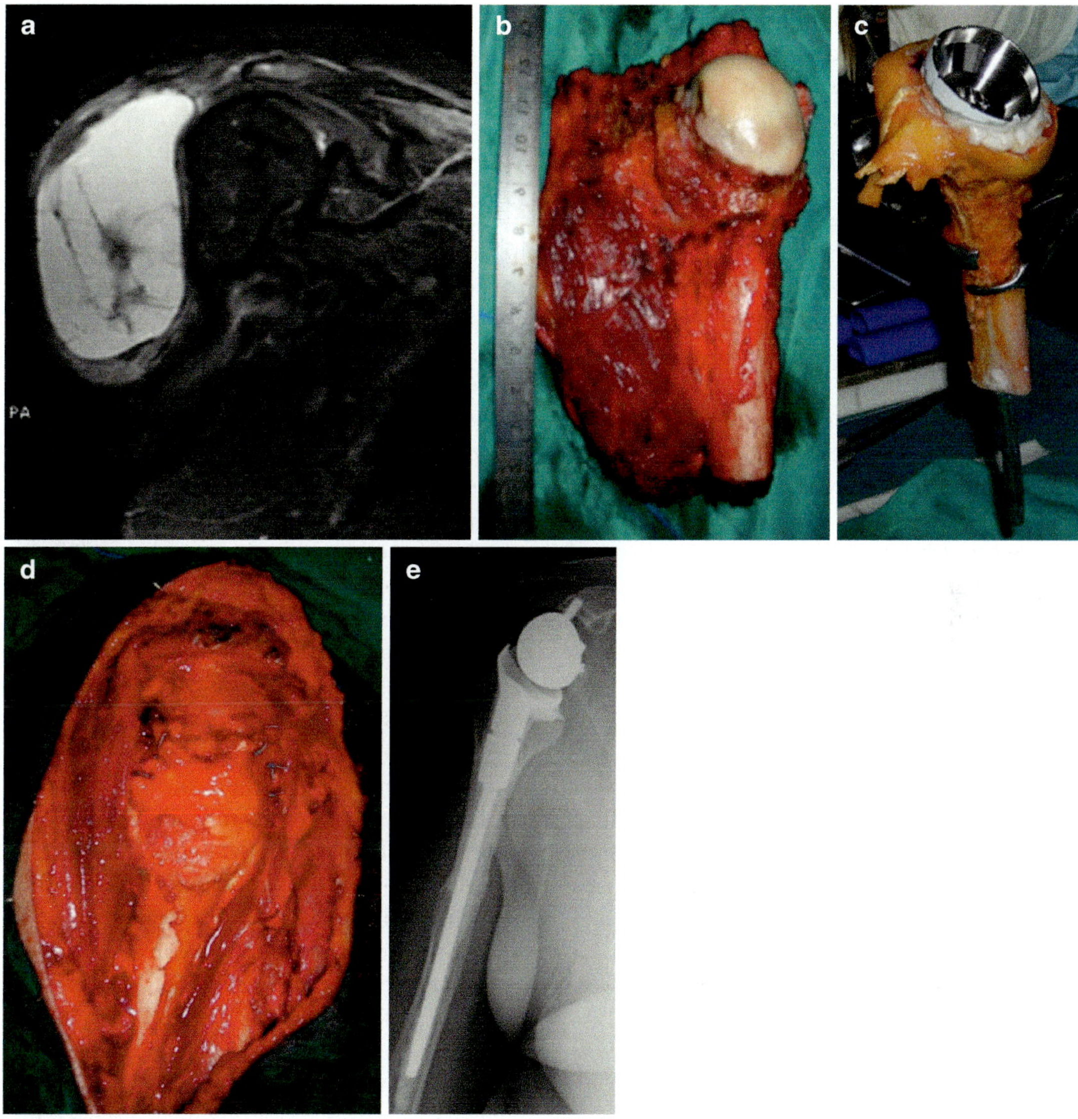

Fig. 24.3 A 64-year-old woman treated for an undifferentiated pleomorphic sarcoma after preoperative chemotherapy and radiotherapy. (**a**, **b**) The lesion starting from the soft tissues is close to the proximal humerus, requiring a bone resection to obtain clear margins. (**c**) Intraoperative pictures showing a long-stemmed humeral component of a RSA previously cemented to an allograft and then to the host bone. (**d**) The transposition of a latissimus dorsi flap completes the reconstruction, since the circumflex nerve has been sacrificed. (**e**) At the last follow-up after almost 10 years, the functionality is moderately limited but painless

As reported above, the partial or complete loss of function of deltoid muscle is not an absolute contraindication to implant a RSA. In fact the only resection of the anterior branch of the axillary nerve leads to the loss of the anterior muscle fibers resulting in a loss of strength in the active forward flexion, but maintaining good function on the other planes. It is reported a better function in patients with RSA and incomplete deltoid function than in patients with a conventional anatomical prosthesis and intact deltoid function [10]. In selected cases the complete absence of the deltoid muscle may be supplied by a latissimus dorsi (LD) muscle transfer either pedicled or as a free flap. Good results were recently reported in non-oncological cases of RSA with LD transfer. A consistent improvement of the active external rotation and an acceptable complication rate have been demonstrated [14, 15].

In limb-sparing surgery, the latissimus dorsi transfer is very useful and could be intended either to restore an acceptable shoulder function or to have a free or pedicled myocutaneous flap to cover the implant after the deltoid muscle resection.

The use of this technique is still debated in oncological orthopedics because the surgeon needs to balance a prolonged surgical time and more potential complications compared to a supposed best functional outcome in a group of patients where the life expectancy is sometimes poor and the residual function is not the primary aim. Probably a more complex surgery could be proposed in young or high-demand patients with a good long-term prognosis.

Postoperative rehabilitation protocol cannot be the same for all patients, but it is adapted to the type of reconstruction. Usually after a RSA implantation, the patients maintain an UltraSling in abduction 60° for 4 weeks allowing sling removal to promote hygiene and elbow active and passive movements. An early careful passive mobilization of the shoulder is recommended but after at least 2 weeks of immobilization. Active range of motion is forbidden until 6–8 weeks followed by an intense physiotherapist-assisted rehabilitation program.

24.5 Advantages of RSA and Potential Complications

It is difficult to assess which is the best approach in terms of functional outcome, implant survival, or complications, because there are no prospective or randomized trials and there are generally no long-term results. Bone and soft tissue sarcomas are rare tumors, as well as metastatic lesions undergoing a resection and reconstruction. Therefore few reference centers deal with these surgical procedures, and the numbers of treated cases are limited.

First of all the oncologic results, in terms of survival and local recurrence, are comparable to those of the conventional prosthesis, as they obviously depend on the quality of tumor excision with adequate margins and on the response to chemotherapy and radiotherapy [16].

There is also no evidence for specific perioperative complications, like major blood loss, or increased surgical time among the different reconstructive options [10].

The reconstruction with a RSA after proximal humerus resection is a safe procedure with an acceptable rate of postoperative complications [17].

In particular, according to the published literature, the rate of instability in RSA is lower than in hemiarthroplasty or total shoulder arthroplasty. While higher rates of instability ranging from 28 to 80% are reported for anatomic shoulder reconstructions, a dislocation rate of up to 30% is reported for RSA.

The most significant advantages from the use of RSA after the resection of the proximal humerus tumors regard the functional results.

De Wilde et al. reported one of the first and largest series of RSA in orthopedic oncology [6].

In this series of 14 patients, excellent results were observed using a composite irradiated autograft. The average active abduction was of 157° after a mean follow-up of 7.7 years. The Authors concluded that RSA has low morbidity and reduces the impairment in the activities of daily living. However the results are much better, compared to other studies, because the detachment of the deltoid muscle was necessary only in two cases. In fact, the resection length itself is not a significant parameter on functional outcome. But the longer the resection, the more muscles should be detached, leading to worse functional results. In their case series composed both of ten patients, Guven et al. [18] described a mean active forward flexion of 96° and a mean active abduction of 88°, while Bonneville et al. [19] reported a mean forward active elevation of 122°.

Both these manuscripts showed worst results in patients after a resection involving the "V" deltoid insertion that was necessary in the majority of these cases.

However, a RSA allows better functional outcomes compared to a conventional anatomical prosthesis. A large series of 83 patients presents a mean active abduction of 41° and a mean active forward flexion of 42° using a conventional prosthesis in patients with the integrity of the axillary nerve [11]. Even patients with a RSA and partial deltoid function show a better function than patients undergoing the implantation of an anatomic prosthesis with intact deltoid function. Therefore, the use of a RSA is recommended in all the patients after a resection with a preservation of the axillary nerve and the deltoid muscle. The deltoid muscle function helps to achieve a wider active range of motion available in the shoulder joint.

The effective joint function is also supported by satisfactory results of functional evaluation scales. Among the different scores examined, the mean Constant-Murley score is ranging from 52 to 80%, the mean Disabilities of the Arm, Shoulder, and Hand (DASH) score is ranging from 26 to 30 points, while the mean Musculoskeletal Tumor Society (MSTS) score is ranging from 67.5 to 80% [10, 18, 19]. However, these values are similar for other types of reconstruction. In a study of 38 consecutive proximal humeral reconstructions using osteoarticular allograft or an endoprosthetic reconstruction, the mean MSTS score is 75.5% [16]. The results of these scores do not reflect the improved function and the increased ability in active abduction, elevation, and rotation. The potential reason is that people compensate with the elbow and hand function that are regularly intact, providing a proper use of the arm in daily activities.

Although functional results are satisfactory, complications are frequent. The greater complexity of the oncologic surgery increases the complication rate compared to non-oncologic RSAs. Most of the postoperative complications after the excision of proximal humerus tumor are related to the type of reconstruction of the humerus.

In general, comparing osteoarticular allografts, allograft-prosthesis composites, and endoprostheses, it has been shown that the use of allografts leads to higher revision rates, but the biologic tendon repair is superior in terms of functional results and stability [20]. This technique is therefore less suitable for patients with low life expectancy and with low functional demands. In both cases, the risk of infection is very high, due to the long duration of surgery and the presence of huge non-biological components. Often patients undergo these surgical procedures after chemotherapy or radiotherapy, with immunodepression and skin closure problems. In addition, antibiotic therapy alone is poorly effective, and complex revisions are often necessary. New coatings (silver-based, iodine) have been recently available to decrease the infection rate, while an accurate soft tissue coverage of the allograft or the prosthesis limits the risk of infection.

Other specific complications associated with APC reconstructions are the possibility of early allograft resorption, the risk of fracture or nonunion between the allograft and the bone host. De Wilde reported radiographic graft resorption in 13 out of 14 patients treated with composite RSA, with the humeral stem suspended with cement alone at the proximal part as a final result [6].

Prosthetic reconstructions generally have more long-term complications associated with prosthetic wear, loosening of the humeral stem, and periprosthetic fractures. Kassab et al. revised two RSAs out of seven for stem fracture or stem loosening after resection of the proximal humerus for tumor at an average follow-up of 85 months [21].

The main complication in oncological reconstruction of the proximal humerus with RSA is the instability. De Wilde et al. reported a rate of 14% of dislocation [6], while other authors reported an instability ranging from 10 to 30% [19, 22]. Guven obtained similar results, with 20% of open reduction for prosthetic dislocation [18].

The rate of instability is certainly higher than in revisions of traditional RSAs [23]. However it remains lower compared to oncological reconstructions using hemiarthroplasty or total shoulder arthroplasty. The main reasons for the predisposition to dislocate are the loss of large segments of the bone and the loss of parts of shoulder musculature and their tendons. These factors often lead to shorter bone reconstructions and consequently to a low tension of the surrounding soft tissues. According to several Authors, the humeral lengthening from 0 to 2 cm, compared to the contralateral arm, looks like the ideal solution to gain a correct pretension of shoulder soft tissues and in particular of the deltoid muscle [24].

This procedure allows to reduce the dislocation rate and to improve the functional outcome. On the other hand, a higher lengthening should be avoided in order not to cause nerve palsies.

The lateralization of the center of rotation is another solution to achieve shoulder stability increasing the compression of the humeral component on the glenosphere and at the same time reducing the risk of impingement.

The use of a synthetic attachment tube associated to an endoprosthesis or a RSA reconstruction is described in several studies as useful to improve joint stability [10, 25].

In particular, when there is a defect of the anterior part of the deltoid, a subscapularis repair is important to avoid anterior instability. The synthetic tube allows the reattachment and the subsequent scar tissue formation even if only a part of the tendon is saved. In addition, the possibility of an easier attachment of the tendons compared to a non-smooth surface such as the prosthesis provides better function of the rotator cuff muscles, in particular recovering the external rotation [18].

24.6 Conclusions

The heterogeneity of clinical patterns makes difficult to define general rules for the surgical treatment of all oncologic patients. The quality of tumor excision is crucial, as it affects patient survival. Advances in surgical techniques, chemotherapy, and radiotherapy have helped to develop more innovative surgical solutions, allowing important improvements in the quality of life and functionality of the operated upper limb. RSA currently represents the most reliable and safe solution for glenohumeral reconstruction. The modern trend is to use RSA when the deltoid muscle and the axillary nerve are saved during the tumor resection. Promising results have been recently described with the use of RSA after the resection of the deltoid muscle and/or the axillary nerve recreating the abduction movement with a latissimus dorsi flap.

References

1. Malawer MM. Overview of resections around the shoulder girdle: anatomy, surgical consideration and classifications. In: Musculoskeletal cancer surgery; 2001.
2. Enneking W, Dunham W, Gebhardt M, Malawar M, Pritchard D. A system for the classification of skeletal resections. Chir Organi Mov. 1990;75(1 Suppl):217–40.
3. Jemal A, Siegel R, Ward E, Murray T, Xu J, Thun MJ. Cancer statistics, 2007. CA Cancer J Clin. 2007;57(1):43–66.
4. Aaron AD. Treatment of metastatic adenocarcinoma of the pelvis and the extremities. J Bone Joint Surg Am. 1997;79(6):917–32.
5. Fottner A, Szalantzy M, Wirthmann L, Stähler M, Baur-Melnyk A, Jansson V, et al. Bone metastases from renal cell carcinoma: patient survival after surgical treatment. BMC Musculoskelet Disord. 2010;11:145.
6. De Wilde L, Boileau P, Van der Bracht H. Does reverse shoulder arthroplasty for tumors of the proximal humerus reduce impairment? Clin Orthop. 2011;469(9):2489–95.
7. Teunis T, Nota SPFT, Hornicek FJ, Schwab JH, Lozano-Calderón SA. Outcome after reconstruction of the proximal humerus for tumor resection: a systematic review. Clin Orthop. 2014;472(7):2245–53.
8. Malawer MM. Tumors of the shoulder girdle. Technique of resection and description of a surgical classification. Orthop Clin North Am. 1991;22(1):7–35.
9. Bus MPA, van de Sande MA, Taminiau AHM, Dijkstra PDS. Is there still a role for osteoarticular allograft reconstruction in musculoskeletal tumour surgery? A long-term follow-up study of 38 patients and systematic review of the literature. Bone Joint J. 2017;99-B(4):522–30.
10. Streitbuerger A, Henrichs M, Gosheger G, Ahrens H, Nottrott M, Guder W, et al. Improvement of the shoulder function after large segment resection of the proximal humerus with the use of an inverse tumour prosthesis. Int Orthop. 2015;39(2):355–61.
11. Cannon CP, Paraliticci GU, Lin PP, Lewis VO, Yasko AW. Functional outcome following endoprosthetic reconstruction of the proximal humerus. J Shoulder Elb Surg. 2009;18(5):705–10.
12. Abdeen A, Healey JH. Allograft-prosthesis composite reconstruction of the proximal part of the humerus: surgical technique. J Bone Joint Surg Am. 2010;92(Suppl 1 Pt 2):188–96.

13. King JJ, Nystrom LM, Reimer NB, Gibbs CP, Scarborough MT, Wright TW. Allograft-prosthetic composite reverse total shoulder arthroplasty for reconstruction of proximal humerus tumor resections. J Shoulder Elb Surg. 2016;25(1):45–54.
14. Sheth M, Ko J-WK, Namdari S. Reverse shoulder arthroplasty and latissimus dorsi tendon transfer. Am J Orthop (Belle Mead NJ). 2017;46(5):E287–92.
15. Wey A, Dunn JC, Kusnezov N, Waterman BR, Kilcoyne KG. Improved external rotation with concomitant reverse total shoulder arthroplasty and latissimus dorsi tendon transfer: a systematic review. J Orthop Surg (Hong Kong). 2017;25(2):2309499017718398.
16. van de Sande MAJ, Dijkstra PDS, Taminiau AHM. Proximal humerus reconstruction after tumour resection: biological versus endoprosthetic reconstruction. Int Orthop. 2011;35(9):1375–80.
17. De Wilde LF, Plasschaert FS, Audenaert EA, Verdonk RC. Functional recovery after a reverse prosthesis for reconstruction of the proximal humerus in tumor surgery. Clin Orthop. 2005;430:156–62.
18. Guven MF, Aslan L, Botanlioglu H, Kaynak G, Kesmezacar H, Babacan M. Functional outcome of reverse shoulder tumor prosthesis in the treatment of proximal humerus tumors. J Shoulder Elb Surg. 2016;25(1):e1–6.
19. Bonnevialle N, Mansat P, Lebon J, Laffosse J-M, Bonnevialle P. Reverse shoulder arthroplasty for malignant tumors of proximal humerus. J Shoulder Elb Surg. 2015;24(1):36–44.
20. Potter BK, Adams SC, Pitcher JD, Malinin TI, Temple HT. Proximal humerus reconstructions for tumors. Clin Orthop. 2009;467(4):1035–41.
21. Kassab M, Dumaine V, Babinet A, Ouaknine M, Tomeno B, Anract P. Twenty nine shoulder reconstructions after resection of the proximal humerus for neoplasm with mean 7-year follow-up. Rev Chir Orthop Reparatrice Appar Mot. 2005;91(1):15–23.
22. Kaa AKS, Jørgensen PH, Søjbjerg JO, Johannsen HV. Reverse shoulder replacement after resection of the proximal humerus for bone tumours. Bone Joint J. 2013;95-B(11):1551–5.
23. Zumstein MA, Pinedo M, Old J, Boileau P. Problems, complications, reoperations, and revisions in reverse total shoulder arthroplasty: a systematic review. J Shoulder Elb Surg. 2011;20(1):146–57.
24. Lädermann A, Walch G, Lubbeke A, Drake GN, Melis B, Bacle G, et al. Influence of arm lengthening in reverse shoulder arthroplasty. J Shoulder Elb Surg. 2012;21(3):336–41.
25. Raiss P, Kinkel S, Sauter U, Bruckner T, Lehner B. Replacement of the proximal humerus with MUTARS tumor endoprostheses. Eur J Surg Oncol. 2010;36(4):371–7.

Failed Total Shoulder Arthroplasty 25

Giuseppe Porcellini, Azad Sait, Giovanni Merolla, and Paolo Paladini

25.1 Introduction

In the last few decades, the advancement in tribology and prosthetic joint design has led to a proliferation in arthroplasties performed all over the world. The number of total shoulder arthroplasties (TSA) performed annually shows a proportionate increase with other major joint arthroplasties. With increasing primary arthroplasty, the need for revision also increases [1, 2]. An intact rotator cuff is essential for a well-functioning TSA. TSA mimics the normal shoulder joint biomechanics in patients with a functioning rotator cuff by generating a balanced force couple that centres the humeral head in the glenoid throughout the range of motion. In the axial plane, the interplay between subscapularis and infraspinatus balances the shoulder joint, while in the coronal plane, supraspinatus counteracts the deltoid vector, thereby maintaining a stable centre of rotation. The success of a total shoulder arthroplasty depends on achieving such a stable centre of rotation that aids the deltoid moment arm to function efficiently [3]. Nonetheless, age-related atrophy, fatty infiltration, tear and subsequent rotator cuff dysfunction are common [4]. This grossly alters the joint biomechanics (Fig. 25.1), thereby placing an eccentric load on the prosthetic joint leading to painful dysfunction and failure.

A proper understanding of the causes of failure of TSA is essential to plan a successful revision. The failed TSA may be grouped broadly into two major categories: aseptic failures and septic failures. Kalandiak et al. have previously classified the complications of TSA leading to failure under three broad categories: (1) failures involving soft tissue problems like instability, stiffness, cuff tear, etc., (2) failure of humeral component and (3) failure of glenoid component [1]. One cause may be complimentary to the other or as a result of another cause; hence, in most cases they are multifactorial. For example, overstuffing of the component may lead to rotator cuff tear. Rotator cuff deficiency may lead to superior instability, which in turn may cause eccentric loading of glenoid and subsequent wear and loosening. However, this anatomical categorisation can be utilised to address the failure in TSA while performing a revision.

Nevertheless, revision of a failed TSA is difficult and challenging. Approximately 11% of TSA ends up in revision [5, 6]. Reverse total shoulder arthroplasty (RTSA) is frequently employed as a salvage for failed TSA. RTSA in a

G. Porcellini · A. Sait (✉) · P. Paladini
Shoulder and Elbow Unit, Cervesi Hospital, AUSL della Romagna Ambito Rimini, Cattolica, Italy

G. Merolla
Shoulder and Elbow Unit, Cervesi Hospital, AUSL della Romagna Ambito Rimini, Cattolica, Italy

Biomechanics Laboratory, Cervesi Hospital, AUSL della Romagna Ambito Rimini, Cattolica, Italy

S. Gumina et al. (eds.), *Reverse Shoulder Arthroplasty*,
https://doi.org/10.1007/978-3-319-97743-0_25

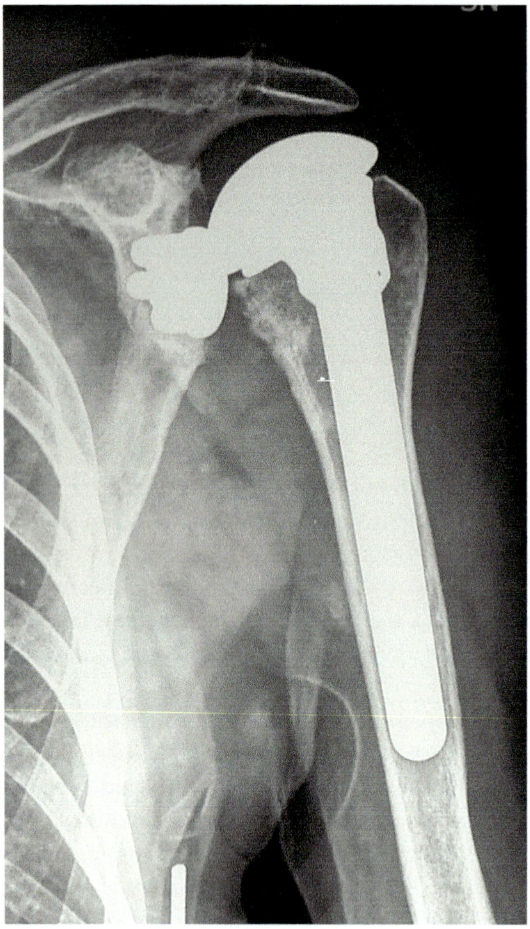

Fig. 25.1 Age-related rotator cuff dysfunction alters the prosthetic joint biomechanics. Note the superior migration of humeral head and decreased acromio-humeral distance

revision setting is complex owing to the frequently encountered humeral and glenoid bone defects as well as the compromised soft tissue around the joint. Although the results of RTSA in a revision setting are inferior to primary RTSA, it predictably decreases the pain and disability and improves function [7, 8].

25.2 Preoperative Planning in Failed TSA

A careful preoperative work-up focused on certain imperative points is essential in planning a revision, which involves a detailed clinical evaluation, imaging and laboratory investigations.

Clinical evaluation in a revision setting is aimed at evaluating the patient's current disability and functional demands. A subjective pain scoring may be recorded by using the visual analogue scale (VAS). A functional scoring using any one of the established standard scoring systems such as Constant score, UCLA, ASES or SST may be done preoperatively [9–12]. This helps to understand the present disability better and may be used in the follow-ups to record the functional improvement. One should specifically look for signs of infection such as an actively draining sinus (Fig. 25.2a), erythema and tenderness, although in most cases the presentation is non-specific with complaints of excessive pain in the shoulder. The functioning of deltoid muscle needs to be ensured through examination (Fig. 25.2b). It may be difficult in painful shoulders to grade the power of deltoid, but one can feel for the contraction of deltoid on attempted shoulder abduction. Deltoid dysfunction may be due to excessive muscle detachment or secondary to neural injury like axillary nerve palsy or brachial plexus palsy during the previous surgery. The reported incidence of neurologic injury is approximately 2% in primary TSA [13]. In the context of a non-functioning deltoid, RTSA also ceases as an option, although theoretically it is possible to combine RTSA with pedicled pectoralis major and trapezius transfers [14]. Whenever in doubt, an electromyography may be obtained to ascertain the deltoid function. The shoulder may be examined for any instability in all directions. Although RTSA with its semi-constrained feature compensates for instability to some extent, the surgeon can be prepared with more constraint designs with offset options for the humeral socket during revision. Preoperative active and passive range of movements should be recorded. Although active elevation can be improved by increasing the deltoid moment arm, one should plan for an implant with lateral offset that tensions posterior deltoid or a concomitant latissimus dorsi and teres major transfer which is suitable for such a condition where the patient's functional improvement demands increased external rotation with arms by the side of the chest.

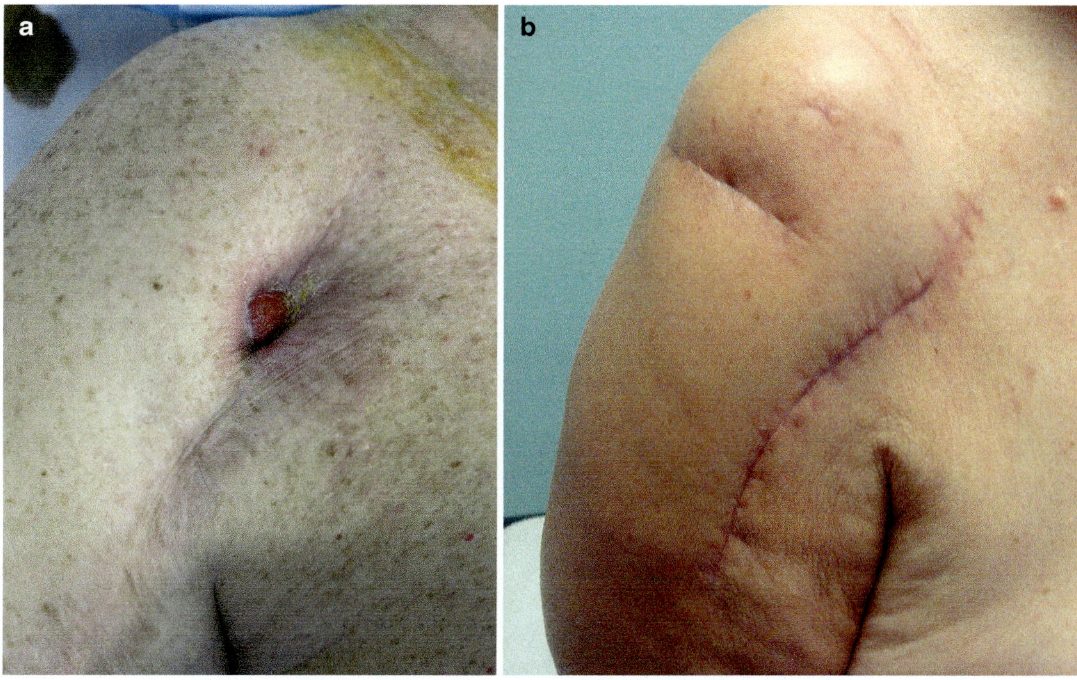

Fig. 25.2 The presence of erythema around the scar and sinus (**a**) suggests the possibility of infection. Functioning of deltoid muscle should be ascertained especially in cases with multiple and unusual scars (**b**)

A detailed interpretation of preoperative images is essential in planning a revision. A routine plain anteroposterior and axillary view radiographs of the shoulder may be obtained. A rough assessment of bone quality and available bone stock for revision fixation may be obtained from the plain radiographs. The humeral metaphyseal and cortical bone thickness in the radiographs throws light on the stress shielding and possibility of uncemented revision. Plain radiographs can give information regarding the direction of instability. Superior migration of the centre of rotation signifies functional inefficiency of the cuff and may be assessed by the decrease in the acromio-humeral distance (Fig. 25.1). Seebauer classified the degree of superior instability into four groups ranging from minimal superior migration to anterosuperior escape [15]. Anterior or posterior subluxation may be assessed in axillary views.

Each component may be separately assessed for the type and quality of fixation, type of implant, component position (version and rotation) and loosening. The humeral component may be a surface replacement prosthesis or a stemmed prosthesis. The stemmed prosthesis can be cemented or uncemented types. Uncemented stems are press-fit stems, and the stem lengths vary from mini stems that rely only on metaphyseal fixation to long stems which depend on distal fixation (Fig. 25.3). The presence of radiolucent lines (RLL) around the humeral component is common in press-fit stems, and this mere presence of RLL doesn't signify component loosening or easy component extraction [16, 17]. Sperling et al. defined radiographic 'at-risk' signs of humeral component as subsidence, tilt or 2-mm RLL around the implant (Figs. 25.4 and 25.13a) [18]. Removal of a well-fixed humeral component is likely to necessitate an osteotomy of the humeral shaft. The length required for the possible osteotomy shall be calculated by the distal level of stem fixation. The removal of the distal cement mantle with the cement restrictor has the possibility to additionally demand a cortical window. The length required for the revision stem, its diameter and type of fixation are perhaps planned accordingly. Not infrequently, the cause of

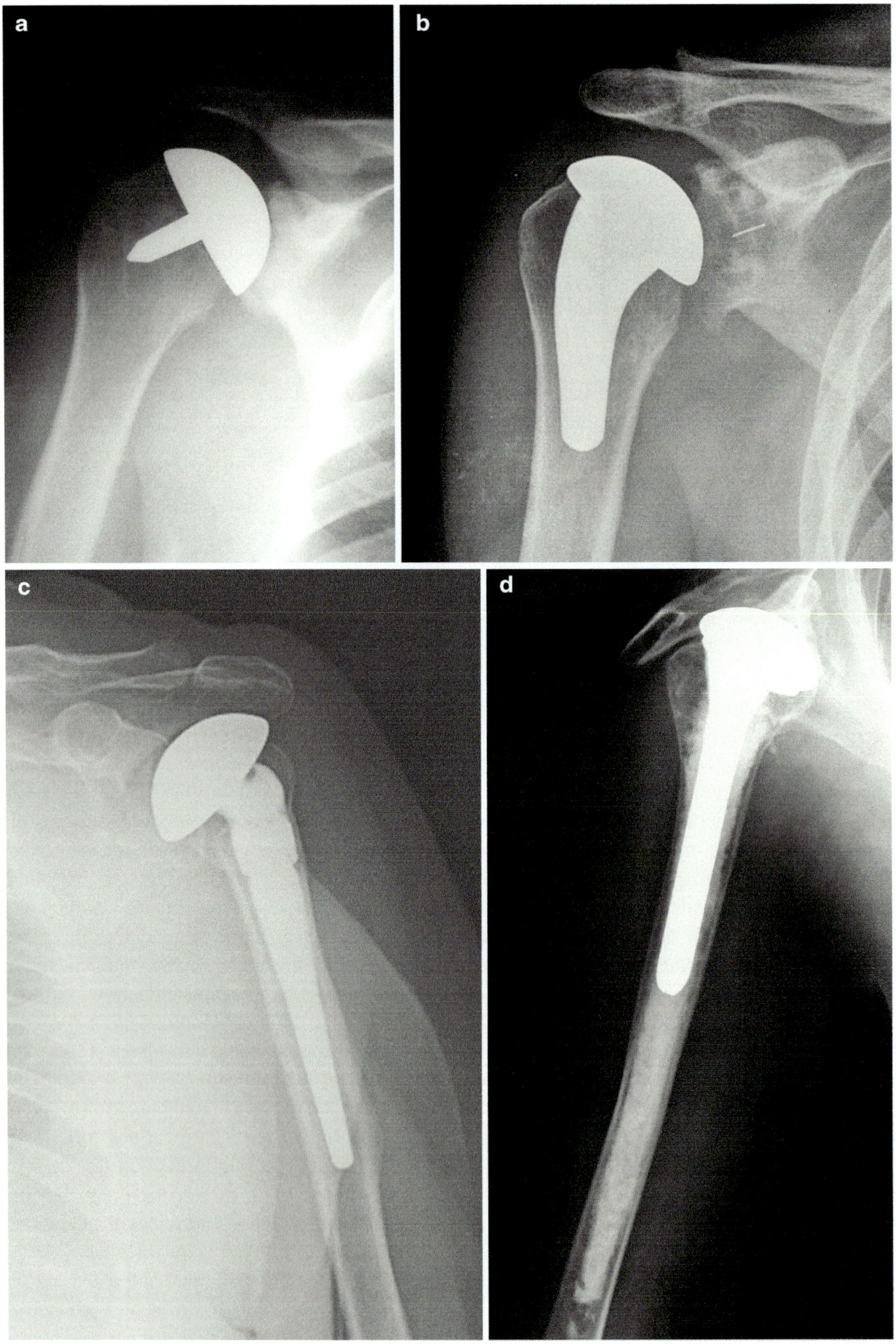

Fig. 25.3 Humeral prosthesis can be surface replacement (**a**), mini stem (**b**), standard uncemented (**c**) or cemented (**d**)

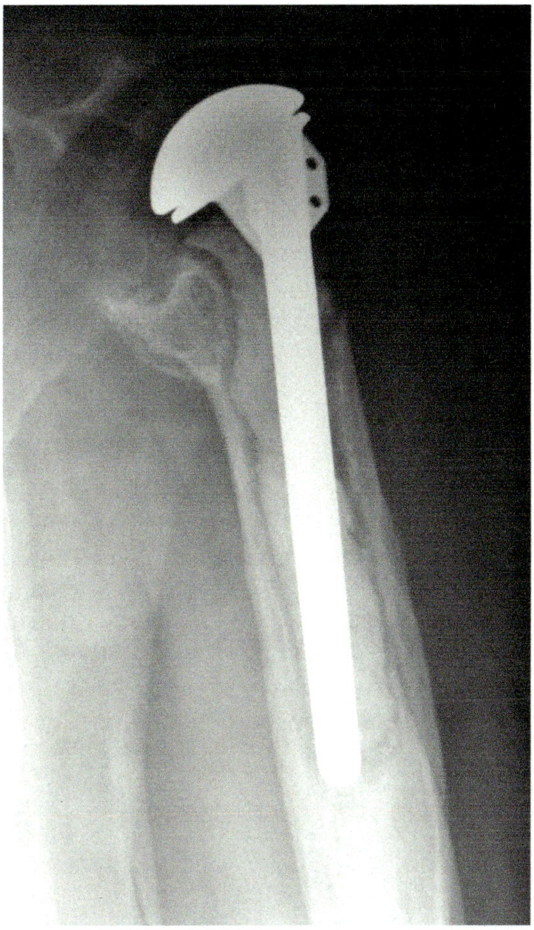

Fig. 25.4 Note the RLL all around the cement-bone interface

revision can be a periprosthetic fracture. The risk of periprosthetic humeral fractures increases with age [19]. Based on fracture location in relation to the humeral stem, Wright and Cofield have classified periprosthetic humeral fractures into three types: (1) type A, spiral fracture centred around the tip of the prosthesis with an extension of more than one third of the humeral stem; (2) type B, fracture centred around the humeral stem with an extension of less than one third of the humeral stem; and (3) type C, fracture well distal to the tip of the prosthesis extending to the distal humeral metaphysis [20]. Worland proposed a classification system taking implant stability also into consideration along with fracture type and location, which is similar to Vancouver classification for periprosthetic femoral fractures in total hip arthroplasty: (1) type A, fracture around the tuberosities; (2) type B, fracture around the stem; and (3) type C, fracture well distal to the tip of the stem [21]. Type B fractures are subclassified into B1, spiral fracture with stable implant; B2, transverse or short oblique fracture about the tip of the stem with stable implant; and B3, fracture around the stem with unstable implant. B2 and B3 fractures require revision to a long-stem prosthesis. In the case of pre-existent rotator cuff dysfunction and preserved glenoid bone stock, revision to a long-stem RTSA should improve shoulder function (Fig. 25.5).

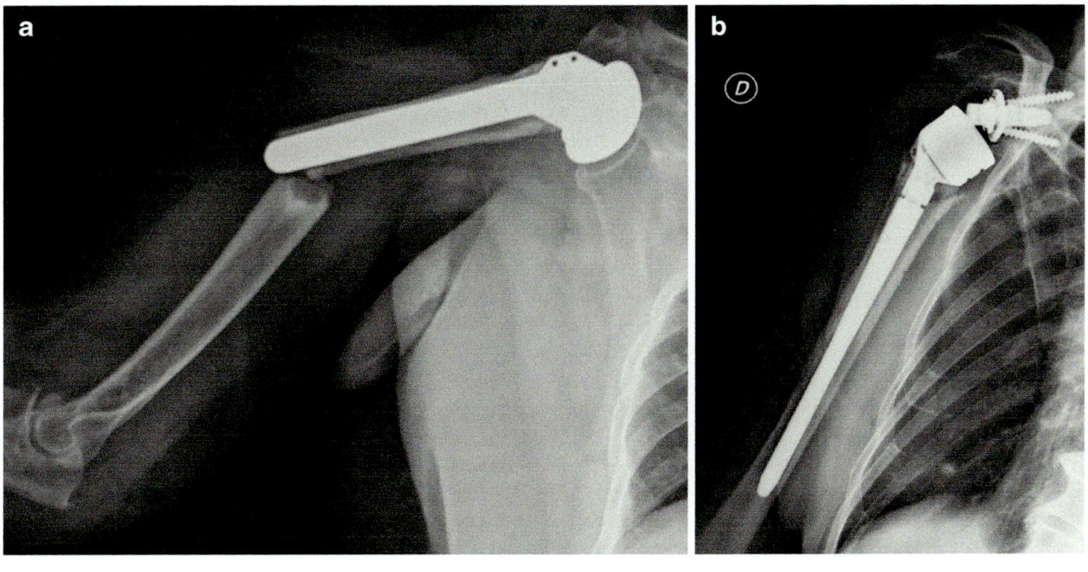

Fig. 25.5 Worland type B2 periprosthetic fracture (**a**) in a patient with rotator cuff dysfunction revised to long-stem RTSA (**b**)

The type of glenoid component can be made out from plain radiographs which may vary from metal-backed component for uncemented fixation to all poly glenoid with either pegs or keel for cemented fixation. Metal-backed components are reported to have higher failure rates and progression of RLL. Osteolysis of the glenoid, dislocation of polyethylene component, glenoid tray fracture and screw breakage are the other reported failures associated with metal-backed glenoid components which may be looked for in the radiographs (Fig. 25.6) [22, 23]. RLL at the cement-bone interface is found in nearly 80% of all polyethylene glenoid components on follow-up radiographs [1]. Component migration, tilt or complete RLL > 1.5 mm, indicates definite loosening of the glenoid component [23]. RLL in immediate post-operative radiographs is commonly found in keeled implants and may be attributed to an incomplete seating of this implant design [24]. The radiolucency about both the keeled and pegged implants shall be graded from 0 (no lucency) to 5 (gross loosening), and the component seating may be graded from A (complete seating) to E (>50% incomplete contact) based on the study by Lazarus et al. [24]. One can compare the initial post-TSA radiographs with the pre-revision radiographs to assess the progress of these grades. Improper version or rotation of the components can predispose to instability, although it is assessed better in CT scans. The role of CT scan is mainly meant to determine the glenoid version and bone defect in anticipation of the need for bone grafting. Prosthetic glenoid version may be measured in a way that is similar for arthritic shoulder by using Friedman's method from an axial CT slice at the tip of the coracoid, which is the angle subtended between a line

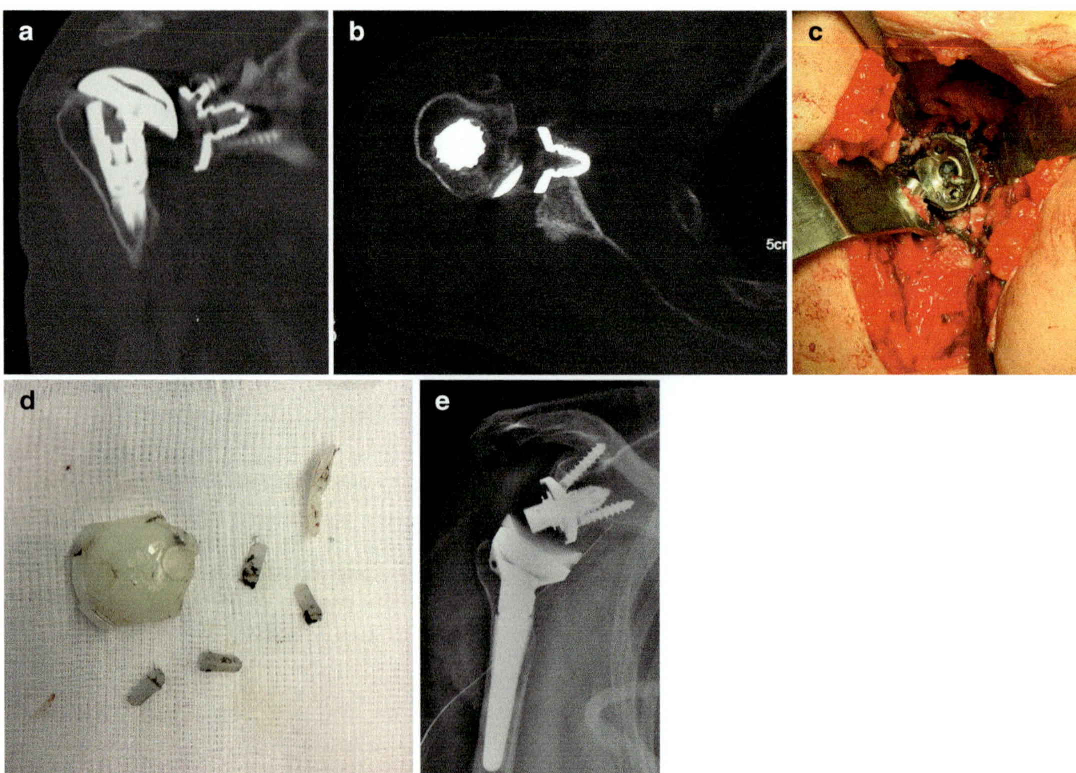

Fig. 25.6 Metal-backed humeral components are associated with higher failure rates. Note the osteolysis in the coronal slice CT (**a**) and glenoid tray loosening with retroversion in the axial slice CT (**b**). Intraoperative pictures show metallosis (**c**) and polyethylene breakage (**d**). Post-operative radiographs after revision to RTSA (**e**). Note the structural bone graft under the glenoid baseplate used to lateralise the glenoid component

joining the anterior and posterior margins of the glenoid bone immediately below the prosthesis and the perpendicular line to the scapular axis (Fig. 25.6b) [25]. In the setting of posterior or superior glenoid defect, an eccentric reaming can be planned for obtaining proper version and inclination of the glenoid baseplate during the revision [26]. If the glenoid erosion has approached too medial near the coracoid, a structural bone graft-baseplate composite needs to be planned to lateralise the baseplate. Over-medialisation of the centre of rotation increases the lateral pull by the deltoid and may predispose to dislocation [3].

Laboratory investigations assume importance in the setting of revision of an infected TSA and fall in line with those for the other major prosthetic joint infections [1]. Blood investigations include total and differential WBC count, ESR, CRP and blood cultures. Joint fluid aspirate analysis and culture also may be done. This will help the surgeon to be prepared with culture-sensitive antibiotics that can be loaded in the cement spacer for a two-staged revision. In certain doubtful situations, a nuclear imaging could be done to differentiate between septic and aseptic loosening [27].

25.3 Surgical Procedure

Surgery is performed in a beach chair position under general anaesthesia. Typically, a deltopectoral approach incorporating the previous surgical scar is utilised which should be extended distally to expose the humeral shaft in case a vertical humeral osteotomy is planned. The tissue planes are likely to be fibrosed and scarred, which brings in the need for a meticulous dissection. Cephalic vein if present guides to the correct interval, but might have been sacrificed in the previous surgery. The direction of the muscles gives an approximate idea of the proper plane. After retracting the deltoid and pectoralis major, identification of coracoid guides further surgical dissection. The conjoint tendon is retracted after clearing its adhesions from the subscapularis. The subdeltoid plane is cleared off all the adhesions to facilitate deltoid retraction. Rotator interval is identified, and the subscapularis may be peeled free or osteotomised with a thin sliver of lesser tuberosity. This exposes the prosthetic joint adequately. The subscapularis is then mobilised medially clearing all the adhesions below it. Axillary nerve is palpated and protected during this step.

The humeral component is delivered into the wound by adduction, extension and external rotation of the arm. The abundant capsular scar tissue may be released all around to facilitate this. Visible metal and polyethylene debris need to be thoroughly cleared off (Fig. 25.6c). After extracting the humeral head in the case of modular implants, the arm should be flexed slightly and teethed Hoffman's retractors be placed anterior and posterior to the glenoid. Scar tissues and capsular remnants are to be circumferentially released around the glenoid to facilitate component removal.

25.4 Humeral Component Revision

It is important to identify the type of humeral stem while planning the revision. Some systems have the versatile humeral stem common for both total and reverse prostheses. In such cases, if the stem is well fixed, the humeral head only needs to be changed for humeral socket. This helps to preserve the humeral bone stock.

Prosthesis Extraction: In case of septic or aseptic loosening, the component extraction may not pose a major challenge. After removing the humeral head, any metaphyseal adhesions are cleared. A mallet used on the bone punch or impactor placed under the medial neck of the prosthesis facilitates its extraction. The removal of a well-fixed humeral component seems difficult by this method. The aim of humeral component removal should be to preserve as much bone stock as possible to support the new prosthesis. A vertical humeral osteotomy (VHO) described by Van Theil et al. may be utilised for extraction of a well-fixed press-fit stem as well as cemented stem [28]. Humeral shaft is exposed between the pectoralis major tendon and deltoid attachment as far distally as needed. The proximal implant/cement-bone interface is interrupted all around using a small thin osteotome. This is to prevent the fracture of the thin tuberosity bone while removing the component. A vertical unicortical osteotomy starting just lateral to the bicipital groove is extended distally up to the tip of the prosthesis. The osteotomy may be performed using a thin power saw to a depth where it touches the implant. The VHO is wedged open by passing multiple osteotomes along the osteotomy track, taking care not to fracture the medial cortex. This 'open book' manoeuvre allows breakage of the bone-implant/cement interface and physical removal of the ingrowth/cement. Additionally, high-speed bone burrs may also be used to debond the interface. Once the implant is sufficiently debonded, it can be hammered out as previously described. It is not uncommon to face difficulty in extracting the humeral stem even after VHO. In these cases, the distal end of the VHO is extended transversely in an L-shaped fashion, and the bone flap is hinged open medially (Fig. 25.7a). Care should be taken during this manoeuvre to avoid fracturing of the diaphysis distally.

Once the prosthesis is removed, the remaining cement mantle can be removed using thin osteotomes, bone rongeurs and burr. Medullary canal may be reamed serially with flexible reamers to remove the residues. The distal cement mantle and restrictor may be drilled using long drill bits to break the mantle and to allow the passage of reamer guide wire. A small end-cutting reamer is used to break down this mantle further. In difficult situations, a distal cortical window is created to ease the removal.

Management of Bone Defect: Deficient bone stock at the proximal metaphyseal region is frequently encountered in a revision setting (Fig. 25.8). This may be secondary to bone loss during component extraction, osteolysis, infection or tuberosity resorption due to previous fracture. Proximal humerus bone loss raises concerns regarding the long-term stability of the revision prosthesis. Proximal bone loss along with deficient soft tissue attachment alters the tension and kinematics of deltoid [29]. In a bone-deficient proximal humerus, stress accumulates at the humeral socket-stem junction and causes component failure [30]. Some authors have suggested the use of a monobloc humeral component to overcome this issue [29, 31]. Native bone augmentation using autografts from the iliac crest or allografts can improve long-term results. Tibial strut allografts are frequently used for small defects (Fig. 25.7b) [7, 29]. An allo-prosthesis composite (APC) or hydroxyapatite mould-prosthesis composite (Fig. 25.9) can be considered in bone defects >5 cm [30]. APC replenishes

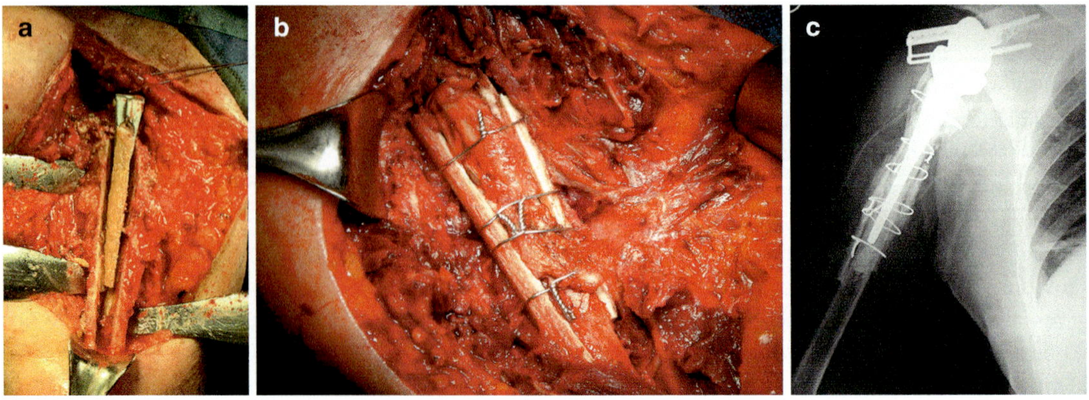

Fig. 25.7 Humeral component removal using a vertical humeral osteotomy extended transversely to open a bone flap (**a**). The osteotomy is closed with tibial strut allograft augmentation using cerclage wires before cementation (**b**). Post-operative radiograph (**c**)

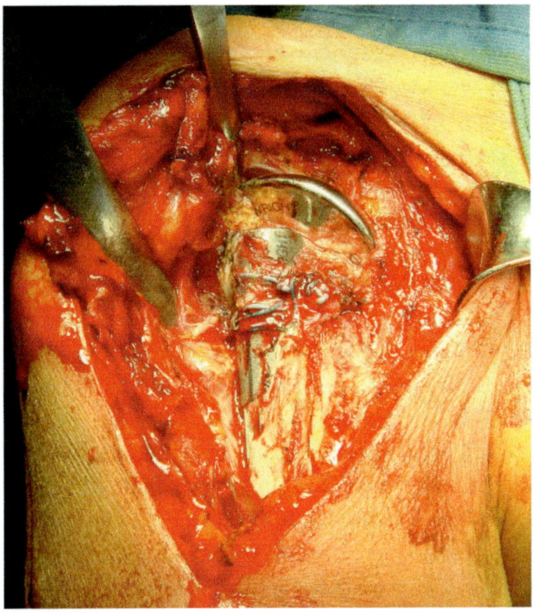

Fig. 25.8 Note the proximal metaphyseal bone defect

the bone stock, improves the deltoid function by recreating the lateral contour of the proximal humerus and decreases the stress concentration on the proximal part of the implant. The complications inherent to the allograft use such as infection, graft resorption, nonunion, etc. are the downsides of APC.

Revision Stem Fixation: One has the option of choosing a cemented or uncemented distal fitting stem. The distal shaft is serially reamed to allow a long stem that extends 2.5 cortical diameters distal to the osteotomy site. The glenoid baseplate and glenosphere are implanted prior to humeral stem implantation. This allows adjustment of height of the humeral component and appropriate soft tissue tensioning while trialling the stem. For uncemented fixation, distal fitting porous-coated stems of different lengths are available. Cerclage wires are tightened over the strut grafts after implanting the stem. For implanting cemented

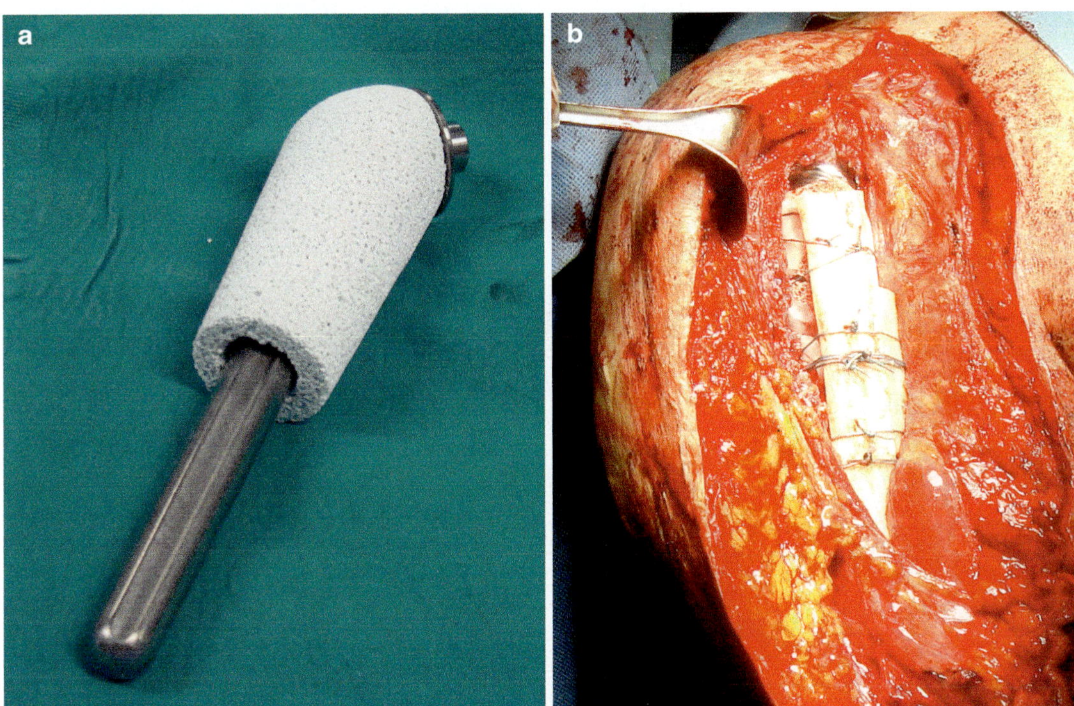

Fig. 25.9 Hydroxyapatite mould-prosthesis composite to address proximal bone deficiency (**a**). Intraoperative pictures after implantation augmented with tibial strut grafts (**b**)

stem, cerclage wires are tightened over allograft struts to create an intact cylinder (Fig. 25.7b, c). A distal cement restrictor is inserted 1.5 cm distal to the tip of the stem. Cemented fixation doesn't require complete removal of the previous cement mantle from the sides. But the distal cement mantle needs to be removed to allow for a long stem. Standard cementation techniques as in hip arthroplasty may be followed. Care should be taken while passing the cerclage wires to avoid radial nerve entrapment in the cerclage. Any intraoperative fracture extending below the tip of the stem may require additional fixation with a cable-plate system (Fig. 25.10).

For implantation of APC, proximal humeral allograft is prepared. The neck cut is made at the desired angle and inclination. Distal transverse cut is made at the desired length. The allograft may be primarily fixed to the native bone using cable-plate devices and the prosthesis be implanted. Alternatively, the prosthesis is implanted to the allograft first and the resulting allo-prosthesis in the native bone. Supplementary fixation is achieved by a cable-plate device.

Management of Intraoperative Periprosthetic Humeral Fractures: Periprosthetic humeral fractures can occur before the prosthesis implantation (during exposure, reaming or trial reduction) while definitive implantation or after implantation (during reduction). Errors in surgical technique like inadequate extension of the humeral shaft while reaming, eccentric reaming causing medial cortical perforation, overzealous rotation of arm and forceful impaction of trial stem may result in fractures before the implantation of prosthesis. This can be managed with a long-stem prosthesis which bypasses the distal end of prosthesis by at least two cortical diameters

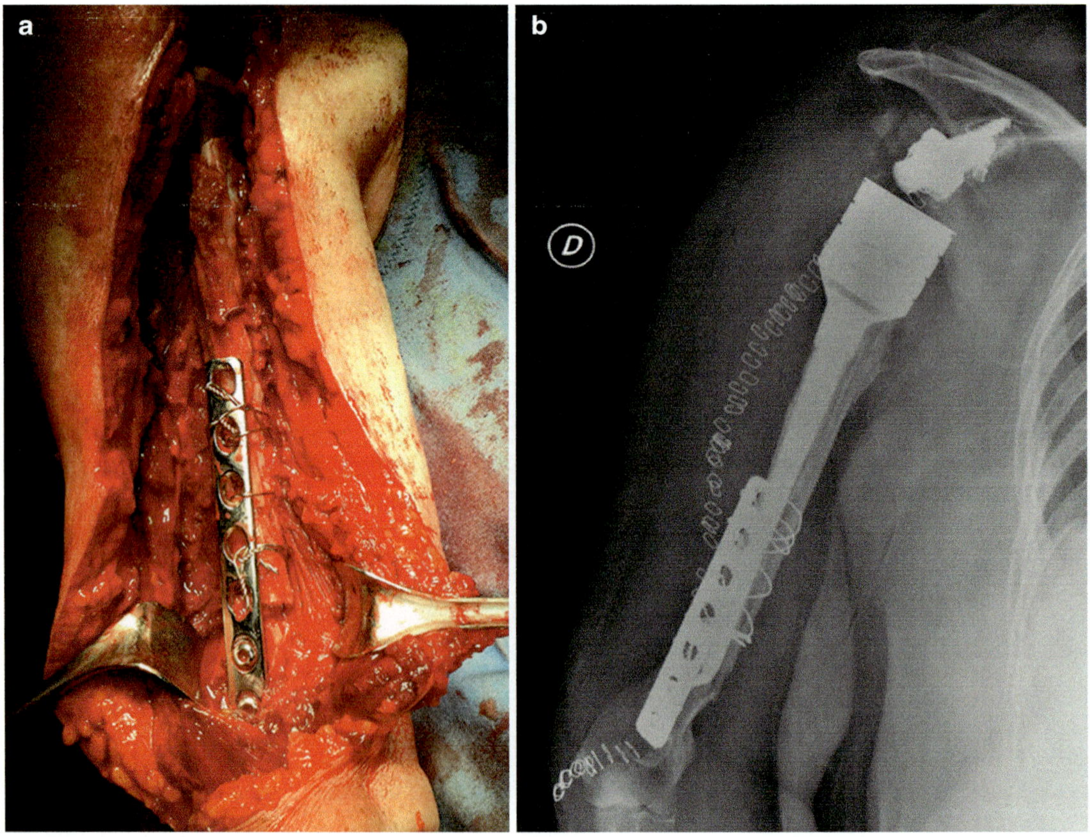

Fig. 25.10 Intraoperative picture (**a**) and post-operative radiograph (**b**) showing fixation of Worland type C periprosthetic fracture with plate and cerclage wires

combined with cerclage wiring. Forced impaction of the definitive prosthesis and rotation manoeuvres during reduction can also result in fractures. In such cases, the management is based on fracture location and implant stability. Worland types A and B1 fractures could be managed by cerclage wiring alone, while type C fractures need to be fixed with a cable-plate device (Fig. 25.10). Type B2 fractures may either be revised with a long-stem prosthesis if the primary implant can be easily extracted or be fixed with a cable-plate system. Type B3 fractures require revision to long-stem prosthesis with additional cerclage wires proximally.

25.5 Glenoid Component Revision

The aim of glenoid component revision is to fix the glenoid baseplate at a proper version, inclination and adequate lateralisation to provide a stable centre of rotation (COR). Establishing a stable COR by its semi-constrained design analogues the function of rotator cuff in a normal shoulder [3]. The deltoid moment arm is effectively increased by the medial placement of COR. Distal placement of COR increases its resting tension. This allows deltoid to effectively elevate the shoulder with less force. By using a hemispherical design of glenosphere, the COR may be placed close to the baseplate. This decreases the shear force on the glenoid baseplate interface and prevents loosening. Glenospheres with built-in offsets lateralise the COR, thereby increasing the rate of loosening [32]. Hence a bone graft-baseplate composite is superior to lateralising glenoid design in a revision setting [33].

Prosthesis Extraction: Removal of the glenoid component by preserving as much bone stock as possible should be the goal. Metal-backed glenoid components may be difficult to remove because of bony ingrowth. Thin osteotomes may be used to gently break the bony ingrowth to facilitate removal. Another problem that might be encountered with these implants is the screw breakage. Broken screw extraction devices are required in some cases. All poly glenoid components may be amputated at the implant-bone interface using an osteotome and removed. The remaining pegs or keels may be curetted out.

Glenoid Defect Management: Glenoid defect may be the result of over-reaming during primary surgery, bone loss while component extraction, osteolysis or infection. Posterior and superior bone losses affect the version and inclination, respectively. Glenoid defect following component extraction has been classified into central, peripheral or combined by Antuna et al. [34]. Depending on the severity of bone loss, each type has further been graded into mild (less than one third of the surface or rim), moderate (one third to two thirds of the surface or rim) and severe (more than two thirds of the surface or rim). Mild-to-moderate central defects can be managed by impaction grafting alone. Mild peripheral defects and combined defects may need asymmetric reaming to correct the version and inclination. Moderate peripheral and combined defects require eccentric reaming and structural bone grafting, because over-medialising the baseplate alters the direction of deltoid pull and predispose to dislocation [35]. The BIO-RSA technique described by Bioleau et al. can be used to lateralise the baseplate [35]. An asymmetric cylindrical structural bone graft is harvested from iliac crest or femoral head allograft with the baseplate to make a bone graft-baseplate composite. The graft is shaped to match the defect. The central peg hole for the baseplate is made in the native glenoid in correct version and inclination. The long peg of bone graft-baseplate complex is directed into the peg hole and is impacted (Fig. 25.11). Larger diameter pegs with trabecular metal are available with some systems which can be utilised for obtaining immediate stability in the cases with larger defects. Trabecular metal is shown to have excellent biocompatibility and osteo-integrative properties [36, 37]. Additional screw fixation improves its stability. However in severe glenoid defects, inadequacy of glenoid bone stock to accommodate the central bone peg may result in failure of fixation of the bone graft-baseplate complex to the native glenoid. In such cases, the possibility of 3D printing could be

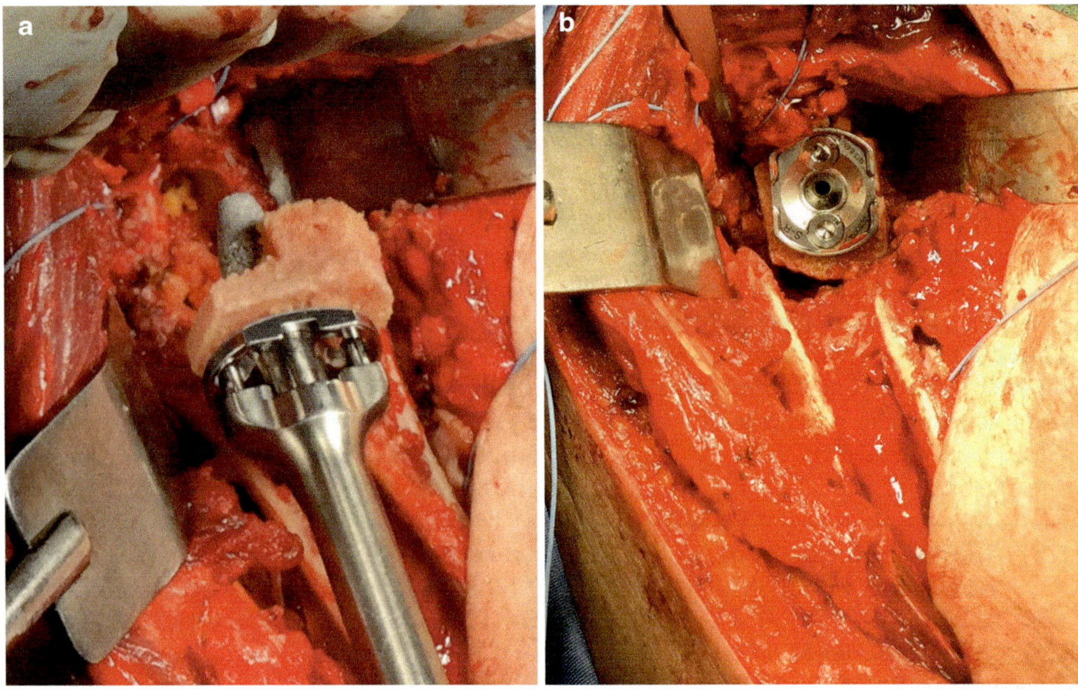

Fig. 25.11 Glenoid reconstruction using bone graft-baseplate composite. Note the asymmetric defect matched bone graft and long trabecular metal peg of the glenoid component that provides immediate post-fixation stability (**a**). Stability is increased by additional screw fixation (**b**)

explored to manufacture custom-made implants (Fig. 25.12). This allows to predetermine the version and inclination, accurate drilling and placement of screws in the best available bone. In cases with extreme glenoid deficiency or complicated with glenoid fracture while component extraction, the salvage option is to revise the humeral component only to hemiarthroplasty, leaving the glenoid unimplanted.

25.6 Soft Tissue Balancing and Management of Instability

Previous instability in the failed TSA may be well balanced by the inherent semi-constrained nature of RTSA. Proper version of the glenoid and humeral components can prevent anteroposterior instability. Decreasing the glenosphere-socket mismatch adds more constrain at the expense of increased wear. Subscapularis repair does not have a definite role in preventing anterior laxity, but it could be done upon feasibility [38]. Inferior laxity in a RSA can be corrected by using a longer humeral stem. Lateral instability can be corrected by using humeral socket of varying thickness and offset. Proper deltoid tensioning is important in maintaining the stability [39]. Newer eccentric glenosphere design places the COR inferiorly, thereby tensioning the deltoid.

25.7 Improving Range of Motion

RTSA decreases the force required for the deltoid to abduct the arm by 30% [40]. This is achieved by increasing the deltoid moment arm and resting tension by the infero-medial placement of COR. A stable COR provided by the semi-constraint implant allows the deltoid to work more efficiently. Improving active shoulder external rotation continues to be a challenge. The loss of active rotation is associated with severe postero-superior

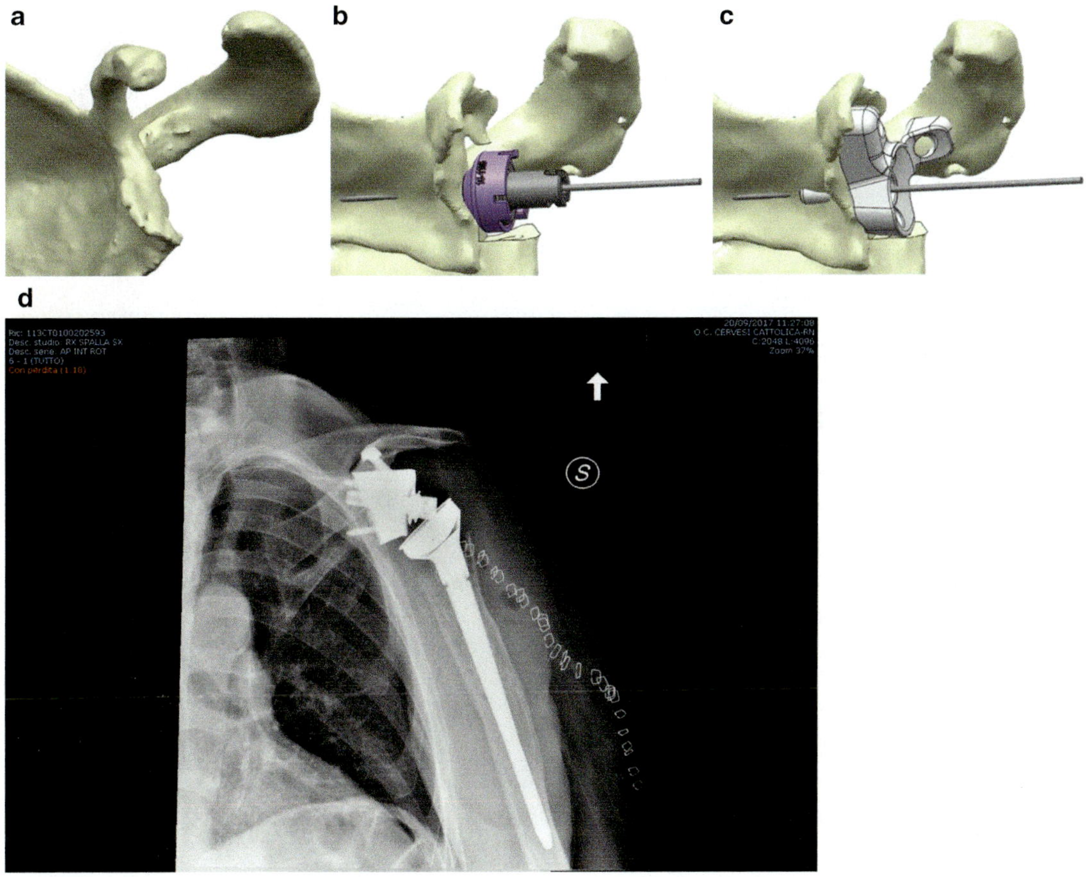

Fig. 25.12 Custom-made glenoid component can be utilised in severe defects. 3D printing (**a**) helps to customise the instrumentation to allow accurate drilling and screw placement in the best possible bone (**b**, **c**). Post-operative radiograph after revising with custom-made glenoid component (**d**)

cuff tear involving teres minor or atrophy and fatty infiltration which cause its dysfunction. This is quite disabling for the patients as they lack the control of spatial orientation of the hand in activities such as handshaking, combing, wearing shirt, etc., when the hand drifts into internal rotation. Traditional Grammont design fails to address this disabling problem. Many authors have suggested concomitant latissimus dorsi and teres major transfer in patients with absent active external rotation preoperatively [41–43]. Newer designs with less medialisation of the COR improve the external rotation by tensioning the posterior deltoid, thus avoiding the need for tendon transfers. This is achieved by using either a glenosphere with lateralised COR or eccentric humeral socket design or a combination of both [44].

Post-operative rehabilitation should be emphasised on improving total active elevation and external rotation. Deltoid and superior portions of the pectoralis major are found to be the active elevators. Posterior deltoid is found to be more recruited in external rotation [45, 46]. Therapy should be focused on strengthening these muscles.

25.8 Revision of Infected TSA

Revising an infected TSA follows the guidelines for revision of other major joints. A two-staged revision is preferred by most surgeons. The usual organisms are *Staphylococcus* and *Propionibacterium* [47]. Antibiotics may be withheld till intraoperative

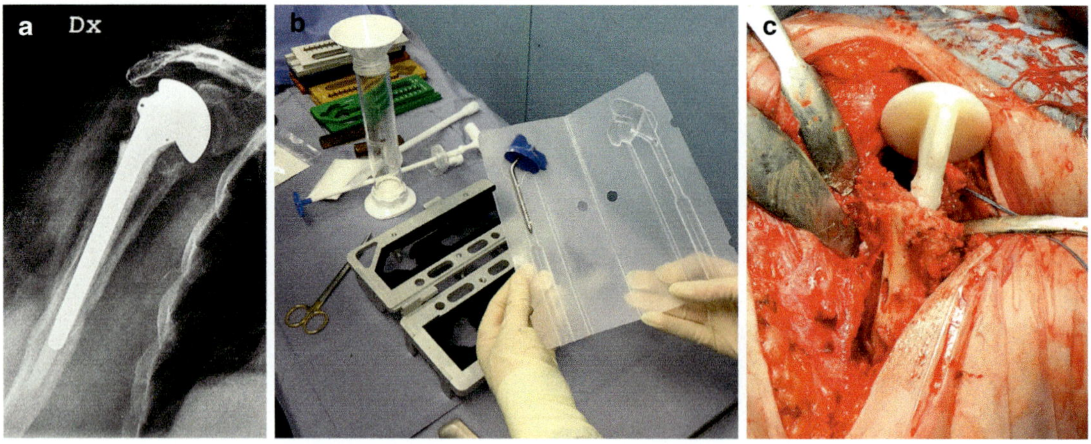

Fig. 25.13 Radiograph of infected prosthesis. Note the radiolucency around the cement-bone interface with subsidence (**a**). Antibiotic-loaded cement spacer insertion in the first-stage revision (**b**, **c**)

cultures are obtained. The cultures need to be held for 2–3 weeks for *Propionibacterium acnes*. During the first stage, implant removal, thorough debridement, removal of all previous bone cement and culture-sensitive antibiotic cement spacer insertion are done (Fig. 25.13). Intravenous antibiotics are continued, and inflammatory markers are followed up. The second stage may be planned after 6–12 weeks once the inflammatory markers come down. The steps and principles of second-stage surgery are the same as those discussed above.

25.9 Conclusion

Although less favourable than primary RTSA, many authors have reported more than 80% patient satisfaction rate in long-term follow-up [8, 48]. The issues concerned with failed TSA are shoulder pain and loss of function that adversely affect the patient's functional abilities. This disabling problem can be addressed by a successful conversion to RTSA in most of the patients. In the patients with preserved glenoid bone stock, the results are often seen better. Hence RTSA remains the current standard of treatment for failed TSA.

References

1. Bohsali KI, Wirth MA, Rockwood CA. Complications of total shoulder arthroplasty. J Bone Joint Surg Am. 2006;88(10):2279–92.
2. Kim SH, Wise BL, Zhang Y, Szabo RM. Increasing incidence of shoulder arthroplasty in the United States. J Bone Joint Surg Am. 2011;93(24):2249–54.
3. Jarrett CD, Brown BT, Schmidt CC. Reverse shoulder arthroplasty. Orthop Clin North Am. 2013;44(3):389–408, x.
4. Tashjian RZ. Epidemiology, natural history, and indications for treatment of rotator cuff tears. Clin Sports Med. 2012;31(4):589–604.
5. Habermeyer P, Magosch P. Strategies in revision shoulder arthroplasty. Orthopade. 2013;42(7):542–51.
6. Gonzalez J-F, Alami GB, Baque F, Walch G, Boileau P. Complications of unconstrained shoulder prostheses. J Shoulder Elb Surg. 2011;20(4):666–82.
7. Kelly JD, Zhao JX, Hobgood ER, Norris TR. Clinical results of revision shoulder arthroplasty using the reverse prosthesis. J Shoulder Elb Surg. 2012;21(11):1516–25.
8. Patel DN, Young B, Onyekwelu I, Zuckerman JD, Kwon YW. Reverse total shoulder arthroplasty for failed shoulder arthroplasty. J Shoulder Elb Surg. 2012;21(11):1478–83.
9. Constant CR, Murley AH. A clinical method of functional assessment of the shoulder. Clin Orthop. 1987;214:160–4.
10. Ellman H, Hanker G, Bayer M. Repair of the rotator cuff. End-result study of factors influencing reconstruction. J Bone Joint Surg Am. 1986;68(8):1136–44.

11. Michener LA, McClure PW, Sennett BJ. American shoulder and elbow surgeons standardized shoulder assessment form, patient self-report section: reliability, validity, and responsiveness. J Shoulder Elb Surg. 2002;11(6):587–94.
12. Godfrey J, Hamman R, Lowenstein S, Briggs K, Kocher M. Reliability, validity, and responsiveness of the simple shoulder test: psychometric properties by age and injury type. J Shoulder Elb Surg. 2007;16(3):260–7.
13. Lädermann A, Lübbeke A, Mélis B, Stern R, Christofilopoulos P, Bacle G, et al. Prevalence of neurologic lesions after total shoulder arthroplasty. J Bone Joint Surg Am. 2011;93(14):1288–93.
14. Elhassan BT, Wagner ER, Werthel J-D, Lehanneur M, Lee J. Outcome of reverse shoulder arthroplasty with pedicled pectoralis transfer in patients with deltoid paralysis. J Shoulder Elb Surg. 2017;27(1):96–103.
15. Visotsky JL, Basamania C, Seebauer L, Rockwood CA, Jensen KL. Cuff tear arthropathy: pathogenesis, classification, and algorithm for treatment. J Bone Joint Surg Am. 2004;86–A(Suppl 2):35–40.
16. Maynou C, Petroff E, Mestdagh H, Dubois HH, Lerue O. Clinical and radiologic outcome of humeral implants in shoulder arthroplasty. Acta Orthop Belg. 1999;65(1):57–64.
17. Matsen FA, Iannotti JP, Rockwood CA. Humeral fixation by press-fitting of a tapered metaphyseal stem: a prospective radiographic study. J Bone Joint Surg Am. 2003;85–A(2):304–8.
18. Sperling JW, Cofield RH, O'Driscoll SW, Torchia ME, Rowland CM. Radiographic assessment of ingrowth total shoulder arthroplasty. J Shoulder Elb Surg. 2000;9(6):507–13.
19. Chin PYK, Sperling JW, Cofield RH, Schleck C. Complications of total shoulder arthroplasty: are they fewer or different? J Shoulder Elb Surg. 2006;15(1):19–22.
20. Wright TW, Cofield RH. Humeral fractures after shoulder arthroplasty. J Bone Joint Surg Am. 1995;77(9):1340–6.
21. Worland RL, Kim DY, Arredondo J. Periprosthetic humeral fractures: management and classification. J Shoulder Elb Surg. 1999;8(6):590–4.
22. Boileau P, Avidor C, Krishnan SG, Walch G, Kempf J-F, Molé D. Cemented polyethylene versus uncemented metal-backed glenoid components in total shoulder arthroplasty: a prospective, double-blind, randomized study. J Shoulder Elb Surg. 2002;11(4):351–9.
23. Martin SD, Zurakowski D, Thornhill TS. Uncemented glenoid component in total shoulder arthroplasty. Survivorship and outcomes. J Bone Joint Surg Am. 2005;87(6):1284–92.
24. Lazarus MD, Jensen KL, Southworth C, Matsen FA. The radiographic evaluation of keeled and pegged glenoid component insertion. J Bone Joint Surg Am. 2002;84–A(7):1174–82.
25. Friedman RJ, Hawthorne KB, Genez BM. The use of computerized tomography in the measurement of glenoid version. J Bone Joint Surg Am. 1992;74(7):1032–7.
26. Mori D, Abboud JA, Namdari S, Williams GR. Glenoid bone loss in anatomic shoulder arthroplasty: literature review and surgical technique. Orthop Clin North Am. 2015;46(3):389–97. x
27. Aksoy SY, Asa S, Ozhan M, Ocak M, Sager MS, Erkan ME, et al. FDG and FDG-labelled leucocyte PET/CT in the imaging of prosthetic joint infection. Eur J Nucl Med Mol Imaging. 2014;41(3):556–64.
28. Van Thiel GS, Halloran JP, Twigg S, Romeo AA, Nicholson GP. The vertical humeral osteotomy for stem removal in revision shoulder arthroplasty: results and technique. J Shoulder Elb Surg. 2011;20(8):1248–54.
29. Chacon A, Virani N, Shannon R, Levy JC, Pupello D, Frankle M. Revision arthroplasty with use of a reverse shoulder prosthesis-allograft composite. J Bone Joint Surg Am. 2009;91(1):119–27.
30. Cuff D, Levy JC, Gutiérrez S, Frankle MA. Torsional stability of modular and non-modular reverse shoulder humeral components in a proximal humeral bone loss model. J Shoulder Elb Surg. 2011;20(4):646–51.
31. Levy J, Frankle M, Mighell M, Pupello D. The use of the reverse shoulder prosthesis for the treatment of failed hemiarthroplasty for proximal humeral fracture. J Bone Joint Surg Am. 2007;89(2):292–300.
32. Merolla G, Tartarone A, Sperling JW, Paladini P, Fabbri E, Porcellini G. Early clinical and radiological outcomes of reverse shoulder arthroplasty with an eccentric all-polyethylene glenosphere to treat failed hemiarthroplasty and the sequelae of proximal humeral fractures. Int Orthop. 2017;41(1):141–8.
33. Merolla G, Wagner E, Sperling JW, Paladini P, Fabbri E, Porcellini G. Revision of failed shoulder hemiarthroplasty to reverse total arthroplasty: analysis of 157 revision implants. J Shoulder Elb Surg. 2017;27(1):75–81.
34. Antuna SA, Sperling JW, Cofield RH, Rowland CM. Glenoid revision surgery after total shoulder arthroplasty. J Shoulder Elb Surg. 2001;10(3):217–24.
35. Boileau P, Moineau G, Roussanne Y, O'Shea K. Bony increased-offset reversed shoulder arthroplasty: minimizing scapular impingement while maximizing glenoid fixation. Clin Orthop. 2011;469(9):2558–67.
36. Christie MJ. Clinical applications of trabecular metal. Am J Orthop (Belle Mead NJ). 2002;31(4):219–20.
37. Bogle A, Budge M, Richman A, Miller RJ, Wiater JM, Voloshin I. Radiographic results of fully uncemented trabecular metal reverse shoulder system

at 1 and 2 years' follow-up. J Shoulder Elb Surg. 2013;22(4):e20–5.
38. Trappey GJ, O'Connor DP, Edwards TB. What are the instability and infection rates after reverse shoulder arthroplasty? Clin Orthop. 2011;469(9):2505–11.
39. Clark JC, Ritchie J, Song FS, Kissenberth MJ, Tolan SJ, Hart ND, et al. Complication rates, dislocation, pain, and postoperative range of motion after reverse shoulder arthroplasty in patients with and without repair of the subscapularis. J Shoulder Elb Surg. 2012;21(1):36–41.
40. Henninger HB, Barg A, Anderson AE, Bachus KN, Tashjian RZ, Burks RT. Effect of deltoid tension and humeral version in reverse total shoulder arthroplasty: a biomechanical study. J Shoulder Elb Surg. 2012;21(4):483–90.
41. Boileau P, Chuinard C, Roussanne Y, Bicknell RT, Rochet N, Trojani C. Reverse shoulder arthroplasty combined with a modified latissimus dorsi and teres major tendon transfer for shoulder pseudoparalysis associated with dropping arm. Clin Orthop. 2008;466(3):584–93.
42. Gerber C, Pennington SD, Lingenfelter EJ, Sukthankar A. Reverse Delta-III total shoulder replacement combined with latissimus dorsi transfer. A preliminary report. J Bone Joint Surg Am. 2007;89(5):940–7.
43. Wey A, Dunn JC, Kusnezov N, Waterman BR, Kilcoyne KG. Improved external rotation with concomitant reverse total shoulder arthroplasty and latissimus dorsi tendon transfer: A systematic review. J Orthop Surg (Hong Kong). 2017;25(2):2309499017718398.
44. Valenti P, Sauzières P, Katz D, Kalouche I, Kilinc AS. Do less medialized reverse shoulder prostheses increase motion and reduce notching? Clin Orthop. 2011;469(9):2550–7.
45. Ackland DC, Richardson M, Pandy MG. Axial rotation moment arms of the shoulder musculature after reverse total shoulder arthroplasty. J Bone Joint Surg Am. 2012;94(20):1886–95.
46. Ackland DC, Roshan-Zamir S, Richardson M, Pandy MG. Moment arms of the shoulder musculature after reverse total shoulder arthroplasty. J Bone Joint Surg Am. 2010;92(5):1221–30.
47. Zavala JA, Clark JC, Kissenberth MJ, Tolan SJ, Hawkins RJ. Management of deep infection after reverse total shoulder arthroplasty: a case series. J Shoulder Elb Surg. 2012;21(10):1310–5.
48. Flury MP, Frey P, Goldhahn J, Schwyzer H-K, Simmen BR. Reverse shoulder arthroplasty as a salvage procedure for failed conventional shoulder replacement due to cuff failure—midterm results. Int Orthop. 2011;35(1):53–60.

Reverse Shoulder Arthroplasty in Patients Younger than 55 Years

26

Michele Ciccarelli, Giuseppe Della Rotonda, Antonio Guastafierro, and Raffaele Russo

Reverse total shoulder arthroplasty (rTSA) was initially developed to treat patients with massive and irreparable rotator cuff tear and after used also in case of four-part proximal humerus fractures, inflammatory arthritis, and revision shoulder arthroplasty. Outcomes are correlated to preoperative diagnosis as reported by Wall et al. [1] with better result in cuff tear arthropathy rather than in post-traumatic and revision cases. At the beginning, the results reported by Grammont [2] in 1987 to treat the cuff tear arthropathy with this prosthesis were object of debate in the United States where most of surgeons used an hemiarthroplasty (HA) in case of eccentric osteoarthritis. Nevertheless, in the last decade, the indications for reverse replacement have widely expanded and finally accepted from most of the orthopedic surgeons [1–3]. Compared to the early Grammont prostheses, latest generation of reverse designs had some biomechanical changes especially for the lateral offset and inferior tilt of the glenosphere to minimize the risk of scapular notching and improve the active range of motion (ROM).

Traditionally, the majority of RSA are performed in old patients with low functional demand to gain two important results: pain decrease and an acceptable ROM [4]. However, the conditions that potentially benefit from an RSA implant are not restricted to an elderly population.

Indication for RSA in young patients (60 years or younger) is actually the most controversial point among shoulder surgeons due to the high functional request in these patients and the potential failures of the implant in terms of instability or mobilizations of glenosphere, humeral component, or screws breaking. It has been shown that patients with complex glenohumeral arthritis younger than 55 years had less predictable outcomes rather than older ones [5–8].

Padegimas and Lazarus [9] showed that the request for shoulder arthroplasties in the United States is increasing with a perspective trend expectation and is likely to continue based on the Nationwide Inpatient Sample (NIS). In the literature, the increase in the number of shoulder arthroplasties for the general population is well reported [5, 9, 10]; there are few studies that analyze the request and the results of this surgery in young patients (55 years old or younger). The purpose of this study is to report the clinical outcomes (range of motion [ROM], strength, patient function) of patients younger than 55 years who underwent a RSA.

M. Ciccarelli (✉) · G. Della Rotonda
A. Guastafierro · R. Russo
Orthopedic Surgery, Pineta Grande Hospital, Caserta, Italy

S. Gumina et al. (eds.), *Reverse Shoulder Arthroplasty*, https://doi.org/10.1007/978-3-319-97743-0_26

26.1 Method

From January 2008 to December 2015, 600 RSAs were implanted: 450 for degenerative diseases, 95 for complex proximal humeral fractures, 15 for fractures sequelae, and 40 for revision surgery. The mean patients' age was 73 years (42–95 years), 11 patients (6%) were less than 55 years (mean age 52.4 years), 10 were male and 1 female, and in 7 cases the dominant arm was involved. In these cases we had two failed rotator cuff repairs, three fractures sequelae (open reduction internal fixation (ORIF)), three failed hemiarthroplasties, one irreparable fracture, and two primary osteoarthrosis with glenoid dysplasia.

We review all the patients at mean follow-up of 4.8–1.5 years, and the clinical evaluation was done according to Constant score associated with X-ray and CT scan studies; in seven cases (63%), the CT scan was done with MAR technique.

All CT examinations were performed since April 2014 with a 64-detector CT scanner (Revolution EVO; GE Medical Systems, Milwaukee, Wisconsin).

Scanning parameters were settled to minimize metals artifact as follows: helical scan type, collimation 64× 0.625, high keV (140), dose modulation of 350 mA, 1 s rotation time, 1 mm helical thickness, and pitch 0.8.

The scan volume begins 1 cm above the AC and extends 2–3 cm below the stems.

The images were reformatted using a MAR (metal artifact reduction), an adaptive filtering to reduce as much as possible the photon starvation, beam hardening, and streak artifacts due to metal implants.

The images were finally reformatted on MPR planes and visualized on a PACS station using the extended CT scale (starting with a window value of 4000 and a center value of 400) [11].

We used in all cases a Lima rTSA (*Lima Corporate Villanova di San Daniele del Friuli, Italy*); in eight patients (72.7%), 36 mm glenosphere was implanted while in three cases (27.3%) a 44 mm and in all cases a no cement humeral stem.

A deltopectoral approach was performed in all cases in order to better expose the glenoid, and the glenosphere was always flushed to the inferior border of glenoid with a baseplate's inclination of 5°–10° inferior tilt. In two cases with glenoid dysplasia, a glenoid bone graft (bio-rTSA) was used. The glenoid dysplasia in a young patient with glenohumeral arthritis usually involves the posterior-inferior part of the glenoid and the scapular neck, often with an enlarged labrum (Fig. 26.1). This condition is rare in the general population (around 14%), but it has been demonstrated to predispose patients to early osteoarthritis [12–14] and in young patients with clear arthritis could be a challenge for surgeons due to glenoid retroversion associated with a decreased glenoid bone stock.

Several studies has been reported good results in this patients treated with r-TSA as published by Allen and Cofield [14] in 20 patients (22 shoulder) treated with total shoulder arthroplasty and hemiarthroplasty, 8 hemiarthroplasties and 14 total shoulder arthroplasties with pain relief and good range of motion. They reported that four shoulders having hemiarthroplasty underwent revision surgery because of painful glenoid arthrosis, two shoulders with total arthroplasty underwent revision for infection, and three underwent revision for glenoid component issues.

For this study, patients with inclusion criteria were contacted for follow-up, and all the preoperative data were collected such as previous procedures, mechanism of injury, diagnosis at the time of surgery, and concomitant procedures. The clinical examination was performed by a trained independent observer based on the Constant -score and to all patients a pain score on a visual analog scale (VAS), Simple Shoulder Test (SST) score and American Shoulder and Elbow Surgeons (ASES) score were submitted. Preoperative and postoperative anteroposterior and axillary shoulder X-rays were evaluated by two independent observers. On the most recent postoperative X-ray, we looked for any evidence of humeral component loosening, glenoid component loosening, scapular notching, osteoarthritis, fracture, and dislocation (Fig. 26.2). In seven cases (63%), a postoperative CT scan study was performed in order to value the glenoid baseplate, the bone graft, and the tuberosities (Fig. 26.3).

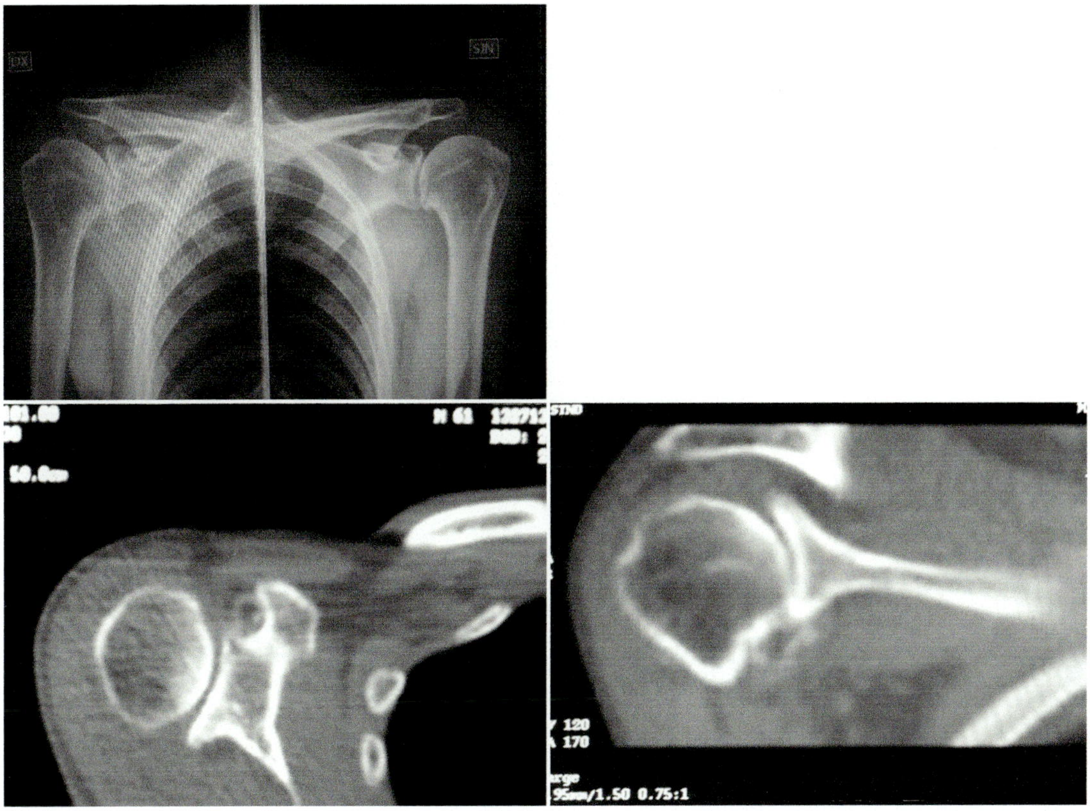

FIG. 26.1 X-ray and CT scan of right shoulder glenoid dysplasia in a 54-year-old man

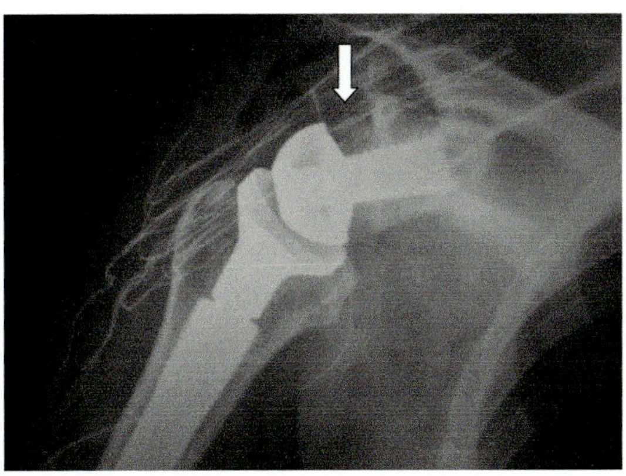

Fig. 26.2 Postoperative X-ray after BIO-RSA: the arrow shows autologous bone graft and Axioma baseplate

The evaluation of the humeral component loosening was based on criteria described by Sperling et al. [15], where a humeral component was deemed "at risk" for loosening if a lucent line greater than 2 mm in width was present in at least three of eight zones or if two of three independent observers identified migration or tilt of the component. Glenoid component loosening was based on the six-part grading scale described by Lazarus et al. [16] The scapular notching was assessed on the four-part grading scale described by Sirveaux et al. [17].

26.2 Results

Demographic cohort information are shown in Table 26.1. At the time of surgery, all the patients were in a work time while at follow-up time eight (72%) of them were still workers, although one had switched to a desk job and currently while two patients, changed their original manual job.

Postoperative, VAS, ASES, and SST scores and forward flexion were all significantly improved from preoperative values. The mean active elevation improved from 59 to 135.

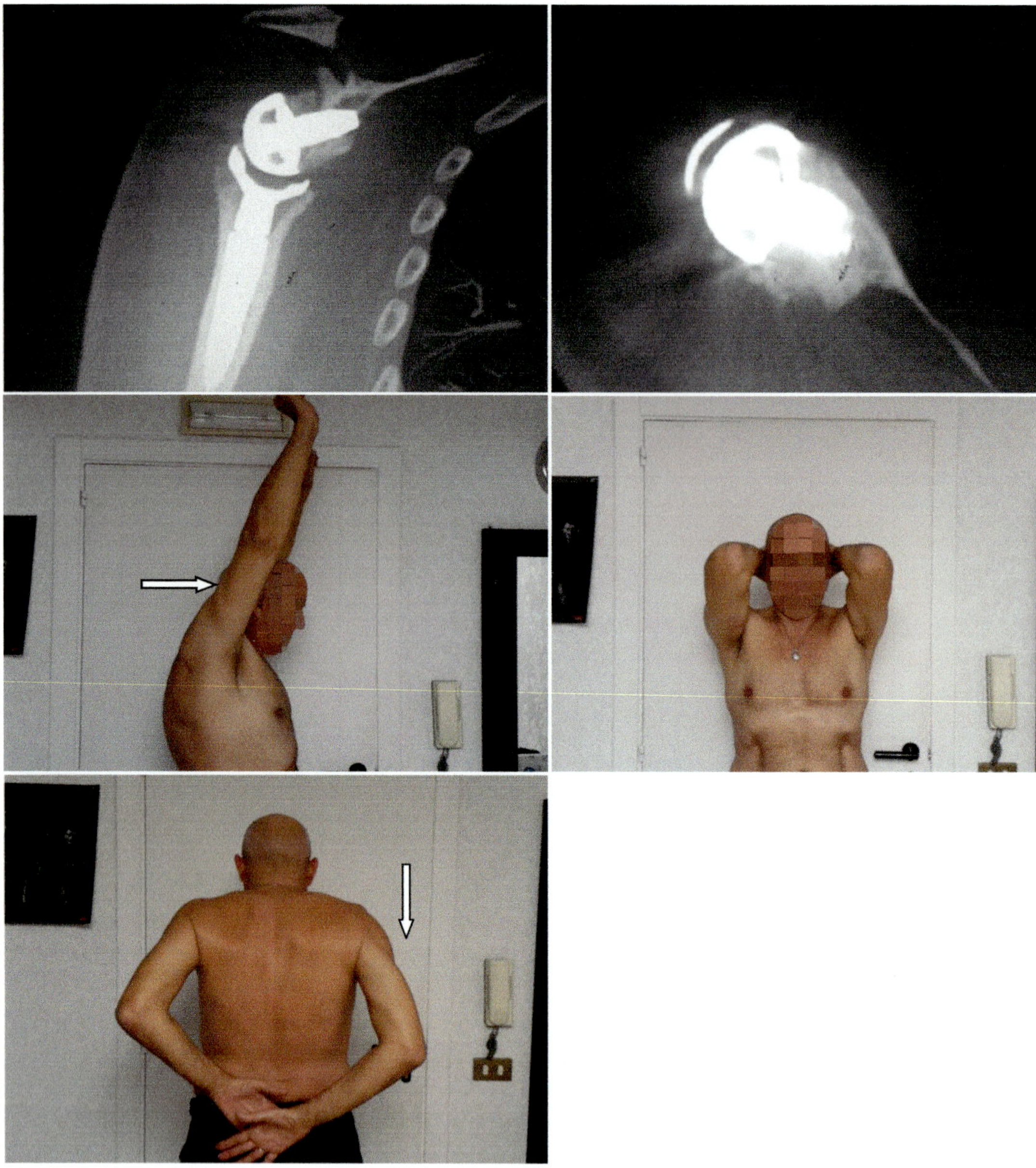

Fig. 26.3 CT scan and clinical examination, with excellent integration of the bone graft

Table 26.1 Patient demographic characteristics

	Data (*n* 11)
Age (years)	52.4 _ 3.8
Male	90%
Dominant arm injury	63.6%
Job injury	21%
Diabetes	20%
Tobacco history	50%
Ethylism and cocaine history	10%

The ASES score significantly improved from a preoperative mean of 31.1 to a postoperative mean of 69.2% (Table 26.2).

Radiographic follow-up imaging (mean 4.8 years) was available for ten patients (90.9%) and showed no patient was found with risk factor of humeral component loosening and glenoid component loosening. Evidence of grade 1 scapular

Table 26.2 Comparison of preoperative and postoperative shoulder function among 11 patients

	Preoperative	Postoperative
VAS score	6.5 ± 2	2.6 ± 2
ASES score	32 ± 15	65.5 ± 2
Constant score	_	58 ± 12
FE	60 ± 25	125 ± 40
FE > 90°	20%	85%

Table 26.3 Scapular notching grades for patients after RSA

	Description	*n* (%)
Grade 0	No defect	
Grade 1	Defect confined to pillar	2 (20%)
Grade 2	Defect in contact with lower screw 0	(0)
Grade 3	Defect over lower screw 0	(0)
Grade 4	Defect extends under baseplate 0	(0)

notching was present in two patients (20%) (Table 26.3).

One patient, with significant history of multiple shoulder surgery, underwent after 1 year to surgical revision due to traumatic dislocation implant and reported glenoid fracture with baseplate rupture and a fracture of the great tuberosity. We treated this case with a Hemy-CTA associated with donor Achilles tendon (IOR Bologna tissue bank) as reinforcement tie to stabilize H-CTA.

The 2-year clinical outcome is not very satisfactory, but the prosthesis is stable and not painful (Fig. 26.4).

26.3 Rehabilitation

The mean time of the immobilization in sling was 26 days, and the patients were allowed to move passively the arm 2 days after surgery. Rehabilitation in water started 4 weeks after surgery in all patients, in the same center following a specific protocol: for the first 2 months, a passive rehabilitation was done to reach the full anterior elevation and then with a protocol to improve the external rotation.

26.4 Discussion

RSA has showed in a long-term follow-up good clinical and radiographic results into the management of cuff tear arthropathy in terms of pain relief and restoration of range of motion and strength [1, 3, 18, 19]. Furthermore, a different study showed good outcomes of RSA in case of severe bone loss, multi-part fractures in the elderly patients, failed fracture fixation, and revision shoulder arthroplasty [3, 20–23]. However in the literature are reported results on elderly patients, and few studies are focused on young patients with degenerative and traumatic problems treated with rTSA [8, 9, 24, 25]. Many surgeons have concerns to implant rTSA in patients younger than 60 years because of the lack of long-term studies on the survivorship of these implants. Few reports have looked at its use in the younger patient with short-term to midterm outcomes [8, 9, 24–26].

This study reports on the clinical and radiographic results at short–midterm follow-up (mean, 3.0 years) in 11 young patients (aged <55 years) treated for various pathologies with an rTSA.

In literature, there have been few reports that directly deal with reverse arthroplasty in a younger patient population, specifically those younger 60 years.

Muh et al. [27] reported on 67 RSAs at a mean age of 52.2 years and a follow-up of 36.5 months. Patients had significant improvements in ROM, ASES score, and visual analog scale score, but there was a lower satisfaction rate compared with older patients.

In Ek et al.'s [26] paper, there is a significant improvement in clinical function but a high complication rate of 37.5%. Twenty-five percent of patients underwent partial or total component exchange, conversion to hemiarthroplasty, or removal. Although patients had improvement in function that was maintained at up to 10 years, there was a high complication and reoperation rate, requiring appropriate patient counseling preoperatively.

Concerning information can be extrapolated from the study by Favard et al. [28] that may have applicability for a young patient. In this report,

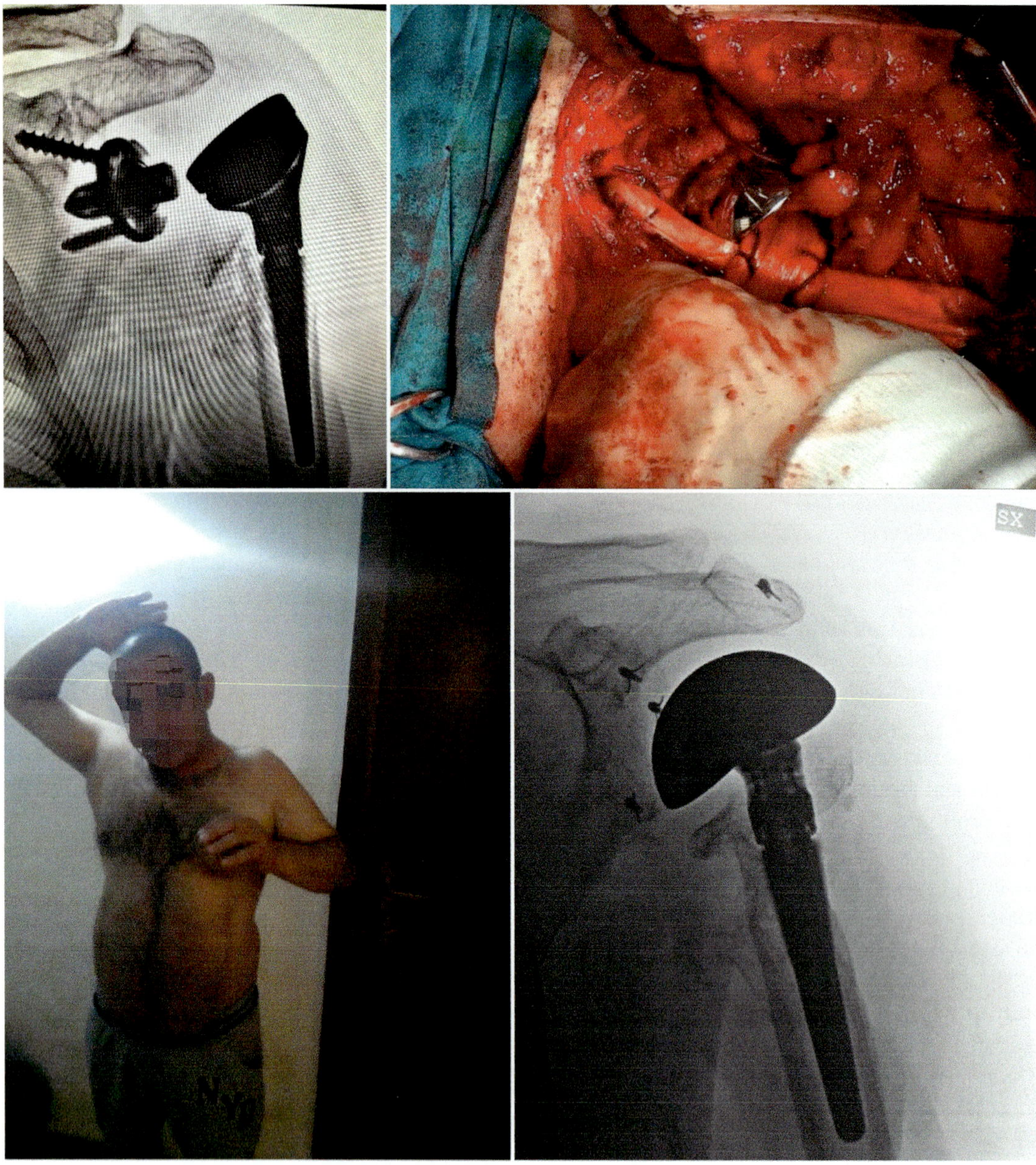

Fig. 26.4 The CTA revision in an alcoholic 44-year-old patient

489 patients with a reverse prosthesis were reviewed with 2, 5, 7, and 9 years' follow-up. The complication rate was 18%, with a 10-year survival rate of 89%.

The authors also showed a relative decline in function with longer follow-up. The Constant-Murley score in patients with more than 9 years' follow-up was significantly lower than that in those with fewer than 5 years' follow-up. Humeral, glenoid, and scapular notching was also present in 39, 32, and 50%, respectively, of patients with more than 9 years' follow-up.

The authors conclude that these results are concerning for the longevity of the reverse prosthesis and it should be used with caution in a younger patient population.

Furthermore, the normalized postoperative Constant score (mean, 58) reported in our study was similar to that in studies by Wall et al. [1] (mean, 59.7), Ek et al. [26] (mean, 57), and Boileau et al. [29] (mean, 55.8).

Likewise, the postoperative ASES score of 65.5 is within the range of scores reported in other studies [2, 30, 31]. Our results for the three patients classified as having irreparable rotator cuff tears without glenohumeral arthritis (VAS score, 1.7; ASES score, 71.8) correspond well with the results of older patients with the same etiology on whom Mulieri et al. [31] reported (VAS score, 1.9; ASES score, 75.4). Furthermore, our results for the three patients treated for failed arthroplasty (VAS score, 1.8; ASES score, 66.4) compare favorably with the results of older patients (mean age, 69 years) with the same etiology in a study by Levy et al. [30] (VAS score, 2.44; ASES score, 52.1).

In our patients, the improvement in active forward flexion (from 60_ to 125_) was similar to or greater than the improvement in the studies by Wall et al. [1] (from 86_ to 137_), Boileau et al. [29] (from 82_ to 123_), Mulieri et al. [31] (from 53_ to 134_), and Levy et al. [30] (from 38_ to 72_).

Our low postoperative rates of gross glenoid or humeral loosening (2.0%) are similar to rates in other studies [26, 29, 30, 31].

The more time from the prosthetic implant increases the incidence of complication; in fact the incidence of scapular notching, grade 1 (20%), is much lower than rates reported by Boileau et al. [29] (74%), Ek et al. [26] at 2–5 years (46%), and Wall et al. [1] (50.7%) but is similar to the rate in the study by Mulieri et al. [31] only looking at patients with preoperative Hamada grades 1, 2, or 3 (13%) [32].

This study has some limitations. The retrospective design prevents a direct comparison between rTSA and other treatments for the included etiologies. All the procedures were performed by experienced shoulder surgeons; less experienced surgeons may not obtain the same outcomes.

In addition, the minimum follow-up duration of 3.3 years (4.8–1.5 years) is relatively short for a reverse total shoulder replacement, and much longer follow-up is required for these young patients.

To our knowledge, this study is one of the few that reported a series of clinical outcomes of rTSA in younger patients. This is a patient population that is growing in both size and importance as the indications for reverse arthroplasty continue to expand. This patient population aged younger than 60 was complex, with very poor function, previous surgery, fractures, and/or instability sequelae. In addition, this population had clinical conditions that combined rotator cuff deficiency, poor active elevation, joint damage, and pain that led to severe shoulder dysfunction. Anterosuperior instability or escape was also present in this group. Functional compromise was significant, and patients desired to use their hand away from their body from waist to chest level for simple activities of daily living. Thus, there are very few options to provide this functional ability besides rTSA, especially in a complex population in which over 50% of patients had previous shoulder surgery.

These patients can be expected to have higher functional levels and require longer implant survival when compared with the more traditional elderly patient. In this study, patients aged younger than 60 had significant functional increases and decreases in pain compared with preoperative scores at a mean follow-up of 3.3 years.

However, of notable concern is that clinical results have been shown to deteriorate after 6–8 years. Thus, although our midterm results show good survivorship (90%), and improved functional scores, longer-term follow-up is certainly necessary in this younger patient population [33, 34].

Reference

1. Wall B, Nove-Josserand L, O'Connor DP, Edwards TB, Walch G. Reverse total shoulder arthroplasty: a review of results according to etiology. J Bone Joint Surg Am. 2007;89:1476–85. https://doi.org/10.2106/JBJS.F.00666.
2. Grammont PM, Baulot E. Delta shoulder prosthesis for rotator cuff rupture. Orthopedics. 1993;16:65–8.
3. Boileau P, Watkinson D, Hatzidakis AM, Hovorka I. Neer award 2005: the Grammont reverse shoulder prosthesis: results in cuff tear arthritis, fracture

sequelae, and revision arthroplasty. J Shoulder Elb Surg. 2006;15:527–40. https://doi.org/10.1016/j.jse.2006.01.003.
4. Berhouet J, Garaud P, Favard L. Evaluation of the role of glenosphere design and humeral component retroversion in avoiding scapular notching during reverse shoulder arthroplasty. J Shoulder Elb Surg. 2014;23:151–8. https://doi.org/10.1016/j.jse.2013.05.009.
5. Day JS, Lau E, Ong KL, Williams GR, Ramsey ML, Kurtz SM. Prevalence and projections of total shoulder and elbow arthroplasty in the United States to 2015. J Shoulder Elb Surg. 2010;19:1115–20.
6. Hattrup SJ, Cofield RH. Osteonecrosis of the humeral head: results of replacement. J Shoulder Elb Surg. 2000;9:177–82.
7. Hovelius L, Sandström B, Saebö M. One hundred eighteen Bristow-Latarjet repairs for recurrent anterior dislocation of the shoulder prospectively followed for fifteen years: study II—the evolution of dislocation arthropathy. J Shoulder Elb Surg. 2006;15:279–89.
8. Dillon MT, Inacio MC, Burke MF, Navarro RA, Yian EH. Shoulder arthroplasty in patients 59 years of age and younger. J Shoulder Elb Surg. 2013;22:1338–44.
9. Padegimas EM, Maltenfort M, Lazarus MD, Ramsey ML, Williams GR, Namdari S. Future patient demand for shoulder arthroplasty by younger patients: national projections. Clin Orthop Relat Res. 2015;473(6):1860–7. https://doi.org/10.1007/s11999-015-4231-z.
10. Kim SH, Wise BL, Zhang Y, Szabo RM. Increasing incidence of shoulder arthroplasty in the United States. J Bone Joint Surg Am. 2011;93:2249–54.
11. Pessis E, Sverzut JM, Campagna R, Guerini H, Feydy A, Drapé JL. Artifact with dual-energy CT: virtual monospectral imaging with fast kilovoltage switching and metal artifact reduction software. Semin Musculoskelet Radiol. 2015;19(5):446–55. https://doi.org/10.1055/s-0035-1569256.
12. Harper KW, Helms CA, Haystead CM, Higgins LD. Glenoid dysplasia: incidence and association with posterior labral tears as evaluated on MRI. AJR Am J Roentgenol. 2005;184:984–8.
13. Sperling JW, Cofield RH, Steinmann SP. Shoulder arthroplasty for osteoarthritis secondary to glenoid dysplasia. J Bone Joint Surg Am. 2002;84-A:541–6.
14. Allen B, Schoch B, Sperling JW, Cofield RH. Shoulder arthroplasty for osteoarthritis secondary to glenoid dysplasia: an update. J Shoulder Elb Surg. 2014;23:214–20.
15. Sperling JW, Cofield RH, O'Driscoll SW, Torchia ME, Rowland CM. Radiographic assessment of ingrowth total shoulder arthroplasty. J Shoulder Elb Surg. 2000;9:507–13.
16. Lazarus MD, Jensen KL, Southworth C, Matsen FA III. The radiographic evaluation of keeled and pegged glenoid component insertion. J Bone Joint Surg Am. 2002;84:1174–82.
17. Lévigne C, Boileau P, Favard L, Garaud P, Molé D, Sirveaux F, Walch G. Scapular notching in reverse shoulder arthroplasty. J Shoulder Elb Surg. 2008;17(6):925–35. https://doi.org/10.1016/j.jse.2008.02.010.
18. Nolan BM, Ankerson E, Wiater JM. Reverse total shoulder arthroplasty improves function in cuff tear arthropathy. Clin Orthop Relat Res. 2011;469:2476–82. https://doi.org/10.1007/s11999-010-1683-z.
19. Sirveaux F, Favard L, Oudet D, Huquet D, Walch G, Mole D. Grammont inverted total shoulder arthroplasty in the treatment of glenohumeral osteoarthritis with massive rupture of the cuff. Results of a multicentre study of 80 shoulders. J Bone Joint Surg Br. 2004;86:388–95. https://doi.org/10.1302/0301-620X.86B3.14024.
20. Bufquin T, Hersan A, Hubert L, Massin P. Reverse shoulder arthroplasty for the treatment of three- and four-part fractures of the proximal humerus in the elderly: a prospective review of 43 cases with a short-term follow-up. J Bone Joint Surg Br. 2007;89:516–20. https://doi.org/10.1302/0301-620X.89B4.18435.
21. Willis M, Min W, Brooks J, Mulieri P, Walker M, Pupello D, et al. Proximal humeral malunion treated with reverse shoulder arthroplasty. J Shoulder Elb Surg. 2012;21:507–13. https://doi.org/10.1016/j.jse.2011.01.042.
22. Cazeneuve JF, Cristofari DJ. The reverse shoulder prosthesis in the treatment of fractures of the proximal humerus in the elderly. J Bone Joint Surg Br. 2010;92:535–9. https://doi.org/10.1302/0301-620X.92B4.22450.
23. Russo R, Della Rotonda G, Cautiero F, Ciccarelli M. Reverse shoulder prosthesis to treat complex proximal humeral fractures in the elderly patients: results after 10-year experience. Musculoskelet Surg. 2015;99(Suppl 1):S17–23. https://doi.org/10.1007/s12306-015-0367-y.
24. Merolla G, Porcellini G. Reverse shoulder arthroplasty in patients aged sixty years old or younger: are we really doing the best? Transl Med UniSa. 2014;9:66–7.
25. Sershon RA, Van Thiel GS, Lin EC, McGill KC, Cole BJ, Verma NN, Romeo AA, Nicholson GP. Clinical outcomes of reverse total shoulder arthroplasty in patients aged younger than 60 years. J Shoulder Elb Surg. 2014;23(3):395–400. https://doi.org/10.1016/j.jse.2013.07.047.
26. Ek ET, Neukom L, Catanzaro S, Gerber C. Reverse total shoulder arthroplasty for massive irreparable rotator cuff tears in patients younger than 65 years old: results after five to fifteen years. J Shoulder Elb Surg. 2013;22:1199–208. https://doi.org/10.1016/j.jse.2012.011.016.
27. Muh SJ, Streit JJ, Wanner JP, Lenarz CJ, Shishani Y, Rowland DY, Riley C, Nowinski RJ, Edwards TB, Gobezie R. Early follow-up of reverse total shoulder arthroplasty in patients sixty years of age or younger. J Bone Joint Surg Am. 2013;95(20):1877–83. https://doi.org/10.2106/JBJS.L.10005.
28. Favard L, Levigne C, Nerot C, Gerber C, De Wilde L, Mole D. Reverse prostheses in arthropathies with

cuff tear: are survivorship and function maintained over time? Clin Orthop Relat Res. 2011;469:2469–75. https://doi.org/10.1007/s11999-011-1833-y.
29. Boileau P, Gonzalez JF, Chuinard C, Bicknell R, Walch G. Reverse total shoulder arthroplasty after failed rotator cuff surgery. J Shoulder Elb Surg. 2009;18:600–6. https://doi.org/10.1016/j.jse.2009.03.011.
30. Levy J, Frankle M, Mighell M, Pupello D. The use of the reverse shoulder prosthesis for the treatment of failed hemiarthroplasty for proximal humeral fracture. J Bone Joint Surg Am. 2007;89:292–300. https://doi.org/10.2106/JBJS.E.01310.
31. Mulieri P, Dunning P, Klein S, Pupello D, Frankle M. Reverse shoulder arthroplasty for the treatment of irreparable rotator cuff tear without glenohumeral arthritis. J Bone Joint Surg Am. 2010;92:2544.
32. Hamada K, Fukuda H, Mikasa M, Kobayashi Y. Roentgenographic findings in massive rotator cuff tears. A long-term observation. Clin Orthop Relat Res. 1990;254:92–6.
33. Guery J, Favard L, Sirveaux F, Oudet D, Mole D, Walch G. Reverse total shoulder arthroplasty. Survivorship analysis of eighty replacements followed for five to ten years. J Bone Joint Surg Am. 2006;88:1742–7.
34. Russo R, Rotonda GD, Ciccarelli M, Cautiero F. Analysis of complications of reverse total shoulder arthroplasty. Joints. 2015;3(2):62–6. https://doi.org/10.11138/jts/2015.3.2.062.

Part VI

Complications

Complications in Reverse Shoulder Arthroplasty: Focus on Comorbidities

27

Roberto Leo, Valentina Fogliata, and Bruno Michele Marelli

Comorbidity: the simultaneous presence of two chronic diseases or conditions in a patient.

(Oxford Dictionary)

The term co-morbidity (then comorbidity) was introduced for the first time by the American epidemiologist Alvan R. Feinstein in an article published in 1970 [1]. He defined this neologism as "the existence or occurrence of any distinct additional entity during the clinical course of a patient who has the index disease under study." In this way, a new term was born to indicate the occurrence of different pathologies in the same individual or, more precisely, the phenomenon for which a patient who is in care for a shoulder arthropathy also presents one or more simultaneous diseases not related to the former. That situation can affect the therapy, the outcomes of the main pathology, the patient's quality of life, and the duration of the hospitalization.

R. Leo (✉) · V. Fogliata
UOS Chirurgia della Spalla e del Gomito, Centro Specialistico Ortopedico Traumatologico Gaetano Pini-CTO, Milan, Italy
e-mail: roberto.leo@asst-pini-cto.it

B. M. Marelli
UOC Ortopedia e Traumatologia 1, Centro Specialistico Ortopedico Traumatologico Gaetano Pini-CTO, Milan, Italy

Specifically, in our clinical practice, we perform a careful study of the comorbidities of each single patient admitted to our Shoulder Surgery Unit. This evaluation should be emphasized for those operations, such as reverse shoulder arthroplasty (RSA), for which these pre-existing and non-modifiable conditions may play an important role in the development of local or systemic complications.

The number of RSA implants is greatly increasing, along with the growing age of the population. Consequently, we should be experiencing, over the years, an ever-increasing number of pathologies that can be considered as comorbidities and must be carefully pondered for the possibility of onset of complications that may be, if provided, in some cases, well manageable. Knowledge of comorbidities is therefore useful in assessing the risk/benefit ratio in the treatment of shoulder arthropathy.

For this reason, we believe it is essential to have an accurate preoperative medical history with a careful evaluation of the patient in order to proceed toward a correct decision-making process trying to avoid as many complications as possible.

S. Gumina et al. (eds.), *Reverse Shoulder Arthroplasty*,
https://doi.org/10.1007/978-3-319-97743-0_27

Over the years, several classification systems have been studied and validated. Those scores are based on statistical and arithmetic analyses and associate the presence of pre-existing pathologies with the increased risk of postoperative complications.

The two most important classification systems are:

- Charlson Comorbidity Index (CCI)
- American Society of Anesthesiologist Physical Status Classification System (ASA Score)

27.1 Charlson Comorbidity Index

In 1987 the so-called Charlson Comorbidity Index was drawn up [2]. Initially it has been introduced to study the probability of readmission to the hospital within a year for each patient not subject to trauma, assessing his comorbidities. For each pathology, scores of 1–6 points were assigned to the patient, and the sum of the scores determined the probability of readmission to the hospital (Fig. 27.1, Table 27.1).

The Charlson Comorbidity Index has been subjected to many revisions and variations over the years and has been transformed into a questionnaire to be submitted to the patient but is still a reference standard in survival clinical trials.

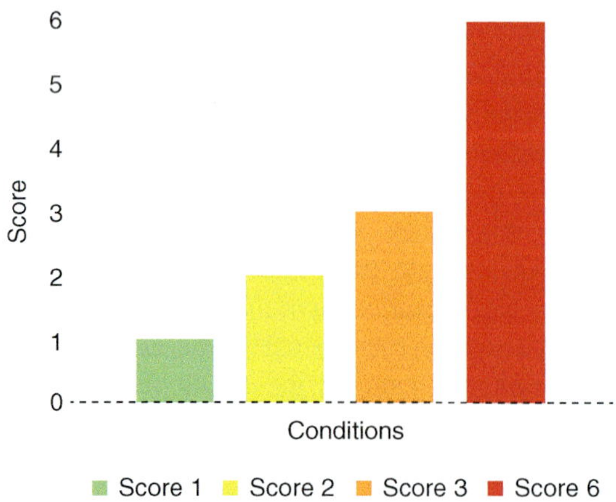

Fig. 27.1 Charlson Comorbidity Index—score representation

The work conducted by Voskuij et al. [3] validates the use of this important score in orthopedic clinical practice and also underlines how this can be useful as a predictor of different types of risk: (1) risk of perioperative transfusions, (2) risk of hospital readmission, and (3) risk of mortality. Regarding the risk of perioperative transfusion, an increase of one point in the CCI has been evaluated to lead to a 0.11% increase of the risk of perioperative transfusion after prosthetic surgery and a 0.45% increase of this risk following trauma surgery. Also in the case of risk of hospital readmission, an increase of one point in the CCI brings a 0.45% probability increase of the risk factor after prosthetic surgery and a 0.63% increase after trauma surgery. Finally, this study shows an increase of 0.25% risk of mortality for each additional point in CCI after shoulder surgery and 0.24% after trauma surgery.

In addition, every year of aging increases risk of mortality by an average of 0.03% for all the surgeries.

An interesting example of using this score is the work of Singh et al. [4] and Chalmers et al. [5] who argue that the CCI is a significant predictor of postoperative complications in their researches. In the first study, an increase of this

Table 27.1 Charlson Comorbidity Index—assigned weights for each condition that a patient has [2]

Score	Conditions
1	Myocardial infarct Congestive heart failure Peripheral vascular disease Cerebrovascular disease Dementia Chronic pulmonary disease Connective tissue disease Ulcer disease Mild liver disease Diabetes
2	Hemiplegia Moderate or severe renal disease Diabetes with end-organ damage Tumor Leukemia Lymphoma
3	Moderate or severe liver disease
6	Metastatic solid tumor AIDS

Index was associated with increased mortality in the following 90 days after shoulder arthroplasty, and in the second study, this score has been indicated as the best predictor for the likelihood of postoperative complications. We therefore believe that CCI can be a useful tool in common clinical practice, which can help the surgeon in the proper therapeutic planning suited to the individual patient.

CCI can help the orthopedic surgeon in the full preoperative patient evaluation, avoiding the risk of just focusing on the shoulder pathology requiring shoulder prosthesis.

27.2 American Society of Anesthesiologist Physical Status Classification System

This classification system was introduced for the first time in 1963 as a patient preoperative classification for anesthetic risk assessment [6], and it is constantly updated by the American Society of Anesthesiologist. The current version is reported in Table 27.2 [7].

The addition of "E" denotes emergency surgery (an emergency is defined as existing when delay in treatment of the patient would lead to a significant increase in the threat to life or body part).

Although it is used in anesthesiological clinical practice, it is not usually taken into account in common orthopedic practice. However, it is important to consider how the increase in the value attributed to the individual patient increases the risk of perioperative complications (Fig. 27.2).

This evaluation is highly important while we are studying the patient, as demonstrated by Ricchetti and collaborators [8] and by Dunn et al. [9] who have shown that the presence of comorbidities leads to ASA III or higher class, corresponding to the following circumstances:

- Longer hospitalization
- Increased risk of mortality in the first postoperative 90 days
- Increased risk of complications after shoulder arthroplasty according to the work of Shields et al. [10]

Table 27.2 ASA score, last approved by the ASA House of Delegates on October 15, 2014 [7]

ASA PS classification	Definition	Examples
ASA I	A normal healthy patient	Healthy, nonsmoking, no or minimal alcohol use
ASA II	A patient with mild systemic disease	Mild diseases only without substantive functional limitations
ASA III	A patient with severe systemic disease	Substantive functional limitations—one or more moderate to severe diseases
ASA IV	A patient with severe systemic disease that is a constant threat to life	
ASA V	A moribund patient who is not expected to survive without the operation	
ASA VI	A declared brain-dead patient whose organs are being removed for donor purposes	

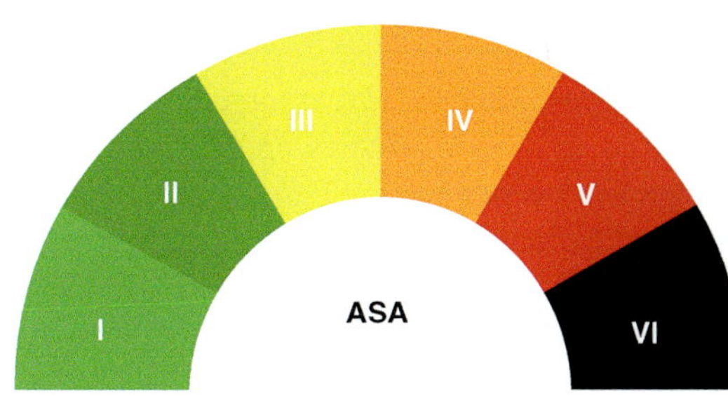

Fig. 27.2 Visual scale that shows how increasing the ASA value attributed to each patient, increases the risk of perioperative complications

Before we systematically approach the discussion of the details of comorbidities that most frequently affect the overall outcome in shoulder prosthesis surgery, we must point out that **aged patients** and **recent traumas** are related to less successful result.

Although **age** itself cannot be considered as comorbidity, it can still play an important role. We think it is impossible to generalize by indicating age as a risk factor, but it must be considered in relation to the complication that can be observed after surgery. For example, an older age increases the risk of a thromboembolic event, but, at the same time, an older age is considered as a protective factor in a patient who needs revision surgery maybe because elderly patients have less functional requirements.

Regarding the risk of postoperative infection, Singh's [11] work shows that a lower age and male sex are associated with a higher risk of developing a periprosthetic infection, whereas an advanced age and female sex are associated with a significantly lower risk of developing these infections. The causes remain unknown. One hypothesis, according to author, might be that younger and male patients are more likely to have developed a traumatic cause. As age increases, as is well known, there is also a depression of the immune system, which is therefore a factor facilitating infections in elderly patients.

In any case as age increases, we record a growth in the number of comorbidities of each patient, stressing the need to carefully evaluate this parameter in our patients.

Regarding **traumas**, we can note how humerus fractures requiring a prosthetic replacement are a predictive factor of a less functional outcome that will not be completely satisfactory if compared to the same prosthesis in elective surgery. In fact, as evidenced by several studies among which we cite the work conducted by Farng's and collaborators [12], undergoing a shoulder prothesis replacement after a proximal humerus fracture predisposes to a greater risk of complications in the first 90 postoperative days.

On the other hand, the same work highlights how the same patients are at a lower risk of requiring long-term revision surgery, evidence that this probably reflects the poor functional demand of this population.

An interesting Davis' et al. paper [13] also analyzes the increase of hospitalization costs in patients who underwent shoulder prosthesis in post-traumatic arthritis, compared to patients undergoing the same surgery in primary osteoarthritis, probably due to the fact that trauma patients require major clinical, diagnostic, and technical dedication. As a matter of fact, the choice of using a reverse shoulder arthroplasty is very complex and is performed on the basis of fracture type and patient characters. The patient to whom a reverse shoulder arthroplasty will be implanted for a fracture, however, as far as our experience is concerned, is still an older patient than the one who is subjected to elective surgery, resulting in lower functional requirements, greater comorbidity, and hence possibility to develop local or systemic postoperative complications.

We did not find in literature a systematic list of comorbidities that most frequently could compromise functional outcome in prosthetic shoulder surgery, but the goal of our work is to clarify this intricate subject.

We must therefore first distinguish different groups of diseases associated with the simultaneous presence of comorbidities in prosthetic shoulder surgery.

27.3 Cardiovascular Diseases

Previous acute cardiac event
Previous thromboembolic event
CAD (coronary artery disease)

Several works associate a previous cardiac and thromboembolic event with an increased risk of complications in the first 90 postoperative days, as evidenced, for example, by Singh et al.'s 2012 work [14], which evaluates in detail the risk of developing cardiological and thromboembolic complications, indicating an incidence of 2.6% for the first and 1.2% for the latter.

Risk factors for cardiac complications are, as it may be intuitive, a previous cardiac event, an advanced age, and an increased CCI.

However, with regard to the single thromboembolic risk, this article indicates that risk factors for the development of this complication are female gender, age older than 70 years, high BMI, traumatic diagnosis, pre-existing thromboembolism, and a high Charlson Comorbity Index. These comorbidities should therefore be considered during the study of patient's history, as well as evaluating how a previous pathological event may play a role in the possibility of developing postoperative complications.

Moreover, concerning CAD, a study by Davis et al. [13] shows how the presence of this and other comorbidities increases the cost of average hospitalization after a shoulder arthroplasty implant, a concept that helps us understand how a patient with this comorbidity may be on average more complex to manage from a clinical point of view during the immediately postsurgery period.

27.4 Respiratory Diseases

27.4.1 COPD (Chronic Obstructive Pulmonary Disease)

This comorbidity has been well analyzed by Davis and colleagues in the aforementioned paper [13], paying attention to the cost of hospitalization as those patients require extraordinary care compared to the others.

This work showed that the presence of chronic obstructive pulmonary diseases increases the cost of hospitalization for a 4.49% compared to baseline.

27.5 Kidney Diseases

27.5.1 CKD (Chronic Kidney Disease)

As in the case of CAD and COPD, we also consider CKD as the point of reference for Davis and colleagues [13] which show that, for a patient with a chronic kidney disease (CKD), the cost of hospitalization is estimated to be even 15.08% higher than the standard cost of a relatively healthy patient. This gives us an idea of how it should be taken into account while correctly managing this type of patients and their shoulder pathology.

27.6 Autoimmune Diseases

27.6.1 Rheumatoid Arthritis

Rheumatoid arthritis is one of the more representative pathology among the autoimmune diseases in our current orthopedic clinical practice. It is an autoimmune disease with important effects on many joints [15], including the shoulder (Fig. 27.3). The involvement of the shoulder has been shown to be present in more than 90% of the affected patients [16]. The characteristic synovitis may involve not only the synovial membrane but also extend itself to the rotator cuff, setting up true tendon injuries due to this persistent inflammatory process [17]. In the cases in which also the cartilage layer begins to be involved, a reverse shoulder prothesis can also be indicated.

Rheumatoid arthritis, however, as it is known, decreases the immunological system, causing an increased risk of infections [11]. This situation is worsened by modern immunosuppressive therapies that often are used by rheumatologists [18].

The preoperative evaluation of bone performed by a CT scan is very important in these patients in which the therapies and the chronic inflammatory response cause a decrease of the bone density.

All these issues do not interfere with the fact that reverse shoulder arthroplasty remains the surgical treatment of choice for glenohumeral arthropathy also in patients with rheumatoid arthritis, a disease that is now, year by year, better controlled by new therapies. In particular, Davis and colleagues [13] point out a rise in the per day cost of hospitalization for this category of patients, although overall there is a decrease in the total cost of average hospitalization compared to the past thanks to an ever better management of this pathology.

27.7 Metabolic Diseases

27.7.1 Diabetes Mellitus

Also, the diagnosis of diabetes has been shown to increase the cost of hospital admissions [13].

It is estimated that about 50% of diabetic patients are over 60 years of age, which is why, due to the significant incidence of this disease, it is necessary to assess the risk, in case of shoulder surgery in this population [19].

The prevalence of diabetics in the population is, unfortunately, increasing, also due to the often sedentary lifestyle and eating disorder. Although

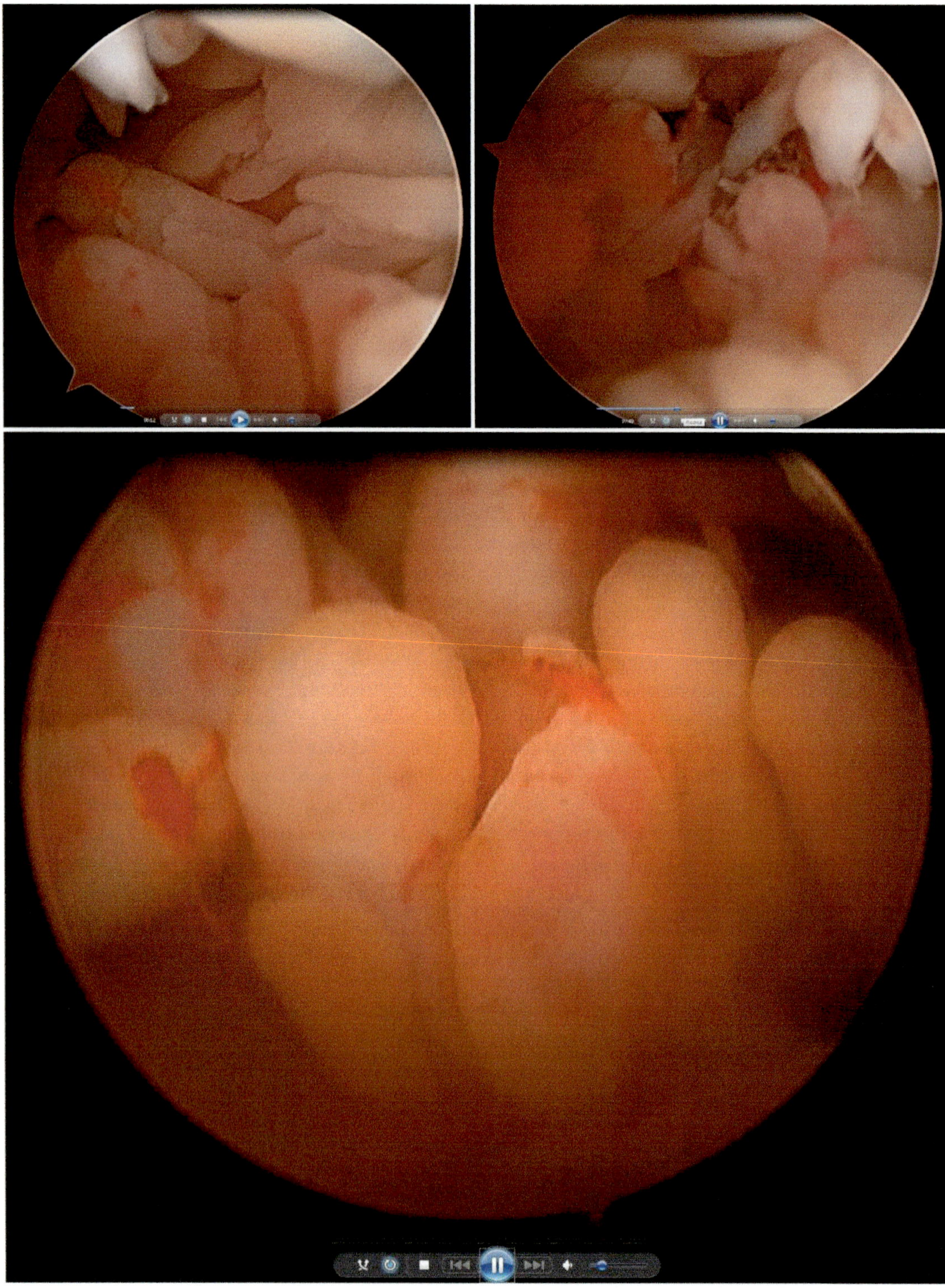

Fig. 27.3 Synovial villi, characteristics for rheumatoid arthritis with shoulder involvement

there is little literature about it, it is now known that diabetic patients have a greater risk of developing complications after joint prosthesis implantation [20].

The 2014 work of Ponce et al. [21] is a reference, regarding diabetes as a comorbidity in the implant of shoulder prosthesis. This work is indicating that the presence of diabetes mellitus is an independent risk factor for (a) perioperative mortality, (b) longer hospitalization, and (c) specific complications such as acute renal failure. Especially for the latter condition, the risk increases so much that a diabetic patient has a probability of 1–5 times greater to develop acute renal failure than a nondiabetic patient. Of course, any medical team, aware of this fact, should pay more attention to factors such as the use of nephrotoxic drugs and the patient's hydration, particularly important in this class of people.

In addition, diabetes has a direct deleterious effect on immune and vascular systems worsening the healing process in common pathologies and trauma; for this reason, we should pay more attention to this category of patients with a tight follow-up [22–25]. Many studies have also suggested that diabetic patients are at a high risk of serious surgical and postoperative systemic complications, including death [26, 27].

27.7.2 BMI: Obesity and Malnutrition

In Singh et al.'s 2011 work [4], it is emphasized that a decrease in BMI corresponds to an increased risk of mortality in the first 90 postoperative days. In fact, the results of this study show how the mortality rate in patients with BMI above 30 kg/m^2 is lower if compared with patients with BMI below 25 kg/m^2.

The abovementioned work is the first observing the association between high BMI and decreased risk of mortality in the first 90 postoperative days in patients undergoing shoulder arthroprosthesis. In this case adipose tissue is considered to be a metabolic organ, a phenomenon we refer as the "obesity paradox." It can be probably explained by the fact that underweight patients usually have a lower amount of energetic reserves than overweight or even obese patients, a condition that makes them susceptible to complications and consequent increased mortality especially in stressful postoperative period. In our opinion, this "paradox" can only be considered true if we compare overweight to really underweight patients (bordering malnutrition) because in our current clinical practice, obesity leads, in general, to greater complications than the normal weight patients.

We find ourselves in agreement with the work [11] that shows that patients with high BMI are subject to the development of more periprosthetic infections, probably due to alterations in the immune system linked to obesity and metabolic syndrome. Regarding the blood loss, some works also show that overweight patients have significantly greater intraoperative blood loss [28] than control groups, while there were no differences in VAS for pain assessment with control groups. This work shows also that obese patients had 35% of various types of complications (such as instability, glenoid loosening, infections) that were much higher than in control groups.

All this information does not necessarily mean that obesity is an absolute contraindication to surgery, but the surgeon must ever carefully consider the risk/benefit ratio for each patient before each procedure.

Malnutrition, on the contrary, is a very important comorbidity to be considered before a shoulder arthroplasty. A study by Garcia and colleagues has highlighted how this is a problem in 7.6% of patients undergoing this surgery [29]. In this work serum albumin level is used as a benchmark for assessing the nutritional status of the patient, pointing out that patients with serum albumin levels below 3.5 g/dL subjected to shoulder prosthesis have a significantly greater risk of developing anemia requiring transfusion compared to patients with higher preoperative values. This study concludes, therefore, that malnourished patients are more likely to develop complications such as anemia requiring transfusion. Malnutrition, in the same work, was also associated with increased length of stay and increased mortality in the first 30 postoperative days.

At the end we agree that an adequate nutritional state is a very important factor as a starting point for a patient undergoing a shoulder prosthesis and, in general, for any other surgery.

27.8 Neurological Diseases

27.8.1 Anxiety, Depression, and Psychiatric Disorders

Anxiety and mood disorder patients are, according to some works, the two major diagnoses at the general population level [30]. Several studies have shown that there is a correlation between the mood and the possibility of developing chronic refractory pain for therapies [31–34], so that it has been proposed to fill a form answering a specific questionnaire to highlight any mood, anxiety, and depression disorders in patients who need a shoulder arthroplasty so that the surgeon may be able to help these patients before the surgical procedure with any support services [35].

An interesting work by Bot et al. [36] suggests that preoperative diagnosis of depression, anxiety, or dementia is associated with a higher risk of adverse events after shoulder arthroplasty surgery. Patients with dementia and schizophrenia, however, according to the same study, are subjected to a higher number of transfusions, probably because they are more likely to be positive for the symptoms of anemia, since symptoms of depression such as asthenia may mimic the symptoms of anemia following surgery. In addition, transfusions can serve as surrogates for nutritional deficiencies that are most prevalent in this class of patients, especially in those with dementia.

Again, according to this study, a reason that can help understand the highest rate of transfusions in psychiatric patients and especially schizophrenic patients is related to the fact that these patients often undergo RSA/TSA surgery for a fracture of the proximal humerus, which is already in itself, as mentioned above, a factor which predisposes for a higher rate of complications and worse outcomes than primary arthrosis.

Our clinical practice fully confirms that there is a difference in postoperative recovery not only in the different perception of pain but also in terms of functionality of the limb, in the approach to rehabilitation and therefore in the timing of returning to daily living activities, which is significantly faster in those who deal with the intervention with a positive mood. We also believe that patients with anxiety and psychiatric illnesses have a lower perception of the quality of the result obtained, as shown by several studies suggesting that symptoms of depression are associated with higher levels of perception of disability and lower threshold of pain accompanied by low levels of satisfaction after surgical therapy [37–40].

27.8.2 Parkinson's Disease

It is a very common condition, with an incidence of 1–2% in the population over 65 years, according to studies conducted in the United States [41, 42]. Despite this, its impact on the shoulder prosthesis is still underestimated, although it is known that this pathology is a very important comorbidity, which can therefore predispose to various kinds of complications, as evidenced in the work of Burrus et al. [43]. Parkinson's disease represents, in some cases, a contraindication in the implant of a shoulder prosthesis.

The upper limbs are much more subordinate, compared to lower limbs, to the dystonic movements characteristic of this pathology, and this increases the probability of trauma in this segment even with low-energy trauma. In those patients, considering the reduced serum level of calcium, typical of this condition, even a low-energy trauma can lead to greater fracture risk. There also seems to exist evidence of higher risk of loosening in the first postoperative period. This hypothesis is supported by works conducted by Kock [44] and Kryzak [45], which account for a 19% need for revision surgery after a shoulder arthroplasty in patients affected by Parkinson's disease due to glenoid or humeral loosening. The mobilization is also supposed to be caused by the increase in the tone of the scapular track with the resulting stiffness characteristic of this pathology.

As a further consequence, the approach to arm mobilization carried out with the aid of a physical therapist leads to additional difficulties in the rehabilitation process, with worse outcomes regarding the postoperative range of motion for the affected shoulder, with less patient satisfaction.

27.9 Tumors

27.9.1 Malignant Tumor

Although it may be clear, we stress that the underlying malignant cancer diagnosis corresponds to a high risk of complications for all surgical interventions, including shoulder arthroplasty implant [4]. This important comorbidity, of course, must be considered both with regard to the pathology itself and the therapies put in place to control it, which are extremely heavy for the body and further lower the immune defenses.

27.10 Infective Diseases

It is obvious to emphasize that the implantation of a shoulder prosthesis a short period after an infectious disease is contraindicated due to the possible presence of a bacteremia (a condition that applies even to recent dental surgery) or to a lower immune system response, still weakened by the recent infection.

HCV falls within this context.

Although for obvious reasons it is not explicitly taken into account in the Charlson Comorbidity Index (only in April 1989, the discovery of HCV virus was published in two articles in the journal *Science*) [46, 47], as underlined by the 2017 Rosas' work [48], a comorbidity that needs to be considered is the presence of Hepatitis C, which has also been shown to have a significant impact on hospitalization costs in postoperative period, as these subjects are exposed to a higher risk of complications including infections, dysplasia, fractures, need for revision surgery, systemic complications, and the need for transfusions.

27.11 Mechanical Factors

Mechanical factors are considered as all those conditions that lead to an overload of the prosthesis that can be dangerous in the immediate postoperative period.

The mechanical energy applied to the shoulder prior to surgery (traumatic energy) or applied after surgery (chronic mechanical overload) represents a negative cofactor on the good functioning of the system, acting as a comorbidity.

Even if these conditions are not comorbidity in the strict sense, there are many situations in which a patient is obliged to mechanically overload the prosthetic implant, for example, patients that require walking with crutches due to advanced age or lower limb pathologies with particular family situations in which the patient, recently operated to the shoulder, needs to help elderly relatives exposing shoulder prosthesis to a nonphysiological mechanical load.

27.12 Conclusions

We can conclude by emphasizing how, in our opinion, for each individual patient waiting for a reverse shoulder implant surgery, both in the case of elective surgery and in the case of trauma surgery, it is compulsory to undertake a deep study of the patient, without limiting the evaluation only to the shoulder. We should examine the presence of any of the pathological conditions abovementioned and summarized as follows (Fig. 27.4).

As it emerged from our discussion, we also do not think the study of comorbidities, strictly speaking, is sufficient, but we think it is necessary to extend our in-depth knowledge also to the patient's living conditions and to all those

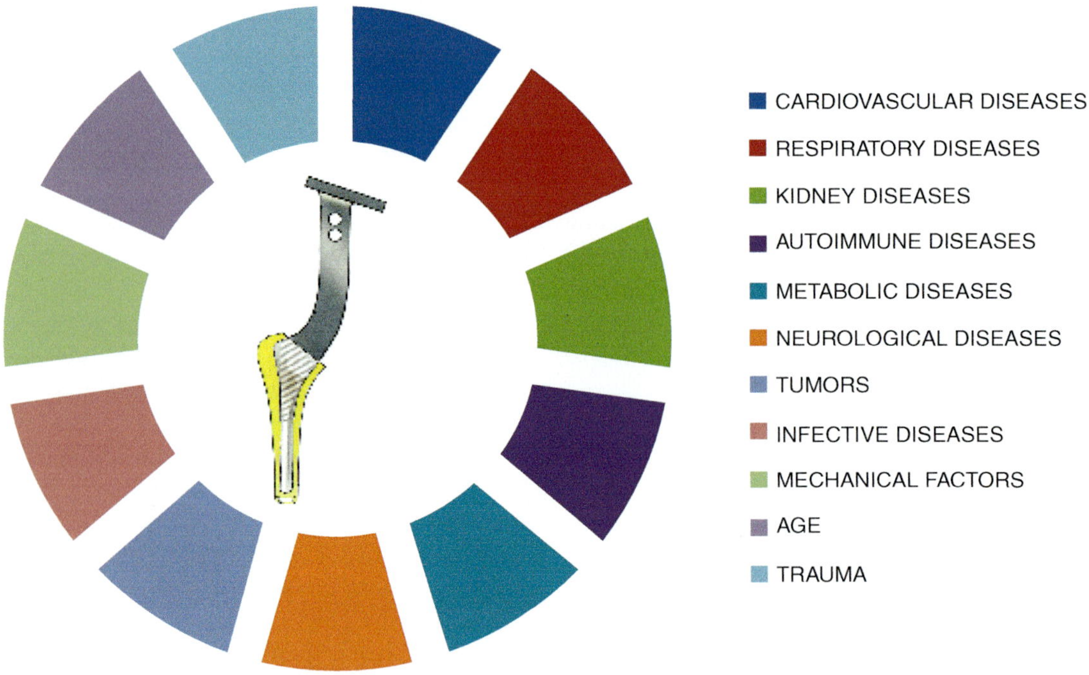

Fig. 27.4 Summary of major comorbidities

pathologies that may affect the immediate post-operative course.

Only in this way, with a 360° view of our patient and with a thorough knowledge of the person we are facing, we can be sure to decide for the correct therapeutic indication, which is not necessarily the surgical one.

References

1. Feinstein AR. The pre-therapeutic classification of co-morbidity in chronic disease. J Chronic Dis. 1970;23(7):455–68.
2. Charlson ME, Pompei P, Ales KL, MacKenzie CR. A new method of classifying prognostic comorbidity in longitudinal studies: development and validation. J Chronic Dis. 1987;40(5):373–83.
3. Voskuijl T, Hageman M, Ring D. Higher Charlson Comorbidity Index Scores are associated with readmission after orthopaedic surgery. Clin Orthop Relat Res. 2014;472(5):1638–44. https://doi.org/10.1007/s11999-013-3394-8.
4. Singh JA, Sperling JW, Cofield RH. Ninety day mortality and its predictors after primary shoulder arthroplasty: an analysis of 4,019 patients from 1976-2008. BMC Musculoskelet Disord. 2011;12(12):231. https://doi.org/10.1186/1471-2474-12-231.
5. Chalmers PN, Gupta AK, Rahman Z, Bruce B, Romeo AA, Nicholson GP. Predictors of early complications of total shoulder arthroplasty. J Arthroplast. 2014;29(4):856–60. https://doi.org/10.1016/j.arth.2013.07.002.
6. Dripps RD. New classification of physical status. Anesthesiol. 1963;24:111.
7. American Society of Anesthesiologists (ASA). ASA Physical Status Classification System. https://www.asahq.org/resources/clinical-information/asa-physical-status-classification-system. [Online].
8. Ricchetti ET, Abboud JA, Kuntz AF, Ramsey ML, Glaser DL, Williams GR Jr. Total shoulder arthroplasty in older patients: increased perioperative morbidity? Clin Orthop Relat Res. 2011;469(4):1042–9. https://doi.org/10.1007/s11999-010-1582-3.
9. Dunn JC, Lanzi J, Kusnezov N, Bader J, Waterman BR, Belmont PJ Jr. Predictors of length of stay after elective total shoulder arthroplasty in the United States. J Shoulder Elbow Surg. 2015;24(5):754–9. https://doi.org/10.1016/j.jse.2014.11.042.
10. Shields E, Iannuzzi JC, Thorsness R, Noyes K, Voloshin I. Postoperative morbidity by procedure and patient factors influencing major complications within 30 days following shoulder surgery. Orthop J Sports Med. 2014;2(10):2325967114553164. https://doi.org/10.1177/2325967114553164. eCollection 2014 Oct
11. Singh JA, Sperling JW, Schleck C, Harmsen WS, Cofield RH. Periprosthetic infections after total shoulder arthroplasty: a 33-year perspective. J Shoulder Elb

Surg. 2012;21(11):1534–41. https://doi.org/10.1016/j.jse.2012.01.006.
12. Farng E, Zingmond D, Krenek L, Soohoo NF. Factors predicting complication rates after primary shoulder arthroplasty. J Shoulder Elb Surg. 2011;20(4):557–63. https://doi.org/10.1016/j.jse.2010.11.005.
13. Davis DE, Paxton ES, Maltenfort M, Abboud J. Factors affecting hospital charges after total shoulder arthroplasty: an evaluation of the National Inpatient Sample database. J Shoulder Elb Surg. 2014;23(12):1860–6. https://doi.org/10.1016/j.jse.2014.04.002.
14. Singh JA, Sperling JW, Cofield RH. Cardiopulmonary complications after primary shoulder arthroplasty: a cohort study. Semin Arthritis Rheum. 2012;41(5):689–97. https://doi.org/10.1016/j.semarthrit.2011.09.003.
15. Davis JM 3rd, Matteson EL, American College of Rheumatology; European League Against Rheumatism. My treatment approach to rheumatoid arthritis. Mayo Clin Proc. 2012;87(7):659–73. https://doi.org/10.1016/j.mayocp.2012.03.011.
16. Cuomo F, Greller MJ, Zuckerman JD. The rheumatoid shoulder. Rheum Dis Clin N Am. 1998;24(1):67–82.
17. Weiss JJ, Thompson GR, Doust V, Burgener F. Rotator cuff tears in rheumatoid arthritis. Arch Intern Med. 1975;135(4):521–5.
18. Germano V, Cattaruzza MS, Osborn J, Tarantino A, Di Rosa R, Salemi S, D'Amelio R. Infection risk in rheumatoid arthritis and spondyloarthropathy patients under treatment with DMARDs, corticosteroids and TNF-α antagonists. J Transl Med. 2014;12:77. https://doi.org/10.1186/1479-5876-12-77.
19. Marchant MH Jr, Viens NA, Cook C, Vail TP, Bolognesi MP. The impact of glycemic control and diabetes mellitus on perioperative outcomes after total joint arthroplasty. J Bone Joint Surg Am. 2009;91(7):1621–9. https://doi.org/10.2106/JBJS.H.00116.
20. Jain NB, Guller U, Pietrobon R, Bond TK, Higgins LD. Comorbidities increase complication rates in patients having arthroplasty. Clin Orthop Relat Res. 2005;435:232–8.
21. Ponce BA, Menendez ME, Oladeji LO, Soldado F. Diabetes as a risk factor for poorer early post-operative outcomes after shoulder arthroplasty. J Shoulder Elb Surg. 2014;23(5):671–8. https://doi.org/10.1016/j.jse.2014.01.046.
22. Toor AS, Jiang JJ, Shi LL, Koh JL. Comparison of perioperative complications after total elbow arthroplasty in patients with and without diabetes. J Shoulder Elb Surg. 2014;23(11):1599–606. https://doi.org/10.1016/j.jse.2014.06.045.
23. Hemmingsen B, Lund SS, Gluud C, Vaag A, Almdal T, Hemmingsen C, Wetterslev J. Targeting intensive glycaemic control versus targeting conventional glycaemic control for type 2 diabetes mellitus. Cochrane Database Syst Rev. 2011;6:CD008143. https://doi.org/10.1002/14651858.CD008143.pub2.
24. Moutschen MP, Scheen AJ, Lefebvre PJ. Impaired immune responses in diabetes mellitus: analysis of the factors and mechanisms involved. Relevance to the increased susceptibility of diabetic patients to specific infections. Diabete Metab. 1992;18(3):187–201.
25. Rask-Madsen C, King GL. Vascular complications of diabetes: mechanisms of injury and protective factors. Cell Metab. 2013;17(1):20–33. https://doi.org/10.1016/j.cmet.2012.11.012.
26. Bolognesi MP, Marchant MH Jr, Viens NA, Cook C, Pietrobon R, Vail TP. The impact of diabetes on perioperative patient outcomes after total hip and total knee arthroplasty in the United States. J Arthroplast. 2008;23(6 Suppl 1):92–8. https://doi.org/10.1016/j.arth.2008.05.012.
27. Soohoo NF, Farng E, Lieberman JR, Chambers L, Zingmond DS. Factors that predict short-term complication rates after total hip arthroplasty. Clin Orthop Relat Res. 2010;468(9):2363–71. https://doi.org/10.1007/s11999-010-1354-0.
28. Beck JD, Irgit KS, Andreychik CM, Maloney PJ, Tang X, Harter GD. Reverse total shoulder arthroplasty in obese patients. J Hand Surg Am. 2013;38(5):965–70. https://doi.org/10.1016/j.jhsa.2013.02.025.
29. Garcia GH, Fu MC, Dines DM, Craig EV, Gulotta LV. Malnutrition: a marker for increased complications, mortality, and length of stay after total shoulder arthroplasty. J Shoulder Elb Surg. 2016;25(2):193–200. https://doi.org/10.1016/j.jse.2015.07.034.
30. Anwar J, Mpofu E, Matthews LR, Shadoul AF, Brock KE. Reproductive health and access to healthcare facilities: risk factors for depression and anxiety in women with an earthquake experience. BMC Public Health. 2011;11:523. https://doi.org/10.1186/1471-2458-11-523.
31. Linton SJ, Halldén K. Can we screen for problematic back pain? A screening questionnaire for predicting outcome in acute and subacute back pain. Clin J Pain. 1998;14(3):209–15.
32. Linton SJ. A review of psychological risk factors in back and neck pain. Spine (Phila Pa 1976). 2000;25(9):1148–56.
33. Magni G, Marchetti M, Moreschi C, Merskey H, Luchini SR. Chronic musculoskeletal pain and depressive symptoms in the National Health and Nutrition Examination. I. Epidemiologic follow-up study. Pain. 1993;53(2):163–8.
34. Magni G, Moreschi C, Rigatti-Luchini S, Merskey H. Prospective study on the relationship between depressive symptoms and chronic musculoskeletal pain. Pain. 1994;56(3):289–97.
35. Bilberg R, Nørgaard B, Overgaard S, Roessler KK. Patient anxiety and concern as predictors for the perceived quality of treatment and patient reported outcome (PRO) in orthopaedic surgery. BMC Health Serv Res. 2012;12:244. https://doi.org/10.1186/1472-6963-12-244.
36. Bot AG, Menendez ME, Neuhaus V, Ring D. The influence of psychiatric comorbidity on perioperative outcomes after shoulder arthroplasty. J Shoulder Elb Surg. 2014;23(4):519–27. https://doi.org/10.1016/j.jse.2013.12.006.

37. Fisher DA, Dierckman B, Watts MR, Davis K. Looks good but feels bad: factors that contribute to poor results after total knee arthroplasty. J Arthroplast. 2007;22(6 Suppl 2):39–42.
38. Ring D, Kadzielski J, Fabian L, Zurakowski D, Malhotra LR, Jupiter JB. Self-reported upper extremity health status correlates with depression. J Bone Joint Surg Am. 2006;88(9):1983–8.
39. Vissers MM, de Groot IB, Reijman M, Bussmann JB, Stam HJ, Verhaar JA. Functional capacity and actual daily activity do not contribute to patient satisfaction after total knee arthroplasty. BMC Musculoskelet Disord. 2010;11:121. https://doi.org/10.1186/1471-2474-11-121.
40. Vranceanu AM, Jupiter JB, Mudgal CS, Ring D. Predictors of pain intensity and disability after minor hand surgery. J Hand Surg Am. 2010;35(6):956–60. https://doi.org/10.1016/j.jhsa.2010.02.001.
41. Kowal SL, Dall TM, Chakrabarti R, Storm MV, Jain A. The current and projected economic burden of Parkinson's disease in the United States. Mov Disord. 2013;28(3):311–8. https://doi.org/10.1002/mds.25292.
42. Leibson CL, Maraganore DM, Bower JH, Ransom JE, O'brien PC, Rocca WA. Comorbid conditions associated with Parkinson's disease: a population-based study. Mov Disord. 2006;21(4):446–55.
43. Burrus MT, Werner BC, Cancienne JM, Gwathmey FW, Brockmeier SF. Shoulder arthroplasty in patients with Parkinson's disease is associated with increased complications. J Shoulder Elb Surg. 2015;24(12):1881–7. https://doi.org/10.1016/j.jse.2015.05.048.
44. Koch LD, Cofield RH, Ahlskog JE. Total shoulder arthroplasty in patients with Parkinson's disease. J Shoulder Elb Surg. 1997;6(1):24–8.
45. Kryzak TJ, Sperling JW, Schleck CD, Cofield RH. Total shoulder arthroplasty in patients with Parkinson's disease. J Shoulder Elb Surg. 2009;18(1):96–9. https://doi.org/10.1016/j.jse.2008.07.010.
46. Choo QL, Kuo G, Weiner AJ, Overby LR, Bradley DW, Houghton M. Isolation of a cDNA clone derived from a blood-borne non-A, non-B viral hepatitis genome. Science. 1989;244(4902):359–62.
47. Kuo G, Choo QL, Alter HJ, Gitnick GL, Redeker AG, Purcell RH, Miyamura T, Dienstag JL, Alter MJ, Stevens CE, et al. An assay for circulating antibodies to a major etiologic virus of human non-A, non-B hepatitis. Science. 1989;244(4902):362–4.
48. Rosas S, Sabeh KG, Buller LT, Law TY, Kalandiak SP, Levy JC. Comorbidity effects on shoulder arthroplasty costs analysis of a nationwide private payer insurance data set. J Shoulder Elb Surg. 2017;26(7):e216–21. https://doi.org/10.1016/j.jse.2016.11.044.

28 Management of Periprosthetic Reverse Shoulder Arthroplasty Infections

Nicola Ivaldo, Tony Mangano, Giovanni Caione, Mario Rossoni, and Giovanni Riccio

28.1 Introduction

Since the time of the reported first shoulder arthroplasty, implanted in 1894 and explanted 2 years later by Jean Péan, periprosthetic shoulder infection (PSI) represents a known severe complication of this kind of surgery, with significant clinical and socioeconomic consequences [1–4]. Published data report infection rates ranging from 1 to 15%, with higher rates after revision surgery than after a primary procedure [5–7] and higher rates after reverse shoulder arthroplasty than after hemiarthroplasty or total shoulder arthroplasty [7, 8]. The hypothesized reasons for this are multifactorial, encompassing the large dead space caused by the reverse configuration of the joint and the fact the arthroplasty is not surrounded and covered by living tissue in the absence of musculotendinous rotator cuff tissue [9]. However, such hypotheses are mostly based on data coming from or involving the older series of patients treated with RSA, and this could bias a realistic estimation of the problem, just considering TSA and RSA were used to manage relatively different pathologic conditions until recent times. Only in the last years, indeed, the indication for RSA implantation has been broadened to include not only salvage situations, and the surgical technique has been sensitively improved. Furthermore, we are currently aware patient-related factors should be better considered while looking for an explanation for higher infection rates, including age, sex, medical comorbidities, and multiple previous operations [10, 11].

The aim of this review is to briefly overview periprosthetic reverse shoulder arthroplasty infections, from diagnosis to treatment and prevention, keeping in mind how difficult could often be to discriminate what is reality and evidence-based data with respect to prejudices or dangerous and erroneous inductions.

28.2 Definition of Periprosthetic Joint Infection

In 2011, the Musculoskeletal Infection Society (MSIS) analyzed the available evidence and proposed a new definition for periprosthetic joint infection (PJI) [12]. During the 2013 meeting in Philadelphia, the International Consensus Meeting Group on PJI slightly modified the 2011

N. Ivaldo · T. Mangano (✉) · G. Caione · M. Rossoni
Unit of Shoulder and Elbow Surgery, Ospedale Humanitas—San Pio X, Milan, Italy

Department of Orthopaedic and Traumatology, Casa di Cura Villa Igea, Acqui Terme, AL, Italy
e-mail: tony.mangano@sanpiox.humanitas.it

G. Riccio
Department of Infectious Diseases and Septic Surgery (MIOS), Ospedale S.M. di Misericordia, Albenga, SV, Italy

S. Gumina et al. (eds.), *Reverse Shoulder Arthroplasty*,
https://doi.org/10.1007/978-3-319-97743-0_28

criteria, by adding the leukocyte esterase test as a minor criterion [13]. Currently we can define PJI exists when:

1. There is a sinus tract communicating with the prosthesis.
2. A (phenotypically identical) pathogen is isolated by culture from at least two separate tissue or fluid samples obtained from the affected prosthetic joint.
3. Three of the following five minor criteria exist:
   (a) Elevated serum erythrocyte sedimentation rate (ESR) *and* serum C-reactive protein (CRP) concentration
   (b) Elevated synovial leukocyte count *or* ++ change on leukocyte esterase test strip
   (c) Elevated synovial polymorphonuclear neutrophil percentage (PMN%)
   (d) Isolation of a microorganism in one culture of periprosthetic tissue or fluid
   (e) Greater than five neutrophils per high-power field in five high-power fields observed from histologic analysis of periprosthetic tissue at 9400 magnification

PJI may be present if fewer than four of these criteria are met.

28.3 Microbiology and Diagnosis

Classically, postoperative infections can be classified into early infection (3–6 months from surgery), delayed infection (4–24 months), and late infection (>24 months), depending on the time of diagnosis after the surgery [14]. This classification is generally related to the microorganism involved and to its virulence.

The microorganisms most commonly isolated in cases of PSI are *Staphylococcus* (*S.*) *aureus*, *S. epidermidis*, and *Propionibacterium* (*P.*) *acnes* [15]. *P. acnes* is a Gram-positive anaerobic bacillus, colonizing the pilosebaceous follicles and strictly correlated to PSI in the last years. It is found both in the skin and in the dermal layer, especially in young male patients [16]. It is often responsible for low-grade infection, presenting as delayed PSI, with mild clinical symptoms, so that many classic clinical patterns do not strictly apply. Despite that it has been isolated in a large percentage of PSI, it is always important to keep in mind that mean duration for culture incubation should not be less than 14 days, and this obviously represents a high risk for culture contaminations. Referring to the MSIS proposal, while isolation of a single virulent organism such as *S. aureus* may represent a PJI, isolation of a single low-virulence pathogen such as coagulase-negative *Staphylococcus*, *P. acnes*, or *Corynebacteria* in the absence of other criteria is not believed to represent a definite infection [12].

In case of low-virulence pathogens, the final diagnosis is often challenging: with respect to other more virulent agents, we cannot usually find swelling, erythema, fever, purulent discharge, or increasing level of biological parameters such as erythrocyte sedimentation rate (ESR), C-reactive protein (CRP), white blood cell count (WBC), and interleukin (IL)-6. Sometimes, we can find a "simple" painful shoulder with reduced range of motion, without clinical signs suggestive for infection or clear radiographic signs of component mobilization.

A diagnostic arthrocentesis with synovial fluid analysis should be performed in all patients with suspected acute PJI, including PSI, unless the diagnosis is clinically evident and surgery is planned and antimicrobials can be safely withheld prior to surgery. Arthrocentesis is also advised in patients with a chronic painful prosthesis in whom there is an unexplained elevated sedimentation rate or CRP level or in whom there is a clinical suspicion of PJI. It may not be necessary if surgery is already planned and the result of the synovial fluid analysis is not expected to alter the final management. Synovial fluid analysis should include a total cell count and differential leukocyte count, as well as leukocyte esterase test and culture for aerobic and anaerobic organisms [13, 17].

Intraoperative deep biopsies from periprosthetic tissues are always needed, and culture from these tissues is still considered a gold standard analysis in a PJI diagnostic workup. In order to optimize the sensitivity and specificity for the diagnosis of a PSI, four to six independent samples should be performed; exchanging the scalpel blade after every sample is taken. The use of intraoperative swabs should be discouraged. The cutoff for a definite diagnostic of infection should be three or more samples positive to the same microorganism [18]. Where the patient is medically stable, withholding antimicrobial therapy for at least 2 weeks prior to collection of synovial fluid for culture and intraoperative culture specimens increases the likelihood of recovering an organism [17]. As already highlighted, the concern is that the growth duration from intraoperative samples is long for *P. acnes*, and every laboratory should be aware that they should not discard the culture samples too early. However, early positive cultures seem to be more predictive of a true infection than a late growth culture, which can be a false-positive result [19].

Intraoperative histopathological examination of periprosthetic tissue samples is a highly reliable diagnostic test, provided that a pathologist skilled in interpretation of periprosthetic tissue is available and tissue sampling does not include the periprosthetic endomedullar membranes (i.e., a site of constant neutrophil-mediated reaction). It should be performed at the time of revision prosthetic joint surgery, if the presence of infection is in doubt and the results will affect management, for example, in deciding between revision arthroplasty or one-stage exchange and two-stage exchange [17]. Furthermore, it represents an important diagnostic resource in the latter situation, following resection arthroplasty or antibiotic-loaded spacer, in order to confirm the absence of residual joint contamination at the time of the second-stage prosthetic implantation.

It is of note, however, we have entered a new era where molecular biomarkers play an increasingly important role in the diagnosis of various conditions and is desirable the use of serum and synovial biomarkers would prove able, in short time, to overcome the current cornerstones of PJI diagnostic workup [20]. Leukocyte esterase is a simple, readily available test, requiring application of synovial fluid to a urine test strip, which is now part of the minor MSIS diagnostic criteria for PJI. High values of sensitivity (93–100%) and specificity (77–89%) have been reported. The synovial fluid α-defensin test has shown promising results, with a sensitivity of 97% and a specificity of 96% for diagnosing PJI [21]. Due to intrinsic features of α-defensin, this test provides reliable results regardless of the organism type, Gram staining, species, or virulence of the organism. Waiting for its final endorsement as a standard diagnostic tool in the evaluation for PJI, it is our opinion its application could likely become ordinary in the setting in which we previously suggested the intraoperative histopathological examination. Further studies in such direction would be warmly advocated.

28.4 Imaging Studies

Standard radiograph of the shoulder still represents the first step of the diagnostic workup together with clinical examination. As in other districts, in the setting of shoulder arthroplasty, periosteal reactions and osteolytic foci or diffuse bone resorption are considered signs of suspicion for PSI (Fig. 28.1a, b) [22]. Furthermore, as suggested by several authors and our experience as well, apparently aseptic loosening should always be suspected to have an infective cause, until finally demonstrated (Fig. 28.1c): this is especially important in relation to infections from low-virulence bacteria (e.g., *P. acnes*, *S. epidermidis*). The same basic X-ray projection is generally useful in order to identify major humeral and glenoid bone loss, signs of instability or component mobilization, presence of periprosthetic fractures, or *loci minoris resistentiae* (Fig. 28.2): all of these data could be used for planning the correct surgery and avoid intraoperative complications.

Ultrasound analysis is a quick, not invasive, and inexpensive tool very useful in defining the presence of abscess or hematoma in the context of soft tissues, especially in the postoperative setting.

Referring to the guidelines of IDSA [17], imaging studies such as bone scans, leukocyte scans, magnetic resonance imaging, computed tomography, and positron emission tomography

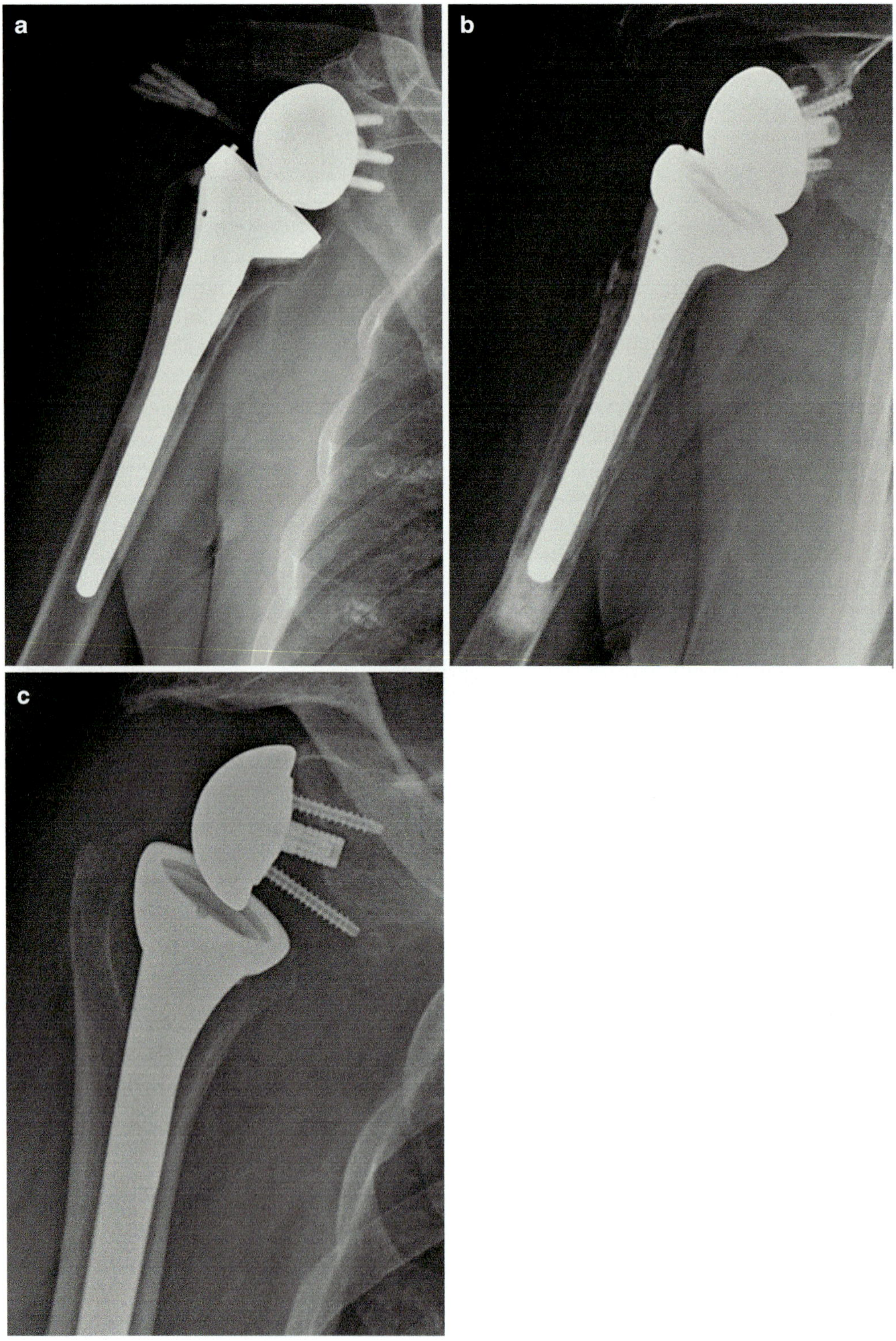

Fig. 28.1 Radiographic signs of suspicion for RSA late periprosthetic infection. (**a**) Periprosthetic multiple osteolytic foci near the humeral stem; (**b**) diffuse periprosthetic bone resorption on the humeral side; (**c**) apparently aseptic glenoid component loosening: subsequent analysis revealed a deep infection from *P. acnes*

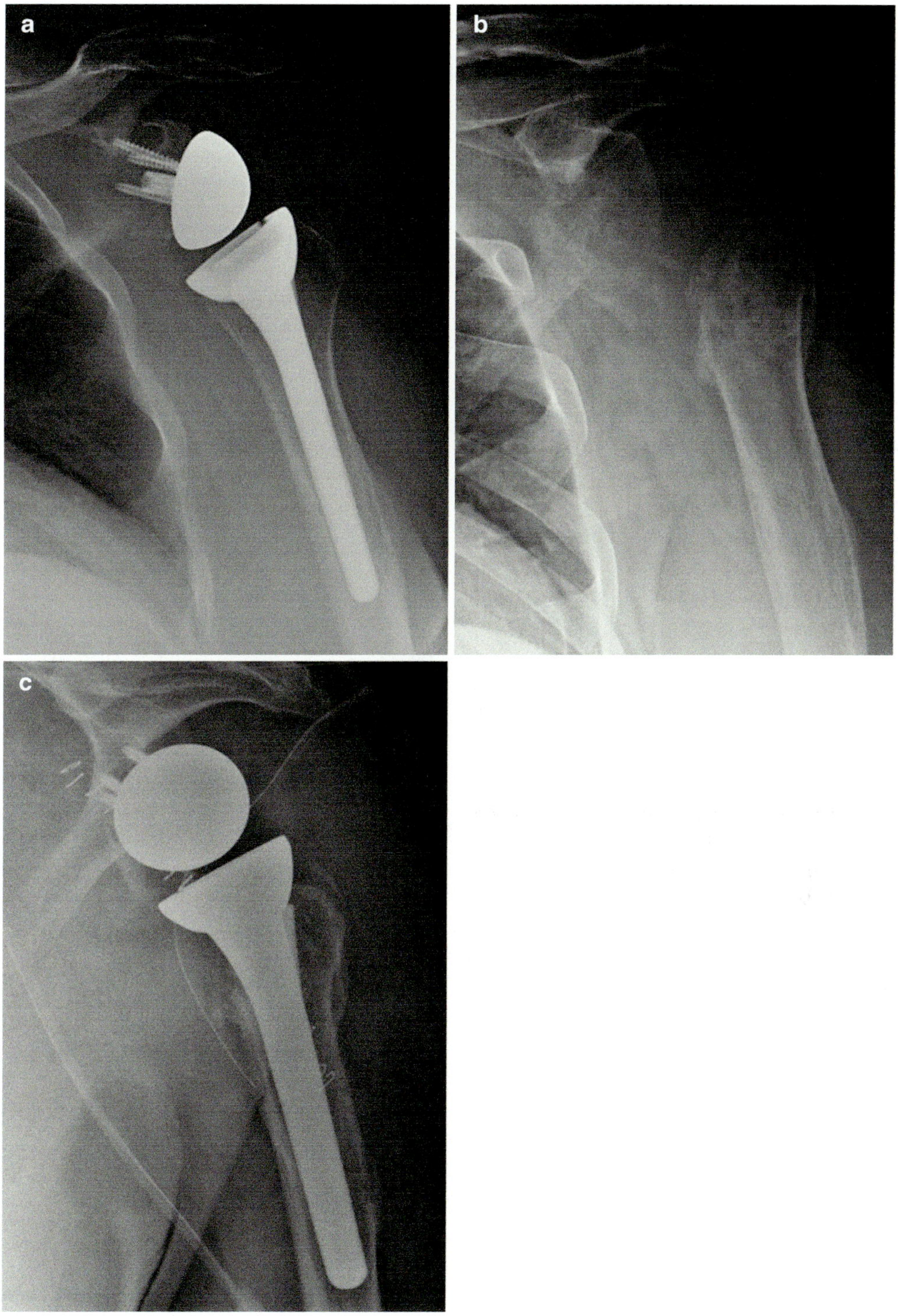

Fig. 28.4 Two-stage revision procedure with temporary resection arthroplasty and final reimplantation with a primary prosthetic RSA implant. (**a**) Radiographic appearance in a case of early deep infection due to *S. aureus*, occurring 4 months after surgery; (**b**) resection arthroplasty radiographic appearance at 3 months after RSA explantation; at this time the patient was judged infection-free and underwent the second surgical stage; (**c**) staged reimplantation with an RSA implant identical to the primary implanted one: early diagnosis and management as well as the choice of temporary resection arthroplasty for the first stage allowed avoidance of glenoid and humeral bone loss and of other complications often associated with delayed diagnosis and with the use of a cement spacer

28.7 Conclusion

Infection after RSA still represents one of the most severe postoperative complications. Early diagnosis and effective treatment can prevent chronic infections and serious damage to the bone and soft tissues. A strict multidisciplinary collaboration between surgeon and infectivologist is highly recommended in order to optimize the diagnostic workup, the antibiotic treatment, and the surgical procedure. With the exception of selected cases, a two-stage exchange strategy is currently considered a gold standard treatment, able to provide eradication of the infection in most of the cases. The use of temporary resection arthroplasty as first stage, instead of a cement spacer, does not seem to decrease the eradication rate, but allows avoiding bone loss and other complications eventually related to the cement spacer itself. Whenever possible, second-stage reimplantation with RSA again leads to good functional results.

References

1. Péan J. Des moyens prosthétiques destinis a obtenir la reparation des parties osseuses. Gaz des Hop Paris. 1894;67:291.
2. Péan J. De la prothèse osseuse. Gaz des Hop Paris. 1897;70:594.
3. Schairer WW, Nwachukwu BU, Lyman S, Craig EV, Gulotta LV. National utilization of reverse total shoulder arthroplasty in the United States. J Shoulder Elb Surg. 2015;24:91–7.
4. Padegimas EM, Maltenfort M, Ramsey ML, Williams GR, Parvizi J, Namdari S. Periprosthetic shoulder infection in the United States: incidence and economic burden. J Shoulder Elb Surg. 2015;24:741–6.
5. Coste JS, Reig S, Trojani C, Berg M, Walch G, Boileau P. The management of infection in arthroplasty of the shoulder. J Bone Joint Surg Br. 2004;86(1):65–9.
6. Sperling JW, Kozak TK, Hanssen AD, Cofield RH. Infection after shoulder arthroplasty. Clin Orthop Relat Res. 2001;382:206–16.
7. Trappey GJ, O'Connor DP, Edwards TB. What are the instability and infection rates after reverse shoulder arthroplasty? Clin Orthop Relat Res. 2011;469(9):2505–11.
8. Richards J, Inacio MC, Beckett M, Navarro RA, Singh A, Dillon MT, Sodl JF, Yian EH. Patient and procedure-specific risk factors for deep infection after primary shoulder arthroplasty. Clin Orthop Relat Res. 2014;472:2809–15.
9. Farshad M, Gerber C. Reverse total shoulder arthroplasty - from the most to the least common complication. Int Orthop. 2010;34:1075–82.
10. Werthel JD, Hatta T, Schoch B, Cofield R, Sperling JW, Elhassan BT. Is previous nonarthroplasty surgery a risk factor for periprosthetic infection in primary shoulder arthroplasty? J Shoulder Elb Surg. 2017;26(4):635–40.
11. Florschütz AV, Lane PD, Crosby LA. Infection after primary anatomic versus primary reverse total shoulder arthroplasty. J Shoulder Elb Surg. 2015;24(8):1296–301.
12. Parvizi J, Zmistowski B, Berbari EF, Bauer TW, Springer BD, Della Valle CJ, Garvin KL, Mont MA, Wongworawat MD, Zalavras CG. New definition for periprosthetic joint infection: from the Workgroup of the Musculoskeletal Infection Society. Clin Orthop Relat Res. 2011;469:2992–4.
13. Parvizi J, Gehrke T. Definition of Periprosthetic Joint Infection. J Arthroplast. 2014;29:1331.
14. Trampuz A, Widmer AF. Infections associated with orthopaedic implants. Curr Opin Infect Dis. 2006;19:349–56.
15. Saltzman MD, Marecek GS, Edwards SL, Kalainov DM. Infection after shoulder surgery. J Am Acad Orthop Surg. 2011;19:208–18.
16. Hudek R, Sommer F, Kerwat M, Abdelkawi AF, Loos F, Gohlke F. Propionibacterium acnes in shoulder surgery: true infection, contamination, or commensal of the deep tissue? J Shoulder Elb Surg. 2014;23:1763–71.
17. Osmon DR, Berbari EF, Berendt AR, Lew D, Zimmerli W, Steckelberg JM, Rao N, Hanssen A, Wilson WR, Infectious Diseases Society ofAmerica. Diagnosis and management of prosthetic joint infection: clinical practice guidelines by the Infectious Diseases Society of America. Clin Infect Dis. 2013;56(1):e1–e25.
18. Zhang AL, Feeley BT, Schwartz BS, Chung TT, Ma CB. Management of deep postoperative shoulder infections: is there a role for open biopsy during staged treatment? J Shoulder Elb Surg. 2015;24:e15–20.
19. Frangiamore SJ, Saleh A, Grosso MJ, Alolabi B, Bauer TW, Iannotti JP, Ricchetti ET. Early versus late culture growth of Propionibacterium acnes in revision shoulder arthroplasty. J Bone Joint Surg Am. 2015;97:1149–58.
20. Shahi A, Parvizi J. The role of biomarkers in the diagnosis of periprosthetic joint infection. EFORT Open Rev. 2017;1(7):275–8.
21. Deirmengian C, Kardos K, Kilmartin P, Cameron A, Schiller K, Parvizi J. Combined measurement of synovial fluid α-Defensin and C-reactive protein levels: highly accurate for diagnosing periprosthetic joint infection. J Bone Joint Surg Am. 2014;96:1439–45.
22. Bauer T, Parvizi J, Kobayashi KV. Diagnosis of periprosthetic infection. J Bone Joint Surg Am. 2006;88:869–82.
23. Gemmel F, Van den Wyngaert H, Love C, Welling MM, Gemmel P, Palestro CJ. Prosthetic joint infections:

radionuclide state-of-the-art imaging. Eur J Nucl Med Mol Imaging. 2012;39(5):892–909.
24. Romanò CL, Borens O, Monti L, Meani E, Stuyck J. What treatment for periprosthetic shoulder infection? Results from a multicentre retrospective series. Int Orthop. 2012;36:1011–7.
25. Zavala JA, Clark JC, Kissenberth MJ, Tolan SJ, Hawkins RJ. Management of deep infection after reverse total shoulder arthroplasty: a case series. J Shoulder Elb Surg. 2012;21(10):1310–5.
26. Klatte TO, Junghans K, Al-Khateeb H, Rueger JM, Gehrke T, Kendoff D, Neumann J. Single-stage revision for periprosthetic shoulder infection: outcomes and results. Bone Joint J. 2013;95-B:391–5.
27. Beekman PD, Katusic D, Berghs BM, Karelse A, De Wilde L. One-stage revision for patients with a chronically infected reverse total shoulder replacement. J Bone Joint Surg Br. 2010;92-B:817–22.
28. George DA, Volpin A, Scarponi S, Haddad FS, Romanò CL. Does exchange arthroplasty of an infected shoulder prosthesis provide better eradication rate and better functional outcome, compared to a permanent spacer or resection arthroplasty? a systematic review. BMC Musculoskelet Disord. 2016;17(1):52–60.
29. Bonnevialle N, Dauzères F, Toulemonde J, Elia F, Laffosse JM, Mansat P. Periprosthetic shoulder infection: an overview. EFORT Open Rev. 2017;2(4):104–9.
30. Cuff DJ, Virani NA, Levy J, Frankle MA, Derasari A, Hines B, Pupello DR, Cancio M, Mighell M. The treatment of deep shoulder infection and glenohumeral instability with debridement, reverse shoulder arthroplasty and postoperative antibiotics. J Bone Joint Surg Br. 2008;90:336–42.
31. Strickland JP, Sperling JW, Cofield RH. The results of two-stage re-implantation for infected shoulder replacement. J Bone Joint Surg Br. 2008;90:460–5.
32. Assenmacher AT, Alentorn-Geli E, Dennison T, Baghdadi YMK, Cofield RH, Sánchez-Sotelo J, Sperling JW. Two-stage reimplantation for the treatment of deep infection after shoulder arthroplasty. J Shoulder Elb Surg. 2017;26(11):1978–83.
33. Farshad M, Grögli M, Catanzaro S, Gerber C. Revision of reversed total shoulder arthroplasty. Indications and outcome. BMC Musculoskelet Disord. 2012;13:160–5.
34. Sabesan VJ, Ho JC, Kovacevic D, Iannotti JP. Two-stage reimplantation for treating prosthetic shoulder infections. Clin Orthop Relat Res. 2011;469(9):2538–43.
35. Anagnostakos K, Wilmes P, Schmitt E, Kelm J. Elution of gentamicin and vancomycin from polymethyl methacrylate beads and hip spacers in vivo. Acta Orthop. 2009;80:193–7.
36. Verhelst L, Stuyck J, Bellemans J, Debeer P. Resection arthroplasty of the shoulder as a salvage procedure for deep shoulder infection: does the use of a cement spacer improve outcome? J Shoulder Elb Surg. 2011;20:1224–33.
37. Ivaldo N, Mangano T, Caione G, Rossoni M, Ligas A. Customized tantalum-augmented reverse shoulder arthroplasty for glenoid bone defect and excessive medialization: description of the technique. Musculoskelet Surg. 2016;100(Suppl 1):13–8.
38. Rispoli DM, Sperling JW, Athwal GS, Schleck CD, Cofield RH. Pain relief and functional results after resection arthroplasty of the shoulder. J Bone Joint Surg Br. 2007;89-B:1184–7.
39. Saltzman MD, Nuber GW, Gryzlo SM, Marecek GS, Koh JL. Efficacy of surgical preparation solutions in shoulder surgery. J Bone Joint Surg Am. 2009;91-A:1949–53.
40. Koh CK, Marsh JP, Drinković D, Walker CG, Poon PC. Propionibacterium acnes in primary shoulder arthroplasty: rates of colonization, patient risk factors, and efficacy of perioperative prophylaxis. J Shoulder Elb Surg. 2016;25(5):846–52.
41. Rezapoor M, Nicholson T, Tabatabaee RM, Chen AF, Maltenfort MG, Parvizi J. Povidone-iodine-based solutions for decolonization of nasal Staphylococcus aureus: a randomized, prospective, placebo-controlled study. J Arthroplast. 2017;32(9):2815–9.

29 Intraoperative Fracture in Reverse Shoulder Arthroplasty

Barbara Melis and Giuseppe Marongiu

29.1 Introduction

Currently, little is known about the incidence, the treatment, and the outcome of intraoperative periprosthetic fractures that occur during reverse shoulder arthroplasty (RSA). Female sex [1–3], revision surgery [2, 4, 5], osteopenia [2], rheumatoid arthritis [2, 6], post-traumatic arthritis [2], surgical approach [2], instability [3], and previous hemiarthroplasty [3] are reported as relative risk factors for intraoperative fractures during RSA. The incidence of intraoperative fractures has been reported between 1.4% [1] and 25% [4] and between 0.9% [5] and 2% [6], respectively, for the humerus and for the glenoid. Humeral and glenoid fractures are the most frequently observed, but further fractures, as acromion or coracoid fracture, can occur. Humeral fractures are classified by their location (greater tuberosity, metaphysis, diaphysis) and displacement. There are multiple classifications, but the Wright and Cofield classification [7] is the most frequently used. This classification was originally created for postoperative fractures, and it is limited to those occurring near the tip of the humeral stem. Later, Campbell [8] proposed a classification system that included tuberosity and metaphyseal fractures, and it is more adequate for intraoperative fractures. Campbell divided these fractures into four types related to the fracture site. Duncan et al. [9] introduced a unified classification system (UCS) addressing the management of all periprosthetic fractures; nevertheless further studies are needed to test the UCS in shoulder periprosthetic fractures.

The treatment depends on the location of the fracture in respect to the prosthetic component and the stability of the component/bone interface. The aims in the treatment of periprosthetic fractures are the preservation of bone stock, successful bony consolidation, and provision of a stable anchoring of the prosthesis with the major goal of restoring the shoulder-arm function.

29.2 Frequency, Risk Factors, and Characteristics of Intraoperative Fractures

29.2.1 Humeral Fractures

Zumstein et al. [5] reported 16 cases of intraoperative humeral fractures (2%) in a systematic review of 782 RSA. Humeral fractures occurred

B. Melis (✉) · G. Marongiu
Unità di Ortopedia e Traumatologia dello Sport, Casa di Cura "Policlinico Città di Quartu", via Silesu 10, 09045 Quartu Sant'Elena, CA, Italy

S. Gumina et al. (eds.), *Reverse Shoulder Arthroplasty*,
https://doi.org/10.1007/978-3-319-97743-0_29

mainly during removal of the primary humeral stem or cement mantle in revision surgery.

Sirveaux et al. [2] reported 44 cases of intraoperative fractures of the greater tuberosity (GT) in a series of 1953 RSA (2.25%). The GT fracture occurred in female in 88% of cases; the mean age of the patients with fracture was not different from the mean age of the entire series (73 years). Fractures were significantly more frequent in the case of fracture sequelae and revision surgery. The incidence of GT fractures was higher if the surgery was performed by deltopectoral than superolateral approach.

García Fernandez et al. [1] reported 3 cases of intraoperative humeral fractures in a series of 203 RSA (1.47%). All fractures occurred in female patients; two cases, involving the metaphysis, occurred during primary RSA, and one case, involving the humeral shaft, occurred in a revision of a hemiarthroplasty, during reaming of the humeral medullary canal.

Chuinard et al. [4] reported 26 cases of intraoperative humeral fractures in a series of 457 RSA (5.7%). Twenty-five of 99 RSA done for revision (25.3%) sustained an intraoperative fracture. Twenty-five fractures occurred during removal of the previous implant or cement; twenty fractures occurred in the diaphyseal region, within the prosthetic zone; five were located at the tuberosity region; and one patient sustained a combined tuberosity and diaphyseal fracture. Twenty-two humerotomies were performed out of a possible 99 revision cases. Seven intraoperative fractures occurred despite humerotomy. The one case of fracture in a primary stem occurred during reaming, representing a breach of the humeral canal.

Wagner et al. [3] reported 36 cases of intraoperative periprosthetic humeral fractures in 224 patients (230 RSA) who underwent to RSA for failed total shoulder arthroplasty (16%). Risk factors for intraoperative fracture included female sex (n = 18 women), history of instability (n = 27), and prior hemiarthroplasty (n = 22). Only 3 fractures were displaced whereas 33 nondisplaced; 30 fractures involved the greater tuberosity, 3 the metaphysis, and 3 the humeral shaft. Eighty-one percent of the fractures occurred during cemented (n = 11) and cementless (n = 25) component removal.

29.2.2 Glenoid Fractures

Zumstein et al. [5] reported seven cases of intraoperative glenoid fractures in a systematic review of 782 RSA (0.9%). Glenoid fractures were related to the initial reaming or fixation technique.

Molé et al. [6] reported 9 cases of glenoid fractures in a series of 457 RSA (2%). In seven cases (1.5%), the fracture was partial, occurring in six cases while reaming and in one case during the removal of periglenoidal osteophytes. The fracture was located at the inferior border in three cases, at the superior border in two cases, and at the posterior border in one case. These fractures were found only in the primary implants, with cuff tear arthropathy as the predominant indication. The average age of the nine patients, compared to the entire series, was 74.3 vs. 72.3 years.

Sirveaux et al. [2] reported 19 complete and 10 partial glenoid fractures in a series of 1953 RSA (1.5%). There were 84% of female compared to 77% of female in the general population without significative difference. The mean age at surgery was the same as in the general population (73 years). The risk was higher when the glenoid was unloaded like in the case of upward migration of the head or prolonged immobilization as in massive cuff tear, acute fractures, rheumatoid arthritis, and tumors. Fracture was more frequent if the surgery was performed by superolateral than deltopectoral approach.

29.2.3 Coracoid Fracture

Sirveaux et al. [2] reported five cases of intraoperative fracture of the coracoid process in a series of 1953 RSA (0.25%). Eighty percent of these fractures occurred in women, and the mean age was 76 years. There were two cases of cuff tear arthropathy Hamada stage 4, two cases of fracture sequelae, and one case of rheumatoid arthritis.

29.2.4 Acromion Fracture

Zumstein et al. [5] reported one case of intraoperative fracture of the acromion in a systematic review of 782 RSA (0.1%). The fracture of the acromion was associated with the transacromial approach.

29.3 Intraoperative Fracture Treatment

29.3.1 Humeral Fractures Treatment

The two proximal metaphyseal fractures reported by García Fernandez et al. [1] were treated with cerclage wiring, but they didn't require changing the cementless stem. The only intraoperative shaft fracture required placement of a long cementless stem and several cerclage wires.

In the series reported by Chuinard et al. [4], 15 of the 20 diaphyseal fractures were treated with a long stem, and 4 of them had supplementary cerclage wiring; 4 were treated with cerclage wiring alone. Four of the five fractures located at the tuberosity region were treated with cerclage wiring. The patient with a combined tuberosity and diaphyseal fracture had an immediate revision of the stem; the one case of fracture in primary implant representing a breach of the humeral canal resulted in cement extrusion.

In the series reported by Wagner et al. [3], intraoperative fractures were treated with stabilization of the prosthetic stem in 28 shoulders (20 press-fit and 8 cemented stem) and adjunctive internal fixation in 8 shoulders. The fractures treated with adjunctive fixation occurred in three patients with minimally displaced greater tuberosity fractures, one combined greater and lesser tuberosity minimally displaced fracture, two nondisplaced metaphyseal fractures, one displaced metaphyseal fracture, and one displaced metaphyseal fracture with extension in the diaphysis. Suture stabilization was used for the three greater tuberosity fractures and the combined greater and lesser tuberosity fracture. The two nondisplaced metaphyseal fractures were stabilized with cerclage wires alone. The two displaced metaphyseal fractures were stabilized using a strut allograft and cables.

29.3.2 Glenoid Fractures Treatment

In the series of Molé et al. [6], partial fractures were reduced by the application of the metaglenoid after drilling the central peg hole, and their fixation was assured by one of the baseplate fixation screws. In two cases, primary stability was improved by the addition of cancellous graft and in one case by the addition of cement. In two cases the fractures were complete but allowed the implantation of a reverse prosthesis glenoid. In one of these cases, the prosthesis was implanted in two steps, after initial cortico-cancellous bone grafting.

In the series of Sirveaux et al. [2], a long peg baseplate was used in four cases to improve the stability of the glenoid implant and by using a 29 mm diameter metaglene in most of the cases. The fracture was managed without graft in 50% of the cases or by using a cancellous autograft in the other cases.

29.4 Complications and Revision

29.4.1 Humeral Fractures

Sirveaux et al. [2] observed further complication in 11 of 44 cases of GT fracture. There were three dislocations, one infection, one hematoma, two humeral loosening, one scapula spine fracture, one humeral disassembly, one glenoid fracture, and one late humeral fracture. Six patients were reoperated: two humeral revisions, one glenoid revision, one hematoma drainage, one revision, and one closed reduction for instability were performed.

A postoperative radial nerve palsy not recovered, which persisted until the latest follow-up (30 months) and will need a tendon transfer surgery, was reported by García Fernandez [1] in the case of intraoperative humeral shaft fracture. All fractures reported in his series healed.

In the series reported by Chuinard et al. [4], all but two fractures healed (one diaphyseal and one tuberosity): the diaphyseal fracture resulted in a postoperative fracture necessitating revision to a long stem; the other went on to develop tuberosity non-union and humeral loosening, but no revision has been made, and no sign of infection was present. Three patients underwent resection arthroplasty because of an associated infection.

Wagner et al. [3] reported 2 postoperative fractures (both treated nonoperatively) in 36 patients who had an intraoperative fracture, and, overall, 3 revision procedures were performed in patients with intraoperative fractures (glenoid loosening ($n = 2$) and instability ($n = 1$)); 2- and 5-year survivorship was not significantly different from results for patients without intraoperative fracture. No patient underwent revision surgery for humeral component loosening.

29.4.2 Glenoid Fractures

Molé et al. [6] reported early loosening in one of the two cases of complete glenoid fractures due to an extension of the fracture, leading to a revision for a hemiarthroplasty. Two cases of glenoid loosening (one septic) were observed in seven cases of partial glenoid fractures.

Sirveaux et al. [2] did not find any postoperative complication related directly to the fracture, but in this group of patients, they observed one plexus palsy, one spine fracture, one acromial fracture, and one humeral fracture; all the implants were still in place, and there was no reoperation for glenoid loosening.

29.4.3 Coracoid Fracture

There was no postoperative complication in the five cases of coracoid fractures reported by Sirveaux [2], except one patient who remained stiff and that was reoperated for an arthroscopic arthrolysis.

Characteristics, risk factors, treatment, and complications of the intraoperative fractures mentioned above are summarized in Table 29.1.

29.5 Clinical and Functional Outcomes After Treatment

Zumstein et al. [5] reported that intraoperative humeral and glenoid fractures influence negatively the final outcome. Sirveaux [2] shown that the average Constant score [10] of the patients who had perioperative GT fracture is significantly lower (47 pts) than those who did not have this complication; equally the active anterior elevation is lower (109° vs. 126°), and the patients loose an average of 10° of active external rotation. Differently, in the case of coracoid fracture, the Constant score averaged 49 points, which was not different with the overall results. Chuinard [4] shown that if a patient sustained a humeral fracture during the procedure, the Constant score is lower than the series without a fracture (42.3 vs. 59.2) and that the range of motion is reduced (forward flexion was 103° vs. 124° and external rotation 0° vs. 9°). Opposite, Wagner [3] reported good postoperative pain relief, improved shoulder abduction, and good functional scores.

Intraoperative glenoid fractures can be considered a severe complication only when they are complete. In this case Molé [6] reported a mean Constant score of 48 points and a rate of glenoid loosening of 33%. The glenoid fracture did not compromise the overall functional results (average Constant score 55 pts) in the series reported by Sirveaux [2].

29.6 Discussion

Intraoperative periprosthetic fractures increase operative time, alter implant choices, and may have a negative effect on postoperative outcomes [2, 4–6]. Women [1–3] have a significantly higher risk of intraoperative fracture as the patients with osteopenia [2], rheumatoid arthritis [2, 6], post-traumatic arthritis [2], and cuff tear arthropathy [2, 6]. Regarding the surgical approach [2], the forces applied on the greater tuberosity by the posterior retractor can explain the higher incidence of GT fracture in the case of deltopectoral approach. Differently, glenoid fracture is observed more

Table 29.1 Intraoperative fractures, characteristics, risk factors, and treatment

Author, number (%), fracture location	Risk factors	Timing of fracture	Fracture stabilization	Complications
Zumstein et al. [5] 16/782 (2%) Humerus	Revision surgery	Removal of the previous implant or cement mantle	–	–
Sirveaux et al. [2] 44/1953 (2.25%) Greater tuberosity	Female sex Fracture sequelae Revision surgery Deltopectoral approach	–	–	Dislocation (3) Infection (1) Hematoma (1) Humeral loosening (2) Scapula spine fracture (1) Humeral disassembly (1) Glenoid fracture (1) Late humeral fracture (1)
García Fernandez et al. [1] 3/203 (1.47%) Metaphysis (2) Shaft (1)	Female sex	Riming the humeral canal	Cerclage wiring (2) Long stem + cerclage wiring (1)	Radial nerve palsy (1)
Chuinard et al. [4] 26/457 (5.7%) Diaphysis (20) Tuberosity (5) Tuberosity + diaphysis (1)	Revision surgery	Removal of the previous implant or cement Riming the humeral canal	Cerclage wiring (8) Long stem (12) Long stem + cerclage wiring (4)	Postoperative fracture (1) Humeral loosening (1) Infection 3
Wagner et al. [3] 36/230 (16%) Greater tuberosity (30) Metaphysis (3) Shaft (3)	Female sex History of instability Prior hemiarthroplasty	Removal of the previous implant	Stabilization of the stem (28) Suture stabilization/ cerclage wires (8)	Postoperative fracture (2) Glenoid loosening (2) Instability (1)
Zumstein et al. [5] 7/782 (0.9%) Glenoid	–	Initial reaming or fixation technique	–	–
Molé et al. [6] 9/457 (2%) Glenoid	Cuff tear arthropathy	Reaming Removal osteophytes	Metaglenoid and baseplate fixation screws ± bone graft	Glenoid loosening (3)
Sirveaux et al. [2] 29/1953 (1.5%) Glenoid	Cuff tear arthropathy Acute fractures Rheumatoid arthritis Tumors Superolateral approach	–	Long peg baseplate (4) Metaglenoid and baseplate fixation screws ± bone graft (25)	Plexus palsy Spine fracture (1) Acromial fracture (1) Humeral fracture (1)
Sirveaux et al. [2] 5/1953 (0.25%) Coracoid	Female Cuff tear arthropathy Fracture sequelae Rheumatoid arthritis	–	–	Stiffness (1)
Zumstein et al. [5] 1/782 (0.1%) Acromion	Transacromial approach	–	–	–

frequent in superolateral approach probably related to the strength applied on the inferior retractor. To avoid fractures, special attention has to be paid to bone quality in primary surgery but especially in revision surgery. In fact, intraoperative humeral fractures occurred in 1.4% [1] of primary RSA reaching 25% [4] during revision of a previous arthroplasty: in revision cases, extraction of a well-fixed stem or cement can lead to humeral fracture or perforation of the diaphysis or fracture of the tuberosities [3–5, 11]. The extremely high rate of intraoperative complications in the revision arthroplasty group makes meticulous preoperative planning paramount. Particular attention must be given to the quality of the humeral bone stock, component surface coating, and the thickness of the humeral cement, especially in elderly females, prior to attempting component extraction. Consideration should be given to utilizing a humeral osteotomy or humeral window [12]. Nevertheless, a planned humerotomy is not always the solution, and, unfortunately, intraoperative fractures occurred in one third of the patients who received a planned humerotomy in the series of Chuinard [4]. Alternatively, the use of cement-within-cement technique and a shorter humeral stem to revise a cemented humeral component in revision RSA can be considered to reduce the risk of distal fractures [13]. The use of convertible or modular shoulder arthroplasty systems could reduce, in the future, the need to remove the stem and the incidence of humeral fractures. Revision shoulder arthroplasty has an intrinsic complication rate significantly higher than primary arthroplasty but not necessarily related to the use of a reverse prosthesis. Athwal et al. [14] reported 1.5% of intraoperative periprosthetic fractures in primary and revision anatomic shoulder arthroplasties.

The treatment of intraoperative humeral periprosthetic fractures depends on the location of the fracture in relation to the prosthetic component and to the stability of the component/bone interface. A systemic approach is necessary to treating these fractures according to the location, displacement, bone quality, and perceived humerus implant stability. In general, intraoperative humeral fractures are located within the stem zone, whereas postoperative fractures are located mainly below the stem. In the case of nondisplaced or minimally displaced fractures, isolated to the greater tuberosity without any extension into the humeral diaphysis, the fixation of the stem or cerclage wire allows to have a good stability of the implant and the consolidation of the fracture. If needed, a long-stem implant or adjunct fixation should be used if the humerus implant stability is in question. Although intraoperative humeral periprosthetic fracture is associated with a high rate of bone healing, there is a substantial rate of associated complications and lower functional result [1, 2, 4, 5, 11]. Differently in the series reported by Wagner et al. [3], the fracture does not appear to affect postoperative outcomes for patients. To avoid complications, the operative planning is mandatory, and, for the performance of revision surgery, modular revision sets including long stems, revision components, as well as plate and cerclage systems or sutures are obligatory besides the explantation instrumentation to deal with the possibility. Furthermore, when removing implants, a systemic approach should be used, starting with an implant-specific removal device and other techniques to separate the proximal implant-bone interface, to help mitigate the risks of intraoperative periprosthetic fractures [13].

Glenoid perforation or fracture during implantation of the baseplate is rare. It is usually focal and small, effectively reduced by the application of the metaglenoid and, if needed, supported by cancellous graft or even by the use of the surgical cement. Partial fractures do not modify the postoperative care, reeducation, and outcome and do not compromise the long-term fixation of the prosthesis. However, in the case of complete intraoperative glenoid fractures, the effects are dramatic and must, absolutely, be avoided. Differently from the humeral fractures, the glenoid fractures occur especially in the primary arthroplasty, when the surgeon might pay less attention than in the revision group [6]. Technical care is required assessing the glenoid. Fracture can occur in the case of cuff tear arthropathy or rheumatoid arthritis when the glenoid is eroded far medially, the bone is brittle, and osteoporosis related to the etiology or to the absence of mechanical loading on the glenoid bone increases the risk of fracture [2]. The danger can be anticipated on standard x-rays; CT scan is always indicated before surgery to obtain precise information concerning orientation of the prosthesis and the relative danger to perforate and break the glenoid. In order to avoid glenoid fracture, care must be taken while reaming the glenoid surface in those patients whose glenoid may not demonstrate the sclerotic changes normally associated with glenohumeral arthritis, such as those patients with cuff tear arthropathy. When glenoid bone is extremely soft or brittle, the use of a hand reamer may be preferable to the use of a motorized reamer [11]. When occur, the fracture can be managed with a standard technique of fixation with or without graft. In a complete unstable situation, conversion to hemiarthroplasty may be preferred.

Future investigation of methods needs to reduce the risk for intraoperative fractures through modification of surgical techniques and to achieve a high fracture union rate with good shoulder function avoiding further complications in case fracture occurred during RSA. Moreover, convertible or modular shoulder arthroplasty systems could reduce the risk of fractures in the future. While these complications cannot be completed avoided, better understanding of their causes and/or patient risk factors may help the surgeon to decrease their frequency.

References

1. García-Fernández C, Lópiz-Morales Y, Rodríguez A, López-Durán L, Martínez FM. Periprosthetic humeral fractures associated with reverse total shoulder arthroplasty: incidence and management. Int Orthop. 2015;39(10):1965–9. https://doi.org/10.1007/s00264-015-2972-7.
2. Sirveaux F, Boudard G, Jacquot A, Molé D. Reverse shoulder prosthesis, intra-operative fractures. In: Shoulder concepts. Reverse shoulder arthroplasty. Montpellier: Sauramps Medical; 2016. p. 397–401.
3. Wagner ER, Houdek MT, Elhassan BT, Sanchez-Sotelo J, Cofield RH, Sperling JW. What are risk factors for intraoperative humerus fractures during revision reverse shoulder arthroplasty and do they influence outcomes? Clin Orthop Relat Res. 2015;473:3228–34.
4. Chuinard C, Trojani C, Brassart N, Boileau P. Humeral problems in reverse shoulder arthroplasty. In: Reverse shoulder arthroplasty. Clinical results—complications—revision. Montpellier: Sauramps Medical; 2006. p. 275–88.
5. Zumstein MA, Pinedo M, Old J, Boileau P. Problems, complications, reoperations, and revisions in reverse total shoulder arthroplasty: a systematic review. J Shoulder Elb Surg. 2011;20:146–57.
6. Molé D, Navez G, Garaud P. Reverse shoulder prosthesis: problems related to the glenoid. In: Reverse shoulder arthroplasty. Clinical results—complications—revision. Montpellier: Sauramps Medical; 2006. p. 289–301.
7. Wright TW, Cofield RH. Humeral fractures after shoulder arthroplasty. J Bone Joint Surg Am. 1995;77:1340–6.
8. Campbell JT, Moore RS, Iannotti JP, Norris TR, Williams GR. Periprosthetic humeral fractures: mechanisms of fracture and treatment options. J Shoulder Elbow Surg. 1998;7:406–13.
9. Duncan CP, Haddad FS. The Unified Classification system (UCS): improving our understanding of periprosthetic fractures. Bone Joint J. 2014;96-B:713–6.
10. Constant CR, Murley AH. A clinical method of functional assessment of the shoulder. Clin Orthop. 1987;214:160–4.
11. Walch G, Wall B, Mottier F. Complications and revision of the reverse prosthesis: a multicenter study of 457 cases. In: Reverse shoulder arthroplasty. Clinical results—complications—revision. Montpellier: Sauramps Medical; 2006. p. 335–52.
12. Sperling JW, Cofield RH. Humeral windows in revision shoulder arthroplasty. J Shoulder Elb Surg. 2005;14(3):258–63.
13. Wagner ER, Houdek MT, Hernandez NM, Cofield RH, Sánchez-Sotelo J, Sperling JW. Cement-within-cement technique in revision reverse shoulder arthroplasty. J Shoulder Elb Surg. 2017;26(8):1448–53. https://doi.org/10.1016/j.jse.2017.01.013.
14. Athwal GS, Sperling JW, Rispoli DM, Cofield RH. Periprosthetic humeral fractures during shoulder arthroplasty. J Bone Joint Surg Am. 2009;91(3):594–603. https://doi.org/10.2106/JBJS.H.00439.

30 Failure of RSA

Raffaele Garofalo and Enrico Ceccarelli

30.1 Introduction

According to Zumstein [1], the definition of complication in reverse total shoulder arthroplasty (RTSA) could be considered any intraoperative or postoperative event that is likely to have a negative influence on the final outcome. We can include in this field fractures, infections, dislocations, nerve palsies, aseptic loosening of humeral or glenoid components, modular stem or polyethylene disassociations, or glenoid screw problems. Such complications can be divided into two distinct categories: those related to a close failure of the prosthesis and its components and the group of complications related to the patient features. However, both may require reoperation including partial or total revision of the prosthetic component to improve clinical situation. Since 1980 there has been a growing interest in using RTSA, and indications continue to expand with regard to the first Grammont prototype designed for the arthritic rotator cuff-deficient shoulders. In recent years the valid clinical outcomes and the increased patient satisfaction with the Grammont semiconstrained prosthesis have led to widening in the use of the RTSA expanding the indication to other conditions with various degrees of cuff deficiency, such as irreparable rotator cuff tears without osteoarthritis [2], inflammatory arthritis [3], fracture sequelae [4], tumor resection [5], failed hemiarthroplasty after fracture [6], failed hemiarthroplasty with cuff deficiency [7], failure after total shoulder arthroplasty [8], and sequelae of septic arthritis [9]. Other indications include the treatment of complex fractures of the proximal humerus in the elderly [10], as well as osteoarthritis with posterior subluxation and a biconcave B2 or C glenoid [11]. Since RTSA is commonly used to salvage complex conditions, not surprisingly the reported complication rate in these particular situations is relatively high [12], increasing failures and consequently the number of reoperations and revisions. On the basis of the Zumstein [1] study published in 2011, the global rates for complications and revisions after RTSA were 24 and 10%, respectively. Although the percentage of reoperation published in literature varied substantially among authors, depending on the criteria adopted for the definition of complication. Moreover it seems to be influenced by the underlying indication and the mix of primary and revision procedures included in each study. Also the component design and the surgeon experience could influence the complication rate. Main complications of RSA are summarized in Table 30.1. Distinguishing intraoperative from postoperative complications, we can state that the former are reported mainly in revision surgery, while in the

R. Garofalo (✉)
Upper Limb Unit, F.Miulli Hospital,
Acquaviva delle Fonti, BA, Italy

E. Ceccarelli
Orthopaedic Department, Casilino Hospital,
Rome, Italy

S. Gumina et al. (eds.), *Reverse Shoulder Arthroplasty*,
https://doi.org/10.1007/978-3-319-97743-0_30

latter, there are mostly prosthetic component problems rather than shoulder problems, and they are frequent in primary surgery.

30.2 Intraoperative Events

Intraoperative fractures can happen on the glenoid or humeral side. In decreasing percentage order, these are humeral, glenoid, and acromion fracture. The humeral fractures are mainly frequent in revision surgery during the removal of the primary humeral stem or cement mantle in up to 24.1% of all revisions [13] (Fig. 30.1). For these reasons, although most early RTSAs were initially designed for cemented fixation of the humeral component, cementless fixation has become more common. Despite this an excessive reaming for the cementless fixation should be avoided, as it may produce a stress riser area at the tip of the reaming area increasing the risk of periprosthetic fracture [14]. Humeral fracture at the metaphysis or the tuberosities can be managed with cerclage fixation or fragment excision. Cerclage fixation should be performed when joint stability or humeral-sided fixation is compromised. Placement of a long-stemmed implant may be considered to avoid future stem loosening resulting from lack of proximal humeral bone (Fig. 30.2). Intraoperative glenoid fractures are

Table 30.1 RTSA complications: intraoperative and postoperative events

Intraoperative events
• Humeral fractures
• Glenoid fractures
• Acromion fractures
Postoperative events
• Infection
• Dislocation
• Acromion fractures
• Scapular fractures
• Mechanical failure
– Aseptic glenoid loosening
– Glenoid disassembly
• Neurologic injury

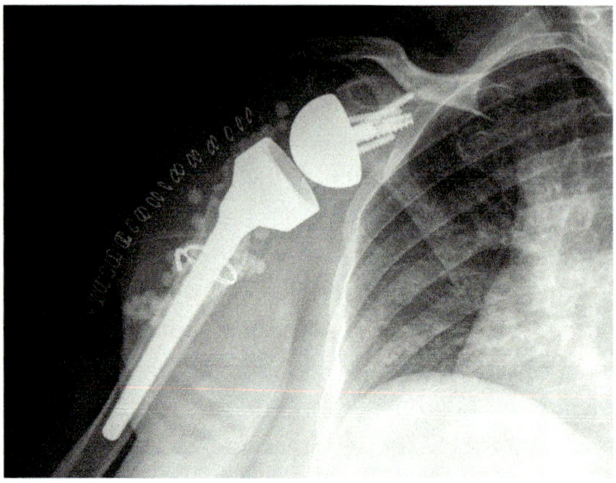

Fig. 30.1 Intraoperative fractures are mainly frequent in revision surgery

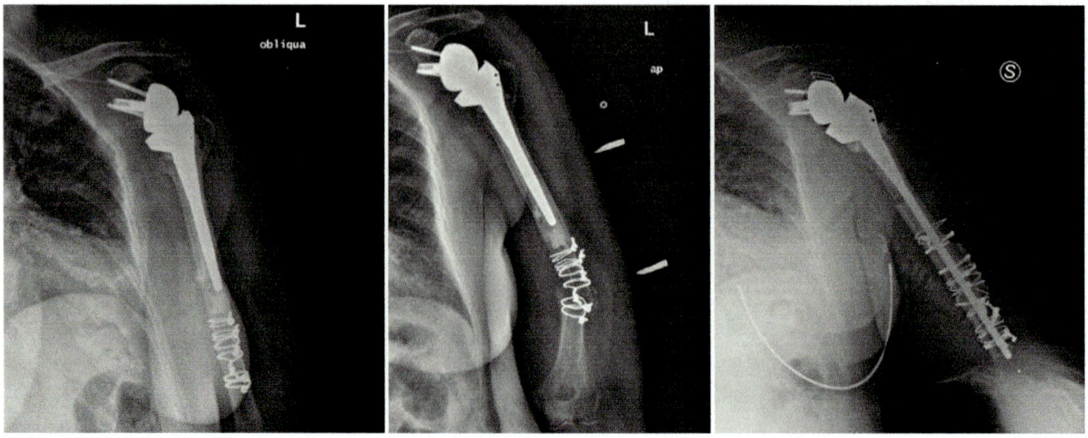

Fig. 30.2 Long-stemmed implant and cerclage fixation should be performed when humeral-sided fixation is compromised

rare and related to the initial reaming or fixation technique [1]. One recommendation, to reduce such incidence, consists to start power reaming prior to placing the reamer on the face of the glenoid and avoidance of over-reaming. Substantial glenoid fractures could make it impossible to achieve component fixation and require intraoperative conversion to a hemiarthroplasty. The intraoperative fracture of the acromion, which is less frequent than the others, is mainly associated with the transacromial approach [15].

30.3 Postoperative Events

Dislocation after RTSA represents a major source of concern (Fig. 30.3). Among the postoperative complications, instability is the most common postoperative complication, with a mean incidence of 4.7%, according to Zumstein meta-analysis [1]. But the percentage varies in literature with rates ranging from 2.4 to 31% according to author indications, type of prosthesis, and surgical approach [16]. Despite the semiconstrained nature of the RTSA, dislocations do happen and sometimes could be extremely difficult to identify causes and mechanisms [17]. RTSA as a concept relies on the effective lever arm of the deltoid to compensate for the absent rotator cuff; this is partially achieved by lengthening the deltoid. Failure to achieve this tension may place the implant at risk of instability. Fracture sequelae, tumor surgery, revision, and instability arthropathy have shown the greatest incidence of prosthetic instability [4, 5, 18]. The primary diagnosis may affect the status of the subscapularis and the rate of impingement and may increase the difficulty of assessing the correct height of the implant on the humeral side; furthermore, version and adequate soft-tissue tension can affect the stability of the implant. In cases of revision or fracture sequelae, intraoperative assessment of deltoid tension can be difficult (e.g., general anesthesia, fibrosis, scar, and retraction of soft tissue), and preoperative templating of the humeral length is essential [17]. To date, preoperative templating with comparison of both arms remains the only objective evaluation to assess for the correct length of the arm at the time of arthroplasty (Fig. 30.4). Intraoperative assessment of stability and impingement is advisable in all cases [19]. Other factors that contribute to postoperative instability include soft-tissue balance, glenosphere diameter, the inclination of the humeral component, erroneous version of the prosthesis, the position of the baseplate, and the axillary nerve/deltoid dysfunction [16]. Also impingement of either bone or soft-tissue structures may contribute to dislocation [17]. Currently, controversy exists regarding the benefit of subscapularis repair. Evidence is lacking to support or refute the assertion that the subscapularis is required to limit instability. Although some authors suggest that repair of the subscapularis may convert it to an adductor and thereby limit motion [20], Edwards et al. [21] suggested that subscapularis reattachment may be beneficial in reducing the rate of dislocation. Conversely, the use of a superolateral approach to avoid violation of the subscapularis appears to be associated with decreased dislocation rates [22]. Frequently, this approach can be performed through the superior rotator cuff defect, thereby minimizing violation of the soft tissue. Disadvantages of subscapularis repair include lack of tendon extensibility, the potential for axillary nerve injury, an increased

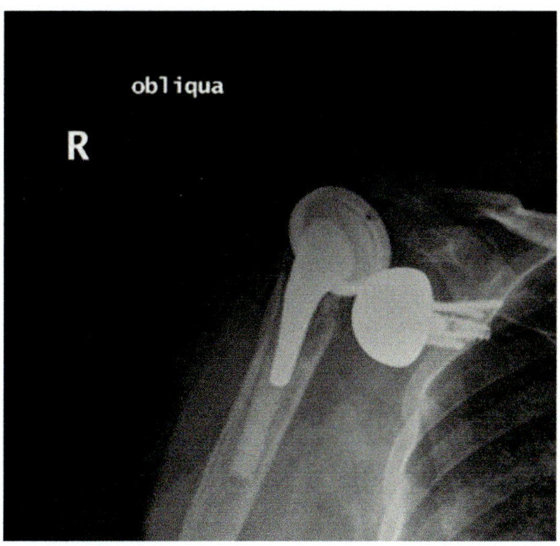

Fig. 30.3 The most common postoperative complication is the instability

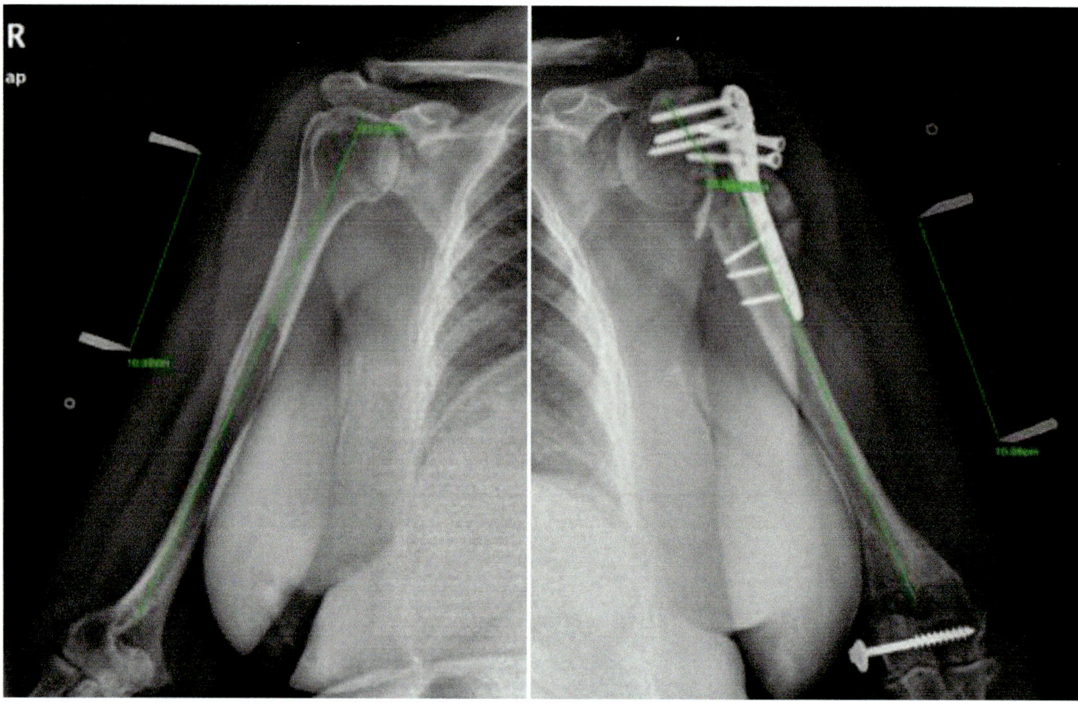

Fig. 30.4 Preoperative templating, with comparison of both arms, for the correct length of the arm

rate of scapular notching resulting from the use of the more difficult inferior exposure, and the potential for deltoid dehiscence postoperatively [23]. When instability happens, it is usually in the first 6 months, and of those, half occurs in the first 3 months [24]. Conservative management can be successful in almost half of patients, and shoulders that remain stable after closed reduction have a similar outcome in terms of pain and motion. On the contrary, recurrent instability may lead to revision surgery, increasing the risk of infection and redislocation [18, 24]. When the dislocation occurs, first-line management typically consists of closed reduction followed by a brief period (6 weeks) of immobilization and avoidance of extension, adduction, and internal rotation. Barring significant trauma, failure to maintain the reduction may necessitate evaluation of implant position, particularly version and height, soft-tissue tension, and surgical technique [16]. Restoration of the anatomic position of the humerus with regard to the lateral offset of the tuberosity-glenoid distance (i.e., lateral-medial tension) and the vertical offset of the acromion-greater tuberosity distance (i.e., superior-inferior tension) seems to be effective in restoring anatomic soft-tissue tension. In patients with humeral or glenoid bone loss, a modified surgical technique may be required, along with bone grafting [25]. Several factors related to prosthesis design and surgical technique have been shown to influence soft-tissue tension, including glenosphere offsets and sizes, humeral neck-shaft angle (i.e., varus or valgus humeral component), and thickness of the humeral insert [26]. Variations in surgical technique include altering the level of the humeral osteotomy, offsetting the placement of the humeral socket, and changing the position of the glenosphere.

30.4 Infection

The reported rate of infection for RTSA is higher than for anatomic shoulder arthroplasty. The reasons are not always clear. The reported incidence in the literature varies from 1 to 10% [16]. In a meta-analysis, Zumstein et al. reported a mean infection rate of 3.8% including primary and revision RTSA, with a higher rate in revision surgery [1]. In particular, the meta-analysis pointed out also that there is an increased rate of infection in the revision group compared with the primary group (5.8 vs 2.9%). As in other shoulder surgeries, low-virulence organisms, such as *Propionibacterium acnes* and *Staphylococcus epidermidis*, are frequently implicated in RTSA infections [1]. As previously mentioned, the large subacromial dead space, the compromised general health of some patients, and the large surgical dissection, especially in revision cases, may predispose to later infection. In patients with a confirmed postoperative infection, antibiotic therapy should be continued postoperatively until the bacteria are identified. Once it is identified, the antibiotic treatment should be tailored to address the sensitivities of specific bacteria. Some species can be identified in 3–4 days; however, slow-growing *Propionibacterium acnes* species may require 10–14 days to ensure proper identification [27]. Acute infection, that is, infection occurring <6 weeks from clinical presentation, can be managed with irrigation, debridement, and polyethylene associated or not with a glenosphere exchange. Chronic infection is best managed with two-stage revision. Stage 1 consists of hardware removal, irrigation and debridement, and the placement of an antibiotic spacer (Fig. 30.5), followed by a minimum 6-week course of parenteral antibiotics. Stage 2, prosthesis reimplantation, should be deferred until blood test results are negative for infections. However, there are evidence that the ideal time to make a reimplantation is between 4 and 8 weeks after debridement time. Before 4 weeks, there is an increase of risk of a new infection;

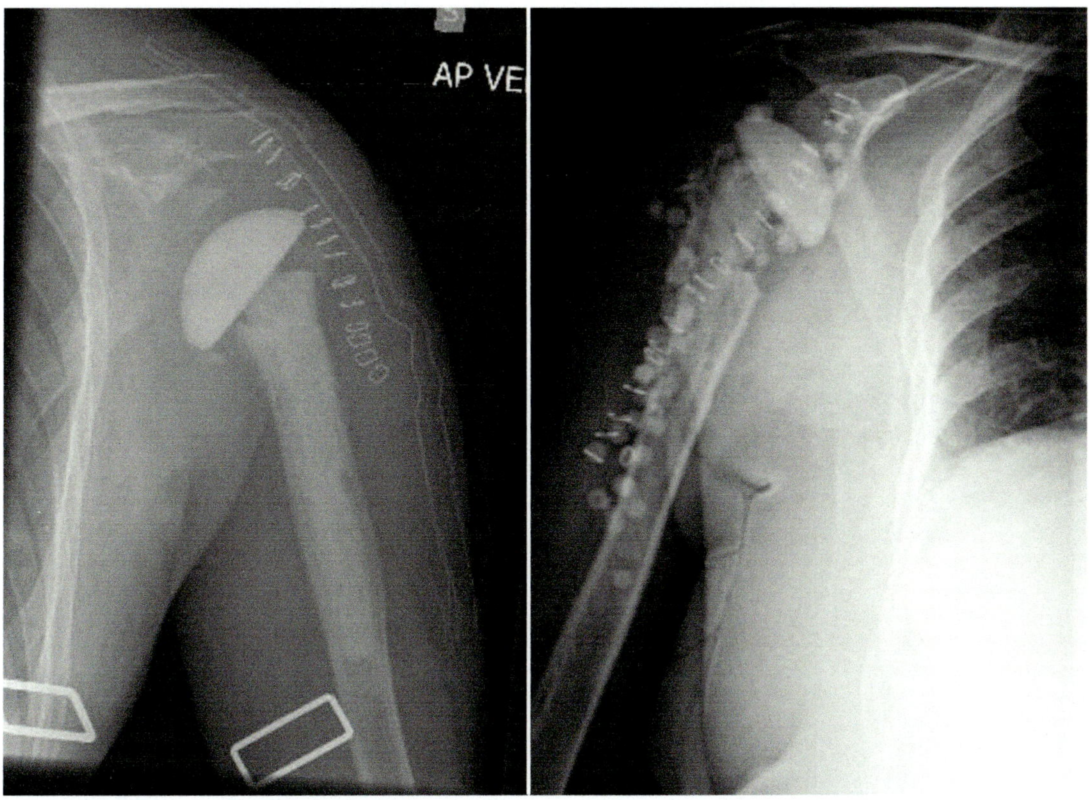

Fig. 30.5 Chronic infection is best managed with placement of an antibiotic spacer

after 11 weeks from the debridement procedure, the risk of stiffness increases. There is also some evidence to suggest that chronic infections can be managed with a one-stage exchange involving irrigation and debridement, reimplantation, and parenteral antibiotics [9].

30.4.1 Acromion and Scapular Fractures

Postoperative fractures of the acromion and scapular spine are rare (1.5% incidence) [9, 28–30]. Postoperative fractures of the acromion often occur spontaneously (Fig. 30.6); it could be correlated to an excessive tensioning of the deltoid that places a weakened acromion at risk of fracture after the implantation of an RTSA. In the case of conservative treatment of an acromion fracture with immobilization, there is no influence on the final outcome reported. However, fractures of the scapular spine or the base of the acromion may require fixation and compromise the final outcome. Acromion fracture can be also treated with skillful neglect and is not a contraindication to a reverse prosthesis. Conversely, postoperative fractures of the scapular spine lead to poor functional outcome and may require osteosynthesis, as reported by Mottier et al. [31].

30.5 Mechanical Failure

30.5.1 Aseptic Glenoid Loosening

Mechanical failure may occur at the humeral or glenoid side. Baseplate failure drove many of the fundamental design changes to early RTSA prostheses. With the initial devices, inadequate fixation coupled with long lever arms led to failure rates between 11.7 and 40% [21, 30]. To avoid loosening, every effort should be made to optimally fix the glenoid component onto good bone stock at the inferior border of the glenoid [22, 33]. Because initial fixation is dependent on the central peg, scapular notching does not seem to predispose to aseptic loosening of the glenoid [33]. The clinical implications of notching are controversial, and some authors have reported no effect over the clinical outcome [12, 34, 35], while others have reported that high grades of notching may be associated with a worse outcome [35, 36]. Eccentric glenospheres with an inferior offset and glenoid component with increased lateral offset (bony

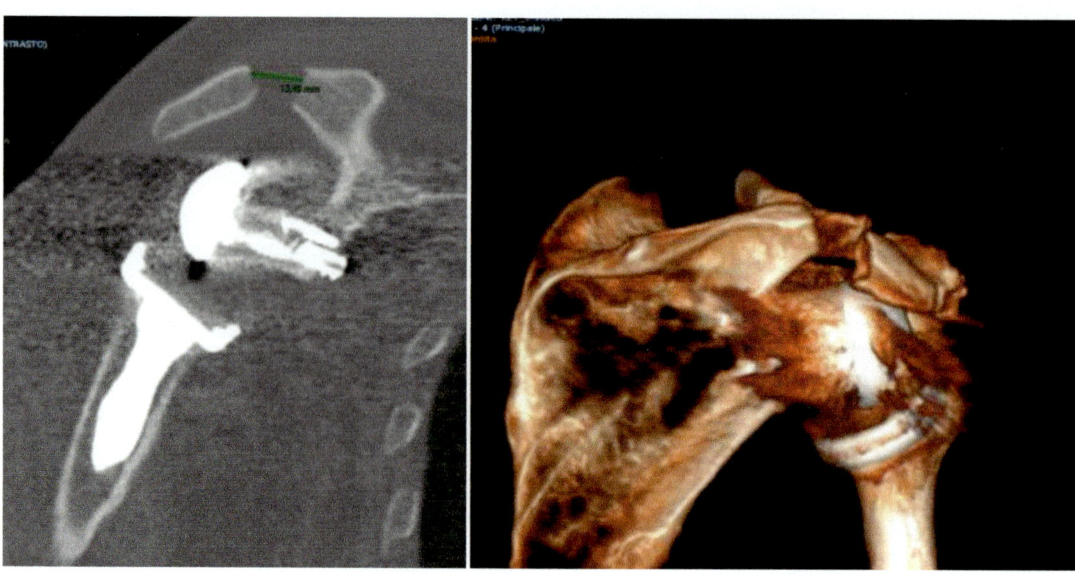

Fig. 30.6 Postoperative fractures of the acromion

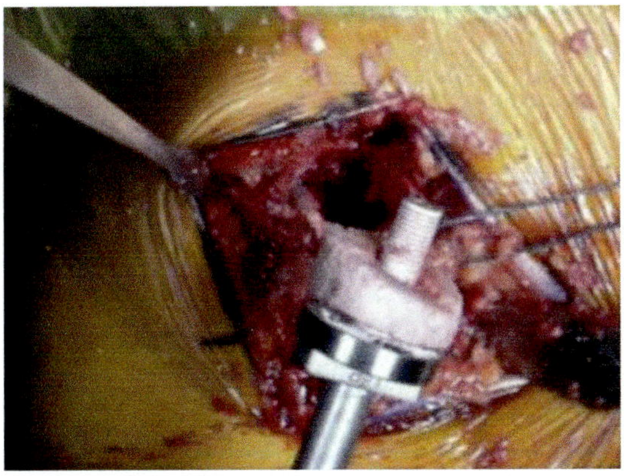

Fig. 30.7 Bio-RSA lateralize the baseplate

or metal) can reduce the rate of notching. Lateralization of the baseplate with the use of a glenoid bone graft taken from the osteotomized humeral head (Bio-RSA) (Fig. 30.7) may theoretically increase the range of motion and reduce the impingement of the humerus on the scapula [37]. According to Frankle study, lack of ingrowth onto the baseplate is associated with baseplate failure, which suggests that bony ingrowth is important in achieving successful long-term outcomes [38]. Significant mechanical stress at the bone-implant interface may influence bony ingrowth and may impact long-term stability. Harman's study sustains that to reduce micromotion below the accepted 150 μm threshold is more relevant to use locking screws rather than offset or screw position [39]. Even though the use of a central screw rather than a peg has been proven to increase the compression of the baseplate to the underlying bone, most current prostheses that use locking screw technology have demonstrated subthreshold micromotion on physiologic loading, increasing the initial mechanical stability [39]. In addition to implant design, also surgical technique seems to be an important variable that influence the rate of glenoid-sided complications. The superior tilt of the glenosphere is correlated with an increased failure rate. Evidence suggests that inferior tilt in combination with locking screws minimizes forces at baseplate-bone interface reducing the rate of failure [26].

Moreover preoperative assessment of glenoid bone stock and careful planning for optimal positioning of the meta-glenoid may be important in preventing loosening [36, 40].

30.6 Glenoid Disassembly

Postoperative glenoid disassembly was rare and was a problem related to the design of the Grammont prosthesis used before 1995. Modification of the Grammont design with a Morse taper central fixation and a new central screw fixation improved the fixation and avoided dissociation of the glenosphere thereafter [28]. Humeral stem disassembly and polyethylene disassociations are also a rare complication in different studies [30, 32, 41, 42]. Humeral stem disassembly did not always need reintervention, and disassociated polyethylene components were revised without clinical impact [30, 32, 41, 44]. According to Melis [34] report evaluating 122 RSTA with 8-year minimum follow-up, cemented stems showed signs of radiolucency without implant migration in 20% of cases. Instead uncemented stems showed proximal bone resorption and signs of stress shielding in 8% of cases, with stem diameter being related to the degree of bone resorption.

30.7 Neurologic Injury

Subclinical neurological injuries with postoperative EMG changes are common after RTSA, while the incidence of clinically evident neurological injury is much less frequent. Since the spontaneous recovery happening in many cases [43], neurologic injury had a negative effect only in the case of incomplete recovery [28]. The most common nerve dysfunction after RSA involves the axillary nerve, although postoperative radial, ulnar, and musculocutaneous nerve palsies have been reported as well [44]. It may be attributed to intraoperative traction, manipulation of the arm, retractor placement, or relative lengthening of the arm. Partial recovery of the axillary nerve may affect the clinical outcome, as it can affect deltoid strength [28]. Whereas axillary nerve palsies are immediate postoperative complications [28], radial nerve palsies are often subsequent to a humeral shaft fracture during follow-up [6, 9, 42]. Also the design of the implant could increase traction at the brachial plexus especially those who require humeral lengthening to provide greater tension on the deltoid to improve stability. Excessive arm lengthening greater than 2 cm has been shown as a potential risk [45]. Anatomical studies show that lateralization is less harmful for the nerve than distalization [46]. The suprascapular nerve and artery may be at risk at the spinoglenoid notch when drilling the posterior screw. Avoiding this complication is important, especially in cases where there is presence of a functional infraspinatus muscle [47].

References

1. Zumstein MA, Pinedo M, Old J, Boileau P. Problems, complications, reoperations, and revisions in reverse total shoulder arthroplasty: a systematic review. J Shoulder Elb Surg. 2010;20:12.
2. Ek ET, Neukom L, Catanzaro S, Gerber C. Reverse total shoulder arthroplasty for massive irreparable rotator cuff tears in patients younger than 65 years old: results after five to fifteen years. J Shoulder Elb Surg. 2013;22(9):1199–208.
3. Holcomb JO, Hebert DJ, Mighell MA, et al. Reverse shoulder arthroplasty in patients with rheumatoid arthritis. J Shoulder Elb Surg. 2010;19:1076–84.
4. Raiss P, Edwards TB, da Silva MR, Bruckner T, Loew M, Walch G. Reverse shoulder arthroplasty for the treatment of nonunions of the surgical neck of the proximal part of the humerus (type-3 fracture sequelae). J Bone Joint Surg Am. 2014;96:2070–6.
5. De Wilde LF, Plasschaert FS, Audenaert EA, Verdonk RC. Functional recovery after a reverse prosthesis for reconstruction of the proximal humerus in tumor surgery. Clin Orthop Relat Res. 2005;430:156–62.
6. Levy J, Frankle M, Mighell M, Pupello D. The use of the reverse shoulder prosthesis for the treatment of failed hemiarthroplasty for proximal humeral fracture. J Bone Joint Surg Am. 2007;89:292–300.
7. Levy JC, Virani N, Pupello D, Frankle M. Use of the reverse shoulder prosthesis for the treatment of failed hemiarthroplasty in patients with glenohumeral arthritis and rotator cuff deficiency. J Bone Joint Surg (Br). 2007;89:189–95.
8. Abdel MP, Hattrup SJ, Sperling JW, Cofield RH, Kreofsky CR, Sanchez Sotelo J. Revision of an unstable hemiarthroplasty or anatomical total shoulder replacement using a reverse design prosthesis. Bone Joint J. 2013;95-b(5):668–72.
9. Cuff DJ, Virani NA, Levy J, et al. The treatment of deep shoulder infection and glenohumeral instability with debridement, reverse shoulder arthroplasty and postoperative antibiotics. J Bone Joint Surg (Br). 2008;90:336–42.
10. Wall B, Walch G. Reverse shoulder arthroplasty for the treatment of proximal humeral fractures. Hand Clin. 2007;23:425–30.
11. Mizuno N, Denard PJ, Raiss P, Walch G. Reverse total shoulder arthroplasty for primary glenohumeral osteoarthritis in patients with a biconcave glenoid. J Bone Joint Surg Am. 2013;95:1297–304.
12. Wall B, Nové-Josserand L, O'Connor DP, Edwards TB, Walch G. Reverse total shoulder arthroplasty: a review of results according to etiology. J Bone Joint Surg Am. 2007;89:1476–85.
13. Weissinger M, Helmreich C, Teumann E. Initial experience using the inverse prosthesis of the shoulder. Acta Chir Orthop Traumatol Cechoslov. 2008;75:21–7.
14. Lee M, Chebli C, Mounce D, Bertelsen A, Richardson M, Matsen F. Intramedullary reaming for press-fit fixation of a humeral component removes cortical bone asymmetrically. J Shoulder Elb Surg. 2008;17:150–5.
15. Baulot E, Chabernaud D, Grammont PM. Results of Grammont's inverted prosthesis in omarthritis associated with major cuff destruction. Apropos of 16 cases. Acta Orthop Belg. 1995;61:112–9.
16. Cheung E, Willis M, Walker M, Clark R, Frankle MA. Complications in reverse total shoulder arthroplasty. J Am Acad Orthop Surg. 2011;19:439–49.
17. Barco R, Savvidou OD, Sperling JW, Sanchez-Sotelo J, Cofield RH. Complications in reverse shoulder arthroplasty. EFORT Open Rev. 2017;1(3):72–80.
18. Trappey GJ IV, O'Connor DP, Edwards TB. What are the instability and infection rates after reverse shoulder arthroplasty? Clin Orthop Relat Res. 2011;469:2505–11.
19. Lädermann A, Edwards TB, Walch G. Arm lengthening after reverse shoulder arthroplasty: a review. Int Orthop. 2014;38:991–1000.
20. Gerber C, Pennington SD, Nyffeler RW. Reverse total shoulder arthroplasty. J Am Acad Orthop Surg. 2009;17:284–95.
21. Edwards TB, Williams MD, Labriola JE, Elkousy HA, Gartsman GM, et al. Subscapularis insufficiency and the risk of shoulder dislocation after revers shoulder arthroplasty. J Shoulder Elb Surg. 2009;18:892–6.
22. Walch G, Wall B, Mottier F. Complications and revision of the reverse prosthesis: a multicenter study of 457 cases. In: Boileau P, editor. Reverse shoulder arthroplasty. Nice: Sauramps; 2006. p. 335–52.
23. Seebauer L. Total reverse shoulder arthroplasty: European lessons and future trends. Am J Orthop (Belle Mead NJ). 2007;36(12 Suppl 1):22–8.
24. Teusink MJ, Pappou IP, Schwartz DG, Cottrell BJ, Frankle MA. Results of closed management of acute

dislocation after reverse shoulder arthroplasty. J Shoulder Elb Surg. 2015;24:621–7.
25. Klein SM, Dunning P, Mulieri P, Pupello D, Downes K, Frankle MA. Effects of acquired glenoid bone defects on surgical technique and clinical outcomes in reverse shoulder arthroplasty. J Bone Joint Surg Am. 2010;92(5):1144–54.
26. Gutiérrez S, Keller TS, Levy JC, Lee WE III, Luo ZP. Hierarchy of stability factors in reverse shoulder arthroplasty. Clin Orthop Relat Res. 2008;466(3):670–6.
27. Zimmerli W, Trampuz A, Ochsner PE. Prosthetic-joint infections. N Engl J Med. 2004;351(16):1645–54.
28. Boileau P, Watkinson D, Hatzidakis AM, Hovorka I. Neer Award 2005: the Grammont reverse shoulder prosthesis: results in cuff tear arthritis, fracture sequelae, and revision arthroplasty. J Shoulder Elb Surg. 2006;15:527–40.
29. Cuff D, Pupello D, Virani N, Levy J, Frankle M. Reverse shoulder arthroplasty for the treatment of rotator cuff deficiency. J Bone Joint Surg Am. 2008;90:1244–51.
30. Frankle M, Siegal S, Pupello D, Saleem A, Mighell M, Vasey M. The reverse shoulder prosthesis for glenohumeral arthritis associated with severe rotator cuff deficiency. A minimum two-year follow-up study of sixty patients. J Bone Joint Surg Am. 2005;87:1697–705.
31. Mottier F, Wall B, Nove-Josserand L, Galoisy Guibal L, Walch G. Reverse prosthesis and os acromiale or acromion stress fracture. Rev Chir Orthop Reparatrice Appar Mot. 2007;93:133–41.
32. Werner CM, Steinmann PA, Gilbart M, Gerber C. Treatment of painful pseudoparesis due to irreparable rotator cuff dysfunction with the Delta III reverse-ball-and-socket total shoulder prosthesis. J Bone Joint Surg Am. 2005;87(7):1476–86.
33. Nyffeler RW, Werner CM, Simmen BR, Gerber C. Analysis of a retrieved delta III total shoulder prosthesis. J Bone Joint Surg Br. 2004;86:1187–91.
34. Melis B, Defranco M, Lädermann A, et al. An evaluation of the radiological changes around the Grammont reverse geometry shoulder arthroplasty after eight to 12 years. J Bone Joint Surg (Br). 2011;93:1240–6.
35. Lévigne C, Boileau P, Favard L, et al. Scapular notching in reverse shoulder arthroplasty. J Shoulder Elb Surg. 2008;17:925–35.
36. Simovitch RW, Zumstein MA, Lohri E, Helmy N, Gerber C. Predictors of scapular notching in patients managed with the Delta III reverse total shoulder replacement. J Bone Joint Surg Am. 2007;89:588–600.
37. Boileau P, Roussanne Y, Brassart N. Bony increased offset reverse shoulder arthroplasty (BIO-RSA): a biologic solution to scapular notching, prosthetic instability and limited shoulder rotation. Presented at: Society of European Shoulder and Elbow Surgeons, 21st Annual Meeting. Brugge, Belgium; 2008. p. 69.
38. Frankle M, Pupello D, Gutierrez S. Rationale and biomechanics of the reverse shoulder prosthesis: the American experience. In: Frankle M, editor. Rotator cuff deficiency of the shoulder. New York: Thieme Medical Publishers; 2008. p. 76–104.
39. Harman M, Frankle M, Vasey M, Banks S. Initial glenoid component xation in "reverse" total shoulder arthroplasty: a biomechanical evaluation. J Shoulder Elb Surg. 2005;14(suppl S):162S–7S.
40. Nyffeler RW, Werner CM, Gerber C. Biomechanical relevance of glenoid component positioning in the reverse Delta III total shoulder prosthesis. J Shoulder Elb Surg. 2005;14:524–8.
41. Boulahia A, Edwards TB, Walch G, Baratta RV. Early results of a reverse design prosthesis in the treatment of arthritis of the shoulder in elderly patients with a large rotator cuff tear. Orthopedics. 2002;25:129–33.
42. Gohlke F, Rolf O. Revision of failed fracture hemiarthroplasties to reverse total shoulder prosthesis through the transhumeral approach: method incorporating a pectoralis-major-pedicled bone window. Oper Orthop Traumatol. 2007;19:185–208.
43. Nagda SH, Rogers KJ, Estokas AK, et al. Neer Award 2005: peripheral nerve function during shoulder arthroplasty using intraoperative nerve monitoring. J Shoulder Elb Surg. 2007;16(suppl):S2–8.
44. Lädermann A, Lübbeke A, Mélis B, et al. Prevalence of neurologic lesions after total shoulder arthroplasty. J Bone Joint Surg Am. 2011;93:1288–93.
45. Favard L, Sirveaux F, Oudet D, Huguet D, Mole D. Hemiarthroplasty versus reverse arthroplasty in treatment of arthropathy with massive rotator cuff tear. Proceeding of the European Federation of National Associations of Orthopaedics and Traumatology (EFORT). J Bone Joint Surg Br. 2004;86.(suppl III:230ff.
46. Liem D, Marquardt B, Witt KA, Steinbeck J. Shoulder arthroplasty: biomechanics and design. Orthopade. 2007;36:1027–36.
47. Loew M, Raiss P, Kasten P, Rickert M. Shoulder arthroplasty following rotator cuff tear: acquired arthropathy of the shoulder. Orthopade. 2007;36:988–95.

Part VII

Rehabilitation

31 Postop Rehabilitation in rTSA

Marco Conti, Valentina Spunton, and Roberto Fenini

In this chapter our goal is to highlight the specific characteristics of a postop rehabilitation program in patients that underwent surgery for the implant of a reverse prosthesis.

These specific characteristics are strictly linked to the deep meaning of such a type of surgery and of its goals.

To manage this topic, we will start from the most important aspects that could push the patient to question or accept this type of surgery, which correctly could be called "rescue surgery".

31.1 The Goals

As explained in a previous chapter of this book, the patient that undergoes this type of surgery could be affected by the following:

- Degenerative or post-traumatic glenohumeral (GH) arthritis
- Massive irreparable rotator cuff tears (RCT)
- Complex fracture of the humeral head
- Need of a revision of a previous failed conventional total shoulder arthroplasty (TSA) for the rupture of the rotator cuff
- Avascular necrosis
- Tumors [1, 2]

Musculoskeletal and systemic comorbidities of these patients strongly influence recovery potential.

Apart from patients with fractures, the majority of patients have reached the third age and in this type of patient the major complaints are pain and functional limitation in activities of daily living (ADL) [3].

The patient that hopes to solve pain and functional limitation must, due to the pathology, face the fact that because it is a complicated salvage surgery the aspects that can "go wrong" are several, starting with the patient acceptation of the implant.

In this scenario, a first critical point for the satisfaction of the patient is the correct relationship between the patient, his reverse prosthesis, the surgeon, and the physiotherapist. This relationship should be based on the thorough, detailed explanation (in the preop phase) of the characteristics of the implant and its limitations, constraints, and possible complications [4]. These can be summarized as:

- Substantial modification of the proprioception of the shoulder that could be perceived by the patient as "different from before" or "different from the contralateral." This modification requires a specific rehabilitation and, sequentially, a specific strategy for the use of the arm [5].

M. Conti (✉)
HumanPerformance & Rehabilitation Lab, MedSport, Como, Varese, Italy

V. Spunton · R. Fenini
Private Practice Office & Castagna Shoulder Team, Milan, Italy

S. Gumina et al. (eds.), *Reverse Shoulder Arthroplasty*,
https://doi.org/10.1007/978-3-319-97743-0_31

- Biomechanical constraint, depending from the type/model of prosthesis chosen by the surgeon, on the basis of his knowledge and capability to implant, and also on the characteristics of the pathology that requires the implant [6–8].
- Intraop specific choices and surgically adapted technical solutions that could be adopted for each patient, implant, and tissue scenario such as major or minor lateralization or bone stock use [9–12].
- Possible postop instability of implant components and/or implant dislocation.
- Final functional result is highly dependent on that the posterior RC is still functional [13].
- Possible hardware failure.
- Possible damage to nervous tissue.
- Possible hematoma with following tissues adherence.
- Infections requiring revision of the surgery [14].

All this information can simplify the acceptance of the procedure and of all subsequent problems during the postop phase, which would be mainly pain and residual functional limitations.

A detailed explanation on limited functionality and limited biomechanics must be reserved for the patient with an active and sportive lifestyle, which requires an extensive use of the arm during the preop daily life.

31.2 Constraints and Complications Relevant for the Rehabilitation

Relevant topics that need to be thoroughly explained to the patient, both before and immediately after the surgery, and that also have to be understood and taken into account by the therapist are the constraints and complications of this kind of surgery.

The rTSA implant (please refer to other chapter of this book for all technical aspects of this implant) is performed in a scenario dominated by the RC absence, mainly by the loss of the supra- and infraspinatus.

Both are responsible for the correct drive and force of the anatomical humeral head in the abduction and forward flexion elevation.

Their loss is the basic requirement to decide to implant a rTSA, but the overall scenario could be further complicated by a subscapularis rupture or by the impossibility to repair it [15, 16].

For all these reasons, the full functionality of the teres minor is at the basis of the residual external rotation capability after rTSA implant, as the full functionality of the deltoid is fundamental for the abduction and forward flexion [17].

The loss also of the teres minor could lead the surgeon to associate a muscle transfer to the rTSA implant to obtain a minimal force in external rotation and elevation. Clearly, this association does not only complicate the length of surgery but also the rehabilitation process.

A second key point is the center of rotation of the "new" reverted GH articulation, which in the implant is medialized and inferiorly positioned, with respect to the original anatomical one. This induces an increase of the deltoid moment arm and deltoid tension, enabling an enhancement of the torque obtainable from the deltoid, as well as the line of pull of the same deltoid.

To obtain the best functional result, the integrity of the deltoid in its anatomical and neurological aspects is mandatory, and for this reason the deltopectoral approach is considered the best for its minimal impact on shoulder anatomy.

The purpose of the rTSA is to obtain the capability of the deltoid to compensate the RC deficit, resulting in the possibility of an active elevation of the arm, often overhead in most patients. This means that if a different surgical approach deeply involving the deltoid is chosen, an early postop activation of the deltoid must be avoided [18].

One typical complication of the rTSA is considered the so-called scapular notching, which occurs due to the impingement of the inferior part of the glenoid bone with the medial humeral part of the implant. This can result in pain and discomfort to the patient, which can be managed by the surgeon by regulating the lateralization of the humeral head and inclination of implant components. No actions of the therapist during the rehabilitation process can change the symptoms and history of this problem, apart from the reduction of movements in adduction in front of the thorax. By recognizing the symptoms of scapular notching, the therapist can be an invaluable help to the surgeon [19].

The instability of the system is another possible complication that could be due to an insufficient deltoid tension or to an incorrect positioning of components, or mobilization of one of them (generally the new baseplate for the inverted humeral head). In this case, the risk of autonomous active movement or passive mobilization by the physiotherapist would be the dislocation.

This problem must be monitored by the therapist alongside the entire rehabilitation process, avoiding all ends of range movement and mobilization, particularly those in full external or internal rotation, while continually stimulating a good deltoid muscle tone.

Periprosthetic soft tissue adherence or an excessive humeral head lateralization could reveal to the therapist a problem of stiff shoulder with a greater scapular compensation than in the majority of prosthetic shoulders. This would become a relevant problem for the therapist and the patient, setting a functional limitation. The sensibility of the therapist is crucial in recognizing a stiffness due to increasing postop adherence or due to mechanical reasons; the feeling alongside the movement and at the end of RoM can help determine the underlying cause for the stiffness.

31.3 The Rehabilitation Process

Because a rehabilitation process is in fact a continuum of progress, to define the stages is not something that corresponds to normal clinical practice. However, it is a useful and widely used system that can better explain the basic cues and the main practices in each phase of the rehabilitation process continuum.

For this reason, we will focus our attention on the following periods of the rehabilitation process: acute postop phase (phase I), post-acute phase (phase II), intermediate phase of shoulder strengthening (phase III), and final phase of functional recovery (phase IV) [18].

31.3.1 Acute Postop Phase (Phase I): Protection Phase

In the immediate postop period, the main issues to be addressed are the healing of tissues around the implant (bone that hosts the implant on both sides, scapula and humeral diaphysis), the stability of the prosthesis that is not protected by muscle activity of the rotator cuff, the integrity of subscapularis tendon if re-sutured to the bone on the humeral side, and the healing of soft tissues of the deltopectoral way of access.

Here, the element to be mainly protected is the reattachment of the subscapularis tendon, and for this reason, phase I could last from 4 weeks (if only soft tissue of the deltopectoral way of access must be considered) to 5–6 weeks (if also the subscapularis must be considered). The 6 weeks of protection by sling is also adopted if muscular transfer is associated with the rTSA implant.

During this period, the immobilization of the arm, to protect it from undue active or passive movements, will be obtained using a sling in abduction of 15–30° and external rotation of 0°. This is mandatory not only for the comfort of the patient but also for the mechanical protection of tissues from abrupt stretching, mainly in external rotation or forward flexion, since these movements stress the subscapularis repair. Movements and positioning in extension, internal rotation, and adduction must be avoided because of the risk of dislocation due to the cuff deficiency.

When the posterior integrity of the capsule is compromised and the quantity and quality of posterior cuff are poor, the use of a sling with 15° external rotation is recommended to reduce the stress on these structures and increase healing potential. The use of a sling also reduces the risk of posterior dislocation following undue internal rotation.

At the same time, a gentle self passive mobilization from 0 to 70° in forward flexion and an internal rotation (elbow at the side) to external rotation from −30° to 0° can be performed, such as active/assisted elbow and wrist and hand mobilization, to avoid stiffness. Simple scapular and neck mobilization are suggested to avoid dyskinesia and wrong postures, which encourage compensatory movements or altered timing of muscle activation.

During this time of immobilization, and only if a deltopectoral approach is performed, submaximal isometric contraction of the deltoid can be performed (beware of stress fracture of the acromion!). Gentle, limited, passive mobilization can also be done by the therapist to reduce the harmful effects of immobilization and to recover the sense of positioning and kinesthesia of the "new" shoulder.

Some rehabilitation teams are used to immediately perform passive mobilization in water, after waterproof protection of the scars. This approach can be pursued if surgery involves a standard rTSA implant. However, if subscapularis reattachment, muscular transfer, and bone stock implant are performed, also the reduced stress applied to the shoulder by the movements in water must be avoided for the first 6 weeks.

31.3.2 Post-acute Phase (Phase II): Mobilization Phase

Phase II will start overlapping the discontinuation of the use of a sling at the 4th–6th week based on the needs of phase I, as previously explained.

This "mobilization phase" will last approximately until the 12th week.

During this phase, the goal will be recovery of passive range of motion (PRoM) and, also in the final weeks, the active RoM (ARoM), using passive, assisted, and/or underwater mobilizations (Figs. 31.1, 31.2, and 31.3).

Attention should be paid, in the early phase of the mobilization, to not apply undue stress to the repaired tendons and to bone/metal interface

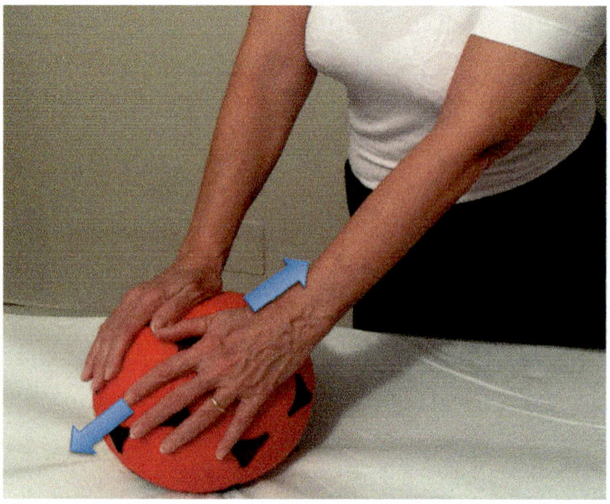

Fig. 31.1 Self-assisted mobilization in flexion and axial compression

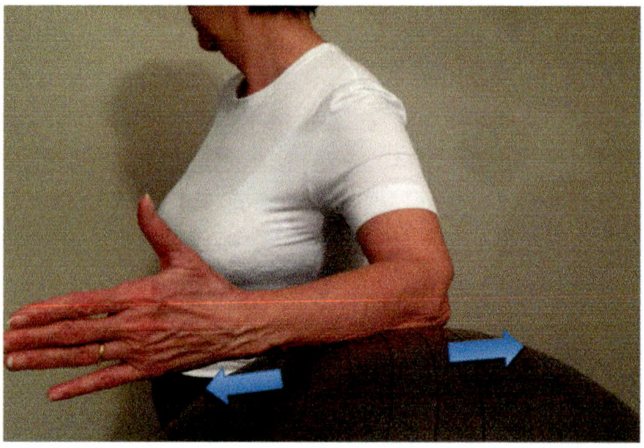

Fig. 31.2 Shoulder flexion-extension self-mobilization partially unloaded by a Swiss ball

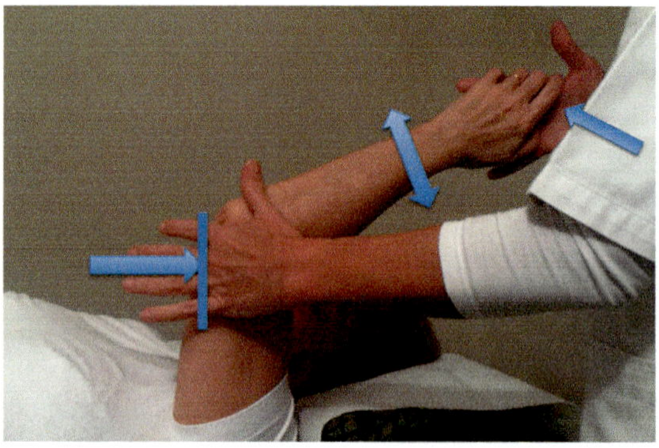

Fig. 31.3 Shoulder isometric stabilization and elbow dynamic control in flexion-extension

mainly at the scapular side. Therefore the mobilization must be on the scapular plane when external, internal, or forward flexion mobilization is performed.

At the same time, exercises in closed kinetic chain can be performed to stimulate the proprioception of the arm, eliciting an initial muscle activation of the rotator cuff and deltoid.

As previously mentioned, the passive and assisted mobilization in water can be performed while including exercises that can elicit not only the RoM recovery but also proprioception and muscles activation.

The core stability and the voluntary activation of scapular stabilizer muscles can also be performed, enhancing the capacity of the patient in recovering the correct posture and scapular positioning and stability. These features are always lost in these patients at the time of the surgery due to the extended history of the glenohumeral joint pathology [20].

During the weeks of phase II, on the basis of the tissue response to the progressive stress in elongation and activation, the PRoM can be increased as well as the quantity of active motion using both specific exercises and daily activity movements, which require the hand control at maximum to the shoulder height (Figs. 31.4 and 31.5).

During isometric conditioning, which should not be started before the 8th week to respect the repaired part of the cuff, sense of force perception should be encouraged.

If the surgeon confirms that no components of the rotator cuff have been repaired, it is possible to initiate isometric conditioning earlier than the 8th week upon the approval of the surgeon.

When PRoM increases, such as the isometric force, a light isotonic strengthening can be started with a low-weight and high-repetition program, using elastic resistance, also in eccentric modality (Figs. 31.6, 31.7, and 31.8).

Cuff and deltoid activity should be progressively promoted from supported to unsupported arm to maximize dynamic stability of the shoulder.

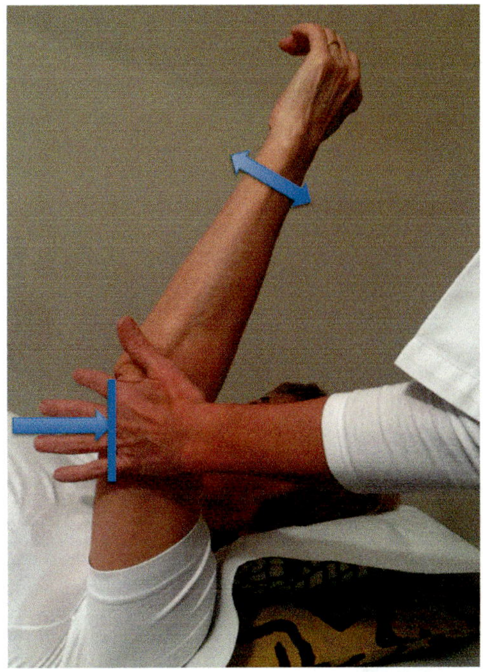

Fig. 31.4 Shoulder isometric stabilization and elbow dynamic control in flexion-extension

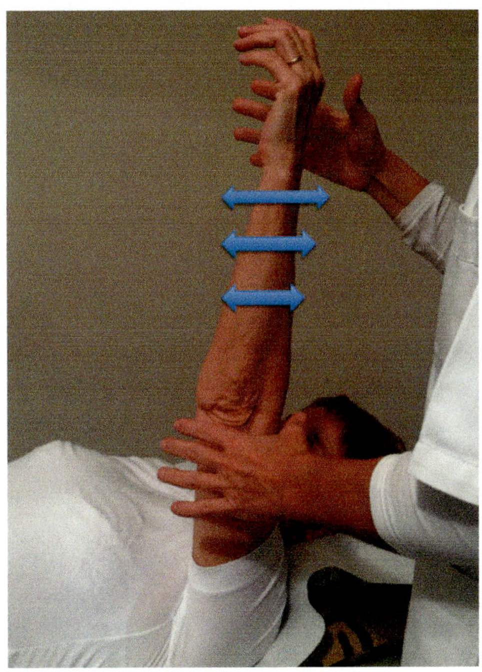

Fig. 31.5 Rhythmic shoulder stabilization with extended arm and low load

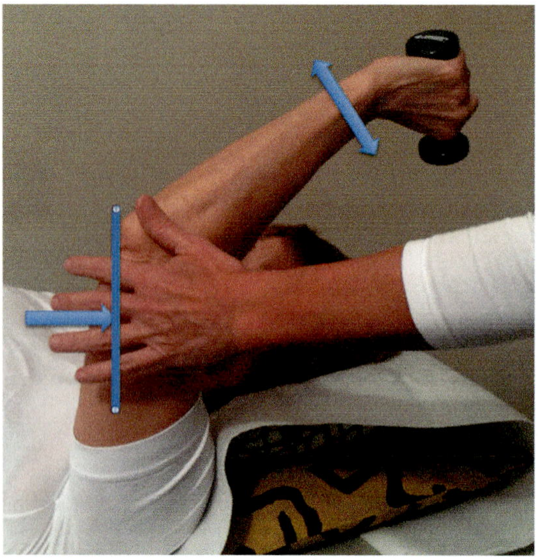

Fig. 31.6 Assisted shoulder stabilization withstanding elbow-loaded extension

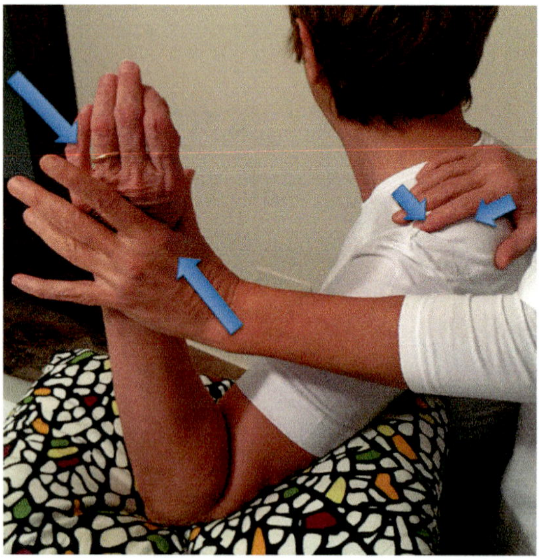

Fig. 31.7 Isometric shoulder external rotation with arm unloaded and compensation control

Be aware that an inferior displacement of the humerus may cause healing problems to the subscapularis [6].

Reducing guarding reactions may be difficult because the residual muscle imbalance, due to posterior cuff deficiency, induces an over-activation of the posterior deltoid, teres minor, and teres major, which are able to limit scaption or elevation.

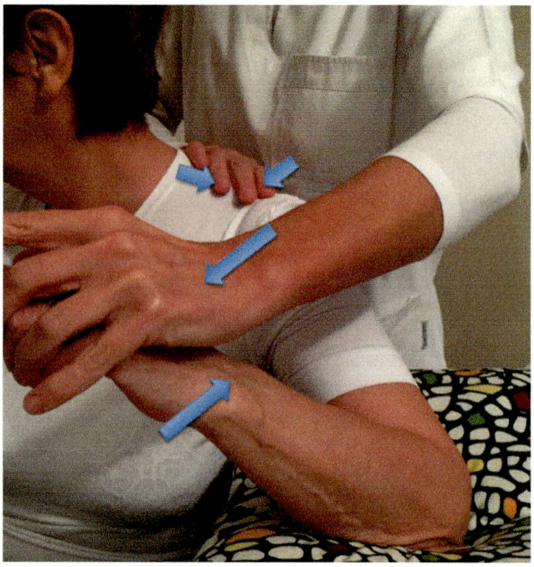

Fig. 31.8 Shoulder external rotation resisted mobilization with arm unloaded and compensation control

Ice and NSAID therapies are always good companions to alleviate the pain and inflammation arising from the mobilization and activation.

If pain and stiffness increase without an acceptable reason, please refer to the surgeon for a check of the inflammatory or infective status of the shoulder.

In a normal progression from 4th to 12th week, a forward flexion of 120° can be attained as well as an external rotation of 45°. Internal rotation can be slowly initiated with no pain provocation.

Since we often have to manage elderly patients, body balance reactions should be encouraged as soon as possible to regain the stability given by the arm.

31.3.3 Intermediate Phase of Shoulder Strengthening (Phase III)

During phase III, starting approximately at the 12th week, given that isometric strength until shoulder height is satisfactory, progression with this kind of force recovery with arm elevation from chest height until maximum is encouraged.

The execution of these exercises should always be closely monitored to avoid compensatory scapular rotation or protraction.

At the same time, there should be progression with the dynamic force recovery under the shoulder level, paying attention to enhancing the shoulder endurance, minimizing the risk of injury/dislocation, and maintaining appropriate pain-free shoulder mechanics.

Particular attention must be paid to the correct periscapular muscle activation and training of the scapula stabilizing muscles to ensure a stable baseplate to the "new" articulation. However, it should be done without considering all upper tilt and protraction movements as pathological, and therefore as something that should be forcefully corrected, as they can be the necessary, obligatory consequence of a forward flexion attempt of a partially stiff or biomechanically unbalanced "new" articulation.

Task-specific activities, repeating daily life movements, should be encouraged as well as progressive increase in ARoM in all directions, moving off progressively from the "safe zone." The scapulohumeral rhythm must always be monitored [21].

A close monitoring of the patient tolerance of exercise and ARoM progression is crucial in this phase [22].

Sudden lifting, pushing, and jerking motions should be avoided indefinitely to minimize the risk of injury/dislocation.

If, to some degree, shoulder stiffness persists, gentle, passive mobilization, managed by a physiotherapist, should be continued.

In the last part of this phase, movements like driving and limited swimming (breaststroke) could be permitted.

31.3.4 Final Phase of Functional Recovery (Phase IV)

After 4 months, the patient should be able to demonstrate functional pain-free shoulder ARoM and be independent with an appropriate strength.

At this stage, a shoulder ARoM is typically 80–120° of elevation, with functional ER up to 60° and 4–7 kg weight lift.

Am home exercise program, possibly remote controlled, must be set up to ensure the progression of recovery or at least the maintenance of the target obtained.

After 6 months, if satisfactory artrocinematic is restored and tissue healing is guaranteed, repetitive arm over shoulder movements, weight lifting, and contact movements can be allowed upon surgeon approval.

At this stage it will be very relevant to compare the outcomes with the initial expectations to be able to manage the reduction/adaptation of daily life functions for a positive physiological balance of the patient. It is imperative that expectations and outcomes match.

rTSA patients can recover to a nearly full ARoM with a reasonable force, compared to the contralateral, also with a dyskinetic scapular compensation that partially absorbs the glenohumeral mobility loss [23]. Therefore, the expectations of the patient could be to also recover full functionality compared to the normal arm. However, the capability of reaching and taking objects is slower and less fluent—most likely due to lesions to the proprioceptive system caused by the implant as well as the detachment of the glenohumeral ligaments [24, 25]—and furthermore, the patient has limited external rotation. All these disabilities reduce the patients' capability of interacting with the surrounding world.

These limitations are not addressed by the surgeons' most used evaluation score system, the Constant score [23].

For this reason, the use of a more comprehensive ADL evaluation system like DASH is strongly suggested.

Patients with initial cuff tear arthropathy have significantly higher improvements in Constant score compared with patients undergoing revision of the prosthesis, post-traumatic osteoarthritis, rheumatoid arthritis, and avascular necrosis.

31.4 Conclusions

As shown in this chapter, the rehabilitation of an rTSA-implanted patient is different from other shoulder rehabilitation processes. On one hand, more attention must be paid to biomechanical issues to obtain a reasonable functional recovery and to avoid risks of implant failure or dislocation. On the other hand, attention must be paid to the psychological aspects to avoid psychological distress of the patient.

A multimodal patient education, tailored to individual preferences and experiences, which may differ according to characteristics such as gender and age, could provide invaluable support in facing all psychological aspects related to the joint replacement; however, it requires a specific training for all caregivers involved.

If addressed correctly, it could be a challenging but gratifying process, giving a "new life" to the patient, thanks to the functional recovery of the arm.

References

1. Samitier G, Alentorn-Geli E, Torrens C, Wright TW. Reverse shoulder arthroplasty. Part 1: systematic review of clinical and functional outcomes. Int J Shoulder Surg. 2015;9:24–31.
2. Alentorn-Geli E, Samitier G, Torrens C, Wright TW. Reverse shoulder arthroplasty. Part 2: systematic review of reoperations, revisions, problems, and complications. Int J Shoulder Surg. 2015;9:60–7.
3. Payne C, Jaggi A, Le Leu A, Garofalo R, Conti M. Rehabilitation for shoulder arthroplasty. Orthop Trauma. 2015;29(5):281–336.
4. Kennedy D, Wainwright A, Pereira L, Robarts S, Dickson P, Christian J, Webster F. A qualitative study of patient education needs for hip and knee replacement. Musculoskelet Disord. 2017;18(1):413.
5. Maier MW, Niklasch M, Dreher T, Wolf SI, Zeifang F, Loew M, Kasten P. Proprioception 3 years after shoulder arthroplasty in 3D motion analysis: a prospective study. Arch Orthop Trauma Surg. 2012;132:1003–10.
6. Boileau P, Watkinson D, Hatzidakis AM, Hovorka I. Neer award 2005: the Grammont reverse shoulder prosthesis: results in cuff tear arthritis, fracture sequelae, and revision arthroplasty. J Shoulder Elb Surg. 2006;15:527–40.
7. Wall B, Nové-Josserand L, O'Connor DP, Edwards TB, Walch G. Reverse total shoulder arthroplasty: a review of results according to etiology. J Bone Joint Surg Am. 2007;89:1476–85.
8. Jarrett CD, Brown BT, Schmidt CC. Reverse shoulder Arthroplasty. Orthop Clin N Am. 2013;23:389–408.
9. De Biase CF, Ziveri G, Delcogliano M, de Caro F, Gumina S, Borroni M, Castagna A, Postacchini R. The use of an eccentric glenosphere compared with a concentric glenosphere in reverse total shoulder arthroplasty: two-year minimum follow-up results. Int Orthop. 2013;37(10):1949–55.
10. Mole D, Wein F, De´zaly C, Valenti P, Sirveaux F. Surgical technique: the anterosuperior approach for reverse shoulder arthroplasty. Clin Orthop Relat Res. 2011;469:2461–8.
11. Walch G, Bacle G, Lädermann A, Nové-Josserand L, Smithers CJ. Do the indications, results, and complications of reverse shoulder arthroplasty change with surgeon's experience? J Shoulder Elb Surg. 2012;21:1470–7.
12. Langohr GD, Giles JW, Athwal GS, Johnson JA. The effect of glenosphere diameter in reverse shoulder arthroplasty on muscle force, joint load, and range of motion. J Shoulder Elbow Surg. 2015;24(6):972–9.
13. Favard L, Levigne C, Nerot C, Gerber C, De Wilde L, Mole D. Reverse prostheses in arthropathies with cuff tear: are survivorship and function maintained over time? Clin Orthop Relat Res. 2011;469:2469–75.
14. Zumstein MA, Pinedo M, Old J, Boileau P. Problems, complications, reoperations, and revisions in reverse total shoulder arthroplasty: a systematic review. J Shoulder Elb Surg. 2011;20:146–57.
15. Routman HD. The role of subscapularis repair in reverse total shoulder arthroplasty. Bull Hosp Joint Dis. 2013;71:S108–12.
16. de Boer FA, van Kampen PM, Huijsmans PE. The influence of subscapularis tendon reattachment on range of motion in reversed shoulder arthroplasty: a clinical study. Musculoskelet Surg. 2016;100(2):121–6.
17. Alta TD, Bergmann JH, Veeger DJ, Janssen TW, Burger BJ, Scholtes VA, Willems WJ. Kinematic and clinical evaluation of shoulder function after primary and revision reverse shoulder prostheses. J Shoulder Elb Surg. 2011;20(4):564–70.
18. Boudreau S, Boudreau E, Higgings LD, Wilcox RB III. Rehabilitation following reverse total shoulder arthroplasty. J Orthop Sports Phys Ther. 2007;37(12):734–43.
19. Terrier A, Scheuber P, Pioletti DP, Farron A. Activities of daily living with reverse prostheses: importance of scapular compensation for functional mobility of the shoulder. J Shoulder Elb Surg. 2013;22:948–53.
20. Walters JD, Barkoh K, Smith RA, Azar FM, Throckmorton TW. Younger patients report similar activity levels to older patients after reverse total shoulder arthroplasty. J Shoulder Elb Surg. 2016;25(9):1418–24.
21. Postacchini R, Paoloni M, Carbone S, Fini M, Santilli V, Postacchini F, Mangone M. Kinematic analysis of reaching movements of the upper limb after total or reverse shoulder arthroplasty. J Biomech. 2015;48(12):3192–8.
22. de Toledo JM, Loss JF, Janssen TW, van der Scheer JW, Alta TD, Willems WJ, Veeger DH. Kinematic evaluation of patients with total and reverse shoulder arthroplasty during rehabilitation exercises with different loads. Clin Biomech. 2012;27:793–800.

23. Cutti AG, Parel I, Pellegrini A, Paladini P, Sacchetti R, Porcellini G, Merolla G. The Constant score and the assessment of scapula dyskinesis: proposal and assessment of an integrated outcome measure. J Electromyogr Kinesiol. 2015;29:81–9.
24. Röijezon U, Clark NC, Treleaven J. Proprioception in musculoskeletal rehabilitation. Part 1: basic science and principles of assessment and clinical interventions. Man Ther. 2015;20(3):368–77.
25. Clark NC, Röijezon U, Treleaven J. Proprioception in musculoskeletal rehabilitation. Part 2: clinical assessment and intervention. Man Ther. 2015;20(3):378–87.

Part VIII
Results

Outcomes of RSA: Review of Literature

32

Daniele Passaretti, Vittorio Candela, and Stefano Gumina

The original indications for reverse shoulder arthroplasty (RSA) were the cuff tear arthropathy, anatomic total shoulder arthroplasty failure, and tumor reconstruction [1, 2]. However, the increasingly widespread use of the RSA leads shoulder surgeons to implant RSA in case of severe proximal humerus fractures, shoulder pseudoparalysis, and massive irreparable rotator cuff tear in absence of cuff arthropathy [2–4].

A recent study [5] analyzed the long-term outcomes of the RSA, with a minimum and mean follow-up of 10 and 12.5 years, respectively. The authors considered 87 implants and concluded that despite a high arthroplasty survival rate and good long-term clinical results, RSA outcomes showed deterioration when compared with medium-term results. The cause of this decrease is probably related to patient aging coupled with bone erosion and/or deltoid impairment over time. In detail, the mean age at the time of surgery was 72.7 years, and Grammont-designed prostheses were used in all patients. At last follow-up, mean absolute and relative Constant-Murley scores (and standard deviations) were 55 ± 16 points and 86 ± 26 points, respectively. Both scores remained acceptable but have decreased significantly compared with the scores at the medium-term follow-up, at a minimum of 2 years (63 ± 14 and 90 ± 21 points, respectively), except for the pain subgroup score. Similarly, anterior active elevation improved significantly after prosthesis implantation but decreased significantly between the medium and long-term follow-up evaluations (138° and 131°, respectively). Rotational range of motion did not diminish between the medium and long-term follow-up assessments.

The complication rate was 29% and only 10% occurred after 2 years. The 73% of the shoulder exhibited scapular notching, 61% of these cases were classified as Sirveaux stage 1 or 2. There were no statistically significant differences in long-term Constant scores between patients without notching or with a lower stage of scapular notching (0, 1, or 2 grade) and those with a higher stage of scapular notching [3 or 4]. Finally, 12% of the patients underwent revision surgery. The 10-year overall prosthetic survival rate using revision as the end point was 93%. Other authors [6, 7] who analyzed the long-term survival of RSA demonstrated similar results.

These studies showed that strength and anterior active elevation decreased, suggesting an impairment of active deltoid power. Muscle con-

D. Passaretti (✉) · V. Candela
Department of Anatomy, Histology, Legal Medicine and Orthopedics, Sapienza, University of Rome, Rome, Italy

Istituto Chirurgico Ortopedico Traumatologico (ICOT), Latina, Italy

S. Gumina
Department of Orthopaedics and Traumatology, Sapienza University of Rome, Rome, Italy

S. Gumina et al. (eds.), *Reverse Shoulder Arthroplasty*,
https://doi.org/10.1007/978-3-319-97743-0_32

tractions of the deltoid tensioned by a lowered and medialized center of rotation correspond to alternating no physiological contraction-stretching cycles. Thus, impaired deltoid efficiency could be the result of muscle senescence coupled with no physiological biomechanical requirements [8–10]. Besides, functional decline varied among the different etiologies leading to the RTSA [5]. Rotator cuff tear arthropathy, primary osteoarthritis, and massive rotator cuff tear were associated with the least long-term deterioration, while failed previous arthroplasty and post-traumatic arthritis were associated with a greater decrease [5].

32.1 RSA in 3–4-Part Proximal Humeral Fractures

Proximal humeral fractures account for about 5% of all fractures [11]; 33% of proximal humeral fractures occurred in the elderly [12, 13] representing the third most frequent fragility fracture.

Among proximal humeral fractures, displaced three- and four-part fractures account for 13–16%, respectively [14–16]. Currently, the main treatments in these patients include nonoperation, open reduction and internal fixation (ORIF), minimally invasive percutaneous pinning, hemiarthroplasty (HA), and RSA. In their recent meta-analysis, Du et al. [17] considered seven studies [18–24] with a total of 347 patients with three- or four-part fractures treated with nonoperation, ORIF, HA, and RSA. The mean age was 75 years and follow-up ranged from 24 to 36 months. The authors concluded that RSA was considered as the best choice for three- or four-part proximal humeral fractures in terms of both functional result and complication rate. The detail about mean Constant scores and reoperation rate in each treatment is shown in Table 32.1. These results are similar to those of previous series [25–28]. In their meta-analysis, Shukla et al. [25] compared RSA to HA stating that RSA was significantly more favorable than HA in terms of forward elevation, abduction, tuberosity healing, and Constant-Murley, ASES, and DASH scores. Only external rotation was clinically worse in RSA. In their prospective cohort study, Klein et al. [27] showed that elderly patients treated with RSA reached a mean of 122.6° of forward flexion and 112.5° of abduction with a mean Constant score of 67.8. In a similar study, Bufquin et al. [28] evaluated the use of RSA for the treatment of three- and four-part fractures in the elderly. Interestingly, the authors stated that tuberosity nonunion only slightly affected external rotation but did not affect any other motion parameter at final follow-up. This study shows that tuberosity nonunion may not significantly affect the final outcome after RSA and that RSA may be the best option for patients with comminuted tuberosity fracture and osteoporosis. Despite these good results, the complication rate ranges from 0 to 68% including instability, complex regional pain syndrome, wound infection, scapular notching, hematoma, nerve injuries, early loosening, and periprosthetic fracture [26].

Table 32.1 Mean Constant-Murley scores and incidence of secondary surgery in each treatment at last follow-up, as showed in Du et al. study [17]

	RSA	HA	Nonoperation	ORIF
Mean CS	56	56	52	50
Reoperation rate	3.2%	13%	3%	16.3%

CS Constant-Murley score, *RSA* reverse shoulder arthroplasty, *ORIF* open reduction internal fixation

Thus, although with the lack of long-term results, compared with HA and ORIF, RSA leads to better short- and mid-term outcomes in elderly patients with osteoporotic comminuted proximal humeral fractures.

32.2 Pseudoparalytic Shoulder

The term *shoulder pseudoparalysis* does not have a uniform interpretation; in medicine *paralysis* means no motion, and it should indicate a no active shoulder elevation with maintained passive elevation. In 2005 Werner et al. [29] correctly defined *pseudoparesis of the shoulder* like a chronic massive rotator cuff tear with active elevation less than 90°, with a free passive elevation.

The mean treatments for this pathology were a nonoperative rehabilitation [30], partial and complete rotator cuff repair [31, 32], RSA [29], and RSA with muscle transfer [33]. All these approaches showed a postoperative improvement of the shoulder scores. Furthermore, cuff repair with augmentation or spanning patches by allograft or xenograft [34–36] and the superior capsular reconstruction (SCR) [37] are recent techniques introduced for these patients.

Analyzing the recent literature [29–34, 38–48], it turns out that the combined RSA-muscle transfer group reached the highest postoperative Constant-Murley score with a final value of 62.

In patients older than 65 years, shoulder arthroplasty is the most studied treatment method for pseudoparalysis in the literature [49]; especially in combination with significant shoulder arthropathy, RSA may be the only reliable approach to improve the range of motion and to restore a pain-free shoulder.

In patients mainly affected by a forward elevation deficiency, RSA showed improved postoperative outcomes regarding active elevation, with mean values ranging from 100° to 126° and a mean postoperative improvement of 47°–67°, higher Constant scores with a mean improvement of 30–37 points, and improved pain scores [49].

Patients affected by a combination of external rotation and forward flexion deficit have been treated with combined RSA and muscle transfer procedures. The latissimus dorsi alone or in association with teres major is the most transferred muscle-tendinous unit [33, 43, 47]. Literature [33, 43, 47] found positive results both for elevation and external rotations; the first one ranged from 126° to 149°, with a mean postoperative improvement of 61°–78°; similarly, postop external rotation improved to 34°–36°.

In the pseudoparalytic patients treated with RSA without muscle transfer, postoperative external rotation (ER) may be a function of prosthetic design; in fact, better ER scores are reported with more lateralized implants. Ek et al. [47] and Werner et al. [29] used a medialized design RSA (Grammont design) and found losses of mean postop ER of 1° and 5°, respectively. In contrast, Valenti et al. [42] reached a mean 15°–30° ER improvement in their group of patients with a lateralized RSA.

In conclusion, RSA in pseudoparalytic patients is associated with the best postop outcomes in terms of Constant-Murley score and forward elevation compared with all the other treatments. Moreover, patients with significant external rotation deficit may be best suited for treatment with either an implant with a lateralized center of rotation or a Grammont-style implant with a combined muscle transfer.

32.3 RSA in Irreparable Massive RCT Without Arthropathy

Patients with massive irreparable rotator cuff tears (MIRCTs) without the presence of osteoarthritis have a high likelihood of achieving a painless shoulder and functional improvements after RSA; Sevivas et al. in their recent meta-analysis [50] reached this conclusion. The authors investigated the six most representative studies [3, 42, 46, 51–53] that assessed the outcomes of RSA in patients with massive irreparable rotator cuff tears (MIRCTs) without osteoarthritis; 266 shoulders were considered, with a mean follow-up of 4 years (range 34–61.4 months). The investigation showed that RSA led to significantly improved shoulder outcomes in patients with MIRCTs. The mean improvement was the gain of 28–36 points in terms of weighted Constant-Murley score and 31–42 points in terms of weighted ASES score. In detail, after RSA treatment the forward flexion yielded a significant improvement (average difference of 41.8°), the same for the external rotation (average difference of 12°) and pain relief (average improvement of −5.2 points) from the preoperative period. The complications rate ranged between 4.1 and 20%: local infections, dislocation, and component failure were the most frequent, and the revision rate ranged from 1.4 to 8.3%.

In patients with isolated loss of active external rotation related to an irreparable posterosuperior cuff tear without osteoarthritis, Boileau et al. [33, 54] advocated that only a tendon transfer (specifically, the authors consider the latissimus dorsi, alone or in association with the teres major) can restore it. In cases with combined loss of active elevation and external rotation, the tendon transfer should be performed with an RSA. Recently, the same conclusions were reached by Hartzler et al. [52] that advocated a mean active external rotation gain of 39° in these patients, when latissimus dorsi transfer was associated to the RSA.

In older patients with symptomatic MIRCTs without osteoarthritis that failed to improve with conservative treatment and presenting signs cuff irreparability, RSA significantly improves shoulder outcomes, such as pain, function, and mobility. However, it should be emphasized that the complication rate can be as high as 1 in each 5 RSAs. Moreover, the revision rate is approximately 1 in each 12 patients at short to medium term. Thus, in these patients, RSA should be recommended.

32.4 Massive Irreparable Rotator Cuff Tears with Arthropathy

Cuff tear arthropathy (CTA) is a well-defined pathology. It was firstly described by Neer et al. [55] as a pathological condition of the shoulder characterized by the association of massive rotator cuff tear and glenohumeral joint degeneration, often accompanied by an anterosuperior migration of the humeral head. In his recent meta-analysis, Petrillo et al. [56] considered seven studies [3, 41, 42, 57–60] regarding patients suffering of CTA that were treated with RSA. Overall, 408 shoulders in 396 patients were enrolled. The mean age at the time of surgery was 71.9 ± 3.2 years (range 34–95 years), and the mean follow-up was 2.9 ± 1 years (range 12–101 months). A statistically significant improvement in all clinical scores and ROM was found comparing the preoperative and postoperative values. A gain in the anterior elevation (mean preop 51° ± 13.2, mean postop 124.4° ± 11.9), abduction (mean preop 41.1° ± 5.7, mean postop 115.4° ± 9.8), and external rotation with the arm in adduction on the side (mean preop 17.1° ± 6.9, mean postop 27.7° ± 13.8) was found. The mean improvement in active external rotation with the arm at 90° of abduction was 28.5°. Similarly, pain (mean preop 6.5 ± 0.4, mean postop 1.8 ± 0.4) and clinical scores (ASES, from 29.4 to 72.2; Constant-Murley, from 31.4 to 60.3; UCLA, from 15.2 to 26.9; SST, from 2 to 7.5) improved after surgery.

Nevertheless, 17.4% of complications occurred; the most frequent was heterotopic ossification, occurring in 6.6% of patients. Revision surgery was necessary in 7.3% of cases.

Considering these results, deltoid can restore anterior elevation and abduction ROM, but it cannot provide appropriate external rotation. Usually, in patients with CTA in which the posterosuperior cuff is deficient, the teres minor (TM) [61] is the only available external rotator muscle. Accordingly, the active external rotation ROM achieved after RSA depends on the condition of this tendon; however, in the elderly population, it is often retracted, atrophied, or fatty infiltrated [62].

Probably, a preoperative accurate MRI evaluation of the TM could be useful to predict the capacity to externally rotate the arm in patients with CTA undergoing RSA, offering also the possibility to plan a tendon transfer procedure in association with RSA [63]. Some authors [64–66] proposed to increase humeral retroversion in order to gain greater active external rotation. In several biomechanical studies, it was reported that placing the humeral component retroversion at 20° [67] or from 20° to 40° [68] increases the degrees of external rotation and impingement-free ROM, reducing scapular notching. On the other hand, better internal rotation ROM can be obtained improving the humeral stem anteversion.

In the Petrillo's series [56], the humeral stem retroversion was 30° in 131 shoulders (32.1%), 20° in 76 shoulders (18.6%), and from 10° to 20° in 141 shoulders (34.5%). However, the degrees of retroversion of the humeral stem (30° vs. 10°–20°of stem retroversion) did not influence the functional outcomes of RSA.

Based on these data, RSA restores pain-free range of motion and improves function of the shoulder in patients with CTA.

32.5 RSA in Patient Younger than 65 Years Old

RSA has classically been reserved for patients older than 65 years, and the more recent literature [5] confirmed that good short-, medium-, and long-term outcomes can be achieved in these patients. Questions remain about the utility of the RSA in younger subjects.

Despite the paucity of data on outcomes in this younger population, improvements in surgical technique and implant design have led to increased use of the RSA in a younger, more active population [48, 69, 70]. Several studies discussed high complication, revision rates and a drop-off in clinical outcomes over time as factors that could limit the successful use of the RSA in younger patients [71–73].

Recently, Samuelsen et al. [74] reviewed the literature and evaluated 67 shoulders with a mean age of 60 years (range, 50–65 years), treated with RSA for cuff tear arthropathy, severe glenohumeral arthritis, and osteonecrosis in 76, 22, and 2% of cases, respectively. The authors stated that patients gain significant improvements in clinical score and range of motion without a large number of early failures; however, the mean follow-up was only 3 years (range, 2–8 years). Patients experienced significant improvements in pain relief and improved active elevation (58° vs. 132°), active abduction (57.5° vs. 132.4°), and active external rotation (20.1° vs. 39.4°) after surgery. At the last follow-up, 90% of patients were satisfied with their result, and 85% felt they were better or much better than before surgery. Complications occurred in 9%: there was an 18% incidence of scapular notching, 3% incidence of dislocation, and no loosening. Finally, the revision-free survival rate was 99 and 91% after 2 and 5 years postoperative, respectively. Post-traumatic instability and deep infection were the mean reason for revision.

These results are comparable to those of previous studies [48, 69, 70] that evaluated patients younger than 65 submitted to RSA. The youngest patients, in each of these series, demonstrated significant improvement in active elevation, pain scores, and ASES and Constant scores [48, 69, 70]. However, the authors reported an overall complication rate ranging from 13.9% [69, 70] to 37.5% [48] and slightly worse 5-year and 10-year reoperation-free survival (88 and 76%, respectively) [48] compared to Samuelsen [74]. Interestingly, Ek et al. [48] found no decline in the subjective shoulder value at the 10-year follow-up in their study of patients younger than 60 years.

32.6 Muscle-Tendinous Transfer and Lateralized Implant

In 2007, Boileau [54] and Gerber [75] stated that in patients with irreparable posterosuperior rotator cuff tears, cuff arthropathy, and loss of active external rotation, RSA in combination with latissimus dorsi transfer (LDT) is reported to restore active abduction, anterior flexion, and active external rotation [54, 75]. Clinical indication to this treatment is based on abduction and/or anterior flexion of no more than 90°, shoulder pain, a positive dropping arm sign, and a horn-blower sign. Usually, patients with sufficient teres minor function will not show an external rotation lag sign or a positive horn-blower sign. Therefore, in the presence of an intact teres minor, most authors advise against a combined procedure.

A recent systematic review [76] analyzed short- and medium-term clinical and radiological outcomes following RSA, combined with the latissimus dorsi transfer (LDT) alone or with teres major, in patients with large irreparable posterosuperior rotator cuff tears, cuff arthropathy, and loss of active external rotation. The authors investigated 7 articles [43, 47, 52, 77–80] with a total of 118 shoulders. The weighted mean follow-up period was ~ 4 years (range, 23–65.4 months), and the weighted mean age at last follow-up was 69.2 ± 2.8 years. All studies reported significant improvement in functional scores, abduction, and external rotation. In particular, the adjusted mean Constant score increased from 38.8% ± 4.2 (range, 26–47) to 81% ± 4.2 (range, 58–93) in the postoperative period. The mean preoperative and postoperative ASES scores were 51 and 73 ± 7.4 points, respectively. The mean SST value was 2 ± 0.8 (range, 1.9–2.5) preoperatively and 7.5 ± 0.9 (range, 7–7.9) postoperatively. The postoperative VAS score decreased to 1.7 ± 0.7 (range, 1.1–1.7), starting from 7.2 ± 0.9 (range, 3.5–8.4). In terms of ROM improvement, the weighted mean pre- and postoperative external rotation was −10° (range, −30°–12°) and 27° (range, −10°–40°), respectively. The pre- and postoperative forward flexion was 64° (range, 40°–100°) and 128° ± 5.9 (range, 100°–170°) and the abduction 64° (range, 31°–87°) and 138° ± 6.5 (range, 92°–149°), respectively.

Regarding the radiologic outcomes, glenoid loosening was found in only one patient; scapular notching was reported in 35% of patients, and it consisted in a grade 1–2 in the majority of cases (73%).

Overall, complications occurred in 26% of patients. The LDT-specific complications (nerve palsies, subluxation, and partial tear) were present in seven subjects, yielding a complication rate of 6%. The highest complication rate was reported in the study of Shi et al. [80], with a complication rate of 43%.

The advantages of lateralization include that the center of rotation and offset more closely approximate those of the normal glenohumeral joint. Such lateralized designs have shown to decrease scapular notching while potentially improving rotation [42, 57]. However, some authors stated that metallic lateralization increases torque and shear forces on the glenoid component, which could lead to glenoid loosening [42, 81, 82]. A recent meta-analysis [83] analyzed 13 recent and significant studies. The authors compared the results of patients treated with a traditional Grammont-designed RSA prosthesis and with a lateralized implant for cuff tear arthropathy and massive irreparable tears. Overall, 349 patients were evaluated, the mean age was 70 years in both groups, and mean follow-up was 3.7 years (41.7 months in the traditional group and 47.6 months in the lateralized group). Lateralized implant significantly improved the external rotation, with a mean gain of 24° in the traditional group and 46° in the lateralized group. The rate of scapular notching and glenoid loosening was lower in lateralized RSA. Notching was noted in 44.9 and 5.4% of patients, respectively, in the traditional and lateralized group. The rate of clinically significant glenoid loosening was 1.8 and 8.8% in traditional and in the lateralized implant, respectively. The total reported complication rate was 15.4% in the traditional group and 22.8% in the lateralized group. Finally, the overall reoperation rate was 7.1 and 10.4%, respectively.

In the traditional group, the mean weighted postoperative Constant-Murley score was 65.5 with a mean Constant pain subscore of 12.2. In the lateralized implant, the mean weighted postoperative VAS score was 1.9; no studies in the lateralized RSA group reported Constant scores. No significant difference was found in terms of postoperative forward elevation (134° in the traditional group and 128° in the lateralized group).

We can conclude that both the traditional Grammont implants and the lateralized offset reverse arthroplasty designs can improve pain and function in patients with cuff tear arthropathy and irreparable rotator cuff tear; a lateralized design can result in increased active external rotation and decreased rates of scapular notching and glenoid baseplate loosening.

32.7 RSA With and Without Subscapularis Repair

Repair of the subscapularis tendon with RSA is controversial. Some studies [84, 85] suggested that the risk of instability increased if subscapularis is not repaired with a prosthetic design that medializes the center of rotation. In particular, Edwards et al. [85] reported a mean 5.1% dislocation rate with the Grammont RSA prosthesis. This value was doubled if the subscapularis was not repaired. In addition, biomechanical studies reported that not repairing the subscapularis requires significantly less force to be generated by the deltoid and the posterior rotator cuff throughout arm abduction [86]. When subscapularis was repaired, the joint reaction force increased by 28%, the required deltoid force increased by 14%, and the required posterior rotator cuff force increased by 34% [87]. Thus, reasons for repairing the subscapularis include anatomic preservation of a functioning rotator cuff muscle and an increased potential for internal rotation. On the other hand, theoretical reasons for not repairing the subscapularis include the following: It may be biomechanically unfavorable for deltoid function because with RSA the subscapularis reacts as an adductor [86–88]; furthermore, it may be biomechanically unfavorable for the posterior rotator cuff, and not repairing the subscapularis minimizes the force required by these muscles to generate external rotation [86–88].

In 2017 Friedman et al. [84] compared 340 patients submitted to the RSA with subscapularis repair to 251 patients without reparation. The mean age was 72.5 years (range, 50–93 years), and the mean and minimum follow-ups were 3 and 2 years, respectively. All patients showed significant improvements in pain and function scores after treatment with RSA. For both cohorts, ASES and Constant-Murley scores significantly improved, as for range of motion. However, the repaired cohort had significantly higher postoperative ASES and Constant scores (from a preoperative mean of 39 to a postoperative mean of 87 points and from 35 to 73, respectively) and significantly more internal rotation score (from 3 to 5 points), whereas the non-repaired cohort had significantly more active abduction (from 75° to 119°) and passive external rotation (from 31° to 50°).

The complication rate was 7.4% (in particular, there was 0% dislocations) for the subscapularis-repaired cohort and 6.8% (with 1.2% dislocations) for the cohort without subscapularis reparation. The RSA subscapularis-repaired cohort had a scapular notching rate of 10.4%, whereas the non-repaired cohort had a rate of 10.7%. No significant differences were noted in the rate of complications and scapular notching.

These results compare favorably with the previous studies published in the literature [57, 59, 89, 90]. Thus, significant clinical improvements were observed for both the subscapularis-repaired and non-repaired cohorts. The repair of the subscapularis did not lead to inferior outcomes as predicted by biomechanical models, and no difference was noted in the complication rates or scapular notching rates, between patients with and without subscapularis repair.

References

1. Bohsali KI, Wirth MA, Rockwood CA Jr. Current concepts review: complications of total shoulder arthroplasty. J Bone Joint Surg Am. 2006;88A:2279–92.
2. Gerber C, Pennington SD, Nyffeler RW. Reverse total shoulder arthroplasty. J Am Acad Orthop Surg. 2009;17:284–95.
3. Mulieri P, Dunning P, Klein S, Pupello D, Frankle M. Reverse shoulder arthroplasty for the treatment of irreparable rotator cuff tear without glenohumeral arthritis. J Bone Joint Surg Am. 2010;92:2544–56. https://doi.org/10.2106/JBJS.I.00912.
4. Cuff DJ, Pupello DR. Comparison of hemiarthroplasty and reverse shoulder arthroplasty for the treatment of proximal humerus fractures in elderly patients. J Bone Joint Surg Am. 2013;95:2050–5.
5. Bacle G, Nové-Josserand L, Garaud P, Walch G. Long-term outcomes of reverse total shoulder arthroplasty: a follow-up of a previous study. J Bone Joint Surg Am. 2017;99:454–61. https://doi.org/10.2106/JBJS.16.00223.
6. Levigne C, Garret J, Boileau P, Alami G, Favard L, Walch G. Scapular notching in reverse shoulder arthroplasty: is it important to avoid it and how? Clin Orthop Relat Res. 2011;469:2512–20.
7. Walch G, Bacle G, Ladermann A, Nove-Josserand L, Smithers CJ. Do the indications, results, and complications of reverse shoulder arthroplasty change with surgeon's experience? J Shoulder Elb Surg. 2012;21:1470–7.
8. Kowalsky MS, Galatz LM, Shia DS, Steger-May K, Keener JD. The relationship between scapular notching and reverse shoulder arthroplasty prosthesis design. J Shoulder Elb Surg. 2012;21:1430–41.
9. Bigorre N, Lancigu R, Bizot P, Hubert L. Predictive factors of scapular notching in patients with reverse shoulder arthroplasty. Orthop Traumatol Surg Res. 2014;100:711–4. https://doi.org/10.1016/j.otsr.2014.06.013.
10. Harman M, Frankle M, Vasey M, Banks S. Initial glenoid component fixation in "reverse" total shoulder arthroplasty: a biomechanical evaluation. J Shoulder Elb Surg. 2005;14(1 Suppl S):162S–7S.
11. Passaretti D, Candela V, Sessa P, Gumina S. Epidemiology of proximal humeral fractures: a

detailed survey of 711 patients in a metropolitan area. J Shoulder Elb Surg. 2017;26:2117–24. https://doi.org/10.1016/j.jse.2017.05.029.
12. Sanders RJ, Thissen LG, Teepen JC, Van Kampen A, Jaarsma RL. Locking plate versus nonsurgical treatment for proximal humeral fractures: better midterm outcome with nonsurgical treatment. J Shoulder Elb Surg. 2011;20:1118–24.
13. Van Den Broek CM, Van Den Besselaar M, Coenen JM, Vegt PA. Displaced proximal humeral fractures: intramedullary nailing versus conservative treatment. Arch Orthop Trauma Surg. 2007;127:459–63.
14. Khatib O, Onyekwelu I, Zuckerman JD. The incidence of proximal humeral fractures in New York State from 1990 through 2010 with an emphasis on operative management in patients aged 65 years or older. J Shoulder Elb Surg. 2014;23:1356–62.
15. Wijgman AJ, Roolker W, Patt TW, Raaymakers EL, Marti RK. Open reduction and internal fixation of three and four-part fractures of the proximal part of the humerus. J Bone Joint Surg Am. 2002;84-A: 1919–25.
16. Platzer P, Thalhammer G, Oberleitner G, Kutscha-Lissberg F, Wieland T, Vecsei V, Gaebler C. Displaced fractures of the greater tuberosity: a comparison of operative and nonoperative treatment. J Trauma. 2008;65:843–8. https://doi.org/10.1097/01.ta.0000233710.42698.3f.
17. Du S, Ye J, Chen H, Li X, Lin Q. Interventions for Treating 3- or 4-part proximal humeral fractures in elderly patient: A network meta-analysis of randomized controlled trials. Int J Surg. 2017;48:240–6. https://doi.org/10.1016/j.ijsu.2017.09.002.
18. Zyto K, Ahrengart L, Sperber A, Törnkvist H. Treatment of displaced proximal humeral fractures in elderly patients. J Bone Joint Surg Br. 1997;79:412–7.
19. Olerud P, Ahrengart L, Ponzer S, Saving J, Tidermark J. Hemiarthroplasty versus nonoperative treatment of displaced 4-part proximal humeral fractures in elderly patients: a randomized controlled trial. J Shoulder Elb Surg. 2011;20:1025–33. https://doi.org/10.1016/j.jse.2011.04.016.
20. Olerud P, Ahrengart L, Ponzer S, Saving J, Tidermark J. Internal fixation versus nonoperative treatment of displaced 3-part proximal humeral fractures in elderly patients: a randomized controlled trial. J Shoulder Elb Surg. 2011;20:747–55. https://doi.org/10.1016/j.jse.2010.12.018.
21. Cai M, Tao K, Yang C, Li S. Internal fixation versus shoulder hemiarthroplasty for displaced 4-part proximal humeral fractures in elderly patients. Orthopedics. 2012;35:e1340–6. https://doi.org/10.3928/01477447-20120822-19.
22. Fjalestad T, Hole MØ, Hovden IA, Blücher J, Strømsøe K. Surgical treatment with an angular stable plate for complex displaced proximal humeral fractures in elderly patients: a randomized controlled trial. J Orthop Trauma. 2012;26:98–106. https://doi.org/10.1097/BOT.0b013e31821c2e15.
23. Sebastiá-Forcada E, Cebrián-Gómez R, Lizaur-Utrilla A, Gil-Guillén V. Reverse shoulder arthroplasty versus hemiarthroplasty for acute proximal humeral fractures. A blinded, randomized, controlled, prospective study. J Shoulder Elb Surg. 2014;23:1419–26. https://doi.org/10.1016/j.jse.2014.06.035.
24. Boons HW, Goosen JH, van Grinsven S, van Susante JL, van Loon CJ. Hemiarthroplasty for humeral four-part fractures for patients 65 years and older: a randomized controlled trial. Clin Orthop Relat Res. 2012;470:3483–91. https://doi.org/10.1007/s11999-012-2531-0.
25. Shukla DR, McAnany S, Kim J, Overley S, Parsons BO. Hemiarthroplasty versus reverse shoulder arthroplasty for treatment of proximal humeral fractures: a meta-analysis. J Shoulder Elb Surg. 2016;25:330–40. https://doi.org/10.1016/j.jse.2015.08.030.
26. Acevedo DC, Vanbeek C, Lazarus MD, Williams GR, Abboud JA. Reverse shoulder arthroplasty for proximal humeral fractures: update on indications, technique, and results. J Shoulder Elb Surg. 2014;23:279–89. https://doi.org/10.1016/j.jse.2013.10.003.
27. Klein M, Juschka M, Hinkenjann B, Scherger B, Ostermann PA. Treatment of comminuted fractures of the proximal humerus in elderly patients with the Delta III reverse shoulder prosthesis. J Orthop Trauma. 2008;22:698–704. https://doi.org/10.1097/BOT.0b013e31818afe40.
28. Bufquin T, Hersan A, Hubert L, Massin P. Reverse shoulder arthroplasty for the treatment of three- and four-part fractures of the proximal humerus in the elderly: a prospective review of 43 cases with a short-term follow-up. J Bone Joint Surg Br. 2007;89:516–20. https://doi.org/10.1302/0301-620X.89B4.18435.
29. Werner CM, Steinmann PA, Gilbart M, Gerber C. Treatment of painful pseudoparesis due to irreparable rotator cuff dysfunction with the Delta III reverse-ball-and-socket total shoulder prosthesis. J Bone Joint Surg Am. 2005;87:1476–86. https://doi.org/10.2106/JBJS.D.02342.
30. Levy O, Mullett H, Roberts S, Copeland S. The role of anterior deltoid reeducation in patients with massive irreparable degenerative rotator cuff tears. J Shoulder Elb Surg. 2008;17:863–70. https://doi.org/10.1016/j.jse.2008.04.005.
31. Denard PJ, Lädermann A, Jiwani AZ, Burkhart SS. Functional outcome after arthroscopic repair of massive rotator cuff tears in individuals with pseudoparalysis. Arthroscopy. 2012;28:1214–9. https://doi.org/10.1016/j.arthro.2012.02.026.
32. Oh JH, Kim SH, Shin SH, Chung SW, Kim JY, Kim SH, et al. Outcome of rotator cuff repair in large-to-massive tear with pseudoparalysis: a comparative study with propensity score matching. Am J Sports Med. 2011;39:1413–20. https://doi.org/10.1177/0363546511399865.
33. Boileau P, Chuinard C, Roussanne Y, Bicknell RT, Rochet N, Trojani C. Reverse shoulder arthroplasty combined with a modified latissimus dorsi and teres

major tendon transfer for shoulder pseudoparalysis associated with dropping arm. Clin Orthop Relat Res. 2008;466:584–93. https://doi.org/10.1007/s11999-008-0114-x.
34. Kokkalis ZT, Mavrogenis AF, Scarlat M, Christodoulou M, Vottis C, Papagelopoulos PJ, et al. Human dermal allograft for massive rotator cuff tears. Orthopedics. 2014;37:e1108–16. https://doi.org/10.3928/01477447-20141124-59.
35. Venouziou AI, Kokkalis ZT, Sotereanos DG. Human dermal allograft interposition for the reconstruction of massive irreparable rotator cuff tears. Am J Orthop. 2013;42:63–70.
36. Badhe SP, Lawrence TM, Smith FD, Lunn PG. An assessment of porcine dermal xenograft as an augmentation graft in the treatment of extensive rotator cuff tears. J Shoulder Elb Surg. 2008;17(Suppl):35S–9S. https://doi.org/10.1016/j.jse.2007.08.005.
37. Mihata T, Lee TQ, Watanabe C, Fukunishi K, Ohue M, Tsujimura T, et al. Clinical results of arthroscopic superior capsule reconstruction for irreparable rotator cuff tears. Arthroscopy. 2013;29:459–70. https://doi.org/10.1016/j.arthro.2012.10.022.
38. Al-Hadithy N, Domos P, Sewell MD, Pandit R. Reverse shoulder arthroplasty in 41 patients with cuff tear arthropathy with a mean follow-up period of 5 years. J Shoulder Elb Surg. 2014;23:1662–8. https://doi.org/10.1016/j.jse.2014.03.001.
39. Birmingham PM, Neviaser RJ. Outcome of latissimus dorsi transfer as a salvage procedure for failed rotator cuff repair with loss of elevation. J Shoulder Elb Surg. 2008;17:871–4. https://doi.org/10.1016/j.jse.2008.04.007.
40. Field LD, Dines DM, Zabinski SJ, Warren RF. Hemiarthroplasty of the shoulder for rotator cuff arthropathy. J Shoulder Elb Surg. 1997;6:18–23.
41. Leung B, Horodyski M, Struk AM, Wright TW. Functional outcome of hemiarthroplasty compared with reverse total shoulder arthroplasty in the treatment of rotator cuff tear arthropathy. J Shoulder Elb Surg. 2012;21:319–23. https://doi.org/10.1016/j.jse.2011.05.023.
42. Valenti P, Sauzieres P, Katz D, Kalouche I, Kilinc AS. Do less medialized reverse shoulder prostheses increase motion and reduce notching? Clin Orthop Relat Res. 2011;469:2550–7. https://doi.org/10.1007/s11999-011-1844-8.
43. Boughebri O, Kilinc A, Valenti P. Reverse shoulder arthroplasty combined with a latissimus dorsi and teres major transfer for a deficit of both active elevation and external rotation. Results of 15 cases with a minimum of 2-year follow-up. Orthop Traumatol Surg Res. 2013;99:131–7. https://doi.org/10.1016/j.otsr.2012.11.014.
44. Goldberg SS, Bell JE, Kim HJ, Bak SF, Levine WN, Bigliani LU. Hemiarthroplasty for the rotator cuff-deficient shoulder. J Bone Joint Surg Am. 2008;90:554–9. https://doi.org/10.2106/JBJS.F.01029.
45. Naveed MA, Kitson J, Bunker TD. The Delta III reverse shoulder replacement for cuff tear arthropathy: a single-centre study of 50 consecutive procedures. J Bone Joint Surg Br. 2011;93:57–61. https://doi.org/10.1302/0301-620X.93B1.24218.
46. Boileau P, Gonzalez JF, Chuinard C, Bicknell R, Walch G. Reverse total shoulder arthroplasty after failed rotator cuff surgery. J Shoulder Elb Surg. 2009;18:600–6. https://doi.org/10.1016/j.jse.2009.03.011.
47. Boileau P, Rumian AP, Zumstein MA. Reversed shoulder arthroplasty with modified L'Episcopo for combined loss of active elevation and external rotation. J Shoulder Elb Surg. 2010;19(Suppl):20–30. https://doi.org/10.1016/j.jse.2009.12.011.
48. Ek ET, Neukom L, Catanzaro S, Gerber C. Reverse total shoulder arthroplasty for massive irreparable rotator cuff tears in patients younger than 65 years old: results after five to fifteen years. J Shoulder Elb Surg. 2013;22:1199–208. https://doi.org/10.1016/j.jse.2012.11.016.
49. Tokish JM, Alexander TC, Kissenberth MJ, Hawkins RJ. Pseudoparalysis: a systematic review of term definitions, treatment approaches, and outcomes of management techniques. J Shoulder Elb Surg. 2017;26:e177–e87. https://doi.org/10.1016/j.jse.2017.02.024.
50. Sevivas N, Ferreira N, Andrade R, Moreira P, Portugal R, Alves D, Vieira da Silva M, Sousa N, Salgado AJ, Espregueira-Mendes J. Reverse shoulder arthroplasty for irreparable massive rotator cuff tears: a systematic review with meta-analysis and meta-regression. J Shoulder Elb Surg. 2017;26:e265–77. https://doi.org/10.1016/j.jse.2017.03.039.
51. Favard L, Berhouet J, Colmar M, Boukobza E, Richou J, Sonnard A, et al. Massive rotator cuff tears in patients younger than 65 years. What treatment options are available? Orthop Traumatol Surg Res. 2009;95:S19–26. https://doi.org/10.1016/j.otsr.2009.03.005.
52. Hartzler RU, Steen BM, Hussey MM, Cusick MC, Cottrell BJ, Clark RE, et al. Reverse shoulder arthroplasty for massive rotator cuff tear: risk factors for poor functional improvement. J Shoulder Elb Surg. 2015;24:1698–706. https://doi.org/10.1016/j.jse.2015.04.015.
53. Wall B, Nové-Josserand L, O'Connor DP, Edwards TB, Walch G. Reverse total shoulder arthroplasty: a review of results according to etiology. J Bone Joint Surg Am. 2007;89:1476–85. https://doi.org/10.2106/JBJS.F.00666.
54. Boileau P, Chuinard C, Roussanne Y, Neyton L, Trojani C. Modified latissimus dorsi and teres major transfer through a single delto-pectoral approach for external rotation deficit of the shoulder: as an isolated procedure or with a reverse arthroplasty. J Shoulder Elb Surg. 2007;16:671–82. https://doi.org/10.1016/j.jse.2007.02.127.
55. Neer CS, Craig EV, Fukuda H. Cuff-tear arthropathy. J Bone Joint Surg Am. 1983;65:1232–44.
56. Petrillo S, Longo UG, Papalia R, Denaro V. Reverse shoulder arthroplasty for massive irreparable rotator

cuff tears and cuff tear arthropathy: a systematic review. Musculoskelet Surg. 2017;101:105–12. https://doi.org/10.1007/s12306-017-0474-z.
57. Frankle M, Siegal S, Pupello D, Saleem A, Mighell M, Vasey M. The reverse shoulder prosthesis for glenohumeral arthritis associated with severe rotator cuff deficiency. A minimum 2-year follow-up study of sixty patients. J Bone Joint Surg Am. 2005;87:1697–705. https://doi.org/10.2106/JBJS.D.02813.
58. Sadoghi P, Vavken P, Leithner A, Hochreiter J, Weber G, Pietschmann MF, Müller PE. Impact of previous rotator cuff repair on the outcome of reverse shoulder arthroplasty. J Shoulder Elb Surg. 2011;20:1138–46. https://doi.org/10.1016/j.jse.2011.01.013.
59. Nolan BM, Ankerson E, Wiater JM. Reverse total shoulder arthroplasty improves function in cuff tear arthropathy. Clin Orthop Relat Res. 2011;469:2476–82. https://doi.org/10.1007/s11999-010-1683.
60. Jobin CM, Brown GD, Bahu MJ, Gardner TR, Bigliani LU, Levine WN, Ahmad CS. Reverse total shoulder arthroplasty for cuff tear arthropathy: the clinical effect of deltoid lengthening and center of rotation medialization. J Shoulder Elb Surg. 2012;21:1269–77.
61. Berton A, Gulotta LV, Petrillo S, Florio P, Longo UG, Denaro V, Kontaxis A. The effect of humeral version on teres minor muscle moment arm, length, and impingement in reverse shoulder arthroplasty during activities of daily living. J Shoulder Elb Surg. 2015;24:578–86. https://doi.org/10.1016/j.jse.2014.08.019.
62. Goutallier D, Postel JM, Bernageau J, Lavau L, Voisin MC. Fatty infiltration of disrupted rotator cuff muscles. Rev Rhum Engl Ed. 1995;62:415–22.
63. Longo UG, et al. Latissimus dorsi tendon transfer for massive irreparable rotator cuff tears: a systematic review. Sports Med ArthroscRev. 2011;19:428–37.
64. Boileau P, Watkinson DJ, Hatzidakis AM, Balg F. Grammont reverse prosthesis: design, rationale, and biomechanics. J Shoulder Elb Surg. 2005;14(Suppl S):147S–61S.
65. Grammont PM, Trouilloud P, Laffay JP, Deries X. Etude et realization d'une novella prothese d'epaule. Rheumatologie. 1987;39:17–22.
66. Grammont PM, Baulot E. Delta shoulder prosthesis for rotator cuff rupture. Orthopedics. 1993;16: 65–8.
67. Gulotta LV, Choi D, Marinello P, Knutson Z, Lipman J, Wright T, Cordasco FA, Craig EV, Warren RF. Humeral component retroversion in reverse total shoulder arthroplasty: a biomechanical study. J Shoulder Elb Surg. 2012;21:1121–7. https://doi.org/10.1016/j.jse.2011.07.027.
68. Stephenson DR, Oh JH, McGarry MH, Rick Hatch GF 3rd, Lee TQ. Effect of humeral component version on impingement in reverse total shoulder arthroplasty. J Shoulder Elb Surg. 2011;20:652–8. https://doi.org/10.1016/j.jse.2010.08.020.
69. Muh SJ, Streit JJ, Wanner JP, Lenarz CJ, Shishani Y, Rowland DY, et al. Early follow-up of reverse total shoulder arthroplasty in patients sixty years of age or younger. J Bone Joint Surg Am. 2013;95:1877–83. https://doi.org/10.2106/JBJS.L.10005.
70. Sershon RA, Van Thiel GS, Lin EC, McGill KC, Cole BJ, Verma NN, et al. Clinical outcomes of reverse total shoulder arthroplasty in patients aged younger than 60 years. J Shoulder Elb Surg. 2014;23:395–400. https://doi.org/10.1016/j.jse.2013.07.047.
71. Cazeneuve JF, Cristofari DJ. Long term functional outcome following reverse shoulder arthroplasty in the elderly. Orthop Traumatol Surg Res. 2011;97:583–9. https://doi.org/10.1016/j.otsr.2011.03.025.
72. Favard L, Levigne C, Nerot C, Gerber C, DeWilde L, Mole D. Reverse prostheses in arthropathies with cuff tear: are survivorship and function maintained over time? Clin Orthop Relat Res. 2011;469:2469–75. https://doi.org/10.1007/s11999-011-1833-y.
73. Guery J, Favard L, Sirveaux F, Oudet D, Mole D, Walch G. Reverse total shoulder arthroplasty. Survivorship analysis of eighty replacements followed for five to ten years. J Bone Joint Surg Am. 2006;88:1742–7. https://doi.org/10.2106/JBJS.E.00851.
74. Samuelsen BT, Wagner ER, Houdek MT, Elhassan BT, Sánchez-Sotelo J, Cofield R, Sperling JW. Primary reverse shoulder arthroplasty in patients aged 65 years or younger. J Shoulder Elb Surg. 2017;26:e13–7. https://doi.org/10.1016/j.jse.2016.05.026.
75. Gerber C, Pennington SD, Lingenfelter EJ, Sukthankar A. Reverse Delta-III total shoulder replacement combined with latissimus dorsi transfer. A preliminary report. J Bone Joint Surg Am. 2007;89:940–7. https://doi.org/10.2106/JBJS.F.00955.
76. Ortmaier R, Hitzl W, Matis N, Mattiassich G, Hochreiter J, Resch H. Reverse shoulder arthroplasty combined with latissimus dorsi transfer: a systemic review. Orthop Traumatol Surg Res. 2017;103:853–9. https://doi.org/10.1016/j.otsr.2017.03.019.
77. Ortmaier R, Resch H, Hitzl W, Mayer M, Blocher M, Vasvary I, et al. Reverse shoulder arthroplasty combined with latissimus dorsi transfer using the bone-chip technique. Int Orthop. 2014;38:553–9. https://doi.org/10.1007/s00264-013-2139-3.
78. Puskas GJ, Catanzaro S, Gerber C. Clinical outcome of reverse total shoulder arthroplasty combined with latissimus dorsi transfer for the treatment of chronic combined pseudoparesis of elevation and external rotation of the shoulder. J Shoulder Elb Surg. 2014;23:49–57. https://doi.org/10.1016/j.jse.2013.04.008.
79. Puskas GJ, Germann M, Catanzaro S, Gerber C. Secondary latissimus dorsi transfer after failed reverse total shoulder arthroplasty. J Shoulder Elb Surg. 2015;24:e337–44. https://doi.org/10.1016/j.jse.2015.05.033.
80. Shi LL, Cahill KE, Ek ET, Tompson JD, Higgins LD, Warner JJP. Latissimus Dorsi and Teres major transfer with reverse shoulder arthroplasty restores active motion and reduces pain for posterosuperior cuff dysfunction. Clin Orthop. 2015;473:3212–7. https://doi.org/10.1007/s11999-015-4433-4.
81. Boileau P, Moineau G, Roussanne Y, O'Shea K. Bony increased-offset reversed shoulder arthroplasty:

minimizing scapular impingement while maximizing glenoid fixation. Clin Orthop Relat Res. 2011;469:2558–67.
82. Middleton C, Uri O, Phillips S, et al. A reverse shoulder arthroplasty with increased offset for the treatment of cuff deficient shoulders with glenohumeral arthritis. Bone Joint J. 2014;96:936–42.
83. Lawrence C, Williams GR, Namdari S. Influence of glenosphere design on outcomes and complications of reverse arthroplasty: a systematic review. Clin Orthop Surg. 2016;8:288–97. https://doi.org/10.4055/cios.2016.8.3.288.
84. Friedman RJ, Flurin PH, Wright TW, Zuckerman JD, Roche CP. Comparison of reverse total shoulder arthroplasty outcomes with and without subscapularis repair. J Shoulder Elb Surg. 2017;2:662–8. https://doi.org/10.1016/j.jse.2016.09.027.
85. Edwards TB, Williams MD, Labriola JE, Elkousy HA, Gartsman GM, O'Connor DP. Subscapularis insufficiency and the risk of shoulder dislocation after reverse shoulder arthroplasty. J Shoulder Elb Surg. 2009;18:892–6. https://doi.org/10.1016/j.jse.2008.12.013.
86. Hansen ML, Nayak A, Narayanan MS, Worhacz K, Stowell R, Jacofsky MC, et al. Role of subscapularis repair on muscle force requirements with reverse shoulder arthroplasty. Bull Hosp Jt Dis. 2015;73(Suppl 1):S21–7.
87. Roche C, Crosby L. Kinematics and biomechanics of reverse total shoulder arthroplasty. In: AAOS orthopaedic knowledge update. #4. Rosemont, IL: American Academy of Orthopaedic Surgeons; 2013. p. 45–54.
88. Roche CP, Diep P, Hamilton M, Crosby LA, Flurin PH, Wright TW, et al. Impact of inferior glenoid tilt, humeral retroversion, bone grafting, and design parameters on muscle length and deltoid wrapping in reverse shoulder arthroplasty. Bull Hosp Jt Dis. 2013;71:284–93.
89. Boileau P, Watkinson DJ, Hatzidakis AM, Hovorka I. NeerAward 2005: the Grammont reverse shoulder prosthesis: results in cuff tear arthritis, fracture sequelae, and revision arthroplasty. J Shoulder Elb Surg. 2006;15:527–40. https://doi.org/10.1016/j.jse.2006.01.003.
90. Lévigne C, Boileau P, Favard L, Garaud P, Molé D, Sirveaux F, et al. Scapular notching in reverse shoulder arthroplasty. J Shoulder Elb Surg. 2008;17:925–35. https://doi.org/10.1016/j.jse.2008.02.010.

Printed by Printforce, the Netherlands